Imaging of
PEDIATRIC CHEST

Imaging of PEDIATRIC CHEST

Second Edition

Editors

Ashu Seith Bhalla MD FICR MAMS
Department of Radiodiagnosis and
Interventional Radiology
All India Institute of Medical Sciences
New Delhi, India

Manisha Jana MD DNB FRCR
Department of Radiodiagnosis and Interventional Radiology
All India Institute of Medical Sciences
New Delhi, India

Co-Editors

Devasenathipathy Kandaswamy MD DNB FRCR
Department of Radiodiagnosis and Interventional Radiology
All India Institute of Medical Sciences
New Delhi, India

Priyanka Naranje MD DNB EBIR
Department of Radiodiagnosis and Interventional Radiology
All India Institute of Medical Sciences
New Delhi, India

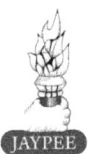

JAYPEE

JAYPEE BROTHERS MEDICAL PUBLISHERS
The Health Sciences Publisher
New Delhi | London

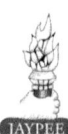 **Jaypee Brothers Medical Publishers (P) Ltd**

Headquarters
EMCA House
23/23-B, Ansari Road, Daryaganj
New Delhi 110 002, India
Landline: +91-11-23272143, +91-11-23272703
+91-11-23282021, +91-11-23245672
E-mail: jaypee@jaypeebrothers.com

Corporate Office
Jaypee Brothers Medical Publishers (P) Ltd.
4838/24, Ansari Road, Daryaganj
New Delhi 110 002, India
Phone: +91-11-43574357
Fax: +91-11-43574314
E-mail: jaypee@jaypeebrothers.com

Overseas Office
JP Medical Ltd.
83, Victoria Street, London
SW1H 0HW (UK)
Phone: +44-20 3170 8910
Fax: +44(0)20 3008 6180
E-mail: info@jpmedpub.com

EU GPSR Authorised Representative
LOGOS EUROPE, 9 rue Nicolas Poussin
17000, LA ROCHELLE, France
Phone: +33 (0) 6 67 93 73 78
Email: Contact@logos europe.eu

Website: www.jaypeebrothers.com
Website: www.jaypeedigital.com

© 2024, Jaypee Brothers Medical Publishers

The views and opinions expressed in this book are solely those of the original contributor(s)/author(s) and do not necessarily represent those of editor(s) or publisher of the book.

All rights reserved. No part of this publication may be reproduced, stored or transmitted in any form or by any means, electronic, mechanical, photocopying, recording or otherwise, without the prior permission in writing of the publishers.

All brand names and product names used in this book are trade names, service marks, trademarks or registered trademarks of their respective owners. The publisher is not associated with any product or vendor mentioned in this book.

Medical knowledge and practice change constantly. This book is designed to provide accurate, authoritative information about the subject matter in question. However, readers are advised to check the most current information available on procedures included and check information from the manufacturer of each product to be administered, to verify the recommended dose, formula, method and duration of administration, adverse effects and contraindications. It is the responsibility of the practitioner to take all appropriate safety precautions. Neither the publisher nor the author(s)/editor(s) assume any liability for any injury and/or damage to persons or property arising from or related to use of material in this book.

This book is sold on the understanding that the publisher is not engaged in providing professional medical services. If such advice or services are required, the services of a competent medical professional should be sought.

Every effort has been made where necessary to contact holders of copyright to obtain permission to reproduce copyright material. If any have been inadvertently overlooked, the publisher will be pleased to make the necessary arrangements at the first opportunity.

Inquiries for bulk sales may be solicited at: jaypee@jaypeebrothers.com

Imaging of Pediatric Chest / Ashu Seith Bhalla

First Edition: 2015

Second Edition: **2024**

ISBN: 978-93-5696-434-1

Contributors

Akshay Baheti MBBS MD
Department of Radiodiagnosis
Tata Memorial Hospital and Homi
Bhabha National Institute
Mumbai, Maharashtra, India

Akshay Kumar Saxena MD FICR FRCR
Department of Radiodiagnosis
and Imaging
Postgraduate Institute of Medical
Education and Research
Chandigarh, India

Amit Gupta MD FRCR
Department of Radiodiagnosis and
Interventional Radiology
All India Institute of Medical Sciences
New Delhi, India

Amarinder S Malhi MD DM
Department of Radiodiagnosis and
Interventional Radiology
All India Institute of Medical Sciences
New Delhi, India

Anisha Garg MD
Department of Radiodiagnosis and
Interventional Radiology
All India Institute of Medical Sciences
New Delhi, India

Ankita Aggarwal MD
Department of Radiodiagnosis and
Interventional Radiology
All India Institute of Medical Sciences
New Delhi, India

Anmol Bhatia MD Fellowship in Pediatric
Radiology
Department of Radiodiagnosis and
Imaging
Postgraduate Institute of Medical
Education and Research
Chandigarh, India

Anuradha Singh MD Fellowship in
Thoracic Radiology Fellowship in Pediatric
Radiology
Department of Radiodiagnosis
Sanjay Gandhi Post Graduate Institute
of Medical Sciences
Lucknow, Uttar Pradesh, India

Aparna Shyamkumar MD FRCR
Department of Radiology
Christian Medical College
Vellore, Tamil Nadu, India

Ashish Dua MD DNB MNAMS
Department of Radiodiagnosis
and Imaging
Postgraduate Institute of Medical
Education and Research
Chandigarh, India

Ashu Seith Bhalla MD FICR MAMS
Department of Radiodiagnosis and
Interventional Radiology
All India Institute of Medical Sciences
New Delhi, India

Ayush Jain MD
Department of Radiodiagnosis and
Interventional Radiology
All India Institute of Medical Sciences
New Delhi, India

Contributors

Deeksha Bhalla MD DNB
Department of Radiodiagnosis and Interventional Radiology
All India Institute of Medical Sciences
New Delhi, India

Devasenathipathy Kandasamy MD DNB FRCR
Department of Radiodiagnosis and Interventional Radiology
All India Institute of Medical Sciences
New Delhi, India

Harshith Gowda MBBS MD
Department of Radiodiagnosis and Imaging
Postgraduate Institute of Medical Education and Research
Chandigarh, India

Iqbal Bashir MD Fellowship in Thoracic Radiology
Department of Radiodiagnosis and Interventional Radiology
All India Institute of Medical Sciences
New Delhi, India

Ishan Gupta MD Fellowship in Thoracic Radiology
Department of Radiodiagnosis and Interventional Radiology
All India Institute of Medical Sciences
New Delhi, India

Kana Ram Jat MD
Department of Pediatrics
All India Institute of Medical Sciences
New Delhi, India

Kushaljit Singh Sodhi MD FICR PhD
Department of Radiodiagnosis and Imaging
Postgraduate Institute of Medical Education and Research
Chandigarh, India

Manisha Jana MD DNB FRCR
Department of Radiodiagnosis and Interventional Radiology
All India Institute of Medical Sciences
New Delhi, India

Nitin Dhochak MD DM
Department of Pediatrics
All India Institute of Medical Sciences
New Delhi, India

Pooja Abbey MD DNB
Department of Radiodiagnosis
Lady Hardinge Medical College
New Delhi, India

Poonam Sherwani DNB Fellowship in Pediatric Radiology MICR
Department of Radiodiagnosis
All India Institute of Medical Sciences
Rishikesh, Uttarakhand, India

Priyanka Naranje MD DNB EBIR
Department of Radiodiagnosis and Interventional Radiology
All India Institute of Medical Sciences
New Delhi, India

Rajendra K Behera MD
Department of Radiodiagnosis and Interventional Radiology
All India Institute of Medical Sciences
New Delhi, India

Rakesh Lodha MD
Department of Pediatrics
All India Institute of Medical Sciences
New Delhi, India

Shruti Badkhane MD
Department of Radiodiagnosis and Interventional Radiology
All India Institute of Medical Sciences
New Delhi, India

Smita Manchanda MD DNB FICR
Department of Radiodiagnosis and
Interventional Radiology
All India Institute of Medical Sciences
New Delhi, India

Sneha Goswami MD
Department of Radiodiagnosis and
Interventional Radiology
All India Institute of Medical Sciences
New Delhi, India

Stuti Chandola MD
Department of Radiodiagnosis and
Interventional Radiology
All India Institute of Medical Sciences
New Delhi, India

Surabhi Vyas MD DNB MNAMS
Department of Radiodiagnosis and
Interventional Radiology
All India Institute of Medical Sciences
New Delhi, India

Sushil K Kabra MD
Department of Pediatrics
All India Institute of Medical Sciences
New Delhi, India

Tany Chandra MD DNB EDiR
Department of Radiodiagnosis
Hamdard Institute of Medical Sciences
and Research
New Delhi, India

Taruna Yadav MD DNB Fellowship in
HPB and IR
Department of Diagnostic and
Interventional Radiology
All India Institute of Medical Sciences
Jodhpur, Rajasthan, India

Vasundhara Patil MD
Department of Radiodiagnosis
Tata Memorial Hospital and Homi
Bhabha National Institute
Mumbai, Maharashtra, India

Preface to the Second Edition

We started our journey in textbook writing with *"Imaging of Pediatric Chest"* in 2015, following which the Clinicoradiological Series was launched in 2016. The aim of this series has been to present a consistent format in each version with relevant clinical as well as imaging information combined into a concise handbook.

The evolution of pediatric pulmonology as a speciality and the growing understanding of common and uncommon conditions that manifest in the pediatric chest, prompted us to consider a revision of the previously published book in an enhanced format. There is comprehensive coverage of various aspects of chest disorders in children, including infections, pediatric interstitial lung diseases, congenital vascular anomalies as well as lung and mediastinal tumors in children. In addition, specifically aimed at postgraduate and superspeciality residents are structured reporting formats for each common disorders with accompanying explanation of application of these, which are sure to simplify comprehension and enhance reporting standards for all readers.

Further, to cater to practicing radiologists as well as pediatric pulmonologists, there are a large number of high-quality illustrations as well as detailed "pattern-based imaging approach" in the form of flowcharts which have been incorporated into this edition. We have also covered recent advances such as the role of interventional radiology and the role of relevant genetic and molecular testing.

We hope this book will be beneficial to practicing radiologists, pediatricians as well as residents, and trainees. We thank our readers for their continuing faith in us, and look forward to their feedback for our latest endeavor.

We would also like to extend our grateful thanks to Shri Jitendar P Vij (Group Chairman), Mr Ankit Vij (Managing Director), Mr MS Mani (Group President), Ms Chetna Malhotra (Senior Director—Professional Publishing, Marketing and Business Development), Ms Nedup Bhutia Pillai (Team Leader—Print Publishing), and other staffs of M/s Jaypee Brothers Medical Publishers (P) Ltd., New Delhi, India, for their efforts and input enabling timely publication of the book.

Ashu Seith Bhalla
Manisha Jana

Preface to the Second Edition

Preface to the First Edition

Although the statement "Children are not little adults" is clichéd it best embodies the fact, that as is true of all organ systems of the body, the spectrum of conditions involving the pediatric chest is distinct from the spectrum seen in the adults. Although there is some overlap, there are several distinct entities which are peculiar to children. Even within the pediatric age group, the differential diagnosis varies as we move from the neonate to the young child and the adolescent.

Imaging plays a vital role in all specialties and chest radiograph is the most commonly performed procedure in most radiology departments. The importance and reliance on imaging is even more in pediatric pulmonology where it forms an integral part of the work-up and management of almost all acute and chronic disorders. An evidence-based algorithmic approach needs to be followed to reach an accurate and prompt diagnosis while incurring minimum cost and radiation burden in this vulnerable group of patients. Basics of radiology are important for the pediatricians also and to this end this book covers the common clinical conditions seen in everyday practice.

Imaging children is challenging and this is especially true for the chest where motion artefacts can play havoc with image quality. Added to these limitations is the immense pressure on the radiologists to answer challenging questions while minimizing the radiation exposure. This effectively implies that every computed tomography (CT) that is performed must be justified not only financially but also in terms of the added radiation burden to the child. To this end, there is an increasing trend towards using ultrasonography and magnetic resonance imaging (MRI) for imaging the chest.

This book is not intended to be a comprehensive text on pediatric chest imaging but we hope that it will help the busy radiologists and pediatricians in interpreting images of the chest in children. This would aid in better management of children with respiratory disorders.

We wish to thank all the contributors, for their efforts in compiling this text.

We would also like to extend our appreciation to Shri Jitendar P Vij (Group Chairman), Mr Ankit Vij (Group President), Mr Tarun Duneja (Director—Publishing) and all the staff of M/s Jaypee Brothers Medical Publishers (P) Ltd., New Delhi, India, for their efforts and input enabling timely publication of the book.

We welcome any feedback on enhancing the content of the book, which can be incorporated in the subsequent editions.

Ashu Seith Bhalla
Arun Kumar Gupta

Contents

Section 1: Imaging Modalities: Basics

1. **Chest Radiograph: Basics and Role** — 3
   Tany Chandra, Priyanka Naranje
   - Radiographic Views 3
   - Fluoroscopy 5
   - Interpretation of Pediatric Chest Radiograph 5
   - Localization of Thoracic Mass Lesion 16

2. **Ultrasound Chest: Basics and Role** — 22
   Amit Gupta, Priyanka Naranje
   - Indications 22
   - Equipment 23
   - Technique 23
   - Normal Ultrasonography Appearances 24
   - Imaging Findings 26
   - Limitations 35

3. **CT Chest: Basics and Role** — 38
   Devasenathipathy Kandasamy
   - Technique 38
   - Radiation Dose 39
   - Imaging Protocols 40

4. **MRI Chest: Basics and Role** — 46
   Surabhi Vyas, Devasenathipathy Kandasamy
   - Indications 47
   - MRI Technique 52
   - Building Block Approach 54
   - Newer MRI Techniques 55

Section 2: Neonatal and Congenital Disorders

5. Neonatal Respiratory Distress — 59
Anmol Bhatia, Ashish Dua, Kushaljit Singh Sodhi
- Medical Causes of Respiratory Distress *59*
- Surgical Causes of Respiratory Distress *62*
- Miscellaneous Causes of Respiratory Distress *67*

6. Congenital Lung Abnormalities — 69
Pooja Abbey, Aparna Shyamkumar
- Nomenclature and Classification *69*
- Embryological Basis and Etiopathogenesis *70*
- Categorization of Congenital Lung Anomalies *70*
- Role of Different Imaging Modalities *90*

Section 3: Chest Infections

7. Bacterial and Viral Chest Infections — 99
Anmol Bhatia, Harshith Gowda, Kushaljit Singh Sodhi, Akshay Kumar Saxena
- Epidemiology *99*
- Role of Imaging *100*
- Viral Pneumonia *100*
- Coronavirus Disease 2019 *102*
- Bacterial Pneumonia *104*
- Round Pneumonia *109*

8. Fungal Chest Infections — 115
Ashu Seith Bhalla, Kana Ram Jat
- Classification of Fungi *116*
- Clinical Features *116*
- Aspergillosis *116*
- Other Fungal Infections *126*

9. Chest Tuberculosis — 136
Taruna Yadav, Sushil K Kabra
- Imaging Modalities *137*
- Choice of Modality *140*
- Imaging Findings *140*
- Signs of Activity *153*
- Specific Situations *153*

10. **Chest Infections in Immunocompromised Host**   156
    Manisha Jana, Nitin Dhochak
    - Primary Immunodeficiency Disorders (PIDs)   *157*
    - Classification of PIDs   *157*
    - Infections in Immunodeficiency   *158*
    - Noninfectious Complications   *160*
    - Specific Primary Immunodeficiency Disorders   *163*
    - Secondary Causes of Immunodeficiency   *173*
    - Approach on Imaging   *174*

Section 4: Diffuse Lung Diseases and Miscellaneous

11. **Diffuse Lung Diseases: Part 1**   179
    Deeksha Bhalla, Priyanka Naranje
    - Pattern-based Approach in Infants   *179*
    - Pattern-based Approach to Classification in Older Children   *184*

12. **Diffuse Lung Diseases: Part 2**   191
    Deeksha Bhalla, Manisha Jana
    - Childhood Interstitial Lung Disease Entities More Prevalent in Infancy   *192*
    - Disorders not Specific to Infancy   *198*

13. **Pulmonary Complications in Congenital Heart Diseases**   217
    Anisha Garg, Amarinder S Malhi
    - Complications Involving Airways   *218*
    - Complications Involving Lung Parenchyma   *224*
    - Complications Involving Pulmonary Vasculature   *229*
    - Complications Involving Pleura and Thoracic Cage   *233*
    - Complications Related to Cardiac Surgery   *234*

Section 5: Airway Imaging

14. **Upper Airway Imaging**   239
    Smita Manchanda, Ankita Aggarwal
    - Classification   *240*
    - Etiological Approach   *241*

15. **Central Airway Imaging**   258
    Iqbal Bashir, Ashu Seith Bhalla
    - Classification   *258*
    - Development and Branching Anomalies of Airways   *259*

- Intrinsic (Intramural) Central Airway Abnormalities 270
- Intraluminal Obstruction 271
- Extrinsic Airway Compression 274

16. Bronchiectasis 279
Stuti Chandola, Smita Manchanda
- Imaging Modalities 279
- Diagnosis 280
- Types of Bronchiectasis 282
- Etiology and Pathogenesis 283
- Complications 284
- Specific Entities 286
- Management 294

17. Small Airway Diseases 296
Priyanka Naranje, Rajendra K Behera
- Introduction/Terminology 296
- Imaging Modalities and Signs 296
- Classification 297
- Asthma versus Small Airway Disease 303

Section 6: Vascular and Lymphatic Disorders

18. Pulmonary Artery Imaging 307
Sneha Goswami, Ashu Seith Bhalla
- Classification 307
- Imaging Modalities 308
- Congenital Anomalies 309
- Acquired Abnormalities 313

19. Pulmonary Veins Imaging 323
Manisha Jana, Ashu Seith Bhalla
- Normal Anatomy 323
- Disorders of Pulmonary Veins 324
- Classification Based on Morphological Changes 324
- Classification Based on Etiology 325
- Congenital Pulmonary Vein Anomalies 325
- Acquired Pulmonary Vein Anomalies 334

20. Lymphatic Anomalies: Imaging and Interventions   337
Ishan Gupta, Priyanka Naranje
- Normal Anatomy *338*
- Imaging *340*
- Management in Lymphatic Malformations in Chest *350*

Section 7: Mediastinum Imaging

21. Approach to Mediastinal Lesions: Part 1   357
Shruti Badkhane, Manisha Jana
- Compartments of Mediastinum *357*
- Role of Imaging *359*
- Mediastinal Masses *362*

22. Approach to Mediastinal Lesions: Part 2   369
Ashu Seith Bhalla, Manisha Jana
- Middle Mediastinal Masses (Visceral Compartment) *369*
- Posterior Mediastinal Masses (Paravertebral Compartment) *372*
- Multicompartmental Masses *373*
- Masses Where Biopsy is not Indicated *375*
- Specific Entities *376*
- Fibrosing Mediastinitis *379*

Section 8: Tumors and Mimics

23. Thoracic Tumors and Mimics: Part 1   385
Deeksha Bhalla, Akshay Baheti
- Spectrum of Pediatric Chest Tumors *385*
- Unique Pediatric Tumors *385*
- Thoracic Tumors with Syndromic Association *386*
- Tumors Presenting in Neonates *387*
- Imaging of Region-specific Tumors in Children *388*

24. Thoracic Tumors and Mimics: Part 2   405
Ashu Seith Bhalla, Vasundhara Patil
- Primary Pulmonary Tumors *405*
- Airway Tumors *413*
- Chest Wall Tumors *417*

Section 9: Chest Wall and Pleural Disorders

25. Chest Wall Imaging — 425
Poonam Sherwani, Ashu Seith Bhalla
- Imaging Modalities 425
- Classification 425
- Specific Entities 426

26. Pleural Disorders: Imaging — 443
Poonam Sherwani, Manisha Jana
- Imaging Modalities 443
- Pleural Pathologies 444
- Nonexpandable Lung After Drainage 460

Section 10: Respiratory Emergencies

27. Hemoptysis: Imaging and Interventions — 465
Priyanka Naranje, Ayush Jain, Ashu Seith Bhalla
- Etiology 465
- Imaging Evaluation 466
- Specific Etiologies 469
- Interventional Radiology Management of Hemoptysis 476

28. Thoracic Imaging in Intensive Care Unit — 479
Surabhi Vyas, Rakesh Lodha
- Imaging Modalities 479
- Parenchymal Abnormalities 480
- Pleural Abnormalities 489
- Airway Abnormalities 491
- Ventilator-associated Air Leak 493
- Lines and Tubes 493

Section 11: Reporting Formats Illustrative Cases and Self-assessment

29. Reporting Formats and Illustrative Cases — 501
Anuradha Singh
- Case 1: Reporting Format for Bronchiectasis 501
- Case 2: Reporting Format for Congenital Lung Abnormalities: Vascular Anomalies 503

- Case 3: Reporting Format for Tuberculosis (TB)   505
- Case 4: Reporting Format for Pediatric Diffuse Lung Diseases (DLD)   507
- Case 5: Reporting Format for Hemoptysis   507

30. **Self-assessment Module**   513
    Anuradha Singh
    - Imaging Modalities   513
    - Congenital Anomalies   516
    - Neonatal Respiratory Distress   520
    - Infections   524
    - Airways   528
    - Interstitial Lung Diseases   530
    - Tumors Including Chest Wall and Pleura   534
    - Interventions   540

Index   541

SECTION 1

Imaging Modalities: Basics

CHAPTER 1: Chest Radiograph: Basics and Role
CHAPTER 2: Ultrasound Chest: Basics and Role
CHAPTER 3: CT Chest: Basics and Role
CHAPTER 4: MRI Chest: Basics and Role

CHAPTER 1

Chest Radiograph: Basics and Role

Tany Chandra, Priyanka Naranje

- ❏ Radiographic views
- ❏ Fluoroscopy
- ❏ Interpretation of pediatric chest radiograph
  - ➢ Effect of age
  - ➢ Technical pearls
  - ➢ Systematic review
- ❏ Localization of thoracic mass lesion
  - ➢ Silhouette sign
  - ➢ Hilar masses
  - ➢ Differentiation of pulmonary from extraparenchymal masses

■ INTRODUCTION

Chest radiographs remain the modality of choice for screening and primary diagnostic workup for respiratory complaints. It uses ionizing radiation and must be used judiciously. It may be done as a single-view or two-view study, depending on the patient cooperation and severity of illness. Radiographic abnormalities should be interpreted after consideration of the age, clinical history, examination findings, laboratory investigation, and previous imaging reports, if available.

■ RADIOGRAPHIC VIEWS

- *Posterior anterior (PA) view*: Standard view which is considered the gold standard is a PA view which includes an erect positioning (standing), posterior irradiation with arms turned out of the field, in full inspiration. The WHO recommends a good quality chest radiography which includes lateral view wherever and whenever possible for evaluation of pediatric pulmonary tuberculosis. Left lateral projection with full inspiration is preferred[1] **(Figs. 1A and B)**. Radiographic views are listed in **Table 1**.

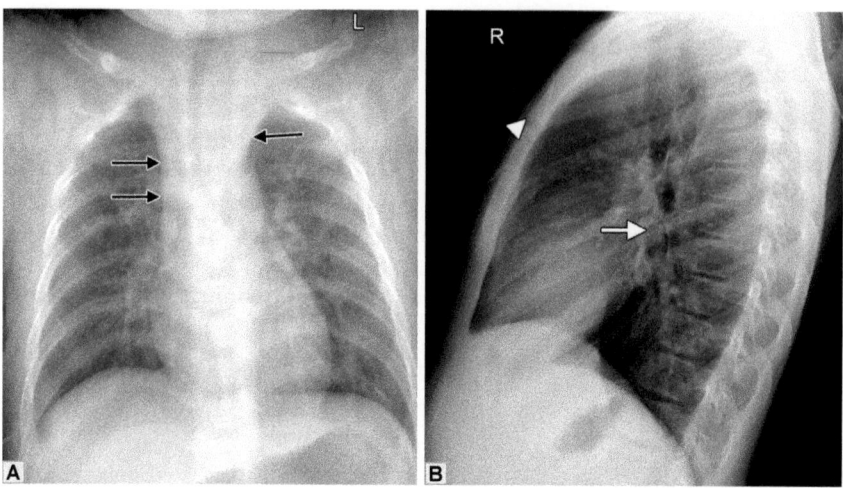

FIGS. 1A AND B: Normal chest radiograph PA (A) and lateral (B) views. (A) Thymic outline (arrows) and (B) hilar structures (white arrow) and radiolucent retrosternal space (arrowhead).

TABLE 1: Radiographic views of chest.	
Type of chest radiograph	**Current utility**
Chest radiograph posteroanterior (PA) view	• Standard technique • Most commonly performed • Most of the measurements and signs described on radiographs apply to this view
Chest radiograph anteroposterior view	Performed when patient cannot be positioned for PA view such as in ICU, bedside and children
Chest radiograph lateral view	Useful ancillary view when CT is not done/not available
Lordotic view (apicogram—if only the apices are included)	Specialized view to demonstrate the apices of lungs which are usually hidden behind the clavicles on routine views
Decubitus view **(Figs. 2A and B)**	• Replaced by US • Can be used in small pleural effusion or pneumothorax
Expiratory radiograph	• Useful in demonstrating air trapping in suspected foreign body aspiration • Can be assessed in fluoroscopy also

- *Anteroposterior view*: It is performed with the patient in supine position or sitting/semierect for critically ill or post-trauma patients, and children (especially neonates).
- *Decubitus view*: Allows us to differentiate between mobile and loculated effusions and for detection of pneumothoraces **(Figs. 2A and B)**.
- *Expiratory radiograph*: Chest radiograph acquired after complete expiration is usually a complimentary study to highlight any air trapping, especially in cases of pediatric endobronchial radiolucent foreign body aspiration **(Figs. 3A and B)**.

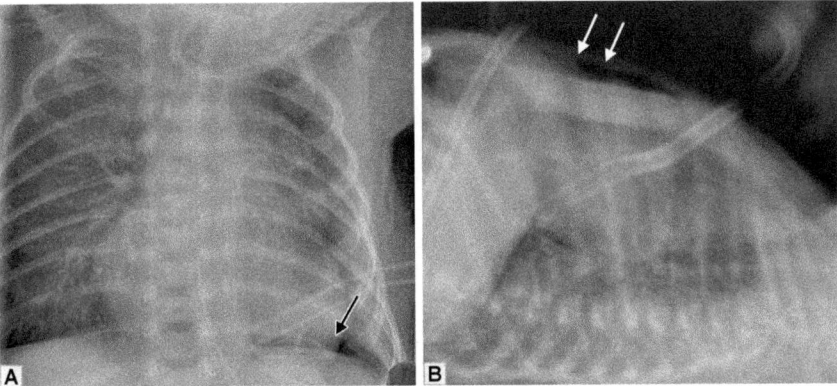

FIGS. 2A AND B: Role of decubitus view in small pneumothorax. (A) Small pneumothorax (arrow) and (B) pneumothorax in nondependent location (arrows).

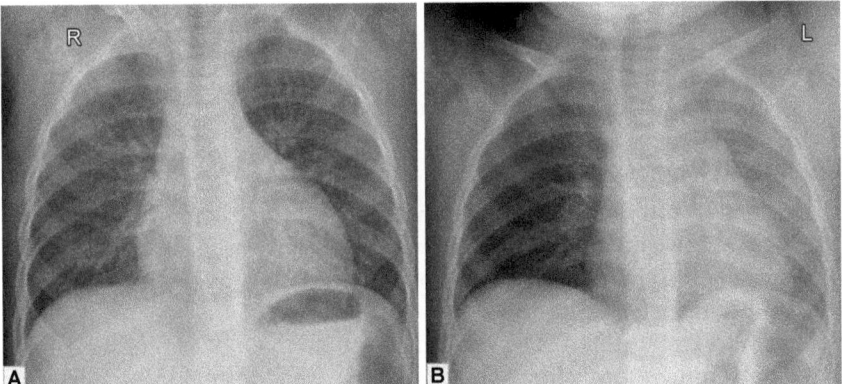

FIGS. 3A AND B: (A) Inspiratory and (B) Expiratory view in suspected foreign body inhalation.
(A) Inspiratory view and expiratory view. Right hemithorax is lucent, suggesting obstruction. Left hemithorax normal, as the density increases.

FLUOROSCOPY

Even in the era of CT, fluoroscopy is useful in evaluation of diaphragmatic excursion, central airway assessment, and lung volume evaluation in short clips.

INTERPRETATION OF PEDIATRIC CHEST RADIOGRAPH

Chest radiographs remain the first line of thoracic imaging and adherence to a systematic approach for interpretation is essential to correctly point to a diagnosis and plan further investigations.

We propose the following steps for a systematic approach to interpret:
- *Check patient particulars (especially age of patient) and the side marker:* Correctly, diagnosing situs is essential and is dependent on the correct marking.

- Note the projection (AP/PA)
- Note the phase of respiration
- Verify the presence of rotation
- Note the presence of artifacts if any
- Analyzing all the structures for abnormalities systematically

Finally, a diagnosis is suggested based on the radiographic findings in *context of the clinical background.*

A few common sources of error in children are discussed below.

Effect of Age

In neonates, young infants, and children, following additional characteristics need to be kept in mind:
- The anteroposterior diameter of the chest is usually more.
- Air bronchogram frequently seen projected in the retrocardiac location in the neonate and young infant.
- If seen more peripherally, considered pathological.
- Anterior aspects of the diaphragms usually are at a higher level and the lower zones may be obscured.
- Thymus and its appearance based on age is discussed later.

Technical Pearls

- As babies and most toddlers are imaged by an AP radiograph, do not forget about cardiac magnification.
- Pleural effusion can give the appearance of increased opacity of a hemithorax, on a supine X-ray.
- Expiratory phase film shows an apparent enlargement of the heart size and prominent bronchovascular markings (in a normal inspiratory film anterior end of 6th rib should be visible above the diaphragm).
- Rotation is the most common cause for unilateral increased or decreased translucency.
- Skin folds may mimic pneumothorax.
- On an oblique or rotated radiograph, sternal ossification centers may mimic lung nodules.

Systematic Review

Discussion of structure-wise approach to a chest radiograph is given below.

Mediastinum

- Tracheal displacement (anterior, posterior, or lateral) should raise suspicion of a mediastinal mass.
- An anterior mediastinal mass is to be suspected when and right border of the cardiac shadow is silhouetted and a lateral radiograph, if performed, shows posterior displacement of trachea **(Figs. 4A to C)**.

CHAPTER 1: Chest Radiograph: Basics and Role

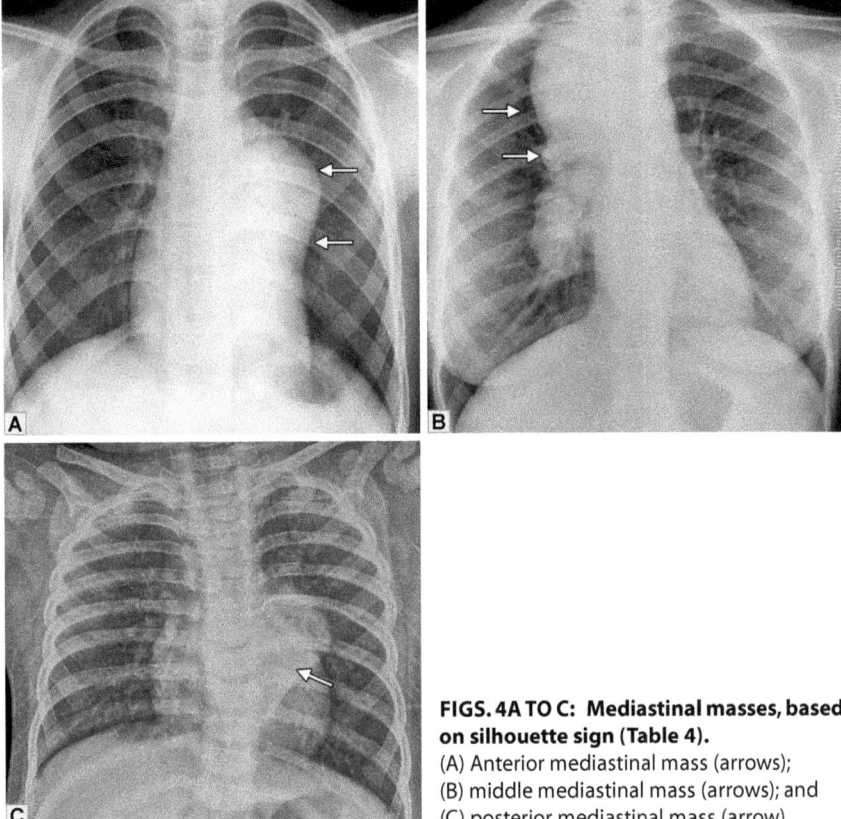

FIGS. 4A TO C: Mediastinal masses, based on silhouette sign (Table 4).
(A) Anterior mediastinal mass (arrows); (B) middle mediastinal mass (arrows); and (C) posterior mediastinal mass (arrow).

- Loss of visualization of the aortic knuckle indicates that the mass lies in posterior mediastinum (adjacent to the aortic arch).
- Lateral deviation of the trachea indicates a middle mediastinal mass (e.g., bronchogenic cyst and lymph nodes).
- Posterior mediastinal mass (e.g., neurogenic tumor) may result in pressure erosion or splaying of the posterior rib ends.
- Acute infection or steroid therapy may cause transient thymic atrophy. However, the possibility of an absent thymus gland must be considered (DiGeorge syndrome), if it is persistently small.
- Rebound thymic hyperplasia and anterior mediastinal tumors may be difficult to differentiate on imaging.
- Also see Chapters 21 and 22.

Thymus
- Prominent anterior mediastinal shadow with the characteristic "sail sign" **(Figs. 5A to D)**
- Begins involuting after 2 years and gradually disappears around 7–8 years of age
- Can appear very prominent in some infants and must be differentiated from a mediastinal mass or consolidation[2,3]
- Relatively less opaque with visualization underlying structure (vis-à-vis pathological opacification)
- Wavy contour (due to ribs) is helpful and sometimes a lateral projection might be of benefit
- Ultrasound shows a characteristic "starry sky appearance".

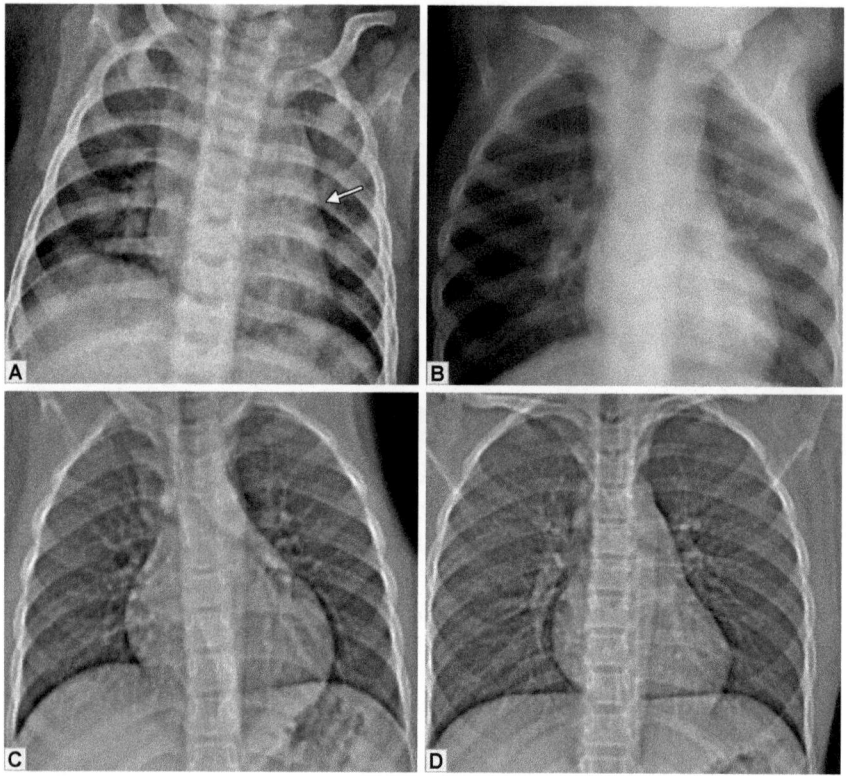

FIGS. 5A TO D: Normal thymus at different ages. (A) Wave sign (arrow) in an infant; (B) 2 years age; (C and D): CT scout images: (C) 7 years age; and (D) 12 years age.

Heart and Great Vessels
- Normal cardiothoracic ratio is 60% in infants **(Fig. 6)**.
- Establish situs by inspection of the bronchial anatomy, gastric bubble, and the ascending and descending aorta.
- Right-sided aortic arch is associated with various congenital heart diseases.
- Closely inspect lungs to assess pulmonary vascularity in any case with cardiomegaly:
  - Visible pulmonary arterial branches in the periphery of the lung, suggests pulmonary plethora (increased blood flow)
  - Nonvisualization of the central pulmonary vessels suggests reduced pulmonary blood flow.
- On chest radiograph, imaging pointers of pulmonary arterial hypertension include peripheral pruning of the pulmonary arteries and enlarged central pulmonary arteries.
- Tracheal position and caliber narrowing on frontal radiographs and anterior bowing of trachea on lateral radiographs can suggest congenital anomalies of pulmonary vasculature which include pulmonary sling and rings.
- While abnormalities in cardiac contour may be useful to diagnose the anatomical cardiac chamber enlargement, the causes of chamber enlargement are wide and nonspecific, which requires full assessment by echocardiography.

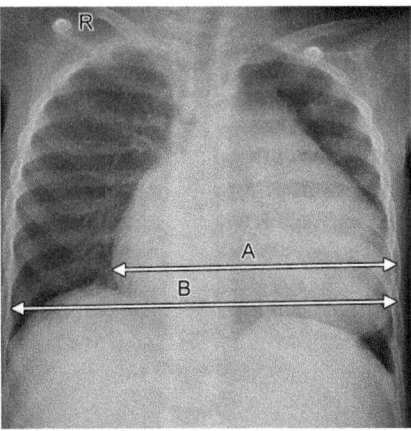

FIG. 6: Increased cardiothoracic ratio (A/B) with straightening and lifting of left heart border.

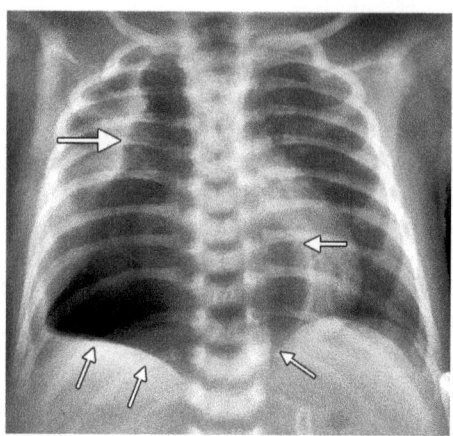

FIG. 7: Pneumomediastinum showing continuous diaphragm sign (arrows), and extra-pleural extension of air (thick arrows).

Pneumomediastinum
- Appearance of central area of increased translucency over the mediastinum
- Increased clarity of the cardiac outline
- Air outlines the lobes of the thymus **(Fig. 7)**.

Lungs

Generalized Increased Translucency of the Thorax
- Large inspiratory effort
- Airway diseases (asthma, bronchiolitis, and cystic fibrosis)
- Upper airway obstruction due to tracheal obstruction (e.g., vascular ring or tracheal foreign body)
- Diffuse bilateral homogenous opacification—neonatal pulmonary disorders including hyaline membrane disease (surfactant deficiency) and transient tachypnea of newborn.

Unilateral Translucency
- Patient rotation probably is the most common cause.
- If there is differential pulmonary vascularity; the side with decreased vascularity is usually abnormal. The side with increased or normal vascularity is normal.
    - Changes in appearance between inspiratory and expiratory films—the side which shows least change on expiration is usually abnormal.
    - Size of the hemithorax—a small opaque hemithorax is usually abnormal.
- In obstructive emphysema, expiratory film will exaggerate disparity between normal and abnormal lung.

- Compensatory emphysema—less marked on expiration.
- Pulmonary hypoplasia—small hyperlucent lung and small caliber of pulmonary artery. Proximal interruption of pulmonary artery is another entity mimicking hypoplasia **(Fig. 8)**.
- Swyer–James–MacLeod syndrome—acquired bronchiolitis obliterans; small lung with hyperlucency, air trapping, and small caliber of pulmonary artery.
- *Poland syndrome*: Absence of pectoralis minor muscle **(Fig. 9)**.

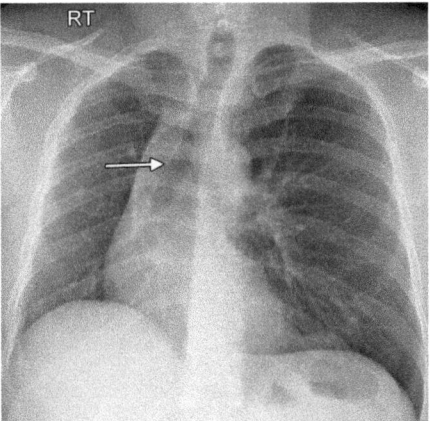

FIG. 8: Unilateral small volume right hemithorax in proximal interruption of pulmonary artery. Normal right main bronchus (arrow), absent/small right hilum; normal left hilum, and reduced pulmonary vascular markings on right side.

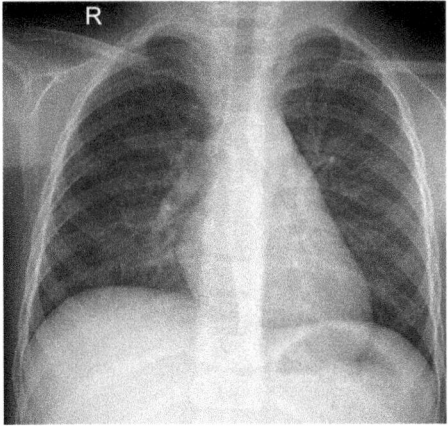

FIG. 9: Unilateral translucent right hemithorax in Poland syndrome.

Increased Pulmonary Opacification
- *Pulmonary infiltrates*: Air space opacities—air bronchograms; consolidation may be segmental or lobar in distribution **(Fig. 10)**.
    - Pulmonary edema, bronchopneumonia, aspiration changes are usually bilateral
    - Interstitial infiltrates: Linear pattern with peribronchial thickening—acute interstitial pulmonary edema or infection (e.g., viral bronchiolitis)
    - Chronic interstitial disease—reticulonodular, nodular, miliary opacities, and a honeycomb appearance
- *Pulmonary collapse*: Area of increased opacity, with loss of lung volume (seen by alteration in the position of the fissures and/or hilar shadows, and mediastinal shift) **(Figs. 11A and B)**
- Pulmonary aplasia and agenesis—small lung volume with increased opacity **(Figs. 12A and B)**
- Large pulmonary/chest wall mass

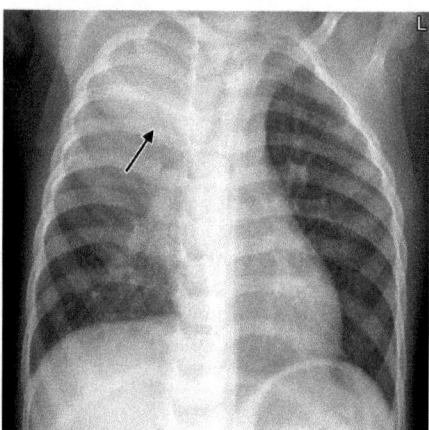

FIG. 10: Community acquired pneumonia presenting radiographically as right upper zone consolidation. Air bronchogram (arrow).

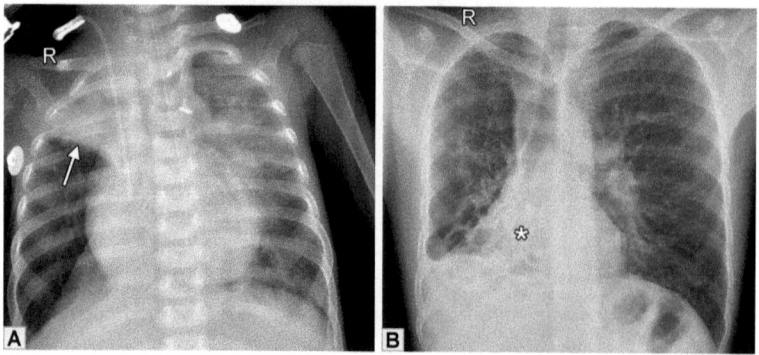

FIGS. 11A AND B: Right upper lobe (A) and combined right middle and lower lobe (B) collapse with cystic bronchiectasis. (A) Upward displacement of minor fissure (arrow) and (B) triangular density (asterisk) silhouetting right cardiac border as well as right hemidiaphragm.

CHAPTER 1: Chest Radiograph: Basics and Role

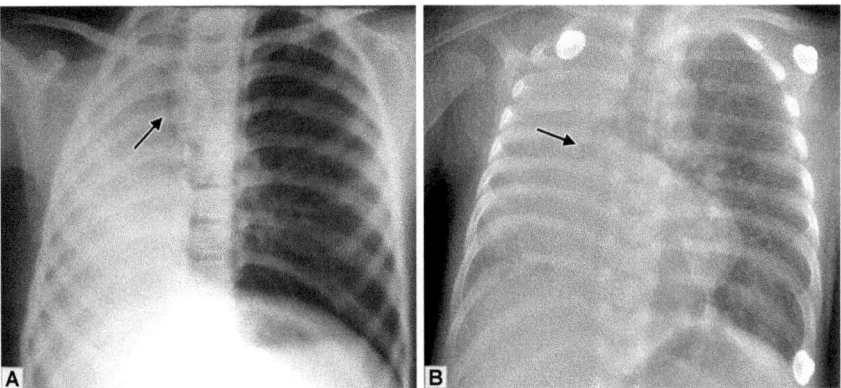

FIGS. 12A AND B. Opaque right hemithorax in right pulmonary agenesis (A) and mucus plug obstruction (B). (A) Ipsilateral mediastinal shift, and nonvisualized right main bronchus (arrow) and (B) Mild ipsilateral mediastinal shift, patent right main bronchus (arrow).

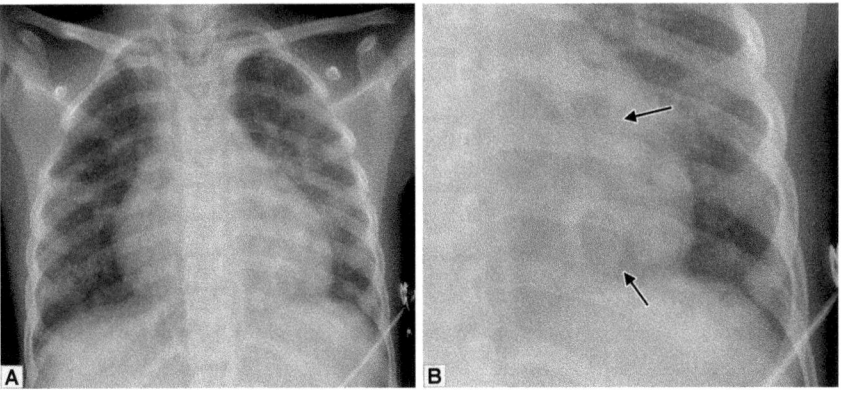

FIGS. 13A AND B: Multiple cavitating nodules (arrows in B) in septic emboli. Chest radiograph PA (A) and magnified view (B).

Pulmonary Nodules
- Wide differential diagnosis.
- Most common cause in childhood is "round pneumonia".
- Multifocal nodules are most commonly infective (septic emboli and miliary nodules), metastases **(Figs. 13A and B)**.
- Solitary nodules can be infective (granuloma and round pneumonia), hamartoma, or metastasis.

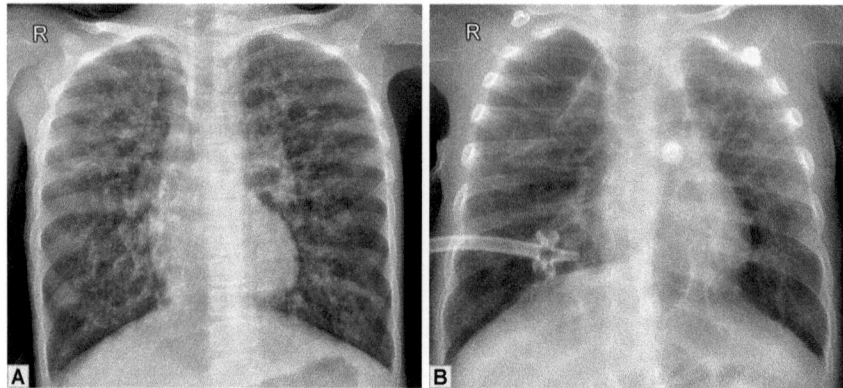

FIGS. 14A AND B: Ring shadows. (A) Bronchiectasis and (B) cysts in Langerhans cell histiocytosis.

Ring Shadows

Ring shadows refer to air-filled cystic lesions with thin wall:
- Bronchiectasis **(Figs. 14A and B)**
- Cystic fibrosis
- Pneumatoceles—staphylococcal and streptococcal pneumonia
- Bronchogenic cyst
- Congenital diaphragmatic hernia
- Cystic adenomatoid malformation
- Bronchopulmonary dysplasia

Pleural Space

Pleural Effusion

Pleural fluid, in supine position, can lead to diffusely increased opacity in hemithorax; in erect position, it leads to blunting of CP angle **(Table 2)**.

Pneumothorax

- Increased translucency of the hemothorax
- Visualization of the lung margin
- Anterior loculation of the pneumothorax may be indicated by the only abnormality of increased clarity of the heart border. Signs on supine and erect radiographs are listed in **Table 3** (also see Chapter 26).

TABLE 2: Signs of pleural effusion on radiograph (Figs. 15A and B).

Signs on erect radiograph	Signs on supine radiograph
Increased density with concave upper margin (meniscus sign)	Increased opacity of hemithorax
Blunting of costophrenic angle	Superior mediastinal widening
Fluid within the fissures	"Apical cap"
	Fluid within the fissures

TABLE 3: Signs of pneumothorax on radiographs (Figs. 16A and B).	
Signs on erect radiograph	Signs on supine radiograph
Lucency having a sharp margin with the underlying lung	Increased lucency of hemithorax
	Deep sulcus sign

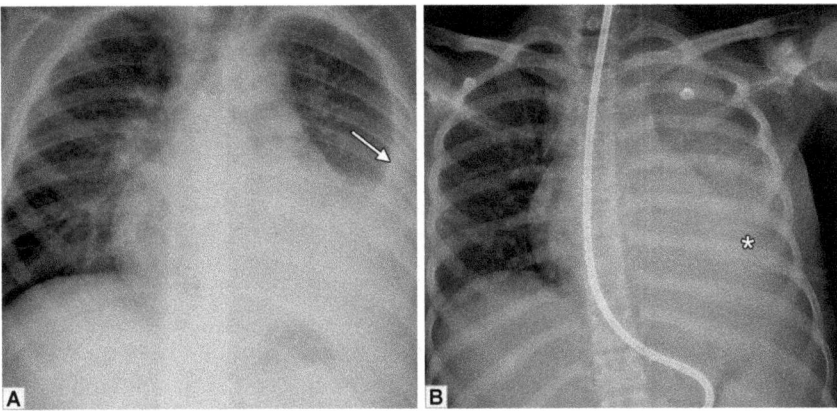

FIGS. 15A AND B: Free pleural effusion on erect (A) and supine (B) radiographs (Table 2). Left costophrenic angle is blunted. Concave upper border which is medially slanting (meniscus sign, arrow in A). Homogeneous increased opacity in the left hemithorax (asterisk in B).

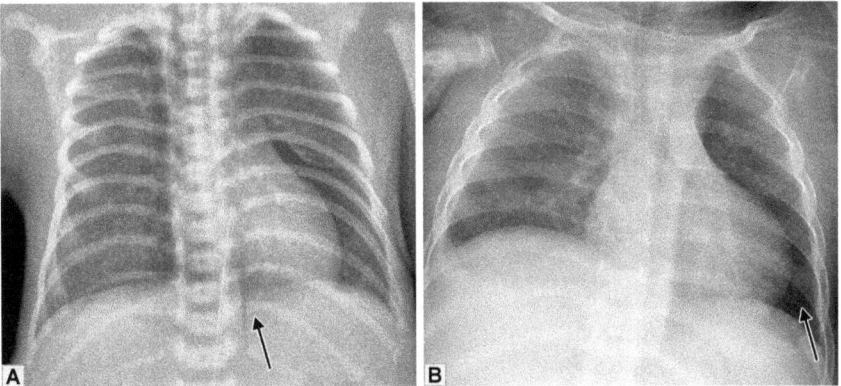

FIGS. 16A AND B: Signs of pneumothorax on supine radiograph. (A) Naclerio's V sign (arrow in A) and (B) increased lucency in left hemithorax (arrow in B).

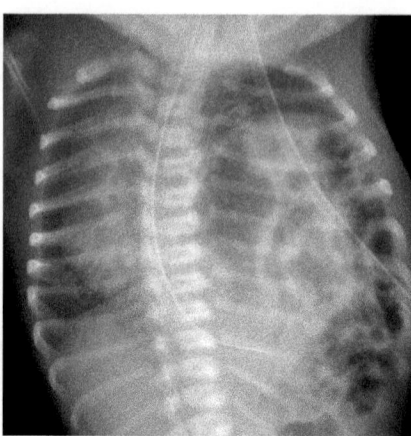

FIG. 17: Congenital diaphragmatic hernia. Bowel loops seen in left hemithorax and contralateral mediastinal shift.

Diaphragms
- *Normal position*: Right hemidiaphragm can normally be higher than left—difference of height > 1.5 cm between the two hemidiaphragms abnormal.
- *Marked elevation*: Loss of lung volume, diaphragmatic paralysis, eventration, congenital diaphragmatic hernia, and subpulmonary effusion **(Fig. 17)**.
- A flattened diaphragm indicates overinflation and loculated subpulmonary pneumothorax.

Special Conditions
- Partial/complete thymectomy generally forms a part, for dissection and approach. Hence, progressive mediastinal widening following surgery must not be attributed to thymic rebound/thymic shadow.
- Barotrauma can be seen in form of pulmonary interstitial emphysema or pneumothorax and pneumomediastinum.

■ LOCALIZATION OF THORACIC MASS LESION

In addition, localization of mass/mass-like lesion on chest radiograph is discussed below.[4]

Silhouette Sign
- Silhouette sign provides anatomic localization of abnormalities on chest radiographs when there is loss of interface between structures in the same anatomic plane.

CHAPTER 1: Chest Radiograph: Basics and Role

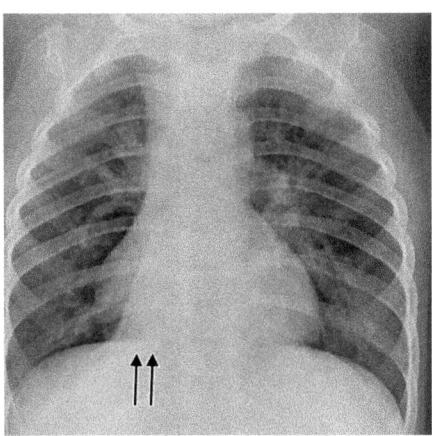

FIG. 18: Silhouette sign in right lower lobe collapse. Obscured right hemidiaphragm margin (arrows) and right cardiac shadow is not silhouetted.

TABLE 4: Silhouette sign and its use in localization.		
Structure silhouetted	**Location of pulmonary lesion**	**Location in mediastinum**
Right heart border	Right middle lobe	Anterior mediastinum
Left heart border	Lingula	Anterior mediastinum
Right hemidiaphragm	Right lower lobe	
Left hemidiaphragm	Left lower lobe	
Aortic knuckle	Left lower lobe	Posterior mediastinum
Descending aorta		Posterior mediastinum

- Consolidation can obliterate the border with an adjacent soft-tissue structure **(Fig. 18)**.
- Consolidation of lingula silhouettes the left-heart border, middle lobe consolidation obscures the right-heart border whereas the ipsilateral hemidiaphragm is silhouetted in lower lobe consolidation **(Table 4)**.

Hilar Masses
- The pulmonary hilum is composed of the pulmonary vessels, bronchi, and lymphatics with the pulmonary artery and vein forming the radiological hilum and the bronchi seen as a radiolucent stripe separating the hilum from the mediastinum.
- Thus, the commonly seen hilar masses arise from lymph nodes, bronchi, and pulmonary vessels **(Table 5; Figs. 19A and B)**. In addition, hilum may get secondarily invaded from adjoining mediastinal structures, e.g., carcinoma esophagus.

TABLE 5: Causes of hilar enlargement based on the structure of origin.	
Structure of origin	Causes
Lymph nodes	Multiple causes of enlargement—nonneoplastic/neoplastic
Bronchi	• Lung carcinoma • Carcinoid tumor
Pulmonary vessels	Pulmonary artery enlargement

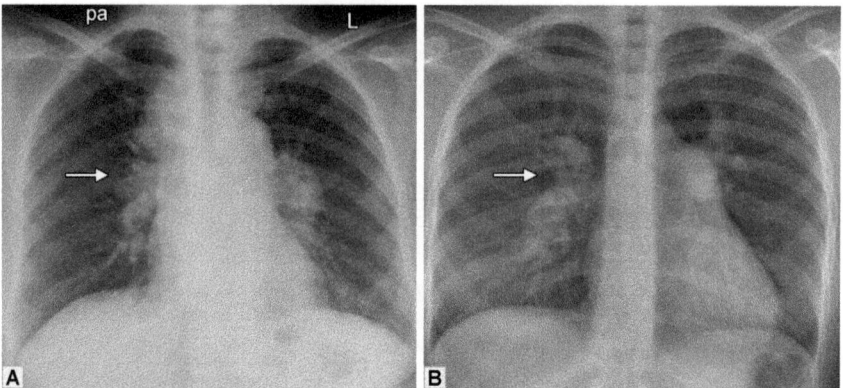

FIGS. 19A AND B: Hilar mass: Structure of origin. (A) Lobulated lymph nodal enlargement (arrow) and (B) enlarged pulmonary arteries converging toward the hilar abnormality (arrow).

- Hilar masses may be true hilar masses or those which are superimposed on the hilum **(Flowchart 2)**.
- On a chest radiograph, an apparent hilar mass may either arise from the structures that constitute the "true hilar" masses, or simply appear as *hilar masses due to overlap on a frontal radiograph*. These masses will display the *"hilum overlay sign"*, i.e., the hilum will be seen through them. Masses that superimpose on the hilum include **(Figs. 19A and B)**:
  ○ Mediastinal masses—anterior or posterior
  ○ Pulmonary masses—apical segment of lower lobes
- *True hilar masses* appear as an enlarged and dense hilum. The normal hilar angle is concave; in the presence of a hilar mass this angle is convex *(Hilar angle sign)*.
- Hilar masses may also *arise from nodes or bronchi of the hilum*. The nodal masses will have lobulated margins and calcification may be seen. The masses of bronchial origin include carcinoma lung (spiculated margins); and carcinoids and salivary gland origin tumors (smooth margins).
- *Hilum convergence sign*: In a juxtahilar mediastinal mass, the pulmonary artery branches are visible through the mass and converge toward the waist of the heart (positive hilum convergence sign). However, if the pulmonary artery branches lead toward the hilar mass, then the opacity is due to an enlarged pulmonary artery (negative hilum convergence sign) **(Figs. 20A and B)**.

CHAPTER 1: Chest Radiograph: Basics and Role

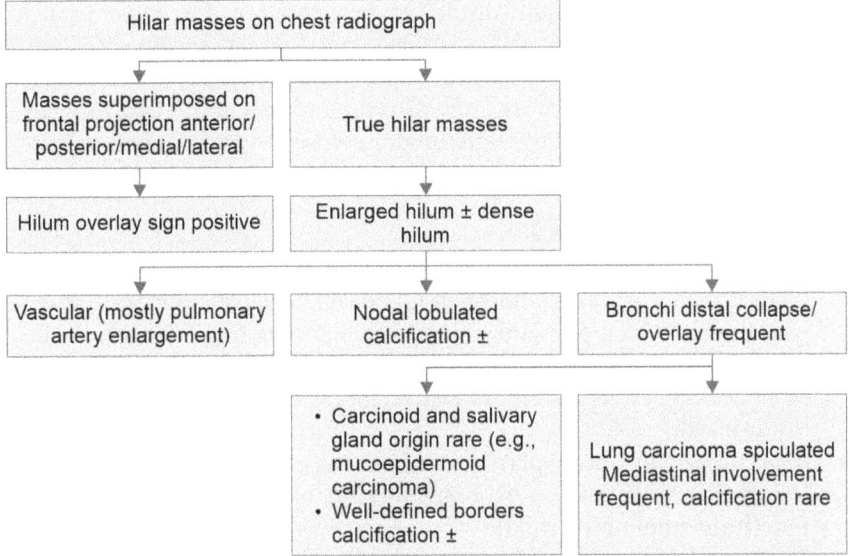

FLOWCHART 2: Approach to Hilar masses on chest radiograph.

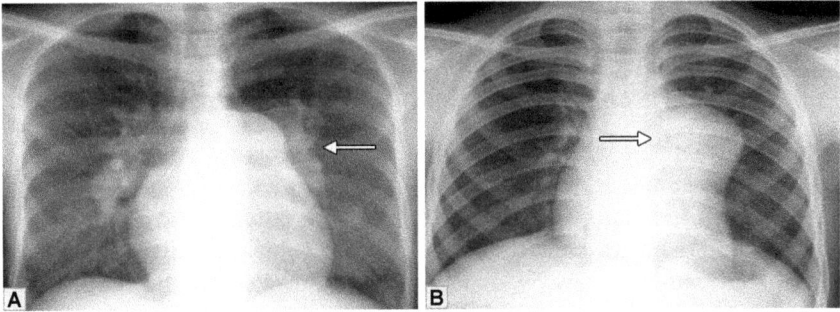

FIGS. 20A AND B. Hilum Convergence Sign. (A) Pulmonary artery branches converge toward the hilar abnormality (arrow) s/o enlarged pulmonary artery and (B) pulmonary artery branches converge toward the heart (arrow) s/o mediastinal mass.

Differentiation of Pulmonary from Extraparenchymal Masses

Pulmonary Lesions

- These are centered in the lung parenchyma and have acute angles with the chest wall and ill-defined margins.[1] Lung parenchymal lesions are surrounded by air on all sides, and hence nodules when present in the lung have complete borders (these borders may be well-defined or ill-defined depending on the nature of the lesion).
- Even when these lesions are about the pleural surface, along costal, mediastinal, or diaphragmatic pleura, they make acute angles with these surfaces.

- In addition, several lesions display air bronchogram, i.e., intact bronchi traverse through them, though these may appear narrow or dilated depending on the type of lesion. Solid components of several invasive tumors, however, compress or involve the bronchi and no air bronchogram is seen. Subsequently with tumor necrosis, however, tumor ruptures into an adjoining bronchus and cavitation develop.

Pleural/Extrapleural Lesions
- These have obtuse angles with tapered margins.
- Pleural lesions will have sharp inner borders, while laterally these merge with the chest wall or mediastinum or diaphragm (depending on which pleural surface is involved). The angles thus formed are obtuse. Laterally, pleural lesions may extend into extrapleural space, and further beyond to chest wall.[1]
- Also, these will not display air within. The presence of air in pleural lesions is a consequence of an intervention, or a bronchial communication (bronchopleural fistula).
- The underlying lung is atelectatic which if normal appears homogenous, and well enhancing. Long-standing pleural thickening can result in round atelectasis in underlying lung.
- Also, when infective pleural effusions heal, small-lobulated collections may remain. Both these situations result in formation of "*pseudomasses*" that can simulate tumors, and should be recognized as such **(Figs. 21A and B)**.
- In addition, the *pleural lesions* change location with respiration and displace extrapleural fat outward.
- *Extrapleural lesions* may arise from extrapleural fat, intercostal muscles, ribs, and neurovascular bundle. These also have obtuse angles with tapered margins, however, extrapleural masses displace the extrapleural fat inward and are more frequently associated with rib erosion.

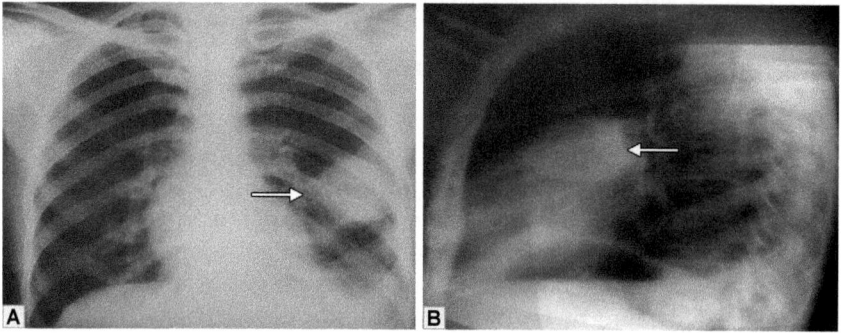

FIGS. 21A AND B: Phantom/vanishing tumor (pseudomass). (A) Well-defined round mass in left lower zone (arrow); (B) Oval shape and orientation along the major fissure (arrow): Loculated effusion.

TABLE 6: Key differentiating features of pulmonary and pleural masses.

Feature	Parenchymal	Extraparenchymal lesion
Shape	Spherical/round/irregular	Oval/longitudinal
Margins	Well-defined/ill-defined/spiculated	Sharply defined, broadly based on pleura
Interface	Acute angle with chest wall and often separated on all aspects	Obtuse angle with chest wall and contiguous in at least 1 projection
Air bronchogram	May be present	Absent
Cavitation, air-fluid level	May be present	Only postintervention, or bronchopleural fistula (rare in setting of neoplasia)
Vessels and airways	Obliterated/destroyed	Displaced
Adjacent lung	No compression Consolidation +/infiltration +	Compression + Consolidation –
Extension into CP angle	–	Sometimes +
Relation to fissures	Usually, do not cross fissures, though can invade when irregular margins are seen	May cross fissures

These differences are highlighted for prototypical pulmonary and pleural masses in **Table 6**. It is important to note that pleural tumors do not always present as masses but more frequently as large effusions/nodules.

■ CONCLUSION

A systematic approach toward pediatric chest radiographs is essential for accurate interpretation.

Other Related Chapters that can be Referred to:
- Chapter 21: Approach to Mediastinal Lesions: Part 1
- Chapter 22: Approach to Mediastinal Lesions: Part 2
- Chapter 26: Pleural Disorders: Imaging

■ REFERENCES

1. Rixe N, Frisch A, Wang Z, Martin JM, Suresh S, Florin TA, et al. The development of a novel natural language processing tool to identify pediatric chest radiograph reports with pneumonia. Front Digit Health. 2023;5:1104604.
2. Gibbs JM, Chandrasekhar CA, Ferguson EC, Oldham SA. Lines and stripes: Where did they go? From conventional radiography to CT. Radiographics. 2007;27(1):33-48.
3. Jana M, Bhalla AS, Gupta AK. Approach to pediatric chest radiograph. Indian J Pediatr. 2016;83(6):533-42.
4. Manchanda S, Bhalla AS, Jana M, Gupta AK. Imaging of the pediatric thymus: Clinicoradiologic approach. World J Clin Pediatr. 2017;6(1):10-23.

CHAPTER 2

Ultrasound Chest: Basics and Role

Amit Gupta, Priyanka Naranje

- ❑ Indications
- ❑ Equipment
- ❑ Technique
  - ➢ Screening and patient positioning
  - ➢ Approaches
- ❑ Normal ultrasonography appearances
- ❑ Imaging findings
  - ➢ Lung
  - ➢ Mediastinum
  - ➢ Chest wall
  - ➢ Diaphragm
  - ➢ Pleura
- ❑ Limitations

■ INTRODUCTION

Traditionally, lung has always been considered as an unsuitable organ to be evaluated by ultrasonography (USG). The reason being that USG cannot traverse through the air within the lung parenchyma. This has limited use of USG in the chest to the diagnosis and drainage of pleural fluid collections.

More recently in the past one or two decades with the advancements of ultrasonographic technology, many newer applications of thoracic USG are being explored. The ready availability of portable USG machines in the intensive care units (ICUs) and wards has only augmented its use in critically ill patients, often as an adjunct or replacement to chest radiograph. The pediatric chest is well suited for USG due to less subcutaneous fat and partially-ossified chest wall that provides additional acoustic windows not available in older children and adults.

■ INDICATIONS

Ultrasonography is informative in several conditions as given in **Table 1**.

TABLE 1: Various indications for chest USG in pediatric patients.	
Lung	• Neonatal point of care USG • Congenital lung lesions • Consolidation • Lung neoplasms
Mediastinum	• Normal thymus/thymic lesions • Mediastinal lymph nodes • Mediastinal masses
Chest wall	• Vascular malformations • Neoplasms • Infections
Diaphragm	Diaphragmatic paralysis
Pleura	• Pleural effusion • Infected pleural fluid collection • Pneumothorax

EQUIPMENT

- Any standard USG scanner with color Doppler is suitable for lung sonography
- Curvilinear low-frequency transducer (2–5 MHz), linear high-frequency transducer (5–12 MHz), phased array probe
- In infants and small children, small footprint linear transducers are more useful.
- For mediastinal lymph node detection, endocavitary or microconvex (5–12 MHz) transducers are essential.

TECHNIQUE

Screening and Patient Positioning

- USG can be performed in supine, prone, or decubitus position depending on area of interest.
- Pneumothorax in an ambulatory patient should be evaluated in a sitting position and the apices are the most important area; anterior area in the basal lungs is the most important area in a supine patient.
- For ambulatory patients who can sit upright, sitting posture is ideal for lung USG.

Approaches

- Acoustic windows available for evaluating pediatric chest include supraclavicular, suprasternal notch, trans-sternal scan, parasternal region, intercostal spaces, transdiaphragmatic approach, and subcostal/subxiphoid scan.
- Parasternal, intercostal, and transdiaphragmatic approaches are good for lung and pleural imaging.
- Supraclavicular, suprasternal, and parasternal views are good to visualize mediastinum.
- For an area of interest detected on either chest X-ray (CXR) or general examination, scanning in different planes (sagittal, transverse, or oblique) should be performed for characterization of the abnormality.
- It can be complimented by M mode and Doppler examination in abnormal areas.
- USG approaches specific to a particular pathology are discussed along with the imaging findings later in the chapter.

■ NORMAL ULTRASONOGRAPHY APPEARANCES

Normal USG signs and artifacts seen in the pediatric chest are summarized in **Table 2** and **Figures 1 and 2**.

TABLE 2: Normal signs and artifacts in pediatric chest USG.

Findings on imaging	Description	Anatomical pathological correlate
Pleural line	Hyperechoic line deep to intercostal muscles	Visceral and parietal pleura
Lung sliding	Back and forth movement of hyperechoic pleural line with respiration	Relative motion between visceral and parietal pleura
Batwing appearance	Posterior acoustic shadowing caused by ribs separated by echogenic pleural line	Ribs separated by pleura in the intercostal space
Seashore sign	Superficial horizontal lines and deep granular appearance on M-mode	Static superficial chest wall and movement of lung deep to it
A-lines	Equidistant parallel echogenic horizontal lines	Reverberation artifacts of pleural line
Z-lines	Short echogenic lines perpendicular to pleural surface, do not erase A lines	Comet-tail artifacts
Starry-sky appearance	Hypoechoic soft-tissue with hyperechoic foci in anterior mediastinum	Normal thymus

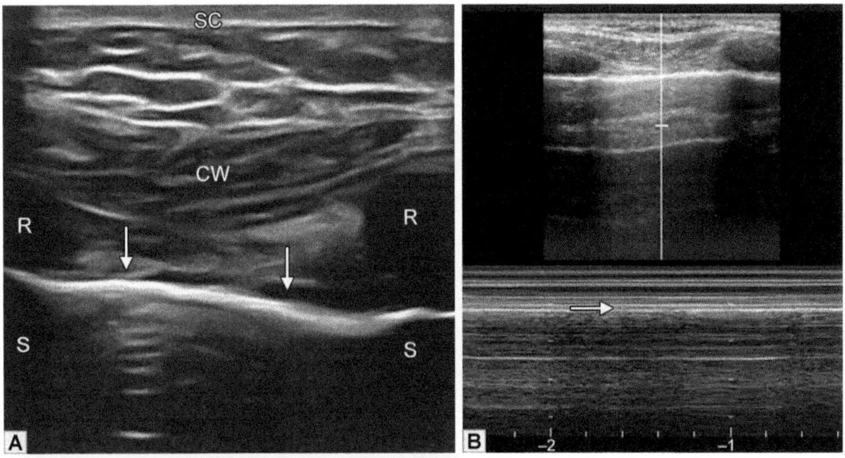

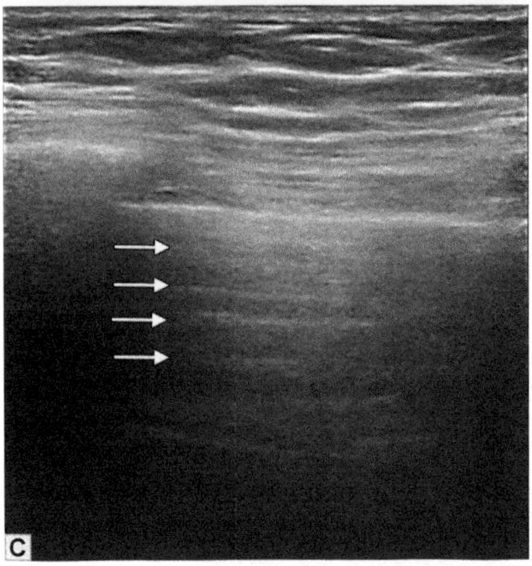

FIGS. 1A TO C: Normal chest USG appearances: A) Echogenic pleural line (arrows). Batwing appearance due to shadowing (S) by the ribs (R). SC—subcutaneous tissue, CW—chest wall muscles; (B) "Seashore sign" (arrow) on M-mode USG; (C) A lines (arrows).

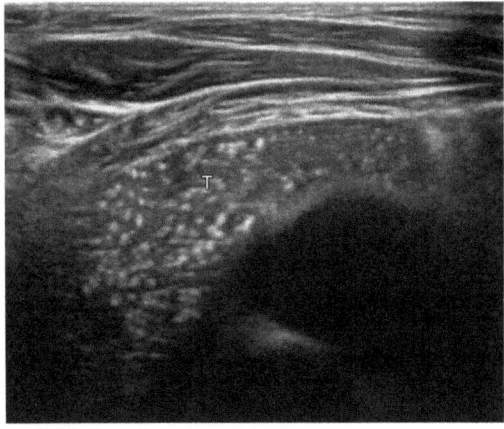

FIG. 2: Normal "starry-sky" appearance of thymus (T).

IMAGING FINDINGS

Various pediatric chest pathologies can be evaluated using USG.

Lung

- USG can be a helpful modality in various lung pathologies.
- Lung USG is performed in a supine, lateral, or prone position in neonates.
- Each hemithorax is divided into anterior, lateral, and posterior regions by the anterior and posterior axillary lines; longitudinal and transverse scans are performed in all areas.[1]
- For the relatively thinner chest walls and smaller thoraces in neonates, a high-frequency linear probe is preferred.

Neonatal Point-of-Care USG

- *Respiratory distress syndrome (RDS):*
  - USG is being utilized as an alternative to radiographs for RDS.
  - Lung consolidations with air bronchograms are the most common USG manifestation of RDS.
  - Few characteristics of consolidations in RDS are more often in posterior part of lungs, subpleural in mild patients with deeper involvement in severe cases, and clear boundary with surrounding lung tissue.
  - Compact, widespread, symmetrical B-lines in bilateral lungs—analogous to "white lung" seen on chest radiographs
  - Thickened, irregular pleural line
  - Absent liver mirror image on subcostal view; replaced by dense B-lines **(Figs. 3A and B)**

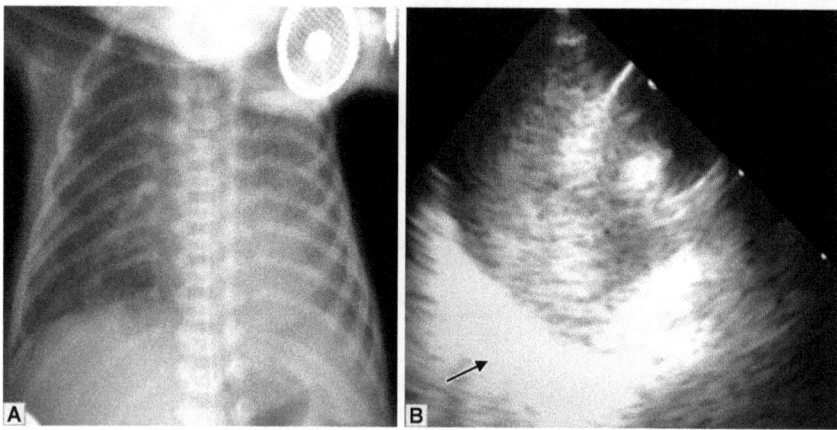

FIGS. 3A AND B: Preterm neonate with respiratory distress syndrome: (A) granular increased density in bilateral lung fields and (B) dense echogenic retrodiaphragmatic shadow (arrow).

- *Grading of RDS on USG:*[2]
  - Mild RDS, "ground glass sign", mild lung consolidation without air bronchogram
  - Moderate RDS, consolidation in some lung zones with "snowflake sign", punctate patchy air bronchogram in a consolidation
  - Severe RDS—consolidation with snowflake sign affecting all lung zones or with complications (hemorrhage, pneumothorax, persistent pulmonary hypertension, and large atelectasis)
- *Follow-up of RDS on USG:*[3]
  - USG can detect improvement in lung findings (consolidations and B-lines) after surfactant therapy.
  - Transition from consolidation to interstitial edema (coalesced B-lines) to normal lung USG pattern can be seen.
  - USG can also help in screening of neonates requiring repeat surfactant or more invasive therapies.
- *Transient tachypnea of newborn (TTN):*
  - Double lung point—more compact B-lines in inferior lung fields
  - B-lines resolve by day 2–3 coinciding with clinical improvement **(Figs. 4A to C)**.
  - Normal pleural line
  - Associated unilateral or bilateral pleural effusion
  - Differentiating features between RDS and TTN on USG are summarized in **Table 3**.

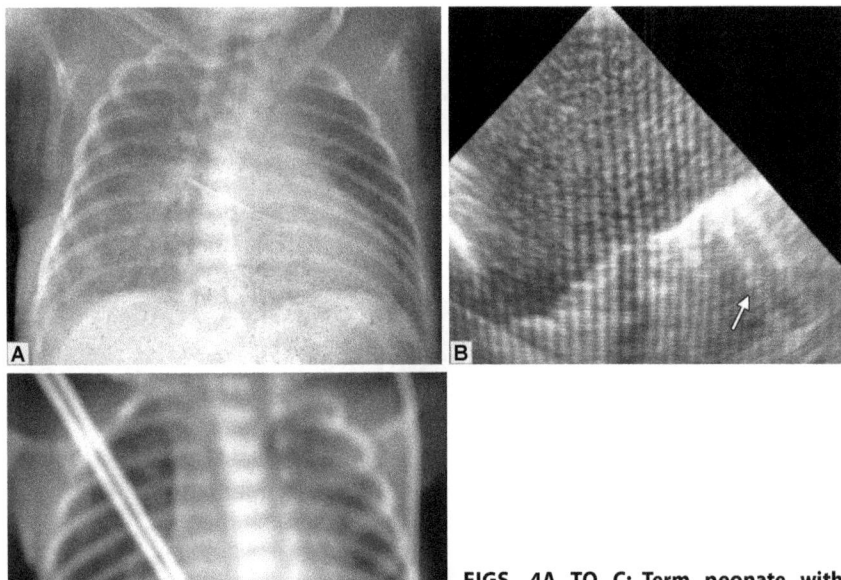

FIGS. 4A TO C: Term neonate with transient tachypnea of the newborn: (A) right lower zone radiopacity with air bronchograms; (B) multiple B lines (arrow); and (C) complete clearing of lung opacity on 48-hour follow-up radiograph.

TABLE 3: Differentiating features of RDS versus TTN on chest USG.		
	RDS	**TTN**
Presentation	Preterm baby with respiratory distress soon after birth	Term baby with respiratory distress; associated with cesarean delivery or maternal diabetes
B-lines	Bilateral diffusely symmetric confluent B-lines	More compact B-lines in inferior lung fields – "double lung point"
Evolution of B-lines	Gradual reduction in number after surfactant therapy	Spontaneous resolution by day 2–3
Pleural line	Thick and irregular	Normal
Consolidation	May be seen	Absent

(RDS: respiratory distress syndrome; TTN: transient tachypnea of newborn; USG: ultrasonography)

- *Other pathologies*:
  - Meconium aspiration syndrome—lung USG can illustrate involvement of lung parenchyma by depicting B-lines indicating presence of interstitial fluid along with associated consolidation.
  - Pulmonary hemorrhage also shows condensed B-lines similar to findings in RDS.

Congenital Lung Lesions
- Most common antenatally detected lung abnormalities include congenital pulmonary airway malformation (CPAM) and pulmonary sequestration.
- A postnatal CXR is must before doing USG examination in such cases.
- Both CPAM and sequestration may be seen as echogenic mass with cystic areas or homogeneous solid mass on USG.
- Anomalous vessel arising from aorta supplying the lung lesion confirms the diagnosis of pulmonary sequestration **(Figs. 5A and B)**.
- *Caveat:* Hybrid lesion can show components of both CPAM and sequestration.

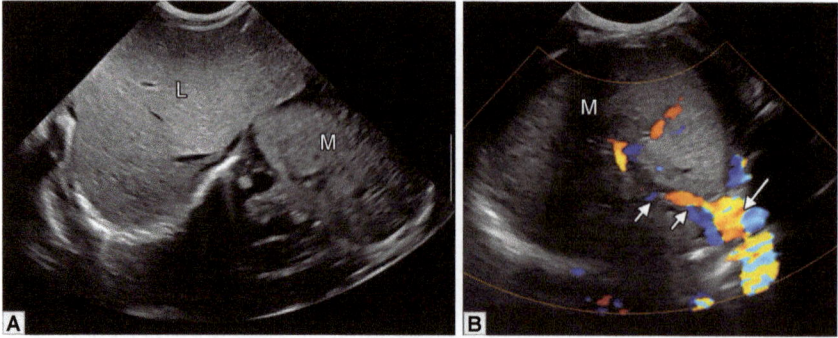

FIGS. 5A AND B: Pulmonary sequestration: (A) echogenic lesion (M) in left lower lobe (L–Liver) and (B) anomalous arterial supply (short arrows) to the lesion from aorta (long arrow) on color Doppler.

Consolidation

- Consolidated airless lung simulates appearance of liver—"hepatization" **(Fig. 6A)**.
- Residual air within the bronchi is seen as branching echogenic foci, "sonographic air bronchogram", usually show movement with respiration—"dynamic air bronchogram" **(Fig. 6B)**.
- Fluid may replace the air within the bronchi—"fluid bronchogram".
- The echogenic pleural line is seen broken into fragments at the area of subpleural consolidation—"shred sign" **(Fig. 6C)**.
- B-lines can be seen along the margin of consolidation. B-lines are vertical (perpendicular) echogenic lines which erase A-lines and extend till the edge of screen **(Fig. 6D)**.
- Consolidated lung shows normal "tree-like branching vascularity" as compared to abnormally oriented vessels in a mass **(Fig. 6E)**.
- USG is helpful for follow-up of pediatric patients with consolidation and monitoring of complications including formation of lung abscess or areas of breakdown in acute necrotizing pneumonia.
- Underlying congenital/acquired cysts (such as hydatid cyst or duplication cyst) can present as nonresolving/recurrent pneumonia. If the consolidation has an area of contact with the lateral thoracic wall, thoracic USG can diagnose the underlying lesion and demarcate the consolidation from the lesion.
- USG can help in characterizing the nature of an area of opacity on a CXR by differentiating among consolidation, mass, and atelectasis. The differentiating features on USG are given in **Table 4**.
- In a child with respiratory distress presenting with opaque hemithorax on CXR, USG can help in differentiating among pulmonary, pleural, and mediastinal pathologies and their characterization.

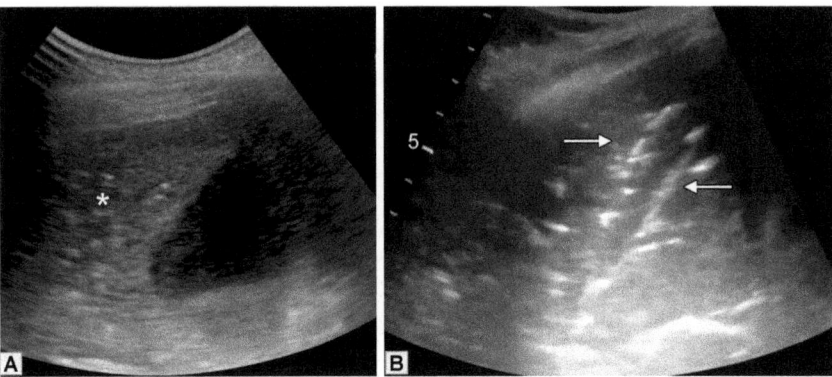

FIGS. 6A TO E: *Continued*

Continued

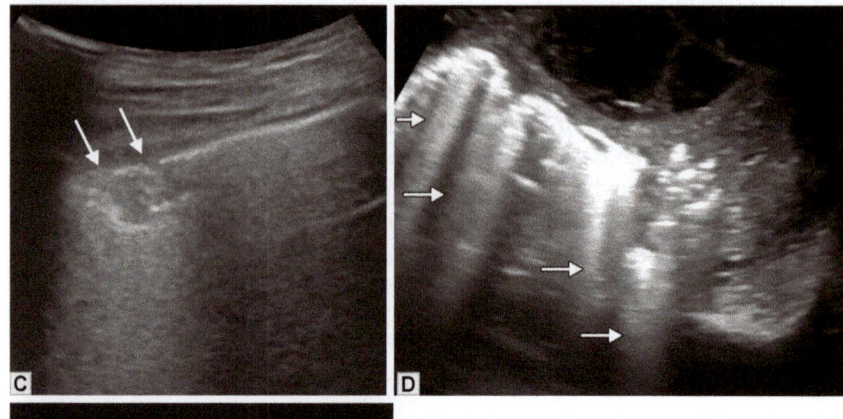

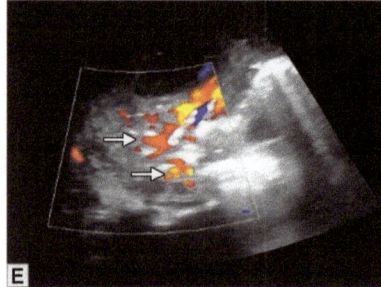

FIGS. 6A TO E: USG appearances of consolidation: (A) tissue-like appearance/hepatization (asterisk); (B) air bronchogram (arrows); (C) shred sign (arrows) in subpleural consolidation; (D) B-lines (arrows) along margin of consolidation; and (E) branching vascularity within consolidation.

TABLE 4: Differentials of pulmonary consolidation.

Imaging features	Consolidation	Mass lesion (neoplasm)	Collapse
Dynamic air bronchogram	Present	Absent	Absent in obstructive collapse
Fluid bronchogram	May be seen	Absent	Seen in obstructive collapse
Pulmonary vessels on color Doppler	Normal distribution and branching	Abnormal orientation, may be reduced or increased	Crowded

Lung Neoplasms
- Pediatric lung neoplasms are rare; but mostly malignant.
- Important differentials in infants include pleuropulmonary blastoma and infantile fibrosarcoma; and in older children include inflammatory myofibroblastic tumors, carcinoids, and respiratory papillomatosis.
- Role of USG is limited to peripheral lung masses for distinction from adjoining consolidation and differentiation of cystic versus solid component.

Mediastinum

Various mediastinal structures and pathologies can be well evaluated on USG.

Normal and Abnormal Thymus

- Normally located in superior mediastinum anterior to the great vessels
- Due to its variable shape and size, thymus can mimic a mediastinal or lung mass on a CXR.
- Characteristic "starry-sky" appearance (hypoechoic with hyperechoic specks) helps in identification of thymic tissue in ectopic location (most commonly neck).
- Normal thymus does not exert any mass effect on adjacent structures and does not show any calcification or necrosis—any of these features are suspicious for pathologies such as lymphoproliferative infiltration or thymic neoplasms.

Mediastinal Lymph Nodes

- Assessment of mediastinal nodes is a relatively new domain of thoracic ultrasound.
- For assessment of right paratracheal and left paratracheal nodes, suprasternal approach using an intracavitary probe and parasternal approaches using small footprint linear probe can be used **(Fig. 7A)**.
- For the prevascular and subcarinal nodes, suprasternal notch approach with an intracavitary/microconvex probe is the most suitable **(Fig. 7B)**.
- Lower mediastinal and posterior mediastinal nodes are usually not visualized using ultrasound.
- Mediastinal nodal enlargement can be defined according to predefined size criteria: >15 mm short axis if single; >10 mm short axis if multiple.[4]

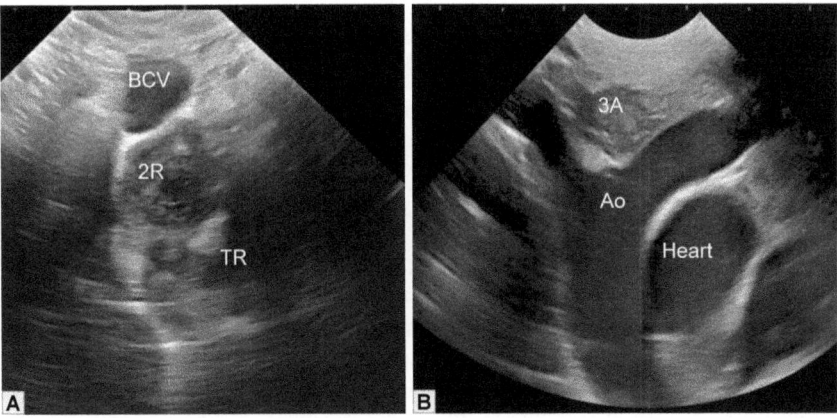

FIGS. 7A AND B: Mediastinal lymphadenopathy: (A) station 2R (anterior and to the right of trachea) lymph node and (B) station 3A (prevascular) lymph node.
(Ao: aorta; BCV: brachiocephalic vein; TR: trachea)

- Necrosis on USG is seen as hypoechoic/anechoic central area in a node.
- Calcifications can be seen as punctate or coarse hyperechoic foci.
- Nonvisualization of the echogenic fat between two nodes signifies matting of lymph nodes, giving a multilocular appearance.

Mediastinal Masses
- USG can determine cystic or solid nature of the mass as well as depict internal areas of vascularity, cavitation, necrosis, or calcifications.
- Cystic mediastinal lesions include developmental cysts (foregut duplication and neurenteric cysts) and venolymphatic malformations.
- Unlike in adults, developmental cysts comprise a significant proportion of mediastinal masses in childhood—high-resolution USG transducer can detect the diagnostic "gut signature" in a duplication cyst.
- Germ cell tumors are usually seen as heterogeneous anterior mediastinal masses with variable presence of calcifications.
- Neurogenic tumors are seen as solid lobulated hypoechoic posterior mediastinal masses with presence of calcific flecks within.
- Mediastinal lymphomas usually appear as homogeneous solid hypoechoic mediastinal masses encasing the mediastinal structures **(Figs. 8A to D)**.

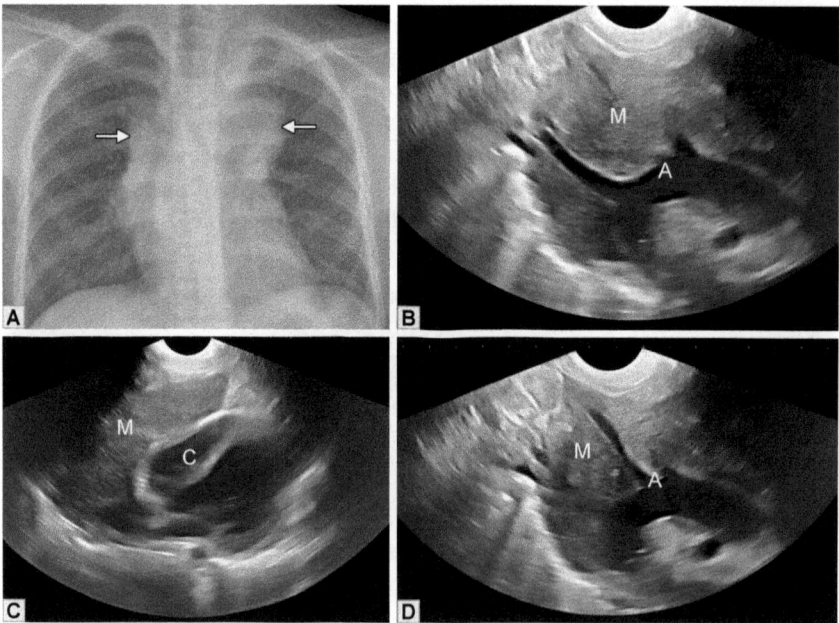

FIGS. 8A TO D: Mediastinal lymphoma: (A) lobulated mediastinal mass (arrows) extending to both sides of midline; (B to D) hypoechoic solid mass (M) lesion encasing the aortic arch (A) and having a broad area of contact with cardiac margins (C).

Chest Wall
- Most nontender palpable chest wall abnormalities in asymptomatic children are due to developmental variants—prominent rib convexities, bifid ribs, asymmetrical costal cartilage, or anterior angulation of xiphoid process—USG can obviate need for further imaging in these cases.
- USG can help in localization of the chest wall lesion and solid versus cystic characterization.

Vascular Malformations
- *Venous malformation*: Compressible anechoic cystic spaces with venous flow on Doppler; phleboliths ±
- *Arteriovenous malformation*: Tangle of vessels (nidus) showing arterial low-resistance blood flow with prominent feeding arteries and draining veins
- Magnetic resonance imaging is better for characterization of extent of the lesion.

Neoplasms
- Benign tumors are more common than malignant.
- *Hemangioma*: Benign vascular tumor; usually hyperechoic with high internal vessel density in proliferative phase.
- Most malignant chest wall tumors are osseous in origin.
- Most common malignant pediatric chest wall masses include small round cell tumors including Ewing sarcoma, rhabdomyosarcoma, and lymphoma.
- USG can depict solid nature of the mass, epicenter (intra- or extrathoracic) of the mass and underlying rib destruction.
- USG-guided biopsy can be done to reach a histopathological diagnosis.

Infections
- Soft-tissue or subperiosteal abscesses can be well-depicted on USG.
- *Empyema necessitans*: Extension of pleural empyema into chest wall; most commonly tubercular in etiology.

Diaphragm
- Diaphragmatic paralysis secondary to phrenic nerve injury is poorly tolerated by infants—early detection is important.
- Subxiphoid approach allows side-by-side comparison of both hemidiaphragms.
- M-mode provides quantitative estimate about diaphragmatic excursion **(Fig. 9)**; <4 mm excursion of one hemidiaphragm or >50% difference in excursion between hemidiaphragms signifies diaphragmatic dysfunction.[5]
- USG can also show juxtadiaphragmatic masses in chest or abdomen that could potentially be responsible for diaphragmatic dysfunction.

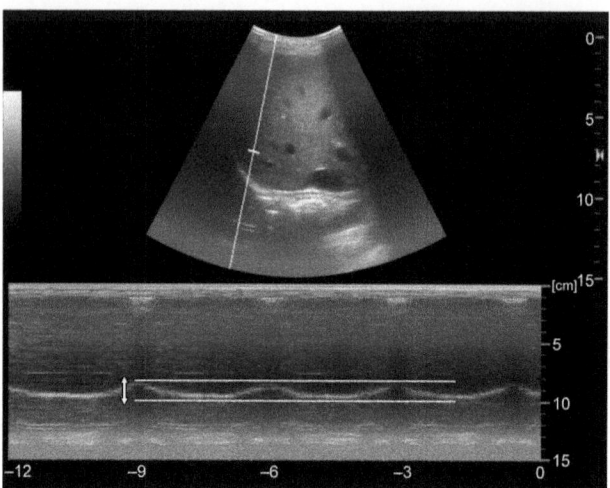

FIG. 9: M-mode USG: Diaphragmatic excursion (double-headed arrow) between peak inspiratory and expiratory diaphragmatic craniocaudal positions (horizontal lines).

Pleura

- Pleural effusion appears as anechoic fluid causing separation of visceral and parietal pleura **(Fig. 10A)**.
- Empyema/infective pleural effusion is diagnosed when the pleural fluid contains mobile echoes with septations **(Figs. 10B and C)**.
- *Quantification on US*: Various formulae are available for estimation of volume of pleural effusion on ultrasound. No specific formula for the pediatric population has been in use. *Goecke 2 formula* measured in erect position of the patient is reported to most closely correlate with actual fluid volume drained.[6] USG image is obtained keeping probe longitudinally oriented along dorsolateral/posterolateral aspect of chest wall, and craniocaudal extent (X cm) and the lung base to mid-diaphragm distance/subpulmonary height [lung to diaphragm distance (LDD) cm] is measured. One can measure the volume of effusion using formula:

$$\text{Estimated volume (EV) in mL} = (X + LDD) \times 70$$

- Pneumothorax is diagnosed when there is an obliteration of the normal "sliding pleura sign". On M mode interrogation, there is presence of a "barcode sign" instead of "seashore sign" **(Figs. 11A and B)**.

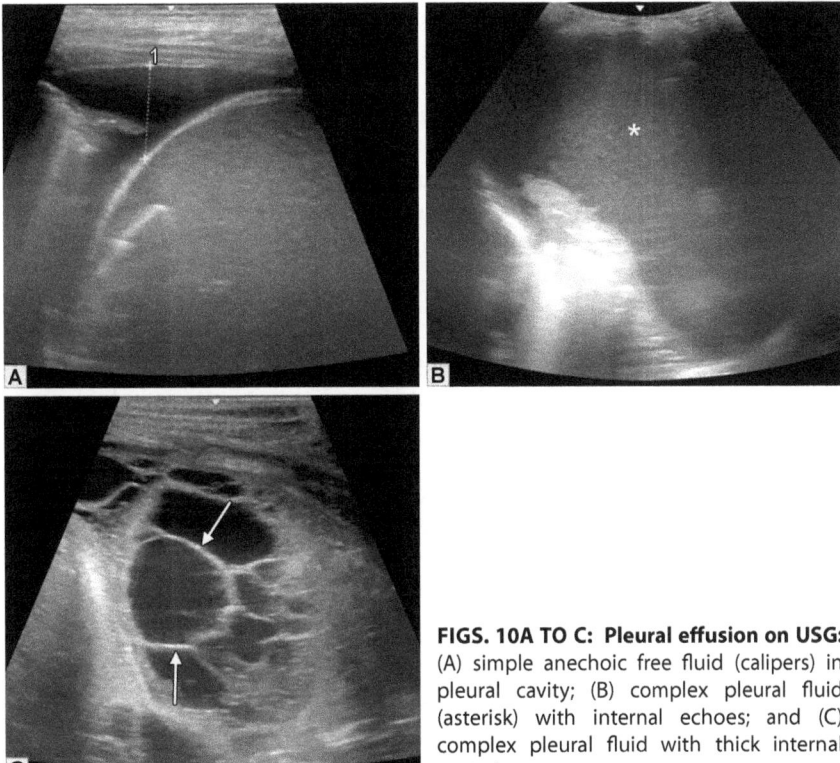

FIGS. 10A TO C: Pleural effusion on USG: (A) simple anechoic free fluid (calipers) in pleural cavity; (B) complex pleural fluid (asterisk) with internal echoes; and (C) complex pleural fluid with thick internal septations.

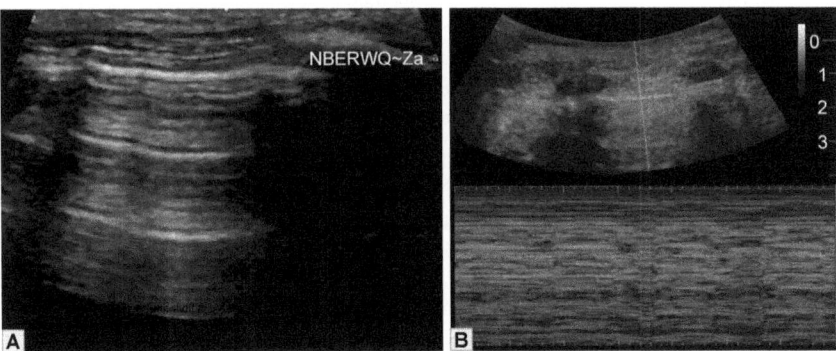

FIGS. 11A AND B: USG findings in pneumothorax: (A) exaggerated horizontal artifacts on B-mode USG. When seen in conjunction with absence of sliding pleura, this is suggestive of pneumothorax. (B) Barcode or stratosphere sign on M-mode USG.

LIMITATIONS

Although USG is a sensitive tool in the detection of pulmonary and pleural pathologies, especially for bedside evaluation, few limitations should be kept in mind.

- Small consolidations away from pleura are invisible to USG.
- In patients with edematous or thick chest wall, visualization of intrathoracic pathology is difficult.
- In subcutaneous emphysema, visualization of intrathoracic pathology is not possible.
- Limited acoustic window (in acute chest conditions with bandages/dressings/tubes; or in empyema and rib crowding).
- Difficult patient positioning in acutely ill patients may preclude detailed evaluation.

CONCLUSION

The various signs and artifacts seen in pediatric chest pathologies are summarized in **Table 5**.

TABLE 5: Pathological signs and artifacts in pediatric chest USG.

Findings on imaging	Description	Anatomical/pathological correlate
Double lung point sign	More compact B-lines in inferior lung fields as compared to superior lung fields	Transient tachypnea of newborn
Subpleural consolidation	Subpleural hypoechoic areas with nonvisualization of overlying echogenic pleural line	Consolidation
Tissue like sign/hepatization	A large subpleural area of lung being replaced by a hypoechoic area which resembles liver	Large area of consolidation
Shred sign	The echogenic continuous pleural line is seen to be broken in multiple discontinuous fragments	Subpleural consolidations
Air bronchogram	Linear or branching echogenic foci within an area of consolidation	Consolidation with air within the bronchi of the segment
Dynamic air bronchogram	Air bronchogram pattern, showing movement during respiration	Consolidation with patent subtending bronchus (inflammatory consolidation/pneumonia)
Static air bronchogram	Air bronchogram pattern, showing no movement during respiration	Passive atelectasis, postobstructive atelectasis, less commonly in infective/inflammatory consolidation
Fluid bronchogram	Hypoechoic branching areas within the hypoechoic area of consolidation	Obstructed bronchus subtending to the area of consolidation
B-lines	Vertical echogenic lines erasing A-lines, extend till edge of the screen	Along the margin of consolidation, also seen with interlobular septal thickening (early fluid overload)

Although USG is a crucial second-line investigation after CXR in the evaluation of intrathoracic pathologies, it has its own limitations. Moreover, it has a long-learning curve and may often lead to overdiagnosis.

Other Related Chapters that can be Referred to:
- Chapter 14: Upper Airway Imaging
- Chapter 26: Pleural Disorders: Imaging

REFERENCES

1. Liang HY, Liang XW, Chen ZY, Tan XH, Yang HH, Liao JY, et al. Ultrasound in neonatal lung disease. Quant Imaging Med Surg. 2018;8(5):535-46.
2. Liu J, Li J, Shan RY. Multi-center prospective study of ultrasonic diagnosis and grading of neonatal respiratory distress syndrome. Chin Pediatr Emerg Med. 2020;27:801-7.
3. Raimondi F, de Winter JP, De Luca D. Lung ultrasound-guided surfactant administration: time for a personalized, physiology-driven therapy. Eur J Pediatr. 2020;179:1909-11.
4. Moseme T, Andronikou S. Through the eye of the suprasternal notch: Point-of-care sonography for tuberculous mediastinal lymphadenopathy in children. Pediatr Radiol. 2014;44:681-4.
5. Epelman M, Navarro OM, Daneman A, Miller SF. M-mode sonography of diaphragmatic motion: description of technique and experience in 278 pediatric patients. Pediatr Radiol. 2005;35(7):661-7.
6. Ibitoye BO, Idowu BM, Ogunrombi AB, Afolabi BI. Ultrasonographic quantification of pleural effusion: comparison of four formulae. Ultrasonography. 2018;37(3):254-60.

CHAPTER 3

CT Chest: Basics and Role

Devasenathipathy Kandasamy

- ❏ Technique
  - ➢ Sedation
  - ➢ Breath hold
  - ➢ Contrast administration
- ❏ Radiation dose
- ❏ Imaging protocols
  - ➢ Noncontrast computed tomography protocols
  - ➢ Contrast-enhanced computed tomography protocols

■ INTRODUCTION

Computed tomography (CT) scan is the most frequent second-line investigation performed in the chest after a chest radiograph. This is due to the inherent contrast that the air in the lungs offers with other tissues, even at low doses. However, there are unique challenges to pediatric chest imaging that are addressed in this chapter.

■ TECHNIQUE

This section addresses the basic techniques while the imaging protocols are discussed subsequently in the chapter.

Sedation

Older children (typically above 5 years) can be done without sedation. Short-term sedation may be required in infants and younger children unable to follow instructions. Explaining the preprocedure instructions such as breath hold will make the child comfortable which will improve the image quality. In small children, the need for sedation can be obviated by using physiological methods such as feed and swaddle, especially for noncontrast examination.

Breath Hold

The default phase of respiration for chest scanning is full inspiration. However, with current rapid acquisition techniques, reasonable diagnostic

TABLE 1: Injection rates for various sized cannula.	
Size of cannula	Rate of injection (mL/s)
24 G	1
22 G	1.5–2
20 G	2–3 *4
16–18 G	3–3.5 *5
* Indicates the maximum rate (the upper limit).	

quality scan can be obtained in free breathing. For CT pulmonary angiogram (CTPA), full inspiration is not advocated, as it impairs good opacification of the pulmonary circulation. Hence, scanning at resting lung volumes is desirable. Paired inspiratory-expiratory scans are indicated for assessing bronchomalacia (central airway) and air trapping (small airways).

Contrast Administration

- Nonionic-iodinated contrast media dose is 1.0–1.5 mL/kg, with an upper limit of 2 mL/kg.
- All general measures regarding assessment of renal functions and allergies need to be followed.
- For angiography techniques, iodine concentration of 300 mg/mL is recommended.
- Size of cannula that can be placed is generally smaller than 22G for children < 5 years and larger cannula for older children.
- Rate of injection of contrast is dependent on the size of cannula in place **(Table 1)**.
- Pressure injectors can be employed for older children with cannula size > 22G, with hand injection sufficing for smaller cannulas (average rate of injection 1 mL/s).
- In children without peripheral intravenous (IV) access, central venous catheters, peripherally inserted central catheter (PICC) lines, or implanted ports can be used for contrast injection. However, it needs to be checked if the implanted PICC line/port is compatible with pressure injectors.

RADIATION DOSE

Children are several times (up to 10 times more so in girls) more sensitive to the ionizing effects of radiation delivered by the CT scanners. Over the last few decades, the usage of CT scans have increased significantly. Studies have shown that up to 2% of cancers in the US are secondary to CT radiation. The harmful effects of radiation are significantly high when the dose exceeds 50 mSv which is not the amount of radiation delivered by a single chest CT scan (which is up to 8 mSv). However, when a child undergoes multiple phases in a study or multiple studies over a period of time the cumulative dose can reach over 50 mSv. The dose-dependent effects of radiation are called deterministic effects and the dose-independent effects are called stochastic effects. The significance of the stochastic effects are uncertain and unclear even in lower dose radiation. Over a period of time, the CT technology has improved significantly. The widespread usage of tube current modulation, iterative reconstruction techniques, improved beam shaping, and detector efficiency along with better awareness about radiation effects among the healthcare professionals have reduced the radiation dose manyfold. In modern scanners, it is possible to obtain a CT of the chest under 1 mSv dose.

IMAGING PROTOCOLS

A CT scan can be informative only if performed with the optimal protocol. The various protocols are enlisted in **Figures 1A to F**.

Noncontrast Computed Tomography Protocols

- *Noncontrast CT (NCCT)*: The term NCCT of chest refers to a default normal dose CT performed in full inspiration **(Figs. 2 and 3)**. The common indications for NCCT are evaluation for pulmonary metastases, bronchiectasis, persistent pulmonary opacities in infections (without mediastinal/pleural component), and unexplained shortness of breath with normal/equivocal chest radiograph. Various reconstructions are useful, in addition to the axial images.[1]
- *High-resolution CT (HRCT)*: HRCT chest in multidetector row CT scanners is not an acquisition protocol but simply a reconstruction algorithm with a specific slice thickness, slice interval (gap), and field of view after a spiral acquisition. Because it is reconstructed from the routine spiral acquisition and there is no dedicated acquisition for HRCT in newer generation scanners, there is no additional dose involved. This is in contrast to the dedicated HRCT protocol in older generation scanners where the thin sequential slices are acquired at a defined interval.
- *Low-dose CT (LDCT)*: LDCT scans refer to chest CT that delivers dose <3 mSv. LDCT can be chosen as the preferred protocol in the scanners. Its widespread applicability is limited by the image quality which is suboptimal for assessing DPLD [diffuse pulmonary lung disease/interstitial lung disease (ILD)] but can be used for nodules/bronchiectasis. In children, LDCT has been employed for the evaluation of infection which was widely used in the era of COVID-19. It is also being employed in children who are on follow-up.
- *Ultralow-dose CT (ULDCT)*: ULDCT refers to scan with radiation dose of <1 mSv. This format is available only in limited high-end scanners because of the need for an iterative image reconstruction algorithm. ULDCT can obtain a diagnostic quality scan in a radiation dose comparable to chest radiographs. The indications of ULDCT are similar to those of LDCT.

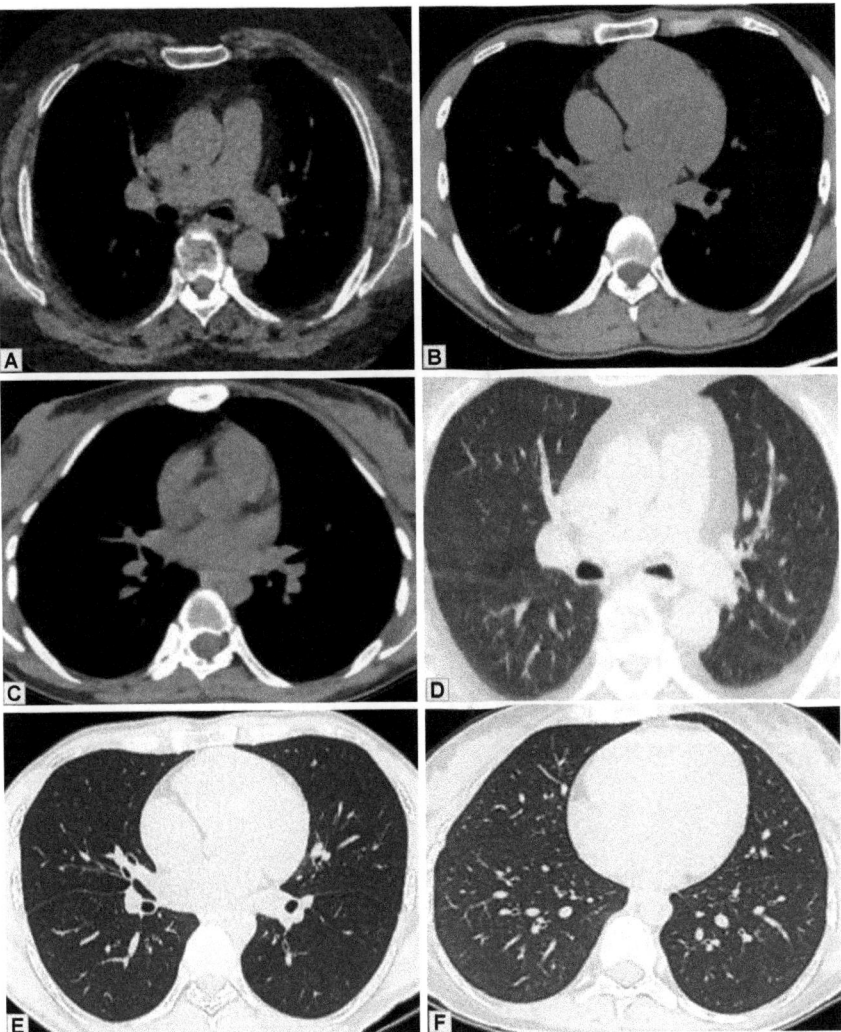

FIGS. 1A TO F: NCCT protocols. *Conventional NCCT images* in mediastinal (A) and lung window (B) performed using routine parameters. Note that the fissures are not clearly demarcated and the images are not crisp compared to the *HRCT images* (C and D). Also, both the major fissures are clearly demarcated. *Low-dose CT images* (E and F) which are performed using low kVp showing diagnostic quality images in spite of low signal to noise ratio.
(HRCT: high-resolution computed tomography; NCCT: noncontrast CT)

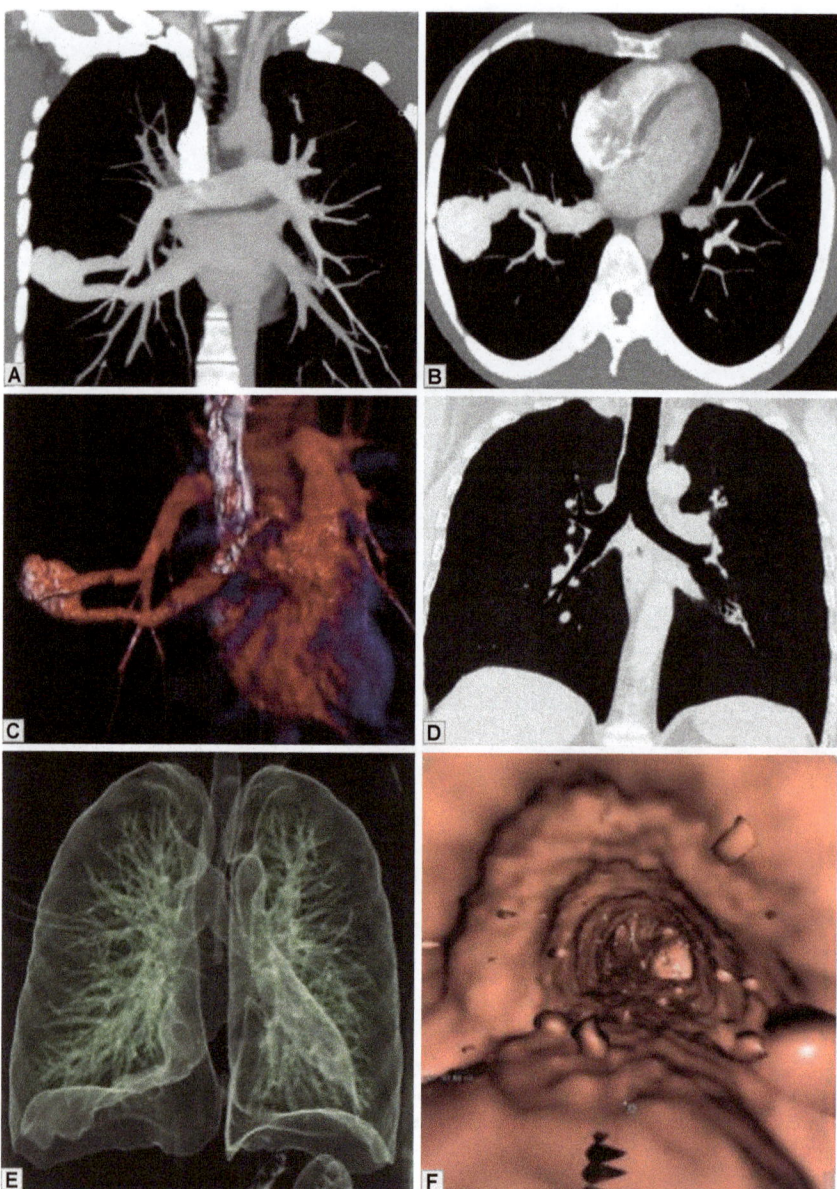

FIGS. 2A TO F: Utility of reconstructions. *Maximum intensity projection (MIP) image* (A and B) of a patient showing a pulmonary arteriovenous fistula. The findings are better demonstrated on a *volume-rendered technique (VRT) image* (C) giving a three-dimensional perspective. *Minimum intensity projection (MinIP) image* (D) showing the airways much better than the conventional coronal reformatted images. *VRT with airway preset and virtual bronchoscopy images* (E and F) demonstrating the three-dimensional view of the airways.

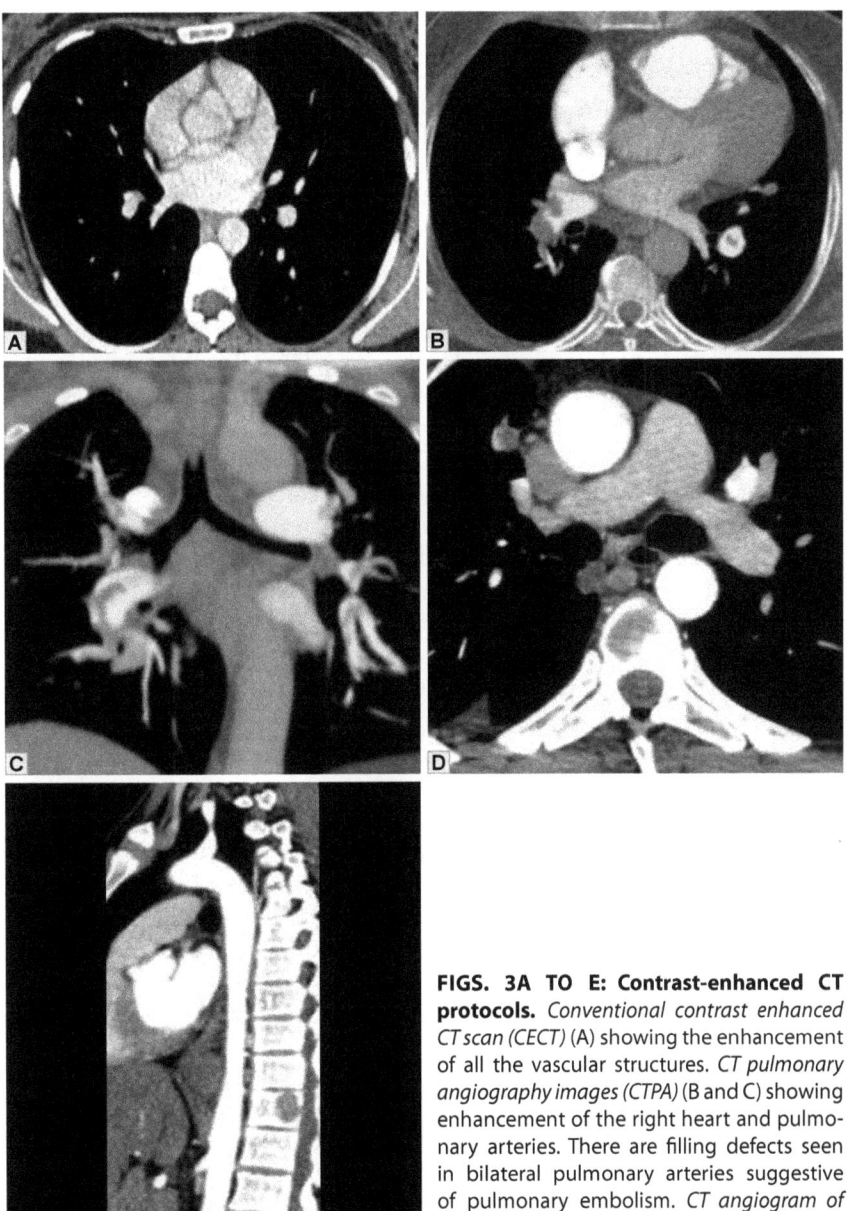

FIGS. 3A TO E: Contrast-enhanced CT protocols. *Conventional contrast enhanced CT scan (CECT)* (A) showing the enhancement of all the vascular structures. *CT pulmonary angiography images (CTPA)* (B and C) showing enhancement of the right heart and pulmonary arteries. There are filling defects seen in bilateral pulmonary arteries suggestive of pulmonary embolism. *CT angiogram of chest* (D and E) showing enhancement of the systemic arterial structures.

Contrast-enhanced Computed Tomography Protocols

- *Contrast-enhanced CT (CECT)*: CECT involves administration of iodinated contrast agent and it is important to evaluate pulmonary neoplasms and infection. It provides valuable information about the mediastinum and chest wall.
- *CT pulmonary angiography (CTPA)*: CTPA is an excellent technique and the modality of choice to evaluate the pulmonary arterial vasculature especially when pulmonary thromboembolism is suspected. If available, CTPA is preferably performed using a dual energy mode. Dual energy protocol can yield additional details about the pulmonary perfusion akin to ventilation perfusion scan. Dual energy CT (DECT) by utilizing the attenuation information on two separate kVps (80/100 and 140 kVp), it can identify various materials in the tissues such as calcium and iodine. This additional capability of DECT comes without any dose penalty, rather there is potential to reduce the dose compared to a single energy CT in certain situations. With more sophisticated techniques of DECT such as photon-counting detectors are coming up the diagnostic yield of scans and quantitative capability will improve with less radiation dose.
- *CT angiography (CTA)*: CTA is performed in situations where thoracic systemic arterial anatomy needs to be evaluated. The acquisition is done in the systemic arterial phase with contrast material injected using a pressure injector.[2,3] It is usually coupled with a venous phase scan which makes it a multiphase study which doubles the radiation dose to the child. To circumvent this increased radiation dose, split bolus technique is preferred where in the contrast material is divided into two parts which are injected sequentially with a calculated time gap. Because of two injections at two separate time points a single-phase split bolus scan will have the features of both the arterial and venous phase. Split bolus has the advantage of dose reduction and it can be combined with a dual energy protocol wherever available.
- The appropriate CT protocol for the common indications are given in the **Table 2** below.

TABLE 2: Investigations depending on clinical indications.

Indications	Appropriate CT protocol
Airway disease	CECT
Interstitial lung disease	CECT
Hemoptysis	• CT angiography • Split bolus
Pulmonary thromboembolism	CT pulmonary angiography (dual energy CT preferable)
Infections	CECT
Tumor	CECT, with arterial phase imaging as well

(CECT: contrast-enhanced computed tomography)

CONCLUSION

Multiple scanning protocols are available for the CT evaluation of pediatric chest disorders. It is important to choose the right protocol depending on the clinical indication to get the desired information. This will significantly reduce the radiation dose to the child without compromising the diagnostic outcome of these investigations.

Other Related Chapters that can be Referred to:
- Chapter 18: Pulmonary Artery Imaging
- Chapter 27: Hemoptysis: Imaging and Interventions

REFERENCES

1. Lee EY, Siegel MJ, Hildebolt CF, Gutierrez FR, Bhalla S, Fallah JH. MDCT evaluation of thoracic aortic anomalies in pediatric patients and young adults: comparison of axial, multiplanar, and 3D images. AJR Am J Roentgenol. 2004;182(3):777-84.
2. Hu XH, Huang GY, Pa M, Li X, Wu L, Liu F, et al. Multidetector CT angiography and 3D reconstruction in young children with coarctation of the aorta. Pediatr Cardiol. 2008;29(4):726-31.
3. Hellinger JC, Daubert M, Lee EY, Epelman M. Congenital thoracic vascular anomalies: evaluation with state-of-the-art MR imaging and MDCT. Radiol Clin North Am. 2011;49(5):969-96.

CHAPTER 4

MRI Chest: Basics and Role

Surabhi Vyas, Devasenathipathy Kandasamy

- ❑ Indications
  - ➢ Established indications
  - ➢ Potential indications
- ❑ MRI technique
  - ➢ Patient preparation sedation/general anesthesia
- ➢ Use of MRI contrast
- ➢ Equipment
- ➢ MRI sequences
- ❑ Building block approach
- ❑ Newer MRI techniques

■ INTRODUCTION

- Chest imaging has historically been synonymous with radiography and computed tomography (CT). However, even with the recent advances in technology, radiation exposure is a cause of concern with these modalities especially in children and young adults. The issue of radiation exposure becomes especially relevant in chronic diseases where repeated imaging and follow-up are required. The search for alternative modalities has pushed for various technological innovations in the field of imaging with magnetic resonance imaging (MRI).
- Chest MRI was traditionally limited by susceptibility to respiratory and cardiac motion artifacts and low proton density in the lungs, both contributing to poor signal. The recent technological advances have made possible the structural assessment of lung comparative to CT in niche indications **(Figs. 1A to D)**. In addition to structural changes, MRI has the potential of functional assessment by means of ventilation and perfusion evaluation.

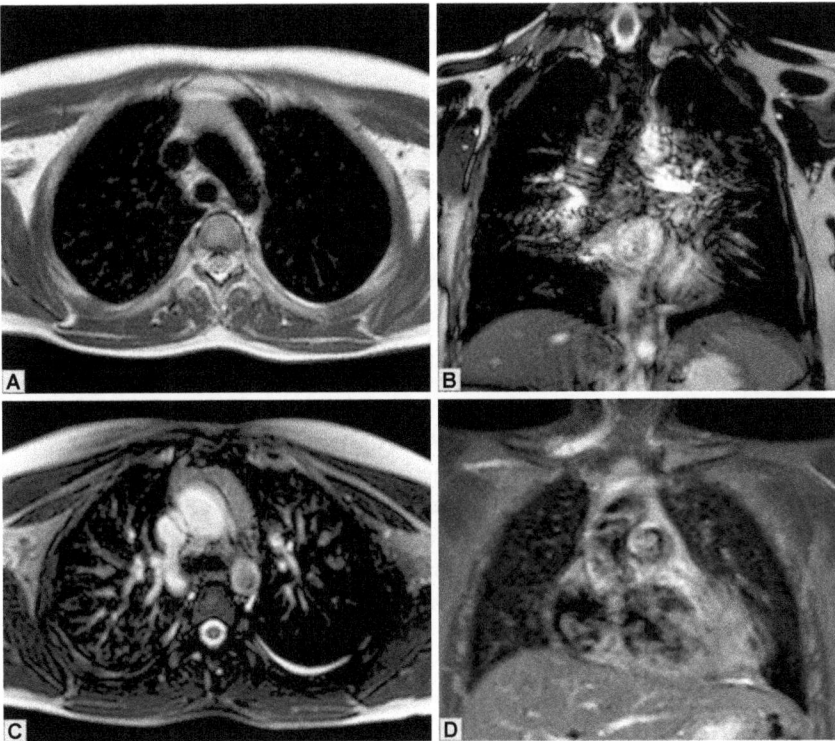

FIGS. 1A TO D: Basic noncontrast lung MRI sequences—(A) axial T2, coronal and axial; (B) coronal SSFP; (C) axial SSFP; and (D) coronal STIR. The images show normal anatomy of lung and mediastinal structures.

(MRI: magnetic resonance imaging; SSFP: steady-state free precession; STIR: short tau inversion recovery)

INDICATIONS

The indications of chest MRI can be divided into established indications and potential areas of indications where ongoing research has shown clinical and diagnostic benefit.

Established Indications

Established current indications are as follows:
- *Airway abnormalities*:
  ○ *Cystic fibrosis (CF)*: Chest MRI has been proven as a contemporary tool for quantification of lung parenchymal abnormality in CF in a radiation free manner. In addition to the structural changes and scarring of the lung, MRI helps differentiate active inflammation from chronic changes and thus guide treatment modalities. Ultrashort echo time (UTE) imaging consistently shows the bronchial wall thickening, bronchial dilatation, mucus plugging, and consolidation changes such that CF-specific MRI scoring systems have been developed functional assessment. Quantitative assessment on UTE imaging is also performed on 3D volumetric imaging without the use of MRI contrast.

- *Allergic bronchopulmonary aspergillosis (ABPA) and bronchiectasis*: MRI has shown to be of value in the diagnosis of altered mucus characteristics seen in ABPA. On T1W and T2W MRI sequences, the "inverted mucoid impaction signal" (IMIS) is described as high T1 signal and low T2 signal, which is a close surrogate for CT high attenuation mucus sign in both CF and non-CF airway abnormalities.[1,2] The IMIS is shown to have a high sensitivity and specificity in diagnosis of CF with ABPA **(Figs. 2A to D)**.
- *Central airway abnormalities*: MRI is also useful in evaluation of central airway abnormality like tracheobronchomalacia in pediatric patients using both 2D and 3D cine MRI, the results have been found to be similar to bronchoscopy and CT.[3]
- *Imaging in immunocompromised host*: MRI has high sensitivity (90%) and specificity (75–100%) in detection of pulmonary parenchymal consolidation in various immunocompromised states such as human immunodeficiency virus/acquired immunodeficiency syndrome (HIV/AIDS) and hematological malignancies.[4,5] The sensitivity is around 75% in diagnosis of ground-glass opacity (GGO) and bronchiectasis in this subset of the population. In chronic pulmonary infections such

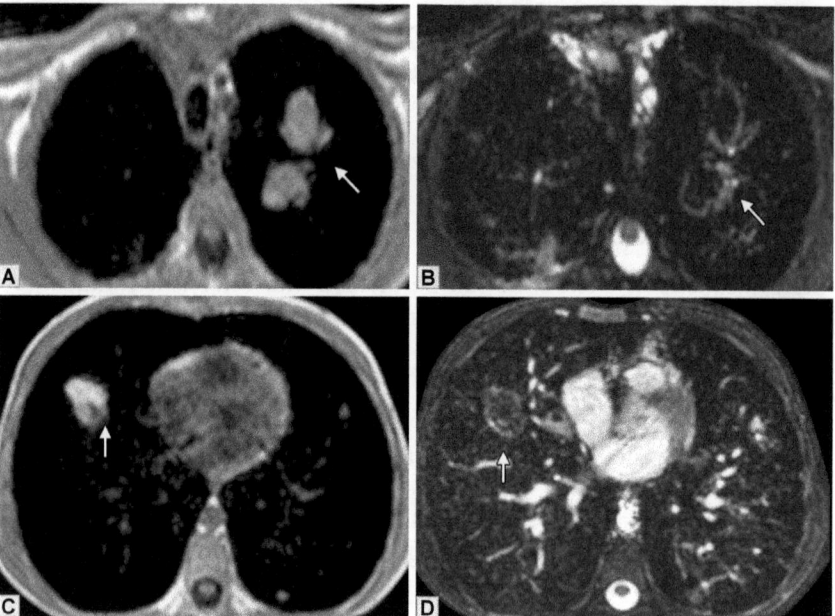

FIGS. 2A TO D: Inverted mucus sign—(A and C) axial T1W—show high-signal intensity within the dilated bronchi (arrow); (B and D) axial T2W—show corresponding hypointense signal (arrow) suggestive of inverted mucus sign, which corresponds to the high-attenuation mucus on CT.

as tuberculosis and fungal infections, the sensitivity is lower than CT, however, it can serve as a viable alternative with a baseline radiography for detection of calcifications.
- *Characterization of masses*:
  - Differentiation of cystic versus solid masses—MRI is extremely useful in diagnosis and differentiation of solid versus fluid containing lesions due to inherently high soft-tissue contrast and also consolidation from lung abscesses by demonstration of restricted diffusion in the later on diffusion-weighted imaging (DWI) **(Figs. 3A to F)**. This is especially useful in centrally located pulmonary lesions which may not be adequately evaluated on ultrasonography. MRI is also more sensitive in depiction of intracystic membranes in hydatid cysts compared to CT.
  - Congenital malformations—MRI and MR angiography have shown usefulness in evaluation of various congenital malformations such as bronchial atresia, sequestration, congenital pulmonary airway malformations, and bronchogenic cysts.

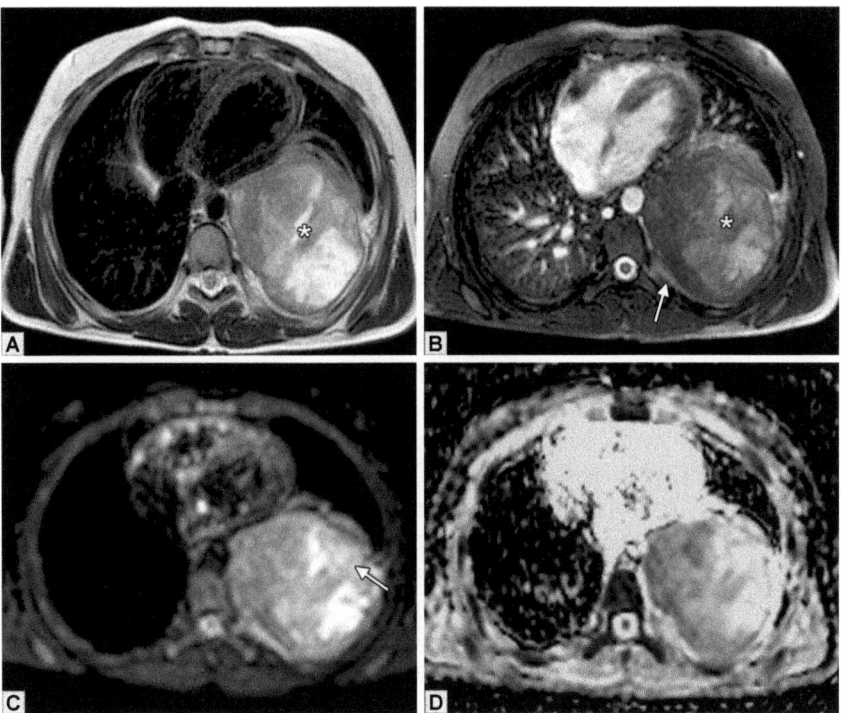

FIGS. 3A TO F: *Continued*

Continued

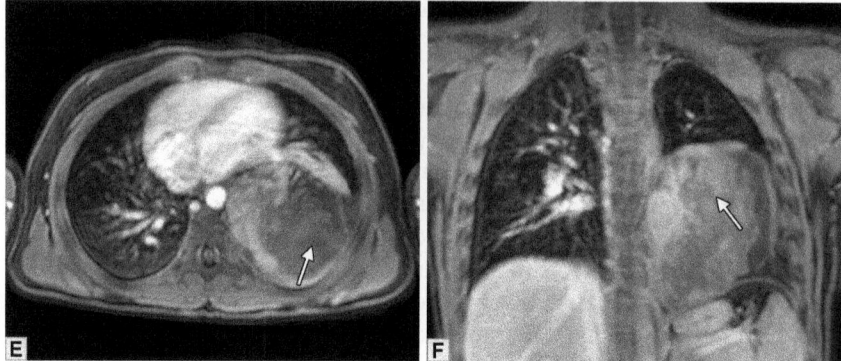

FIGS. 3A TO F: Mesenchymal neoplasm. (A and B) Axial T2 and axial SSFP show a well-defined heterogeneously hyperintense left hemithoracic mass (*), abutting the pericardium, causing passive atelectasis of the adjacent lung (arrow). (C and D) Axial DWI and ADC map image show patchy areas of restricted diffusion within (arrow), which show suppression on corresponding ADC image. (E and F) Axial and coronal fat suppressed postcontrast T1 images show heterogeneous areas of enhancement within the mass.

(ADC: apparent diffusion coefficient; DWI: diffusion-weighted imaging; SSFP: steady-state free precession)

Potential Indications

Potential areas of usefulness of MRI are as follows:
- *Acute versus chronic infections*: DWI is also helpful in differentiation of acute from chronic infections as acute active consolidation shows a higher diffusion coefficient, whereas pus shows lower diffusion coefficient. This feature can be utilized in resolution and evolution of infective changes.
- *Interstitial lung diseases (ILDs)*: MRI sequences especially T2W, short tau inversion recovery (STIR), balanced turbo field echo (BTFE) and multivane sequences very well demonstrate coarse fibrosis, cystic changes, and honeycombing, however, differentiation of GGO from consolidation is limited. In addition to structural changes, MRI perfusion, ventilation, and stiffness have a potential for functional analysis of the lung parenchyma. Most active abnormalities such as edema show high signal on T2W images and fibrotic processes depict hypointense signals on both T1W and T2W images. The available literature is limited to adult subjects, however, the use of MRI in pediatric ILDs shows promise.
- *Metastasis*: MRI can be used as an alternative for detection of pulmonary nodules/metastasis in the younger population with malignancy especially considering the long follow-up and repeated imaging.
- *Lung perfusion*: Perfusion imaging used for mapping areas of reduced perfusion following vascular and airway pathologies make use of

gadolinium-based contrast or alternatively T1 mapping, blood oxygenation level dependent (BOLD) imaging, hyperpolarized helium, and xenon-129. By using Fourier decomposition, lung ventilation and perfusion can be assessed without employing intravenous contrast and/or gaseous agents. These methods are under research for clinical use.

- *Congenital malformations*: MRI chest, especially aided by use of contrast has proven efficiency in detection of congenital pulmonary airway malformations, lobar overinflation, sequestration, bronchial atresia, diaphragmatic hernia, duplication cysts, and hybrid lesions. Use of MR angiography [with contrast or noncontrast techniques such as arterial spin labeling (ASL) and Fourier decomposition], perfusion and Cine MRI may be added in selected cases to improve detection rates.
- *Nodal and mediastinal masses detection*: MRI has shown promise in follow-up of mediastinal lymphadenopathy in infective and noninfective causes, thus obviating the need of repeated CT **(Figs. 4A to C)**. In mediastinal masses, MRI helps in characterization by demonstration of fat and blood products and by signal intensity changes on various sequences **(Figs. 5A and B)**.

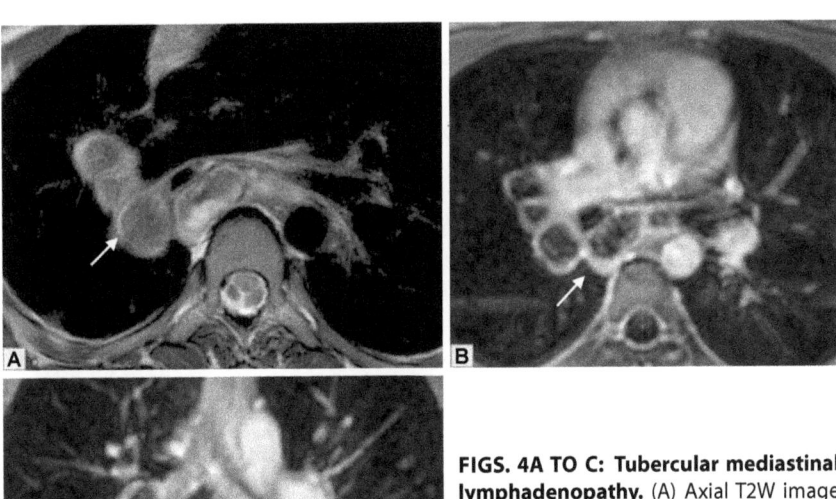

FIGS. 4A TO C: Tubercular mediastinal lymphadenopathy. (A) Axial T2W image shows hypointense enlarged lymph nodes (arrow) in the right hilum and the subcarinal location. (B and C) Axial and coronal T1 fat suppressed postcontrast images show rim enhancement of the enlarged lymph nodes. Histopathology revealed caseating granulomas, consistent with tubercular etiology.

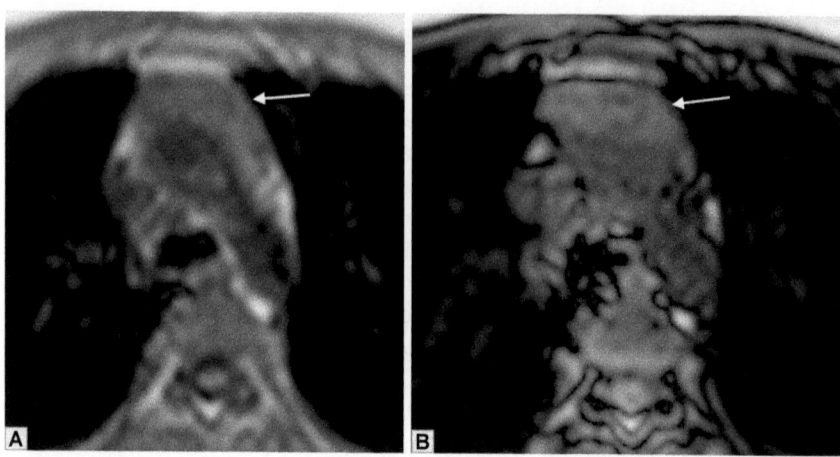

FIGS. 5A AND B: Thymic evaluation. (A) Axial T1 in phase image shows triangular hyperintense T1 signal in the anterior mediastinum corresponding to thymus. (B) Axial T1 opposed phase image shows uniform signal suppression. This feature is seen in normal thymus and thymic hyperplasia signifying utility of chemical shift imaging.

■ MRI TECHNIQUE

Patient Preparation Sedation/General Anesthesia

- It is imperative to understand that anesthesia and sedation are not entirely devoid of risk for the patient. Short-term effects of anesthesia include hemodynamic instability, obstructive sleep apnea, laryngospasm, and bronchospasm. Evidence of long-term adverse effects is less well established and obtained from animal studies, which include neurocognitive risks of anesthetic agents. Generally, efforts are made to minimize repeated anesthesia/sedation and to evaluate risk versus benefit for children.[6,7]
- For neonates and young infants, sedation can be avoided by employing nonpharmacological methods such as feed and wrap or feed and swaddle technique. Other methods that can be employed are sleep manipulation which involves mild sleep deprivation so that the infant sleeps during examination. Use of noise cancelling earmuffs can also be tried. For older children who can understand and follow breathing instructions, appropriate instructions, and demonstration of breathing maneuvers prior to the MRI is usually sufficient. In most cases of imaging with children, presence of parent or guardian during the instructions and the examination is helpful for alleviating anxiety.
- For children between the two age groups, who cannot adhere to the instructions, sedation or anesthesia is required for optimum imaging quality. A respiratory gating by means of motion feedback and motion trigger can also be utilized, however, the examination duration is prolonged by these.

Use of MRI Contrast
Macrocyclic contrast agents such as gadobutrol (Gadovist) and gadoterate (Dotarem) at a dose of 0.1 mL/kg are preferred, especially in children.

Equipment
- Both 1.5T and 3T systems can be used for lung MRI. The advantage of 1.5T is reduced signal loss due to susceptibility in conventional sequences and that of the 3T system is better performance at higher gradients especially in 3D gradient-recalled echo (GRE) sequences **(Table 1)**.
- Multichannel torso or head coil with 16 or 32 channels is most commonly used, depending on the size of the thorax and area of interest.

MRI Sequences
Magnetic resonance imaging sequences—commonly used MRI sequences and their indications are summarized in the **Table 2**.

TABLE 1: Summary of MRI system requirements.

System strength	1.5T/3T
Coil	Torso/head/neck/surface (airway)
Pulse sequence	• Free breathing sequences (PROPELLER, UTE, ZTE) • Breath hold sequences • Functional imaging • MRA and MR perfusion • Dynamic imaging • Lung ventilation
ECG gating	Employed for pathologies in RML and lingula

(ECG: electrocardiogram; MRA: magnetic resonance angiography; MRI: magnetic resonance imaging; PROPELLER: periodically rotated overlapping parallel lines with enhanced reconstruction; UTE: ultra-short echo-time imaging; ZTE: zero echo-time)

TABLE 2: Commonly employed MRI sequences and their indications in chest.

Sequences	Indications
Conventional MRI	Basic characterization and evaluation of extent of abnormality
Diffusion-weighted MRI	• Characterization of fluid containing lesions • Differentiation of cysts from abscess • Characterization of cellular tumors • Response evaluation • Pleural deposits and lymph nodal involvement

Continued

Continued

Sequences	Indications
Perfusion MRI–time resolved/first pass MRA	• Evaluation of pulmonary vasculature, e.g., PTE • Generation of perfusion parameters such as pulmonary blood flow and blood volume • Postchemotherapy response evaluation and follow-up
Cine MRI	• Evaluation of central airway • For chest wall • Diaphragmatic mechanics • Mediastinal invasion
Cardiac MRI (double inversion recovery sequences, cine MRI)	For cardiac invasion

(MRA: magnetic resonance angiography; MRI: magnetic resonance imaging; PTE: pulmonary thromboendarterectomy)

■ BUILDING BLOCK APPROACH

A building block approach is used in chest MRI examination **(Box 1 and Table 3)**.

BOX 1 | **Basic MRI chest sequences.**

- T1 TSE
- T2 TSE
- Steady-state free precession
- Post contrast fat saturated 3D GRE sequence (dynamic contrast enhanced MRI can an optional sequence)

(GRE: gradient-recalled echo; MRI: magnetic resonance imaging; TSE: turbo spin echo)

TABLE 3: Additional MRI sequences based on the indication of examination.

Indication	MRI sequences
Chest wall mass	• FSE T2 fat saturated or STIR • T1 fat saturated postcontrast
Mediastinal mass	• FSE T2 fat saturated or STIR • T1 fat saturated postcontrast
Consolidation/lung nodules	• Gradient-recalled echo sequences—2D or 3D, short or ultrashort • Spoiled gradient echo sequences • *Postcontrast*: 3D gradient recalled T1 fat sat
ILD	• Balanced turbo field echo • MvXD (multiVane XD) • FSE T2 fat saturated or STIR
Airway abnormality	• Spoiled gradient echo sequences • *Postcontrast*: 3D gradient recalled T1 fat sat

(FSE: fast spin echo; ILD: interstitial lung disease; MRI: magnetic resonance imaging; STIR: short tau inversion recovery)

NEWER MRI TECHNIQUES

- *Rapid lung MRI*: A rapid lung MRI protocol was recently proposed for children to overcome the long scanning times which comprises nonrespiratory and non-ECG-gated sequences namely half-fourier acquisition single-shot turbo spin-echo, a PROPELLER, a true fast imaging with steady-state free precession (SSFP), and a volumetric interpolated breath-hold examination (VIBE) sequence. The total duration of the scanning protocol is 14–20 minutes with magnet time of 2 minutes.[5,8]
- *Real-time MRI:* Real-time MRI is based on fast imaging rates of up to 50 frames per second using fast low-angle shot technique 2.0 (FLASH 2.0). With such high frame rates, the effects of physiological motion and bulk motion can be curtailed. Originally used in cranial imaging, the technique has been studied in pediatric chest MRI in nonsedated free breathing subjects and has shown promising results, including scanning the entire lung in 25–30 seconds.

CONCLUSION

Use of MRI chest in the evaluation of pediatric chest conditions is on the rise owing to improved hardware and software technologies. The traditionally described indications of MRI chest for chest wall and mediastinal masses are being supplemented by various infective and noninfective conditions such as lung abscess, ABPA, congenital anomalies, metastasis detection, and perfusion studies as described above. However, the longer scan time and expense with use of MRI in resource constrained settings may prevent widespread use of MRI. With continuing research, MRI has the potential of complementing and replacing CT in niche indications, which is especially relevant in younger patients.

Other Related Chapters that can be Referred to:
- Chapter 9: Chest Tuberculosis
- Chapter 16: Bronchiectasis

REFERENCES

1. Dournes G, Berger P, Refait J, Macey J, Bui S, Delhaes L, et al. Allergic bronchopulmonary aspergillosis in cystic fibrosis: MR imaging of airway mucus contrasts as a tool for diagnosis. Radiology. 2017;285(1):261-9.
2. Garg MK, Gupta P, Agarwal R, Sodhi KS, Khandelwal N. MRI: A new paradigm imaging evaluation of allergic bronchopulmonary aspergillosis? Chest. 2015;147:e58-9.
3. Liszewski MC, Ciet P, Lee EY. MR imaging of lungs and airways in children: past and present. Magn Reson Imaging Clin N Am. 2019;27:201-25.
4. Liszewski MC, Görkem S, Sodhi KS, Lee EY. Lung magnetic resonance imaging for pneumonia in children. Pediatr Radiol. 2017;47:1420-30.

5. Sodhi KS, Khandelwal N, Saxena AK, Bhatia A, Bansal D, Trehan A, et al Rapid lung MRI—paradigm shift in evaluation of febrile neutropenia in children with leukemia: a pilot study. Leuk Lymphoma. 2016;57:70-5.
6. Hirsch FW, Sorge I, Vogel-Claussen J, Roth C, Gräfe D, Päts A, et al. The current status and further prospects for lung magnetic resonance imaging in pediatric radiology. Pediatr Radiol. 2020;50(5):734-49.
7. Kapur S, Bhalla AS, Jana M. Pediatric Chest MRI: A Review. Indian J Pediatr. 2019;86(9):842-53.
8. Sodhi KS, Ciet P, Vasanawala S, Biederer J. Practical protocol for lung magnetic resonance imaging and common clinical indications. Pediatr Radiol. 2022;52(2):295-311.

SECTION 2

Neonatal and Congenital Disorders

CHAPTER 5: Neonatal Respiratory Distress
CHAPTER 6: Congenital Lung Abnormalities

CHAPTER 5

Neonatal Respiratory Distress

Anmol Bhatia, Ashish Dua, Kushaljit Singh Sodhi

- ❑ Medical causes of respiratory distress
  - ➤ Respiratory distress syndrome
  - ➤ Transient tachypnea of the newborn
  - ➤ Neonatal pneumonia
  - ➤ Meconium aspiration syndrome
  - ➤ Pneumothorax
- ❑ Surgical causes of respiratory distress
  - ➤ Congenital lobar overinflation
  - ➤ Congenital pulmonary airway malformation
  - ➤ Congenital diaphragmatic hernia
  - ➤ Esophageal atresia with tracheoesophageal fistula
- ❑ Miscellaneous causes of respiratory distress

■ INTRODUCTION

- Neonatal respiratory distress is characterized by presence of any two of following at the time of presentation on clinical examination:
  i. Respiratory rate of >60/min
  ii. *Presence of chest retractions*: Intercostal, subcostal, sternal, or suprasternal
  iii. *Wheezing, stridor, or grunting*: Suggestive of noisy breathing
- It can be seen in up to 15% of live births and has been seen predominantly in premature babies with gestational age <30 weeks.
- Neonatal respiratory distress can be broadly categorized into:
  ○ Medical causes
  ○ Surgical causes

■ MEDICAL CAUSES OF RESPIRATORY DISTRESS

Respiratory Distress Syndrome
- Also known as surfactant deficiency disease (SDD), hyaline membrane disease (HMD), and lung disease of prematurity.
- Most important and most common cause of respiratory distress in premature babies especially babies with gestational age <29 weeks.[1]
- Main pathophysiology is lack of surfactant production by type 2 pneumocytes. Hence, hyaline membrane forms within the alveoli.

- Chest X-ray (CXR) reveals generalized bilateral symmetrical lung consolidation along with decreased expansion of lungs.[1]
- Reticulogranular opacities **(Fig. 1)** might be present secondary to collapsed alveoli, infiltration of pulmonary interstitium by fluid and air-filled bronchioles. Ultrasound (USG) will[2] show whiteout lungs due to confluent B-lines **(Fig. 2)**.
- Maximum severity of HMD is at 12–24 weeks of birth.
- Surfactant administration is critical in the treatment of HMD. Surfactant along with positive pressure ventilation causes decrease in the lung consolidation and improvement in lung aeration.
- Rarely, positive pressure ventilation may cause dissection of air into peribronchovascular interstitium with resultant pulmonary interstitial edema (PIE) which can subsequently lead to subpleural blebs and eventually pneumothorax as well.

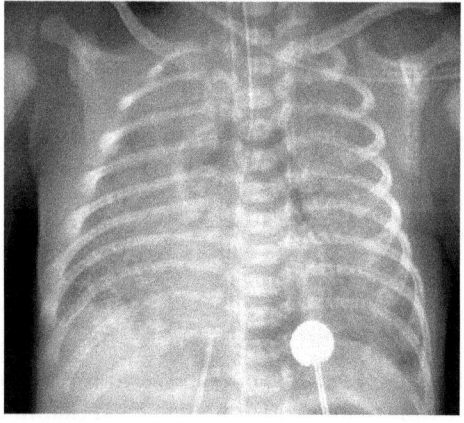

FIG. 1: Hyaline membrane disease. Chest X-ray showing bilateral whiteout lungs with diffuse reticulonodular opacities.

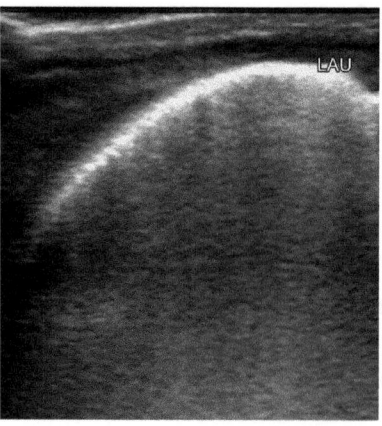

FIG. 2: Ultrasound showing whiteout lung due to confluent B-lines in a neonate with hyaline membrane disease.
(LAU: left anterior upper quadrant)

Transient Tachypnea of the Newborn

- Also known as wet lung disease, this is seen only in term neonates.
- During fetal life, fluid is present within the lungs which get cleared off after delivery by the lungs getting squeezed passing through the birth canal, and lymphatic drainage of lung.
- Delayed clearance of this fluid causes respiratory distress.[1]
- It is a self-liming disease and resolves within 24 hours of life.
- CXR is suggestive of prominent interstitial markings mainly in the perihilar location along with mild hyperinflation and small pulmonary effusion.[1]
- Lung USG can show a characteristic double lung point which is the differential echogenicity between the upper and lower lobes of lung.[3] This sign is characteristically absent in the healthy babies and babies with HMD, pneumonia, or pneumothorax.

Neonatal Pneumonia

- It can occur due to transplacental spread, nonmaintenance of asepsis while performing delivery, secondary to aspiration of amniotic fluid or as a hospital-acquired infection during prolonged hospitalization.
- Predominantly, it has a bacterial etiopathogenesis.
- CXR suggests pulmonary opacities **(Fig. 3)** and may show parapneumonic effusion which can help to differentiate this condition from HMD, transient tachypnea of the newborn (TTNB), and meconium aspiration syndrome (MAS).[4]

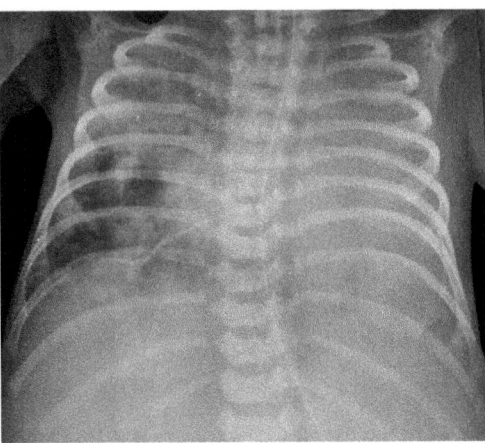

FIG. 3: Neonatal pneumonia. Chest X-ray shows inhomogeneous opacities in the right lung with areas of breakdown.

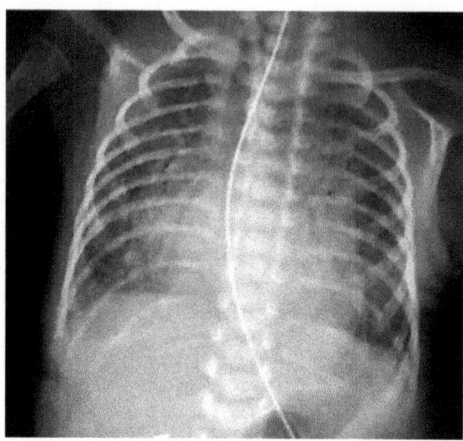

FIG. 4: Meconium aspiration syndrome. Chest X-ray in a neonate showing hyperinflated lungs with coarse nodular opacities.

Meconium Aspiration Syndrome

- It is a pathology of term and post-term babies.
- Intrauterine fetal hypoxia can result in deep gasping respiration attempts by the fetus along with intrauterine passage of meconium.
- Though meconium is sterile, it is a local irritant. Aspiration into the fetal airways can lead to obstruction of small airways.
- CXR appearance can be variable.[1] Incomplete obstruction of bronchioles may lead to overinflation of lung fields while complete obstruction can cause patchy atelectatic changes **(Fig. 4)**.

Pneumothorax

- Though uncommonly seen, it can be spontaneous or secondary to lung infection, aspiration of meconium, or barotrauma due to ventilator.
- Spontaneous pneumothorax is mainly seen in premature neonates **(Fig. 5)**.
- CXR might miss pneumothorax as air accumulates mainly in the anteromedial region and in the subpulmonic recess.
- Subpulmonic pneumothorax can be seen as a radiolucency in the right or left hypochondriac region or might present only as a deep lateral costophrenic angle.[5]

■ SURGICAL CAUSES OF RESPIRATORY DISTRESS

These conditions require surgical correction. Some of these conditions can be seen antenatally, while others present after the neonatal period. Some may not be detected at birth and present later in life.

Congenital Lobar Overinflation

- It is a focal abnormality of the lung airway and can be secondary to bronchomalacia, abnormal vessel crossing, kinks, and webs. These result in impaired function and secondary hyperinflation of pulmonary lobe.
- Most commonly involved segment of lung is left upper lobe followed by the right middle lobe.
- Most babies become symptomatic by first week of life.
- CXR reveals a hyperinflated lobe of lung with splaying of pulmonary vasculature **(Fig. 5)**. There is resultant adjacent lung atelectasis and mediastinal shift to the contralateral side.[6-8]
- CT suggests decreased aeration of the involved part of lung and attenuated vascular markings in the involved lobe(s) **(Figs. 6A to C)**.

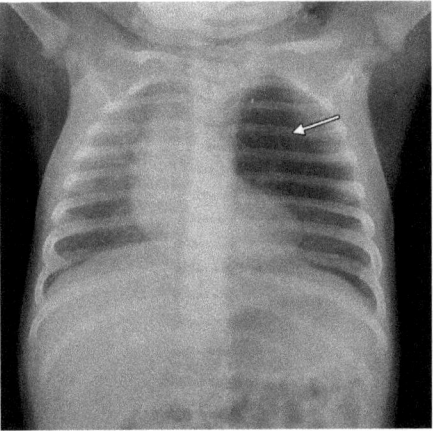

FIG. 5: Congenital lobar overinflation. Chest X-ray in a neonate showing an area of increased lucency involving the left upper lobe (arrow) with reduced vascular markings.

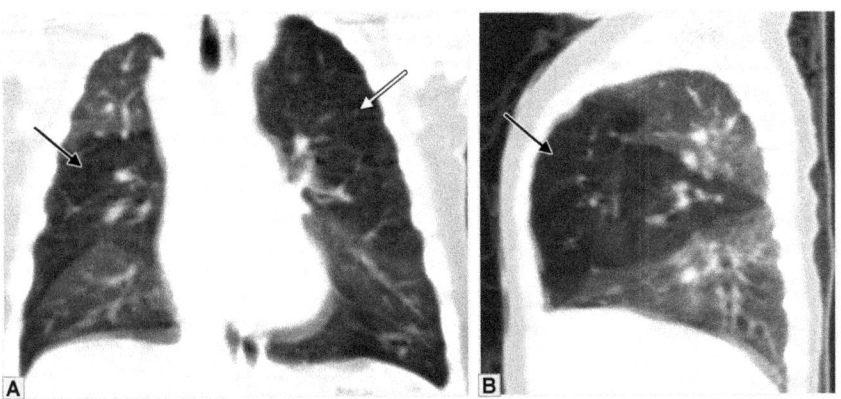

FIGS. 6A TO C: *Continued*

Continued

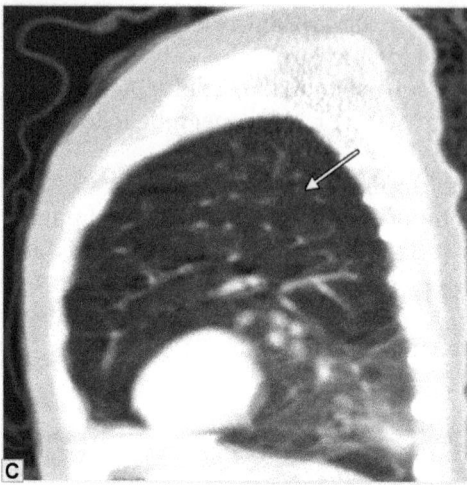

FIGS. 6A TO C: Congenital lobar overinflation. Computed tomography images in lung window showing reduced attenuation of the right middle lobe (black arrows in A and B) and left upper lobe (white arrows in A and C) with reduced vascular markings.

Congenital Pulmonary Airway Malformation

- It is a hamartomatous lesion and is seen due to failure of transformation of pulmonary mesenchymal tissue into the normal bronchovascular tissue.[6-8]
- Radiologically, five types of congenital pulmonary airway malformation (CPAM) are seen:[6-8]
  - *Type 0:*
    - Bilateral acinar dysgenesis
    - Fatal
  - *Type I:*
    - Seen in 50% of patients
    - Single large cyst or multiple large cysts are noted which might communicate with the tracheobronchial tree **(Figs. 7A and B)**, with largest cyst >2 cm in size.
  - *Type II:*
    - Seen in 40% of patients
    - Shows multiple small cysts (largest cysts is <2 cm size) with communication with the tracheobronchial tree **(Figs. 8A and B)**.
  - *Type III:*
    - Seen in <10% patients
    - Shows multiple small cysts (<0.5 cm) which look solid on imaging.
  - *Type IV:*
    - Rarest (<1%) type
    - Shows large cysts **(Figs. 9A and B)** which cannot be distinguished from cyst seen in type 1 pleuropulmonary blastoma.
- CPAM lesions can be easily detected on antenatal USG as well.
- Close differential diagnosis is pneumatoceles which usually show interval resolution post-treatment. Resolution is not seen in patients with CPAM.

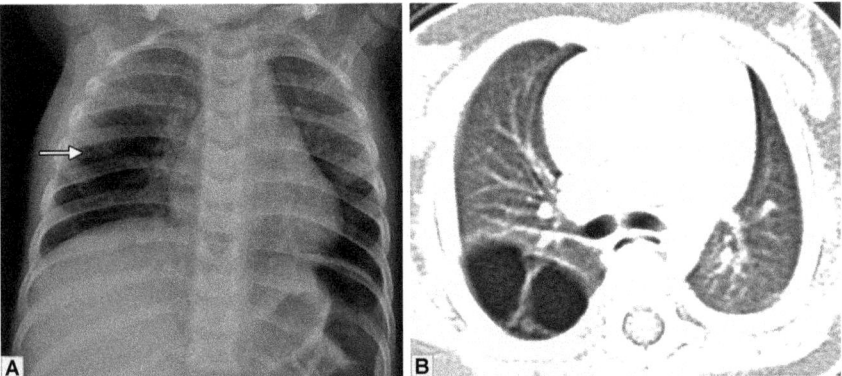

FIGS. 7A AND B: Congenital pulmonary airway malformation (type 1). Chest X-ray (A) shows an ill-defined radiolucent lesion in the right lower lobe (arrow) with septations inside. Axial image of computed tomography scan in lung window (B) shows air filled large cystic lesions in the right lower lobe.

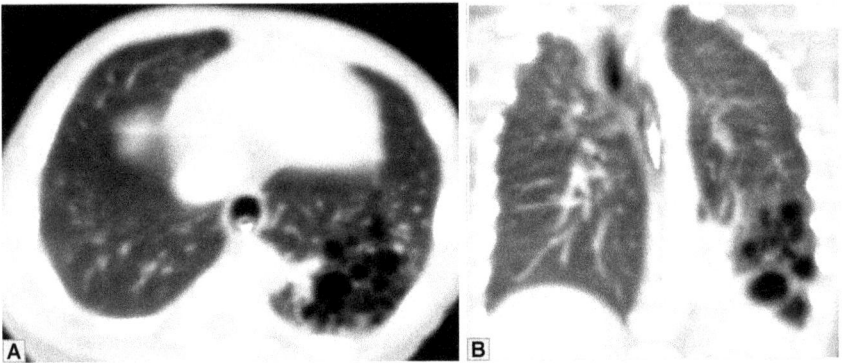

FIGS. 8A AND B: Congenital pulmonary airway malformation (type 2). Computed tomography images in axial (A) and coronal plane (B) show multiple clustered small air-filled cysts in the left lower lobe.

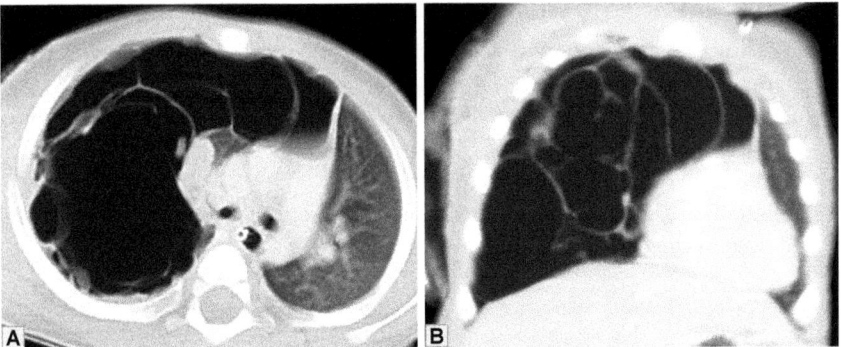

FIGS. 9A AND B: Congenital pulmonary airway malformation (type 4). Computed tomography images in axial (A) and coronal plane (B) show multiple large air-filled cysts with septations replacing the right lung. Histopathological examination showed features of congenital pulmonary airway malformation (CPAM).

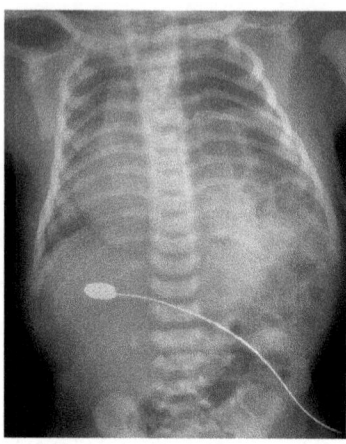

FIG. 10: Congenital diaphragmatic hernia. Chest X-ray shows herniated loops on the left side with mediastinal shift to the right side.

Congenital Diaphragmatic Hernia

- It is a result of intrathoracic herniation of the abdominal contents secondary to a diaphragmatic defect.[6-8]
- Diaphragmatic defect can be anteromedial (known as Morgagni hernia), posterolateral (known as Bochdalek hernia), or can be central.
- The herniation results in pulmonary hypoplasia and congenital diaphragmatic hernia (CDH) can also be associated with other anomalies such as persistent pulmonary hypertension of the neonates and hypoplastic left heart syndrome (HLHS).
- Antenatally, it can be easily detected with abdominal contents seen in thorax and with ipsilateral pulmonary hypoplasia.
- CXR shows abdominal contents like bowel or stomach in the thorax along with contralateral trachea-mediastinal shift **(Fig. 10)**.

Esophageal Atresia with Tracheoesophageal Fistula

- It is the most common surgical cause of respiratory distress requiring neonatal ICU admission.
- Baby pours out excessive secretions postdelivery and can develop respiratory distress secondary to aspiration of these secretions.
- Antenatally, USG reveals polyhydramnios.
- Postdelivery, an attempt of putting orogastric tube might result in coiling of tube in the upper esophageal region **(Fig. 11)**.

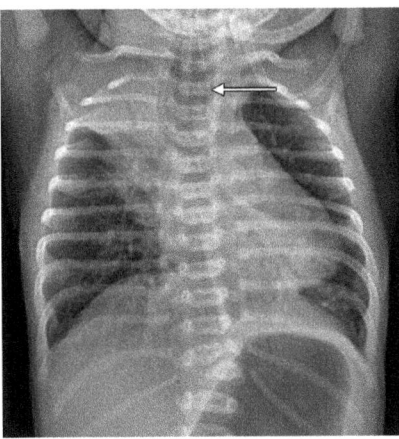

FIG. 11: Chest X-ray of a neonate showing coiled up orogastric tube in the upper thorax (arrow). In addition, collapse of right upper lobe is also seen.

■ MISCELLANEOUS CAUSES OF RESPIRATORY DISTRESS

- Congenital lesions such as bronchogenic and esophageal duplication cysts can cause mass effect on surrounding structures[9,10] and result in respiratory distress **(Figs. 12A and B)**.
- Congenital heart diseases such as transposition of great arteries and tetralogy of Fallot can also cause respiratory distress. Echocardiography is diagnostic for these diseases.
- Other miscellaneous causes include hematological abnormalities, metabolic acidosis, hyperthermia, skeletal abnormalities, etc.

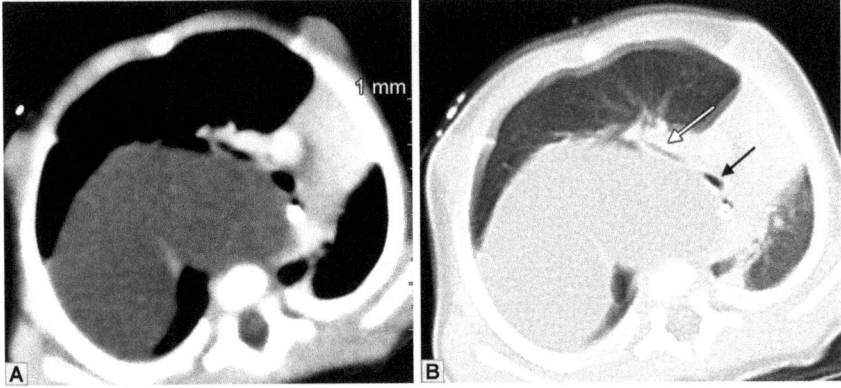

FIGS. 12A AND B: Bronchogenic cyst. (A) A large fluid-filled cystic lesion in the midline and extending on the right side. It is seen to displace the mediastinal structures to the left side with compression on the right (white arrow in B) and left (black arrow in B) main bronchi.

■ CONCLUSION

Neonatal respiratory distress has medical and surgical causes. Plain radiographs remain the first imaging modality, and CT the problem solving tool.

Other Related Chapters that can be Referred to:
- Chapter 2: Ultrasound Chest: Basics and Role
- Chapter 6: Congenital Lung Abnormalities

■ REFERENCES

1. Agrons GA, Courtney SE, Stocker JT, Markowitz RI. From the archives of the AFIP: Lung disease in premature neonates: radiologic-pathologic correlation. Radiographics. 2005;25(4):1047-73.
2. Gregorio-Hernández R, Arriaga-Redondo M, Pérez-Pérez A, Ramos-Navarro C, Sánchez-Luna M. Lung ultrasound in preterm infants with respiratory distress: experience in a neonatal intensive care unit. Eur J Pediatr. 2020;179:81-9.
3. Copetti R, Cattarossi L. The "double lung point": An ultrasound sign diagnostic of transient tachypnea of the newborn. Neonatology. 2007;91(3):203-9.
4. Newman B. Imaging of medical disease of the newborn lung. Radiol Clin North Am. 1999;37(6):1049-65.
5. Gordon R. The deep sulcus sign. Radiology. 1980;136(1):25-7.
6. Lee EY, Dorkin H, Vargas SO. Congenital pulmonary malformations in pediatric patients: review and update on etiology, classification, and imaging findings. Radiol Clin North Am. 2011;49:921-48.
7. Thacker PG, Rao AG, Hill JG, Lee EY. Congenital lung anomalies in children and adults: current concepts and imaging findings. Radiol Clin North Am. 2014;52(1):155-81.
8. Lee EY, Boiselle PM, Cleveland RH. Multidetector CT evaluation of congenital lung anomalies. Radiology. 2008;247(3):632-48.
9. Minkner K, Alamo L. Pre- and neonatal imaging of gastrointestinal complications in congenital diaphragmatic hernia. Abdom Radiol (NY). 2018;43(3):574-82.
10. McAdams HP, Kirejczyk WM, Rosado-deChristenson ML, Matsumoto S. Bronchogenic cyst: Imaging features with clinical and histopathologic correlation. Radiology. 2000;217(2):441-6.

CHAPTER 6

Congenital Lung Abnormalities

Pooja Abbey, Aparna Shyamkumar

- ❏ Nomenclature and classification
- ❏ Embryological basis and etiopathogenesis
- ❏ Categorization of congenital lung anomalies
  - ➤ Parenchymal/airway anomalies
  - ➤ Airway anomalies
  - ➤ Vascular anomalies
- ➤ Pulmonary vein anomalies
- ➤ Combined parenchymal and vascular anomalies
- ➤ Foregut anomalies
- ❏ Role of different imaging modalities
  - ➤ Antenatal diagnosis
  - ➤ Postnatal evaluation

■ INTRODUCTION

Congenital lung anomalies (CLAs) are a group of malformations that may involve the airway, pulmonary parenchyma, pulmonary artery, or veins in various permutations and combinations. They exist as part of a continuum with abnormal lung/airway and normal vasculature on one end of the spectrum, and abnormalities of vasculature without parenchymal abnormality on the other. Overall, incidence is reported to be approximately 1 in 2,500. Congenital anomalies are an important diagnostic consideration in certain clinical situations, such as respiratory distress (RD) in neonates and infants, and recurrent infections in the same lung lobe in children. Imaging findings are quite varied and exhibit significant overlap between different entities. A high index of suspicion, along with knowledge about the basic embryology, etiopathogenesis and imaging findings, is the key to making the correct diagnosis.

■ NOMENCLATURE AND CLASSIFICATION

- A number of terms have been used to describe CLAs. Pryce coined the term "sequestration" in 1946, to describe abnormal lung tissue disconnected from normal bronchial connections and having systemic arterial supply. As variants were discovered, he later classified sequestration under three types—Pryce types I, II, and III.

- In 1974, Sade used the term "sequestration spectrum" to include various anomalies. The term "malinosculation" (mal-abnormal, osculum-mouth) was also described in 1987 to describe anomalous communications between the various components of the lung, parenchyma, airway, arteries, and veins, in the various CLAs.
- As CLAs exist as a spectrum, patients often show a combination of findings. Lesions may involve only the lung parenchyma and/or airway, the pulmonary artery and/or veins, or have both parenchymal and vascular components.
- Rather than trying to fit the abnormality into a specific terminology, it is more important for radiologists to follow a systematic approach while describing these lesions, and look for possible involvement of components of the lung parenchyma, airway, and vessels and also actively look for other associated anomalies.

EMBRYOLOGICAL BASIS AND ETIOPATHOGENESIS

The airway and lungs develop from the lung bud, which is an outpouching from the foregut. The lung bud divides into branches, which give rise to the primary, secondary, tertiary, and further bronchial divisions. Lung development occurs in an orderly fashion in successive stages, namely, the pseudoglandular stage (5-16 weeks), canalicular stage (16-26 weeks), terminal sac stage (26 weeks till birth), and alveolar stage (32 weeks-8 years). Any deviation from the norm can give rise to various CLAs.

It is postulated that airway obstruction or vascular insult/abnormality and genetics may play a role in pathogenesis of CLAs.

CATEGORIZATION OF CONGENITAL LUNG ANOMALIES

The various CLAs may be broadly categorized as parenchymal/airway anomalies, vascular anomalies, and combined anomalies,[1] as enumerated in **Table 1**.

Parenchymal/Airway Anomalies

Congenital Lobar Hyperinflation (or Overinflation)
- Previously known as congenital lobar emphysema (CLE)—this is a misnomer as there is no destruction of alveolar walls in this condition (unlike in emphysema).
- Two types—classical (normal/reduced number of alveoli) and poly-alveolar (increased number of alveoli).
- Seen in infants, 50% of cases present in first month of life. Uncommon (only 5%) after age of 6 months.
- Important cause of neonatal RD. May need emergent surgical resection to alleviate symptoms.
- Progressive hyperinflation of affected lobe can lead to significant mass effect on normal lobes and mediastinum.

TABLE 1: Congenital lung anomalies—categorization as parenchymal, vascular, or combined.	
Predominantly lung parenchymal/airway abnormalities	• Congenital lobar hyperinflation (CLH) • Congenital bronchial atresia (BA) • Congenital pulmonary airway malformation (CPAM) • Laryngeal atresia/stenosis • Tracheal atresia/stenosis • Tracheal bronchus
Predominantly vascular anomalies involving	
Pulmonary artery	• Pulmonary agenesis-aplasia-hypoplasia complex • Proximal interruption of pulmonary artery • Pulmonary artery sling • Isolated systemic supply to normal lung/pseudo-sequestration
Pulmonary vein	• Anomalous pulmonary venous drainage • Pulmonary vein stenosis • Venous varix • Meandering pulmonary vein/pseudo-scimitar
Pulmonary artery and vein	• Pulmonary arteriovenous malformation (AVM)
Combined parenchymal and vascular anomalies	• Pulmonary sequestration (intralobar and extralobar sequestration) • Hybrid lesions • Scimitar syndrome/hypogenetic lung syndrome
Foregut anomalies	• Bronchogenic cyst • Neurenteric cyst • Esophageal duplication cyst

- Most commonly affects one lobe. Left upper lobe is most often involved (42%), followed by middle lobe (35%), and right upper lobe (21%). Lower lobe involvement is uncommon—<1% each.
- Hyperinflation is thought to occur due to airway narrowing and a "ball-valve" effect due to intrinsic cartilage defect, intraluminal mucosal folds, or extrinsic mass effect. No cause may be found in at least half the cases.
- Diagnosis should be suspected in an infant with RD with chest radiograph [chest X-ray (CXR)] showing focal hyperlucency, usually with mass effect **(Fig. 1A)**. Margin of collapsed lower lobe may be seen.
- Computed tomography (CT) confirms the diagnosis **(Figs. 1B to D)** by showing the hyperinflation of involved lobe(s). It is advisable to do a contrast-enhanced CT to look for any lesions [like bronchogenic cysts (BCs)] or vascular anomalies which may be causing bronchial compression and also to look for associated vascular anomalies.
- Involvement of more than one lobe, though uncommon, may be seen **(Figs. 2A to C)**.

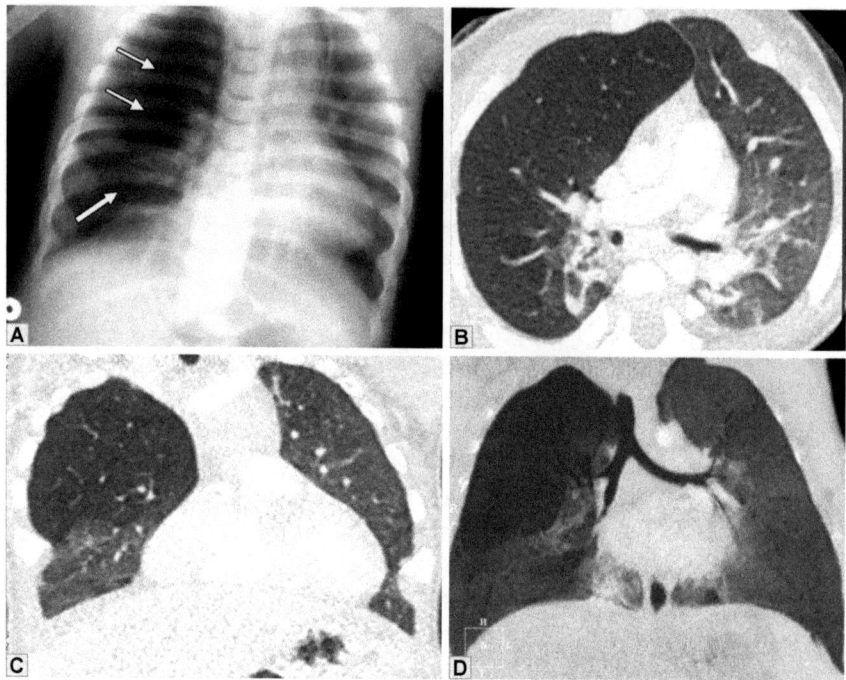

FIGS. 1A TO D: A 6-month-old male with congenital lobar overinflation. Chest X-ray (CXR) (A) shows large area of hyperlucency in the right upper and mid zones (thin arrows), with paucity of vascular markings in this area, associated mass effect with partial collapsed lung seen in right paracardiac region (thick arrow), and contralateral mediastinal shift. CT axial, coronal, and minimum-intensity projection (B to D) images confirm overinflation of right upper lobe.

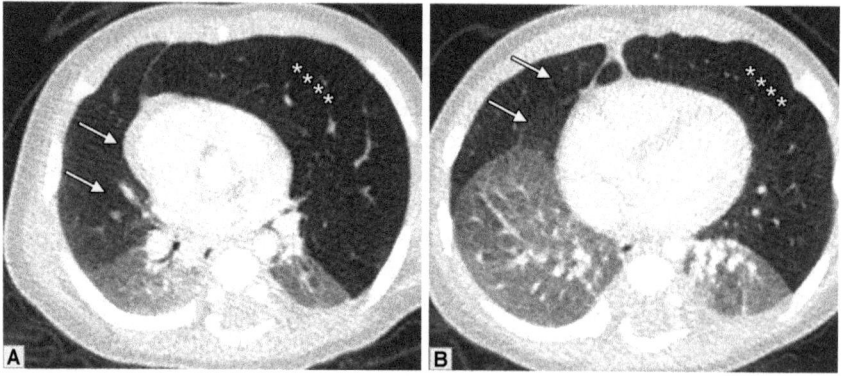

FIGS. 2A TO C: *Continued*

Continued

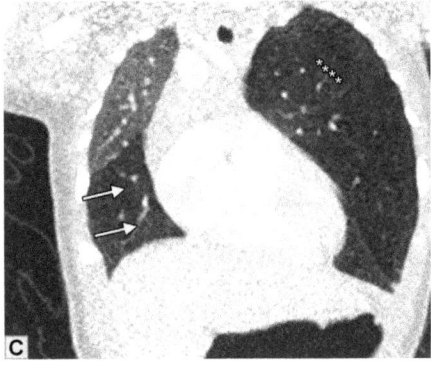

FIGS. 2A TO C: Bilateral congenital lobar overinflation (CLO) in a 3-month-old male with respiratory distress. CT shows overinflation affecting the left upper lobe (****) as well as the right middle lobe (arrows).

Congenital Bronchial Atresia

- It refers to focal interruption of a bronchus, with normal development of distal airways.
- It can affect a lobar, segmental, or subsegmental bronchus.
- Distal to the atretic segment, inspissation of secretions leads to formation of bronchocele.
- Collateral air drift through pores of Kohn and canals of Lambert often leads to air-trapping and hyperinflation of the involved lung segments.
- Isolated cases are often asymptomatic.
- Bronchial atresia (BA) may be associated with other CLAs such as pulmonary sequestration (PS) and congenital pulmonary airway malformation (CPAM).
- CXR may demonstrate focal hyperlucency, which corresponds to air-trapping on CT. Bronchocele may be seen on CXR and CT as a branching, tubular, nonenhancing opacity **(Figs. 3A to C)**.
- In older patients, it is advisable to look for any small endobronchial obstructing lesion which may be causing the bronchocele.

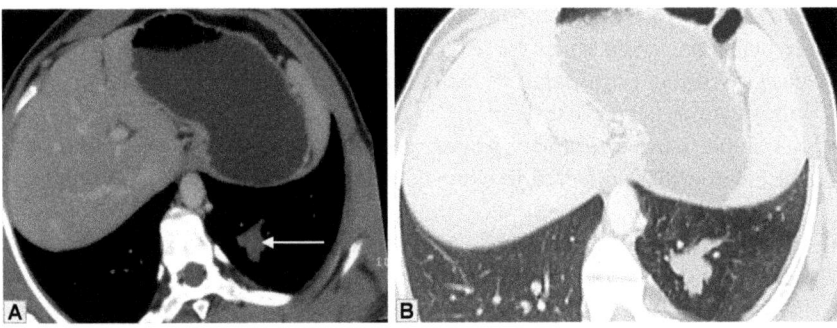

FIGS. 3A TO C: *Continued*

Continued

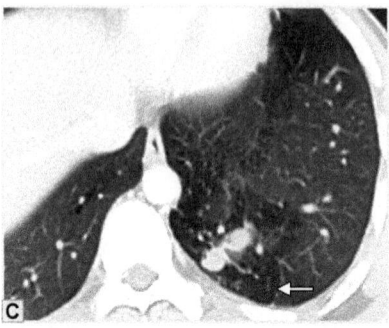

FIGS. 3A TO C: Bronchial atresia affecting the posterior basal segment of left lower lobe in a 17-year-old male. CT reveals a bronchocele—tubular, hypodense branching opacity (arrow), showing no enhancement on the mediastinal window (A). The surrounding lung shows hyperinflation (short arrow) on the lung window images (B and C).

Congenital Pulmonary Airway Malformation

- Congenital pulmonary airway malformations (CPAMs) are a group of congenital cystic lung lesions that result from disorganized growth of the primary bronchioles, which have a communication with the bronchial tree.
- Previously, they were called congenital cystic adenomatoid malformations (CCAM).
- Stocker initially described three types—(1) type 1 CPAM (most common, seen in 60% cases) comprises single or multiple large cysts, size >2 cm, (2) type 2 (15-20% cases)—smaller cysts <2 cm but >0.5 cm, and (3) type 3 (5-10% cases) comprises microcysts <0.5 cm and these may appear pseudosolid on imaging.
- Later two more types were added in the updated Stocker classification—(4) type 0 is the rarest, results from bilateral acinar dysgenesis, and is fatal. (5) Type 4 (10-15% of CPAM) is large cysts (like type 1) of distal acinar origin.[2]
- Types 1 and 4 cannot be differentiated on imaging from cystic type of pleuropulmonary blastoma.[2]
- 95% of cases involve a single lobe of lung. There is no lobar predilection.
- Antenatal ultrasonography (USG) may detect a cystic lung lesion with varying sized fluid-filled cysts **(Fig. 4A)**. Due to bronchial communication, soon after birth the lesion shows air within it. CXR may show focal hyperlucency or a lung cyst **(Figs. 4B and 5A)**. CT confirms a cystic lung lesion with air (compared to bronchogenic cyst which is fluid-filled and air is usually seen postinfection).
- CT depicts the size and number of cysts **(Figs. 4C to F and 5B to E)**, associated mass effect, and signs of secondary infection (air-fluid levels, thick walls).
- Hybrid lesions may be seen, CPAM (often type 2) may exist along with PS, and show a systemic arterial supply.
- Majority (85%) of cases become symptomatic in infancy with RD, or in early childhood with recurrent pneumonia in the same lobe.
- Complications include secondary infection, pneumothorax, and there is a small risk of development of malignancy (risk of malignancy is more in type 4 lesions).

- CPAMs are usually managed by surgical resection. But, some prefer observation in asymptomatic low-risk patients as some of them may even spontaneously resolve.³

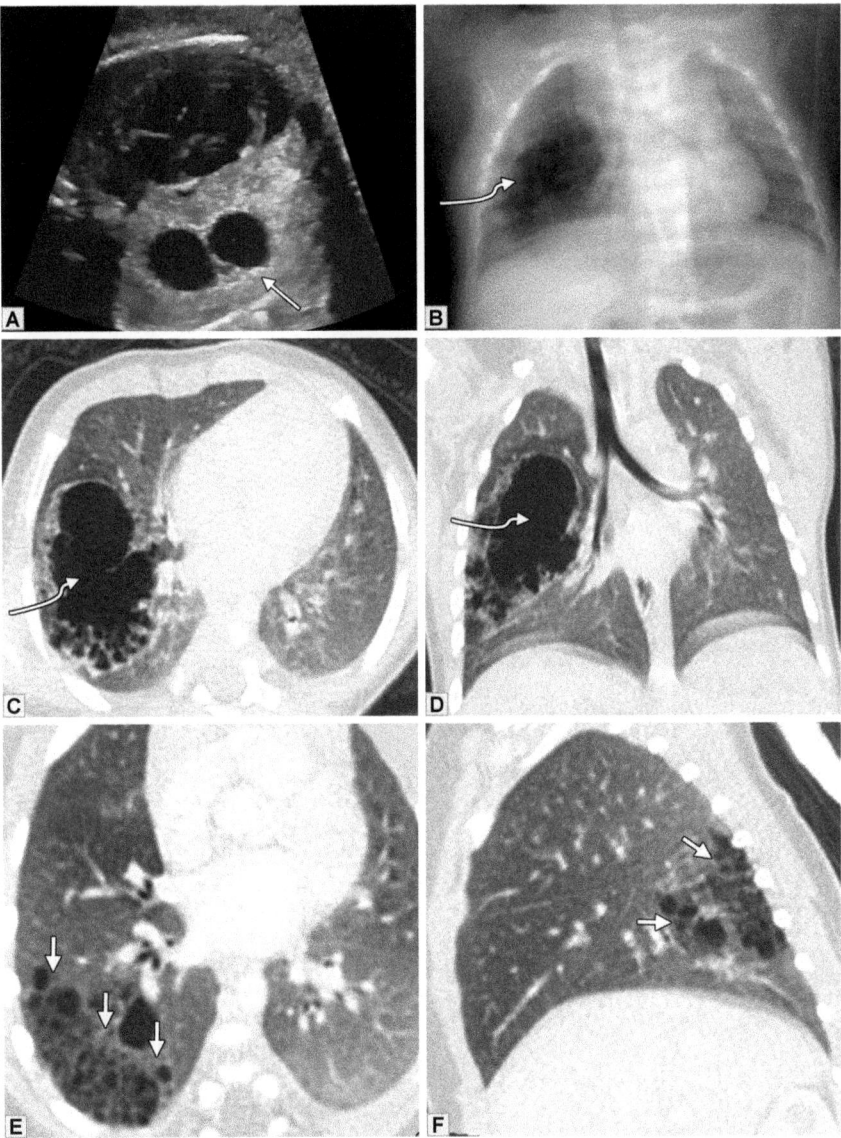

FIGS. 4A TO F: Two cases of CPAM detected antenatally. Antenatal USG (A) shows a right lung lesion containing multiple large anechoic fluid-filled cysts (arrow) causing mediastinal shift to opposite side. Postnatal CXR (B), CT (C and D) at 1 month of age confirms a type 1 CPAM (curved arrows) in the right upper lobe, with minimal mass effect. Axial and sagittal CT (E and F) chest in lung window in a different patient (antenatal USG not shown) at day 7 of life reveals a type 2 CPAM in the right lower lobe (short thick white arrows) with smaller cysts 0.5–1 cm in size.
(CPAM: congenital pulmonary airway malformation; CT: computed tomography; CXR: chest X-ray; USG: ultrasonography)

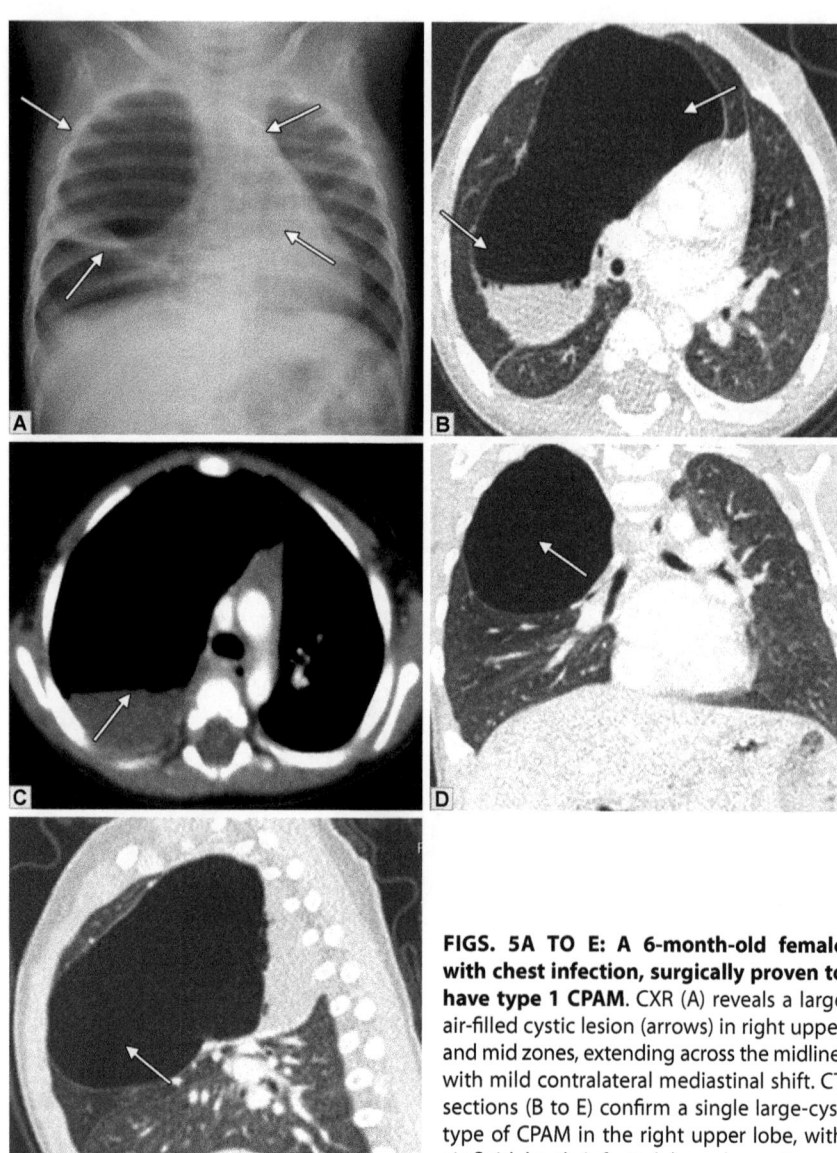

FIGS. 5A TO E: A 6-month-old female with chest infection, surgically proven to have type 1 CPAM. CXR (A) reveals a large air-filled cystic lesion (arrows) in right upper and mid zones, extending across the midline, with mild contralateral mediastinal shift. CT sections (B to E) confirm a single large-cyst type of CPAM in the right upper lobe, with air-fluid level. Infected bronchogenic cyst can look similar on imaging.

(CPAM: congenital pulmonary airway malformation; CT: computed tomography; CXR: chest X-ray)

Airway Anomalies

Laryngeal Atresia/Stenosis: Congenital High Airway Obstruction Syndrome

- Congenital high airway obstruction syndrome (CHAOS) is a rare, lethal condition in which there is a complete/near-complete obstruction of the fetal upper airway.
- Complete laryngeal atresia may be seen with/without-associated tracheoesophageal fistula. Some cases may show near-complete stenosis.
- On pathology, pulmonary hyperplasia is seen distal to the airway obstruction.
- Antenatal USG reveals bilateral enlarged and echogenic lungs, which cause mass effect upon mediastinum and diaphragm. Distal to obstruction, fluid-filled trachea, and bronchi are seen. Fetal ascites and hydrops may eventually develop.

Tracheal Atresia/Stenosis

- Tracheal atresia is a rare condition with congenital absence of the trachea. Antenatal USG findings resemble those of CHAOS.
- Congenital tracheal stenosis usually presents in early life with stridor or wheeze. Three main types are—(1) generalized hypoplasia, (2) funnel-shaped narrowing, or (3) segmental stenosis. It is often associated with other anomalies such as tracheoesophageal fistula or vascular slings.

Tracheal Bronchus

- Tracheal bronchus is a variant—anomalous or accessory bronchus arising directly from supracarinal trachea and supplying whole/part of right upper lobe **(Fig. 6A)**.
- Most often detected incidentally. Coronal CT sections in lung window or minimum-intensity projections (MinIP) **(Fig. 6B)** best demonstrate the anomaly.

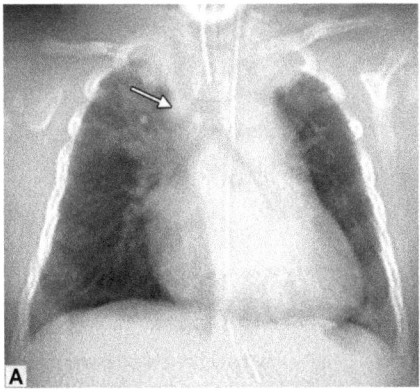 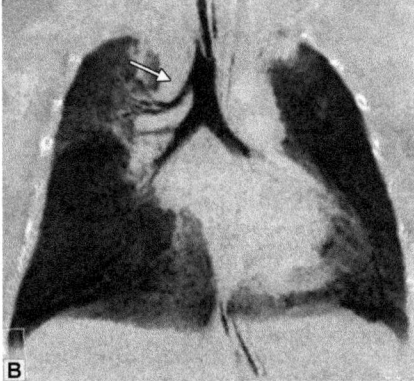

FIGS. 6A AND B: A 3-month-old male with chest infection. CXR (A) and coronal MinIP (minimum-intensity projection) CT image (B) reveal a tracheal bronchus (arrows) supplying part of the right upper lobe.
(CT: computed tomography; CXR: chest X-ray)

Vascular Anomalies

Pulmonary Agenesis-aplasia-hypoplasia Complex

- This is a spectrum of pulmonary underdevelopment disorders. Pulmonary agenesis implies complete absence of lung tissue, absent bronchus, and pulmonary artery. In aplasia, only a rudimentary bronchus is seen, with absent pulmonary artery and lung tissue. Cases with pulmonary hypoplasia show a rudimentary bronchus, small pulmonary artery, and small amount of lung tissue **(Table 2)**.
- CXR will show thoracic asymmetry with volume loss of affected side with ipsilateral mediastinal shift. CT can differentiate between these three entities **(Figs. 7A to D)**.

TABLE 2: Comparison between pulmonary agenesis, aplasia, and hypoplasia.

	Lung tissue	Bronchus	Pulmonary artery
Pulmonary agenesis	Absent	Absent	Absent
Pulmonary aplasia	Absent	Rudimentary	Absent
Pulmonary hypoplasia	Small	Rudimentary	Small

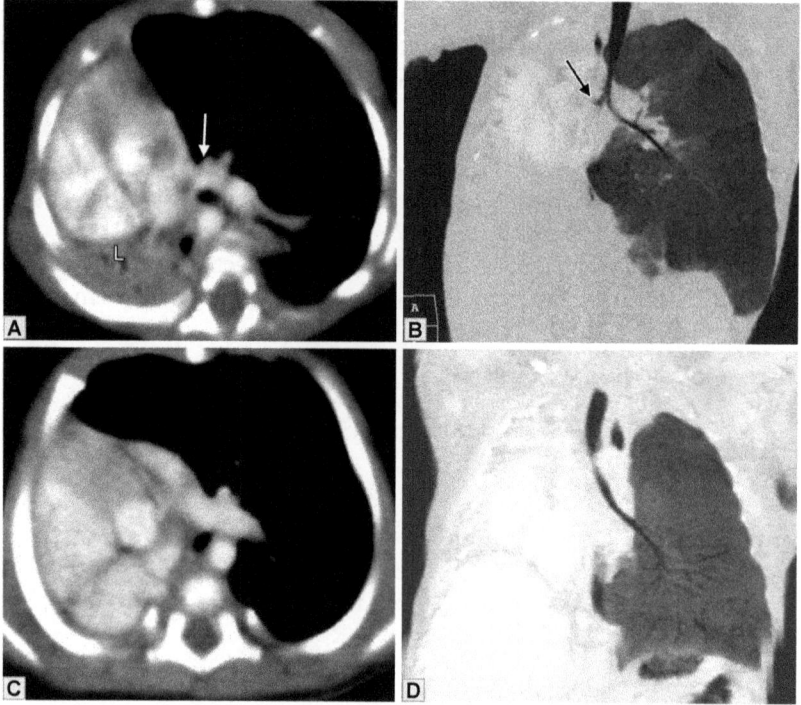

FIGS. 7A TO D: Two different cases of 3-month-old children with right-sided pulmonary hypoplasia (A and B) and right lung agenesis (C and D). In pulmonary hypoplasia, a hypoplastic right pulmonary artery (white arrow) and rudimentary right bronchus (black arrow) are visible on CT along with a small amount of lung tissue (L). The case of pulmonary agenesis (C and D) shows no rudimentary bronchus, absence of ipsilateral pulmonary artery and lung tissue.

Proximal Interruption of Pulmonary Artery

- This rare anomaly results from failure of development of the proximal portion of the pulmonary artery, with associated pulmonary hypoplasia. It is more common on right side usually affects the side opposite to the side of aortic arch.
- Distal pulmonary vasculature is intact and receives blood through systemic arterial collaterals. These collaterals may be transpleural giving rise to subpleural reticular opacities.
- CXR **(Fig. 8A)** shows a small hemithorax with small hilum and reduced vascularity. CT confirms the diagnosis **(Figs. 8B to E)** and can demonstrate the systemic collateral arterial supply.
- Patients may be asymptomatic or present with recurrent chest infections (lack of arterial blood flow may impair body's immune response to affected region), pulmonary hypertension, or hemoptysis.

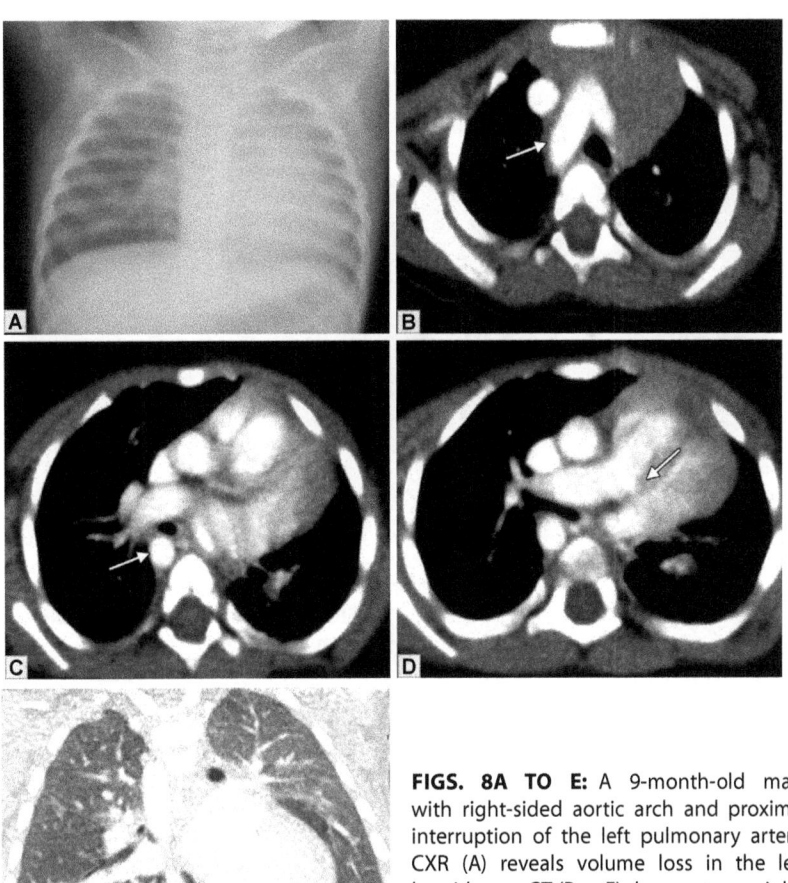

FIGS. 8A TO E: A 9-month-old male with right-sided aortic arch and proximal interruption of the left pulmonary artery. CXR (A) reveals volume loss in the left hemithorax. CT (B to E) demonstrates right-sided aortic arch and descending aorta (white arrows) and interruption of left pulmonary artery (white arrow), along with a small left lung.

(CT: computed tomography; CXR: chest X-ray)

Pulmonary Artery Sling
- In this anomaly, the left pulmonary artery has an anomalous origin and course, arising from the proximal right pulmonary artery and crossing toward the left, passing between the trachea and esophagus, and forming a sling around the lower trachea.
- There are two types. Type 1 has carina at normal position (T4–T5), while type 2 **(Figs. 9A to C)** is associated with a low-lying carina (T6), along with other anomalies such as bridging bronchus, tracheal stenosis, and congenital heart disease.

Isolated Systemic Supply to Normal Lung/Pseudosequestration
- In this entity, there is systemic arterial supply to lower lobe of the lung, in the absence of pulmonary arterial supply **(Figs. 10A to D)**.
- The involved segment shows normal communication with the tracheobronchial tree, hence it is also called pseudosequestration.
- It needs to be differentiated from a condition where there may be dual arterial supply to normal lung—involved lung shows both systemic and pulmonary arterial supply.

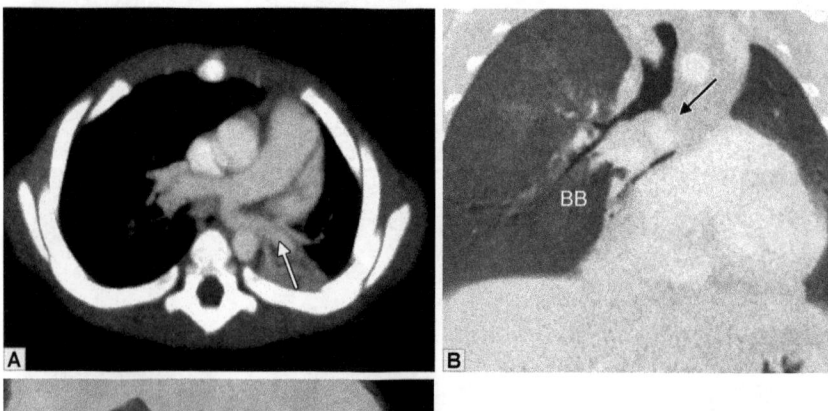

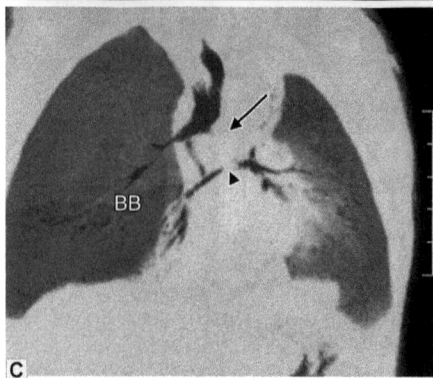

FIGS. 9A TO C: A 7-month-old male with persistent wheeze. CT reveals a type 2 pulmonary artery sling, with left pulmonary artery arising from the proximal right pulmonary artery (A). Coronal lung window and MinIP images (B and C) reveal narrowing of the intermediate left bronchus at the carina (black arrows) and formation of a pseudocarina (arrowhead) at level of T6, with a bridging bronchus (BB) supplying the right middle and lower lobes.

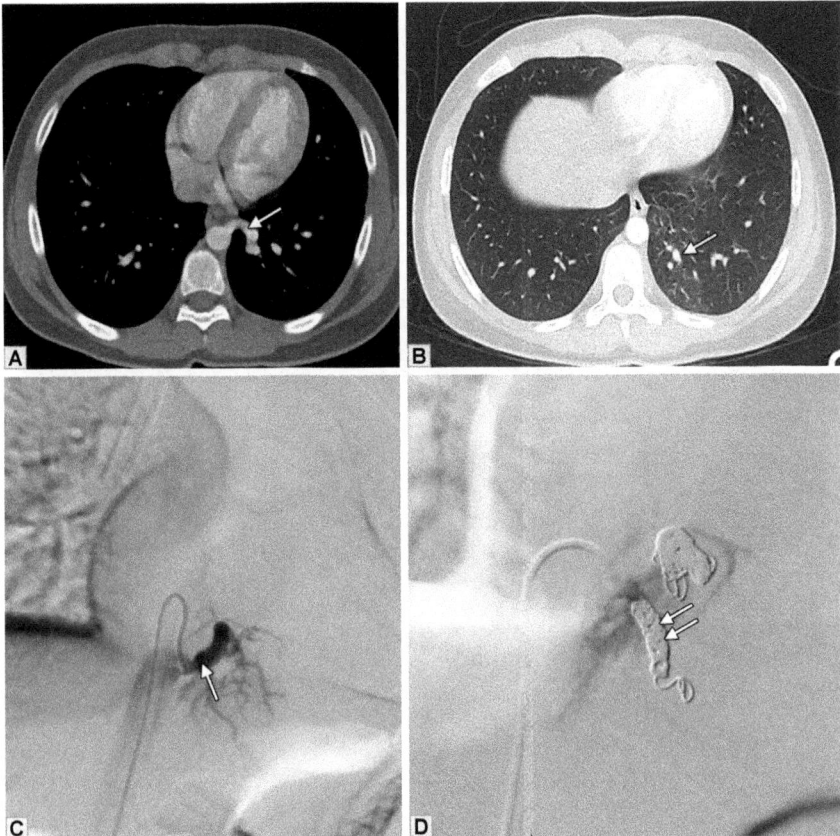

FIGS. 10A TO D: Isolated systemic supply to normal lungs (ISSNL) in a 10-year-old girl with hemoptysis. Axial CT sections in mediastinal and lung windows (A and B) show the anomalous systemic artery (arrow) arising from the descending thoracic aorta supplying the posterior basal segment of the left lower lobe; the lung is otherwise normal. Selective angiogram of the anomalous vessel (arrow) is shown in C which was coil embolized (double arrows in D).

Pulmonary Vein Anomalies

Anomalous Pulmonary Venous Drainage
- It may be partial or total.
- In partial anomalous pulmonary venous connection (PAPVC), one/some pulmonary vein(s) do(es) not drain into the left atrium **(Figs. 11A to E)**.
- In total anomalous pulmonary venous connection (TAPVC), all four pulmonary veins do not drain into left atrium. TAPVC may be supra-cardiac, cardiac, or infracardiac.
- On imaging, any focus of obstruction should be looked for in the anomalous vein, especially where the vein crosses the diaphragm.

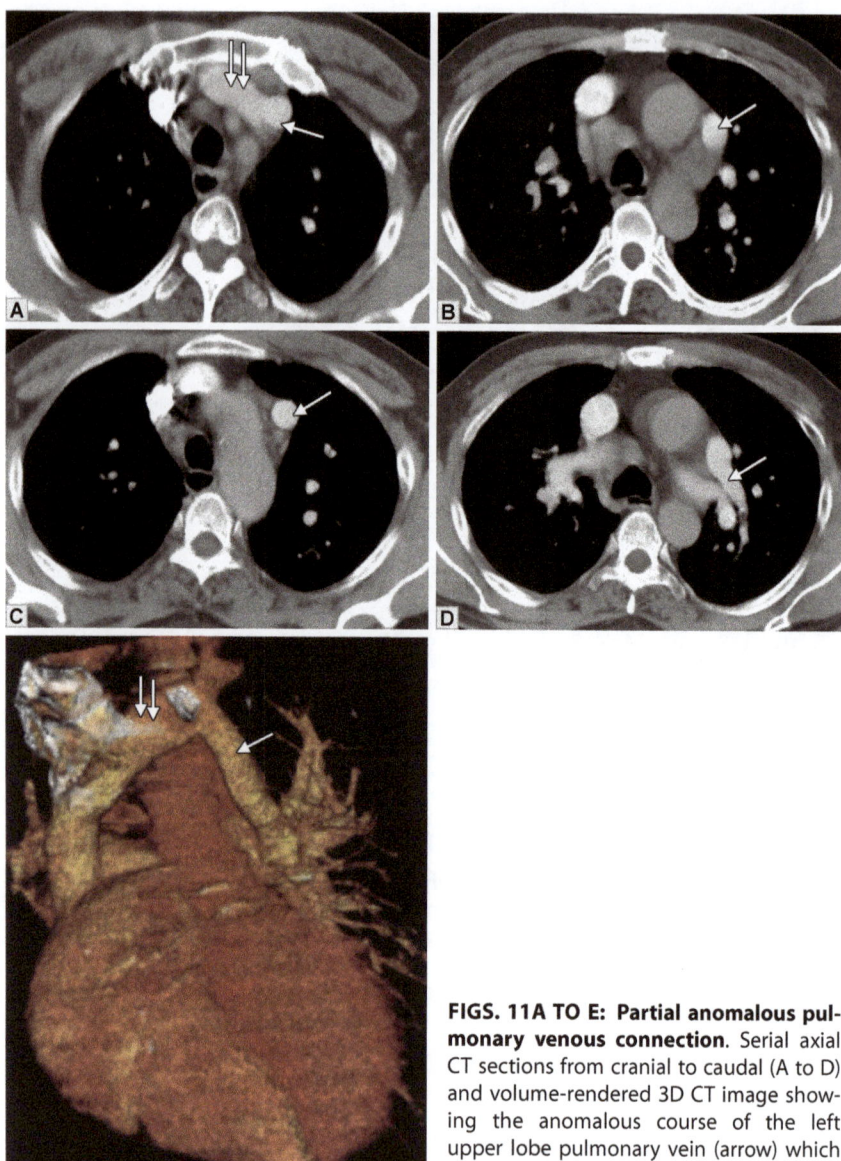

FIGS. 11A TO E: Partial anomalous pulmonary venous connection. Serial axial CT sections from cranial to caudal (A to D) and volume-rendered 3D CT image showing the anomalous course of the left upper lobe pulmonary vein (arrow) which connects to the left brachiocephalic vein (double arrows).

Pulmonary Vein Stenosis

It may occur in isolation, or in association with PAPVC or congenital heart disease.

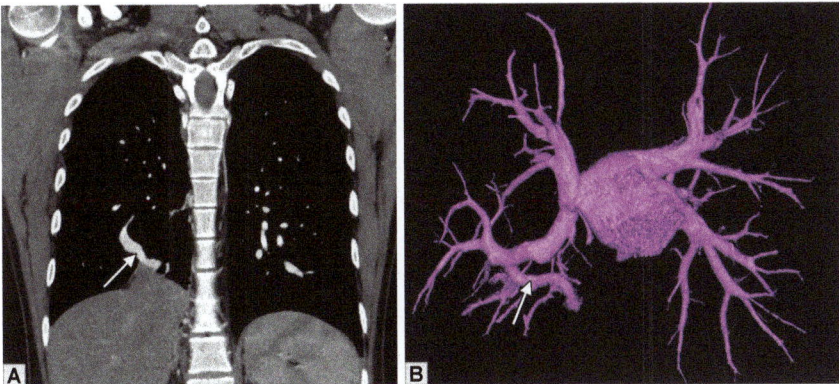

FIGS. 12A AND B: Meandering pulmonary vein. Coronal CT (A) and volume-rendered image (B) showing right inferior pulmonary vein (arrow).

Venous Varix
- A pulmonary varix is a dilated pulmonary vein in the absence of a feeding artery or nidus [c.f. arteriovenous malformation (AVM)].
- Patients are usually asymptomatic.
- It may mimic AVM or pulmonary nodule on CXR.

Meandering Pulmonary Vein/Pseudo-scimitar
- In this condition, an inferior pulmonary vein may show anomalous course and follow a circuitous course **(Figs. 12A and B)** through the lung. It then opens normally into the left atrium.
- On CXR, this may be confused with a scimitar vein [scimitar vein opens into the inferior vena cava (IVC)].

Pulmonary Arteriovenous Malformation
- Pulmonary AVMs show abnormal communication between pulmonary arteries and veins **(Figs. 13A to D)**. Most often location is subpleural, in the lower lobes (50–70% cases).
- They may be single or multiple; multiple often associated with Osler-Weber-Rendu syndrome/hereditary hemorrhagic telangiectasia.
- It may be classified as "simple" AVM—single feeding artery or "complex" AVM—multiple feeding vessels.
- Embolization is the mainstay for treatment, as it is less invasive than surgery and can be performed repeatedly in patients with multiple AVMs.[4]
- The important indications for embolization include prevention of neurological complications (stroke, cerebral abscess), avoiding hemoptysis and for improvement in exercise tolerance.
- Embolization may be done using coils, balloons, or vascular plugs.

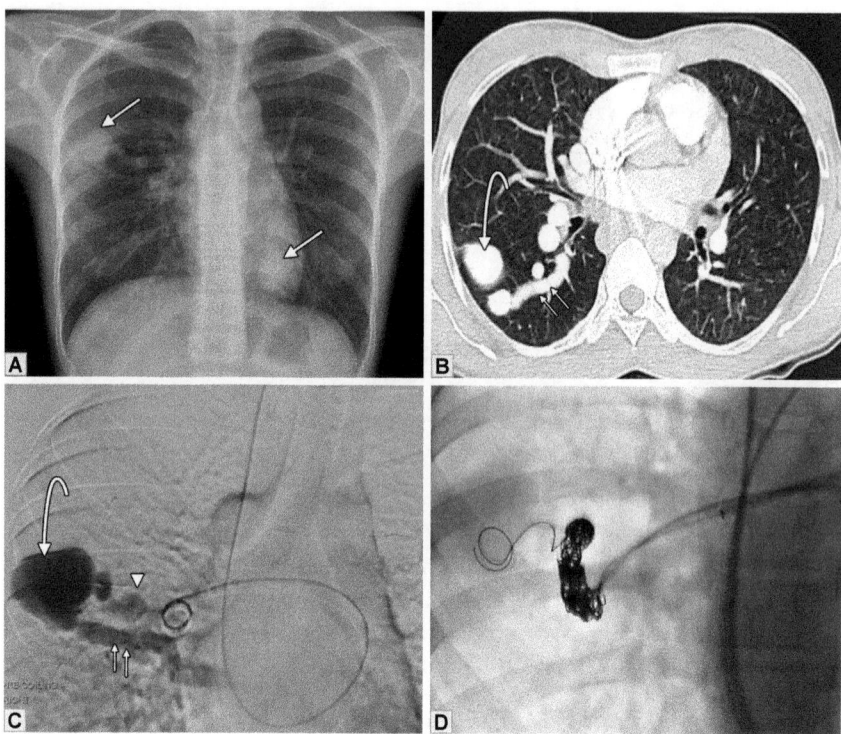

FIGS. 13A TO D: Pulmonary AVMs. CXR (A) shows multiple ovoid nodular opacities in right mid zone and left retrocardiac regions (arrows). Axial CT section (B) shows an aneurysmal dilatation (curved arrow) at the site of the AVM with dilated draining vein (double arrows). Selective angiogram of right lower lobe pulmonary artery (C) showing dilated supplying pulmonary arterial branch (arrowhead), aneurysmal dilatation at the site of the AVM (curved arrow) and dilated early draining vein (double arrows). This was subsequently coil embolized (D).

(AVM: arteriovenous malformation; CT: computed tomography; CXR: chest X-ray)

Combined Parenchymal and Vascular Anomalies

Pulmonary Sequestration

- The term "sequester" means to isolate or hide away. PS refers to non-functioning lung tissue that lacks a normal communication with the tracheobronchial tree, and derives its blood supply from systemic arteries.
- Two types of PS are described—(1) intralobar sequestration (ILS) (75-85% cases) and (2) extralobar sequestration (ELS) (15-25% cases). ILS refers to a sequestered portion of lung that shares the visceral pleural covering of normal lung. ELS has its own separate pleural envelope.
- Both ILS and ELS have systemic arterial supply, however, venous drainage of ILS is usually through pulmonary veins, whereas of ELS is through systemic veins. Mixed patterns may occur.

- Systemic arterial supply to sequestered lung is usually from lower thoracic or upper abdominal aorta, but may be from other systemic arteries including intercostal arteries and internal thoracic artery. Multiple supplying vessels may be present.
- ELS is most commonly located between the left lower lobe and diaphragm, or just below the left hemidiaphragm.
- 98% of ILS occur in the lower lobes of lung (left >> right) involving the posterior/medial basal segments.
- Both ILS and ELS may, rarely, show a communication with the foregut (esophagus/stomach).
- ELS does not show air within it unless it has associated communication with gastrointestinal (GI) tract.[3] Majority are associated with other congenital anomalies, including congenital diaphragmatic hernia. Diagnosis is often made in infancy.
- ILS usually presents in older children with recurrent infections **(Figs. 14A to E)**. It can show a variety of imaging appearances. The sequestered region may show fibrosis, consolidation, and cystic changes and may contain air. Surrounding lung may show overinflation.

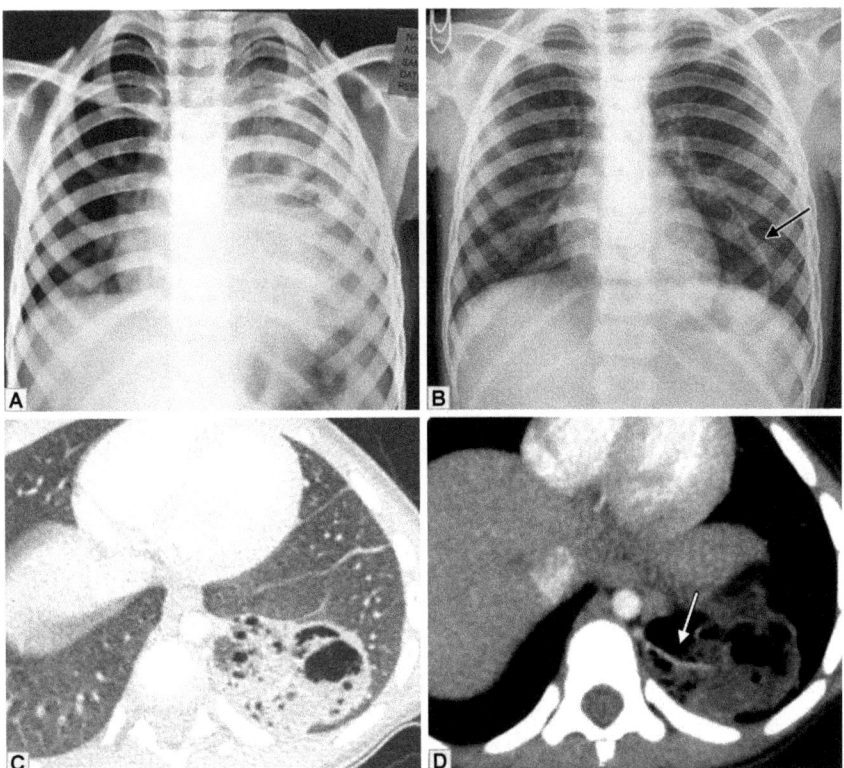

FIGS. 14A TO E: *Continued*

Continued

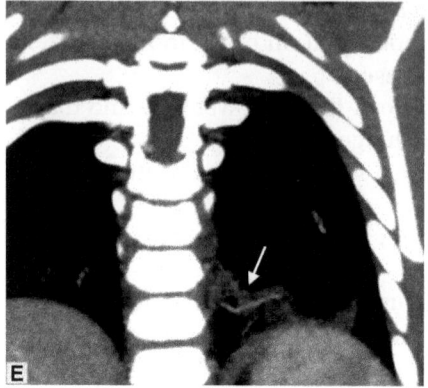

FIGS. 14A TO E: Intralobar sequestration in a 5-year-old male with recurrent chest infections. Chest X-ray (CXR) at presentation (A) shows extensive patchy consolidation in the left lower and mid zones. Follow-up CXR (B) reveals a persistent cystic lesion in the left lower zone (black arrow). (C to E) CT demonstrates the pulmonary sequestration showing intralesional cystic changes and systemic arterial supply (white arrows).

- In a child with recurrent lower lobe pneumonia, any persistent radiographic opacity should be suspected to be PS, and investigated further with contrast-enhanced CT (CECT) to look for the anomalous systemic artery which will help to clinch the diagnosis.
- Surgical resection, segmental resection or lobectomy, is usually required for ILS.[4] ELS may not need surgery, or may be surgically removed without removing normal lung—sequestrectomy. Endovascular (coil) embolization has also been tried in selected cases.
- The important differences between ILS and ELS are summarized in **Table 3**.

TABLE 3: Features of intralobar and extralobar sequestration.

	Intralobar sequestration	Extralobar sequestration
Pleural covering	Shares the visceral pleural covering of normal lung	Separate pleural covering
Tracheobronchial communication	No But, may contain air	No Usually does not contain air, unless it communicates with the GI tract
Arterial supply	Systemic	Systemic
Venous drainage	Pulmonary veins	Systemic veins
How often	75–85% of the cases	15–25% of the cases
Associated anomalies	Diagnosis is made later in life due to repeated infections in the same lobe	Majority are associated with other congenital anomalies, including congenital diaphragmatic hernia. Diagnosis is often made in infancy due to the associated anomalies
Treatment	Usually needs excision	May not always need surgery

Hybrid Lesions
- Pulmonary sequestration may occur in association with CPAM as a hybrid lesion, most often with type 2 CPAM. This may be suspected on imaging appearances, but can be confirmed only on surgery.
- Bronchial atresia is also frequently seen to exist along with PS and CPAM **(Figs. 15A to C)**.

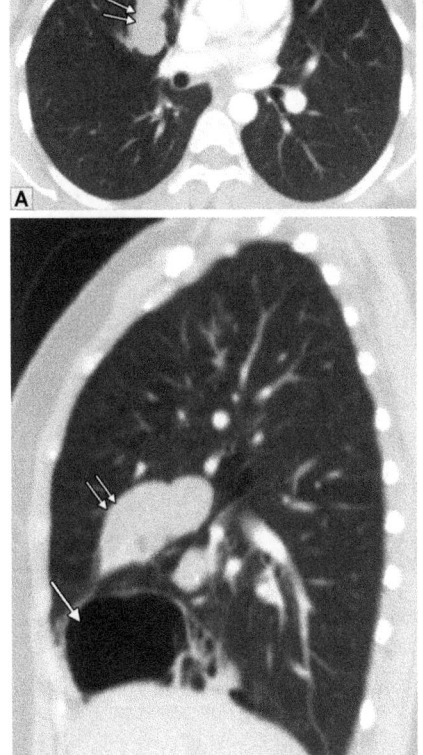
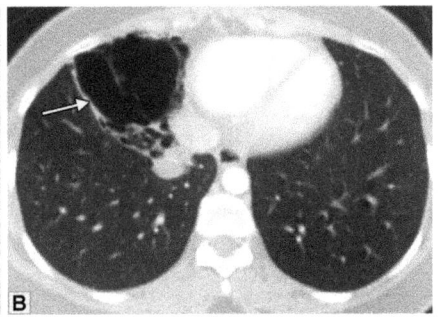

FIGS. 15A TO C: Hybrid lesion with coexisting bronchial atresia and CPAM in the right middle lobe in the same patient. Serial axial CT sections in lung window (A and B) and sagittal CT (C) showing thin-walled cystic lesion with smaller surrounding cysts in the right middle lobe (single arrows), suggestive of CPAM. There is also a bronchocele related to bronchial atresia (double arrows) just superior to the CPAM.
(CPAM: congenital pulmonary airway malformation; CT: computed tomography; CXR: chest X-ray)

Scimitar Syndrome/Hypogenetic Lung Syndrome
- This is a type of PAPVC affecting the right lung, associated with lung hypoplasia and other anomalies.
- The anomalous vein most often drains into the IVC **(Figs. 16A to D)**—this creates a curvilinear opacity on CXR which resembles a "scimitar" (or curved Turkish sword).
- Less commonly, the anomalous drainage may be into right atrium, superior vena cava, portal vein, or hepatic vein.

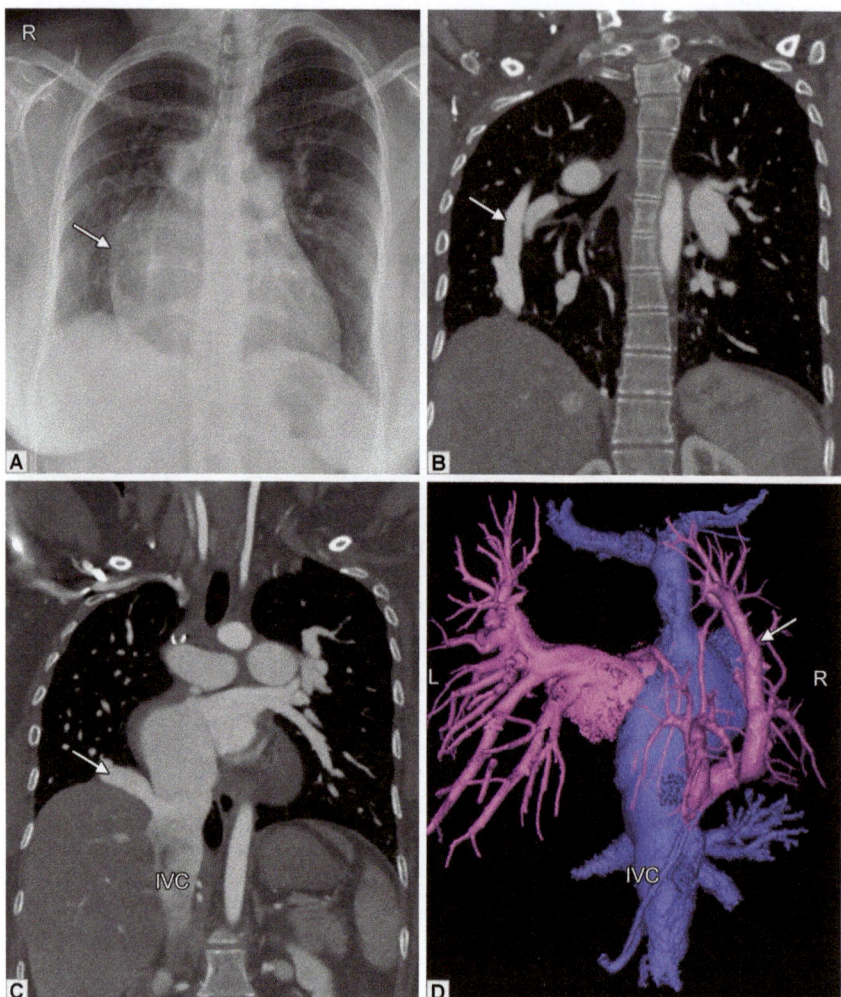

FIGS. 16A TO D: Scimitar syndrome. Chest X-ray (CXR) (A), serial coronal CT sections (B and C) and volume-rendered 3D image (D) as viewed from posterior aspect show smaller size of the right lung, anomalous sickle-shaped vein in the right lung (arrow) which drains into the IVC.

- Associations include hypoplasia of lung and pulmonary artery, systemic arterial supply to right lower lobe, horseshoe lung, diaphragmatic defects, cardiac dextroversion, and congenital heart disease (atrial septal defect, ventricular septal defect, patent ductus arteriosus, and tetralogy of Fallot).
- Symptoms depend on the degree of left to right shunting and vary in severity from no symptoms to heart failure in infancy. Prognosis is often determined by associated cardiac defects.

CHAPTER 6: Congenital Lung Abnormalities

Foregut Anomalies

Bronchogenic Cyst

- Bronchogenic cysts are a part of the spectrum of foregut duplication cysts (DCs) (along with neurenteric cysts and esophageal DCs).
- These cysts most often are mediastinal in location (65–90%). Intrapulmonary location is less common.
- Intrapulmonary BCs may be indistinguishable from type 1 CPAM on imaging. A purely fluid containing congenital lung cystic lesion is suggestive of BC. Once infected, air-fluid levels may be seen, like in CPAM.
- Mediastinal cysts most often occur in subcarinal or right paratracheal region. They may cause pressure effects on airway, resulting in lung overinflation or collapse **(Figs. 17A to D)**.
- CXR may demonstrate the lung or mediastinal cyst, or secondary lung changes.

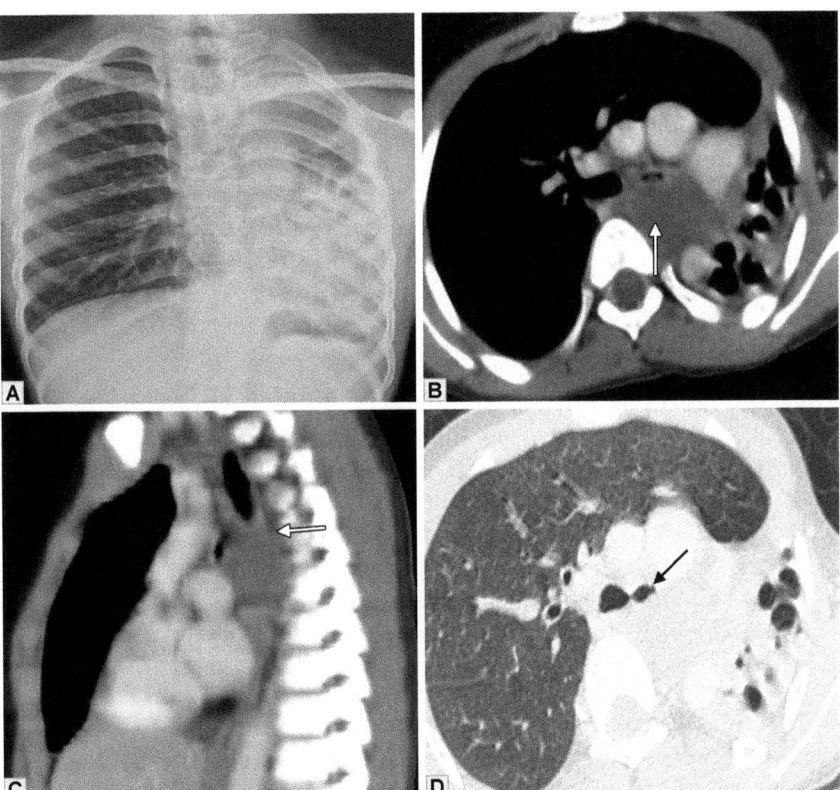

FIGS. 17A TO D: Subcarinal bronchogenic cyst causing left lung collapse in a 9-year-old female with recurrent chest infections. Chest X-ray (CXR) (A) shows volume loss in the left hemithorax, with cystic air lucencies in the left lung. CT axial (B and D) and sagittal (C) images reveal a subcarinal cyst (white arrow) causing severe narrowing of the left main bronchus (black arrow) and chronic left lung collapse.

- The lesion often appears hyperdense on noncontrast CT (NCCT), due to high protein content.
- CT findings may overlap with esophageal DC. Close association with esophagus, elongated, tubular configuration, or abdominal extension through esophageal hiatus may favor diagnosis of esophageal DC.
- Final diagnosis is confirmed on histopathology—BC shows respiratory epithelium lining the cyst (c.f. esophageal/gut mucosal lining in DC).

ROLE OF DIFFERENT IMAGING MODALITIES

Antenatal Diagnosis

- USG is the modality of choice for antenatal detection of CLAs, and provides information about the size and laterality of the lesion as well as presence of cysts within. Doppler imaging may detect systemic arterial supply in PS. Hypervascularity on Doppler is a feature of congenital overinflation detected in utero.
- USG is also useful to assess degree of mass effect, associated lung hypoplasia, features of hydrops fetalis, and any associated malformations.
- Fetal magnetic resonance imaging (MRI) may be employed for further characterization, and is useful in select cases.
- The antenatal behavior of CLAs is variable. Serial USG are useful in assessing any progression in size of lesion or associated complications which may need intervention. Sometimes, the lesion may regress in size after 28–30 weeks of gestation.[3] However, postnatal evaluation is recommended to evaluate the lesion and decide the course of management.

Postnatal Evaluation

Chest Radiography

- CXR is the initial imaging modality. Various radiographic imaging appearances may be seen in different CLAs,[1] as detailed in **Table 4**.
- Due to overlap of imaging appearances between different congenital as well as acquired conditions, it is imperative to correlate with the clinical history and also to compare findings on serial radiographs. It is especially important to review any chest radiographs taken soon after birth/in infancy, which will help in diagnosing the congenital nature of these lesions.

Ultrasonography

Ultrasonography has a limited role in postnatal evaluation. It may be helpful in evaluation of fluid-filled cystic lesions such as bronchogenic and DCs. It may also reveal the parenchymal abnormality, and Doppler imaging can be used to look for systemic arterial supply from the abdominal aorta (**Figs. 18A and B**).

CHAPTER 6: Congenital Lung Abnormalities

TABLE 4: Imaging appearances of CLAs on antenatal USG and CXR.

Imaging modality	Remarks	Imaging appearances of various CLAs	Other important D/Ds
USG/Doppler	In utero detection of CLA—modality of choice	Focal echogenic lung lesions ± mass effect, may have associated polyhydramnios: • CPAM—cysts + (except in microcystic form) • PS—systemic arterial supply + (may not always be detected) • CLH—no cysts, hypervascularity ± • CHAOS syndrome—bilateral enlarged, echogenic lungs	Congenital diaphragmatic hernia (CDH)
Chest radiograph	Initial imaging modality for postnatal evaluation	Focal hyperlucency ± mass effect: • CLH (rarely involve lower lobes) • CPAM • BA • PS (majority in lower lobes, left> >right)	• Loculated pneumothorax • Pneumatocele
		Air/fluid-filled cystic lesions: • CPAM (may be fluid-filled soon after birth, later on contain air) • Bronchogenic cyst (usually fluid filled, air-fluid-levels if infected)	• Hydatid cyst • Lung abscess • Loculated hydropneumothorax
		Thoracic asymmetry: • Pulmonary agenesis-aplasia-hypoplasia complex • Proximal interruption of pulmonary artery • Scimitar syndrome	• Lung collapse • Pneumothorax • Foreign body aspiration • Swyer–James syndrome
		Vascular abnormality: • Pulmonary AVM • Scimitar vein • Total anomalous pulmonary venous connection • Systemic arterial supply to PS	
		Airway abnormality: • Tracheal bronchus • Low-lying carina	

(AVM: arteriovenous malformation; BA: bronchial atresia; CLA: congenital lung anomaly; CLH: congenital lobar hyperinflation; CPAM: congenital pulmonary airway malformation; CXR: chest X-ray; PS: pulmonary sequestration; USG: ultrasonography)

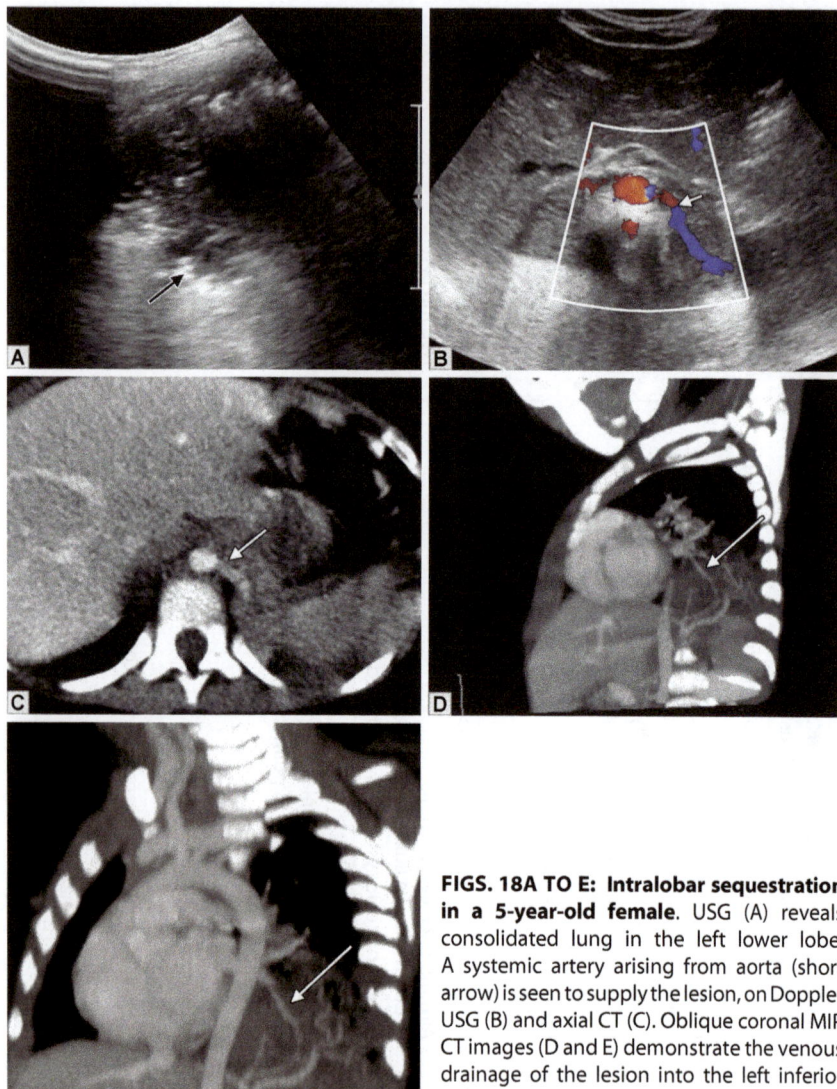

FIGS. 18A TO E: Intralobar sequestration in a 5-year-old female. USG (A) reveals consolidated lung in the left lower lobe. A systemic artery arising from aorta (short arrow) is seen to supply the lesion, on Doppler USG (B) and axial CT (C). Oblique coronal MIP CT images (D and E) demonstrate the venous drainage of the lesion into the left inferior pulmonary vein (long arrows).

(CT: computed tomography; MIP: maximum-intensity projection; USG: ultrasonography)

Role of Computed Tomography

- CT is the current imaging modality of choice for the detailed characterization of CLAs.
- To enable a comprehensive evaluation of any potential vascular component of the anomaly, a CECT should be done.
- The principles of ALARA (as low as reasonably achievable) and "image gently" should be followed in order to limit the radiation dose to the child. Multiphasic postcontrast imaging is not required, and should not be done.

- Multiplanar reconstructions (MPRs), MinIP, and volume-rendered images are helpful in evaluation of various components of the CLA—parenchyma/airway, arterial, and venous systems.[5]
- Thin sections in the mediastinal window are necessary to look for small caliber systemic arterial vessels. Maximum-intensity projections (MIP) in various planes are useful in depiction of vascular anomalies and anatomy **(Figs. 18C to E)**.
- CECT helps in providing a "vascular roadmap" as well as depiction of the parenchymal/airway involvement which is essential for surgical planning. It also depicts the degree of mass effect, and any complications including features of infection or pneumothorax.
- For evaluation of airway abnormalities, lung window and MinIP images are helpful.
- It is important to follow a systematic checklist and look for all components of the CLA, and also for any associated anomalies.

Role of MRI

- Currently, MRI lacks CT's ability to depict finer details of lung parenchyma. Longer scan times than CT also increases the need for sedation, especially in small children.
- However, MRI has the advantage of being a radiation-free modality. As experience with lung MRI is increasing, it is being used more and more for evaluation of CLAs.
- Dynamic contrast-enhanced MRI has been used to detect bronchopulmonary anomalies, which are seen as perfusion defects during the phase of peak pulmonary enhancement. Angiographic images can also be obtained.[6]
- MRI is especially useful in evaluation of mediastinal abnormality, large cystic lesions **(Figs. 19A to C)**, and vascular anomalies. It is also helpful in follow-up imaging of many CLAs.

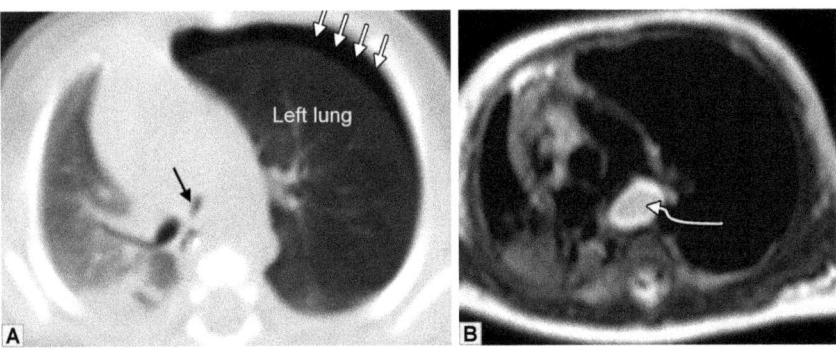

FIGS. 19A TO C: *Continued*

Continued

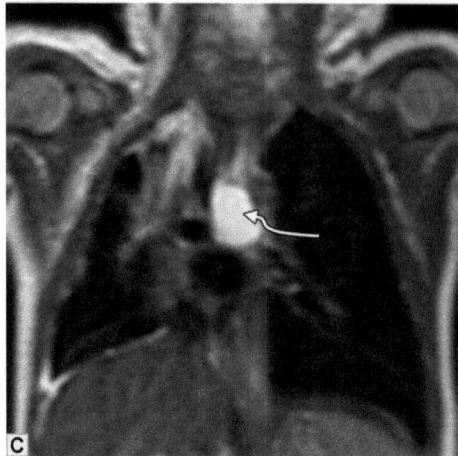

FIGS. 19A TO C: Bronchogenic cyst causing bronchial compression and hyperinflation of left lung. Axial CT section (A) showing narrowing of left main bronchus (black arrow), hyperinflation of left lung and small left pneumothorax (multiple small white arrows). T2-weighted axial (B) and coronal (C) MRI images show a cystic lesion (curved arrows) in subcarinal region, suggestive of a bronchogenic cyst which is causing the left main bronchial compression.

Role of Digital Subtraction Angiography

Angiography is usually done as a part of therapeutic endovascular embolization in pulmonary AVMs, isolated systemic supply to normal lung (ISSNL), and ELS.

■ CONCLUSION

Congenital lung anomalies exist as a spectrum, with varying degrees of involvement of the lung parenchyma, airway, pulmonary arteries, and veins. They may be detected incidentally, or present with neonatal RD, recurrent pneumonias in childhood, hemoptysis, cardiac failure, or other symptoms. Imaging features may show overlap, especially on antenatal USG and on chest radiography. CT, and in some instances MRI, helps in detailed evaluation and surgical planning. A systematic imaging approach and reporting checklist should be followed to document all the components of the anomaly and also to look for other associated congenital abnormalities.

Other Related Chapters that can be Referred to:
- Chapter 5: Neonatal Respiratory Distress
- Chapter 15: Central Airway Imaging
- Chapter 18: Pulmonary Artery Imaging
- Chapter 19: Pulmonary Veins Imaging

REFERENCES

1. Lee EY, Dorkin H, Vargas SO. Congenital pulmonary malformations in pediatric patients: review and update on etiology, classification and imaging findings. Radiol Clin North Am. 2011;49:921-48.
2. Annunziata F, Bush A, Borgia F, et al. Congenital lung malformations: Unresolved issues and unanswered questions. Front Pediatr. 2019;7:239.
3. Newman B. Congenital bronchopulmonary foregut malformations: concepts and controversies. Pediatr Radiol. 2006;36:773-91.
4. Liechty KW, Flake AW. Pulmonary vascular malformations. Semin Pediatr Surg. 2008;17(1):9-16.
5. Lee EY, Boiselle PM, Cleveland RH. Multidetector CT evaluation of congenital lung anomalies. Radiology. 2008;247(3):632-48.
6. Kellenberger CJ, Amaxopoulou C, Moehrlen U, Bode PK, Jung A, Geiger J. Structural and perfusion magnetic resonance imaging of congenital lung malformations. Pediatr Radiol. 2020;50(8):1083-94.

SECTION 3

Chest Infections

CHAPTER 7: Bacterial and Viral Chest Infections
CHAPTER 8: Fungal Chest Infections
CHAPTER 9: Chest Tuberculosis
CHAPTER 10: Chest Infections in Immunocompromised Host

CHAPTER 7

Bacterial and Viral Chest Infections

Anmol Bhatia, Harshith Gowda, Kushaljit Singh Sodhi, Akshay Kumar Saxena

- ❑ Epidemiology
- ❑ Role of imaging
- ❑ Viral pneumonia
  - ➢ Agents
  - ➢ Pathology
  - ➢ Imaging features
  - ➢ Complications
  - ➢ Conditions mimicking viral pneumonia
- ❑ Coronavirus disease 2019
  - ➢ Chest radiography in pediatric patients with suspected or known COVID-19: Imaging findings and recommendations
  - ➢ Chest CT in pediatric COVID-19 patients: Imaging findings and recommendations
- ❑ Bacterial pneumonia
  - ➢ Lobar pneumonia
  - ➢ Bronchopneumonia
  - ➢ Bacterial versus viral pneumonia
  - ➢ Complications
- ❑ Round pneumonia
  - ➢ Progressive pneumonia
  - ➢ Fulminant pneumonia
  - ➢ Chronic pneumonia
  - ➢ Recurrent pneumonia
  - ➢ Aspiration syndrome

■ INTRODUCTION

Chest infections are one of the frequent reasons for children to seek medical attention. Pediatric population requires special concern in terms of imaging as most of the times history is not always reliable and clinical evaluation is also challenging. Most often the first investigation will be a chest radiograph and only selected group of children requiring cross-sectional imaging for further evaluation.

■ EPIDEMIOLOGY

- *Neonates*: Bacterial > viral
- *Less than 2 years*: Viral > bacterial
- *More than 2 years*: Bacterial > viral. Infections such as mycoplasma pneumonia increase in incidence (~30%).

ROLE OF IMAGING

- *Radiographs*: Both frontal and lateral (better evaluation of hyperinflation) radiographs are used often to look for signs of infection.
- *Computed tomography (CT)*:
  - When radiographs are not suggestive of infection but there is high clinical suspicion
  - To look for complications
  - To look for sequalae of chronically ill patient
  - To guide histopathological sampling/drainage procedures.
- *Ultrasonography*: Predominantly used to look for associated effusions and follow-up. It is also used as guide for drainage/histopathological sampling procedures.

VIRAL PNEUMONIA

Agents
Respiratory syncytial viruses (most common) are parainfluenza, rhinovirus, and adenovirus.[1]

Pathology
Typically causes inflammation of mucosa of smaller airways resulting in blockage and thus air trapping. Therefore, hyperinflation is usually the most common feature in viral pneumonia.

Inflammation may spread to adjacent tissue—peribronchiolar inflammation.

Imaging Features
Radiographs
As explained above, features of hyperlucency are usually seen:
- *Frontal radiographs* (**Fig. 1**):
  - Level of diaphragm at the level below the 6th anterior (or 10th posterior) rib
  - Widening of intercostal spaces
  - Flattening of diaphragms
- *Lateral radiographs*:
  - Flattening of hemidiaphragms
  - Increased anteroposterior diameter
  - Increased retrosternal space

Additional features like multifocal wedge-shaped opacities due to segmental atelectasis. This is caused by airway edema and inspissated secretions blocking the smaller airways.

Peribronchiolar inflammation is seen in the form of peribronchial cuffing and increased perihilar shadow (**Fig. 2**).

CHAPTER 7: Bacterial and Viral Chest Infections

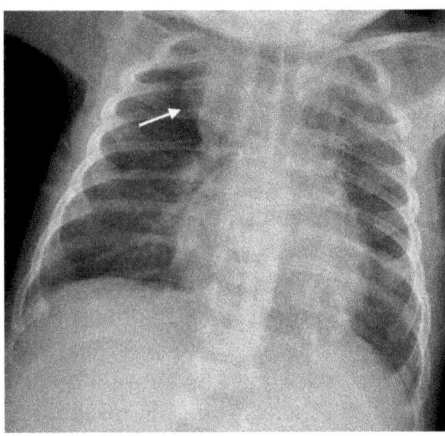

FIG. 1: Viral pneumonia. Chest radiograph in an infant shows hyperinflated lungs with widening of intercostal spaces and flattened hemidiaphragms. Collapse of right upper lobe also seen (arrow).

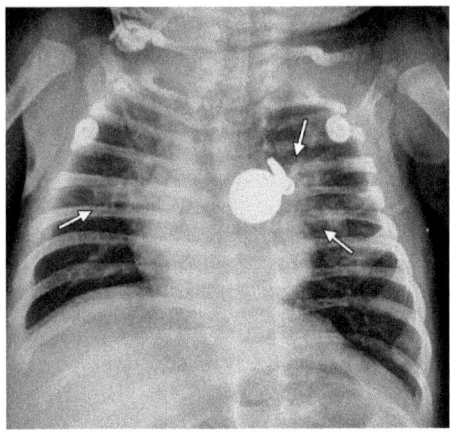

FIG. 2: Viral pneumonia. Chest radiograph in an infant shows hyperinflated lungs with widening of intercostal spaces, flattened hemidiaphragms, and increased perihilar shadows (arrows).

Cross-sectional Imaging/Computed Tomography

- Infections with similar pathogenesis have similar imaging patterns. However, typical imaging patterns are not always seen.
- Respiratory syncytial virus replicates in the nasopharyngeal epithelium and causes bronchiolitis when they reach lungs. Epithelial cells of distal airways are damaged and sloughed. Usually, the imaging reveals multifocal patchy consolidation along with ground-glass opacities (GGOs) and centrilobular nodules. Bronchial thickening may be seen in the form of doughnut/tram track lines radiating from the hilum. Similar

imaging features can be seen in human parainfluenza virus (HPIV) and human metapneumovirus (HMPV) as their pathogenesis is relatable.
- Influenza virus can produce consolidation on imaging. They can cause diffuse alveolar damage and necrotizing bronchitis, which is responsible for the imaging features.
- Adenovirus mostly causes bronchiolitis as they affect terminal bronchioles. necrotizing bronchopneumonia can sometimes be seen as an accompanying feature.
- Herpes simplex virus (HSV) produces both airspace opacities and peribronchial consolidation. This is explained by the fact that it affects both alveoli and airways. The GGOs seen on imaging correspond to the alveolar damage. Histopathological diagnosis is aided by the intranuclear inclusions which can be seen in lung tissue obtained through biopsy. Bronchoalveolar fluid can also reveal same finding on examination.
- Cytomegalovirus (CMV) shows AIP (acute interstitial pneumonia) pattern with diffuse alveolar edema. Multifocal nodular infiltration is seen corresponding to the infected areas. Interstitial fibrocytes, alveolar epithelial cells, and endothelial cells are likely the target of these viruses.
- Pleural effusion and enlarged lymph nodes are not typically seen.

Complications
- Bronchiolitis obliterans
- Swyer–James syndrome

Conditions Mimicking Viral Pneumonia
- Multifocal consolidation in bacterial pneumonia may mimic segmental atelectasis in viral pneumonia.
- Expiratory films can show pseudothickening of bronchioles.
- Pertussis (rare)

■ CORONAVIRUS DISEASE 2019

Coronavirus disease 2019 (COVID-19) is a viral infection caused by the severe acute respiratory syndrome (SARS) coronavirus 2. It belongs to the β-coronavirus cluster of enveloped single-stranded RNA viruses. It became known first in December 2019 as a series of unexplained cases of pneumonia.[2]

Chest Radiography in Pediatric Patients with Suspected or Known COVID-19: Imaging Findings and Recommendations
- *Imaging*: Chest radiographs are less sensitive than CT for detecting lung parenchymal abnormalities in pediatric COVID-19 patients. Findings may be in the form of peripheral and lower lung zone predominant patchy opacities **(Fig. 3)**.
- American College of Radiology (ACR) appropriateness criteria **(Table 1)**.

CHAPTER 7: Bacterial and Viral Chest Infections

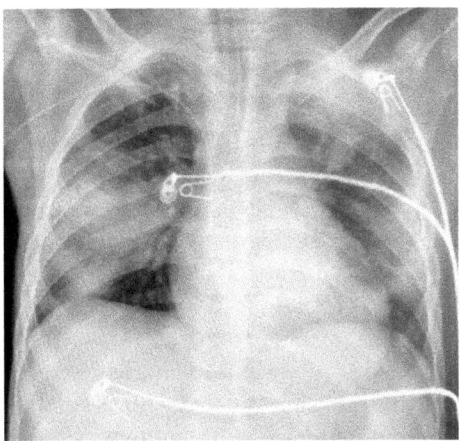

FIG. 3: COVID-19. Chest radiograph in a child showing peripheral patchy opacities in bilateral lungs.

TABLE 1: American College of Radiology (ACR) appropriateness criteria.

Chest radiography not indicated	Chest radiography indicated
Immunocompetent patients ≥ 3 months of age who do not require hospitalization and are clinically well enough	• Child requiring hospitalization • Not responding to outpatient management • Hospital-acquired pneumonia suspected

- Therefore, chest X-rays (CXRs) are not warranted in patients with mild symptoms just as in the case of other viral pulmonary infections. However, in the case of moderate-to-severe acute respiratory symptoms, CXR should be considered.
- *Drawbacks*:
  ○ Limited sensitivity and specificity
  ○ Negative chest radiograph does not exclude pulmonary involvement in patients with laboratory-confirmed COVID-19.
  ○ It does not indicate the absence of COVID-19 infection in cases of suspected COVID-19 infection not yet confirmed by using reverse transcription-polymerase chain reaction (RT-PCR) testing.
- Serial chest radiography may be beneficial in patients with known COVID-19 who showed positive findings on initial radiographs to assess response to treatment or to monitor disease progression.

Chest CT in Pediatric COVID-19 Patients: Imaging Findings and Recommendations

Imaging

- The most common imaging presentation is in the form of multifocal peripheral and/or subpleural GGOs seen bilaterally. They are distributed predominantly in posterior and/or lower lobe. Consolidation may or may not be seen. However, these are usually seen and described in adult population.
- Around half of the cases show focal consolidation with a rim of GGO termed a "halo sign" which aid in diagnosis.
- There are three phases of evolution in pediatric COVID-19 patients showing "halo" sign. Halo sign is usually observed in early phase. These progress to GGOs in progressive phase and further into consolidations in developed phase.
- Peribronchial thickening and inflammation along the bronchovascular bundle are seen in children in increased frequency compared to adults. Fine mesh reticulations and "crazy paving" sign may also be seen; however, these are less commonly reported. As mentioned earlier, pleural effusion and lymphadenopathy are rare.
- RT-PCR test is considered to be the standard of reference for the diagnosis of COVID-19 pneumonia as it has been shown to have comparable (high COVID-19 prevalence areas) to superior sensitivity (low COVID-19 prevalence areas) and overall better specificity compared with chest CT.
- *ACR recommendation*: Chest CT should not be used as first-line screening test in diagnosing COVID-19. It can be used for hospitalized symptomatic patients with certain indications such as excluding pulmonary embolism.

BACTERIAL PNEUMONIA

It can manifest as lobar/airspace pneumonia or bronchopneumonia. Pathology and etiological agents[3,4] are as follows:

Lobar Pneumonia

It is usually considered to be associated with specific bacterial infections such as *Haemophilus influenzae* type b (Hib), *Streptococcus pneumoniae*, and *Klebsiella pneumonia*.

Pathology

Features on CXRs are a nonsegmental, homogenous consolidation predominantly involving one lobe with air bronchograms (large bronchi remain patent and air-filled in contrast to the adjacent nonaerated lung) **(Fig. 4)**. Multilobar pneumonia can occur with several different bacteria and is associated with more severe disease.

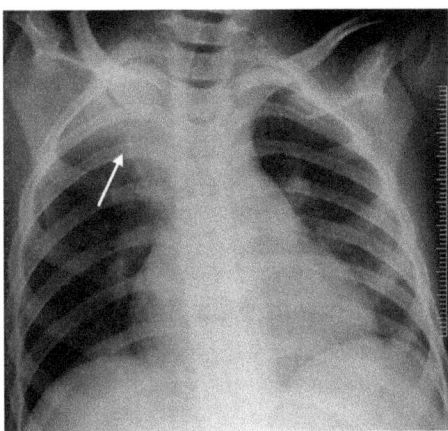

FIG. 4: Lobar pneumonia. Chest radiograph in a 4-year-old boy showing consolidation in the right upper lobe with air bronchograms (arrow).

Bronchopneumonia

It is thought to be usually associated with infections due to gram-negative bacteria, *Staphylococcus aureus,* and some fungi.

Pathology

The radiological appearance of bronchopneumonia varies depending on the severity of disease. Mild disease can manifest as peribronchial thickening and poorly defined air-space opacities **(Fig. 5)**; inhomogeneous patchy

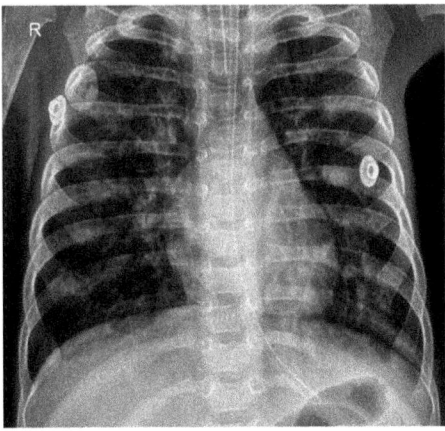

FIG. 5: Bronchopneumonia. Chest radiograph in an infant showing poorly defined air-space opacities in bilateral lungs.

areas of consolidation involving several lobes reflect more severe disease. When confluent, bronchopneumonia may resemble lobar pneumonia.

Pandey et al. showed that the anatomical site of the left both upper and lower with respect to the bacterial cause shows statistical insignificant association, while in the right lung it shows statistically significant association with the bacterial cause.[4] The consolidation on CXR showed statistically significant association with right upper lobe in *S. pneumoniae* cases, while *S. aureus* showed statistically significant with right lower lobe.

Bacterial versus Viral Pneumonia

- It is seen that most children with an alveolar pneumonia, especially those with lobar infiltrates, have laboratory evidence of a bacterial infection. However, up to half of the children with interstitial infiltrates as the sole radiographic finding can have bacterial infection. So, it may be prudent to say that interstitial infiltrates are not a reliable indication of solely viral pneumonia. Conversely, most viral pneumonias show interstitial infiltrates.
- White blood count (WBC), erythrocyte sedimentation rate (ESR), and C-reactive protein (CRP)—all of which may be available to a clinician when deciding on treatment are not so beneficial in deciding upon the differential diagnosis. A serum CRP concentration of >80 mg/L was found to be the most practical laboratory test for bacterial pneumonia.[5]

Complications

Children with pneumonia can present with severe illness characterized by combinations of local complications (e.g., parapneumonic effusion, empyema, necrotizing pneumonia, and lung abscess) and systemic complications (e.g., bacteremia, metastatic infection, multiorgan failure, acute respiratory distress syndrome, disseminated intravascular coagulation, and, rarely, death).[6]

- *Pleural complications*:
  - Pleural complications are more frequently encountered in bacterial pneumonia than viral pneumonia. Initially, there is pleuritis adjacent to the involved subpleural lung which progresses to fluid accumulation (parapneumonic effusion) mostly due to increased permeability of visceral pleura and influx of inflammatory cells. This may progress to fibrinous septations and later pus formation.
  - Chest radiographs are usually the initial imaging available and may reveal blunting of costophrenic angle. In severe cases, there may be complete white out of involved side with contralateral mediastinal shift. Moderate effusion may be seen as meniscus tracking along the lateral chest wall **(Fig. 6)**.
  - Mild-to-moderate cases of effusion may be missed on supine films and can only be inferred from the diffuse haziness of affected side compared to normal side.

- Ultrasonography enables efficient detection, localization and follow-up of effusions. It is the most commonly used imaging modality in guided aspirations. Ultrasound can also depict reduced lung movement adjacent to the thickened pleura suggestive of entrapment (fibrinous pleural septations).
- CT and magnetic resonance imaging are used in specific conditions such as unsuccessful drainage, associated lung parenchymal, and mediastinal changes, and assess tube placement accurately. Pleural thickening and enhancement with lenticular collection can be seen in cases of empyema and "split pleura" sign is accepted as a reliable sign of empyema **(Figs. 7A and B)**.

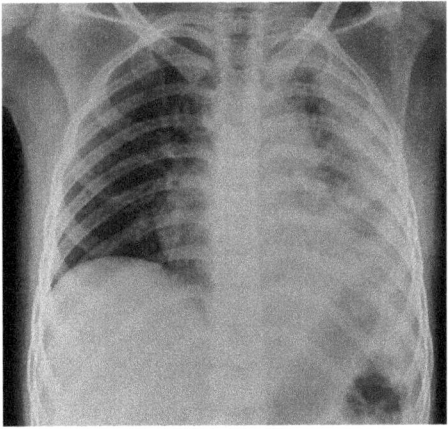

FIG. 6: Empyema. Chest radiograph in a 6-year-old boy showing soft tissue opacity along the left lateral chest wall with blunting of left costophrenic angle.

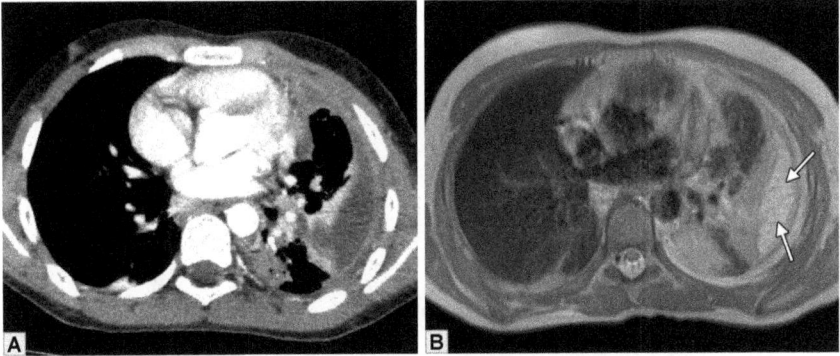

FIGS. 7A AND B: Empyema. Axial contrast-enhanced computed tomography image (A) and T2 turbo spin echo magnetic resonance image (B) in a 6-year-old boy showing loculated collection along the lateral aspect of the pleural cavity with multiple internal septae (arrows in B). Areas of consolidation are seen in left lung.

- *Lung parenchymal complications*:
  - Cavitating necrosis is most seen in pediatric population. It is in the form of cystic areas within necrotic area. This is seen as an ill-defined area with loss of normal lung architecture and decreased enhancement on CT. However, on radiographs, it is difficult to differentiate between infected congenital pulmonary airway malformation (CPAM) and cavitating necrosis. Comparison/serial radiographs might be of benefit in this regard. Moreover, cavitary necrosis can be seen well on radiographs if there is air entry via bronchial communication.
  - Some cases of cavitating necrosis may progress to form a lung abscess which is usually the case in immunodeficient individuals. They are generally round shaped. It is seen as thick-walled cavity with irregular luminal surface **(Fig. 8)**. Air fluid or fluid may be seen within, and surrounding consolidation may be seen.
  - Pulmonary gangrene is the most severe from with complete necrosis and thrombosis of vessels. Entire lobe may be involved with bulging fissures. It often requires surgical intervention.
  - Pneumatoceles are considered milder form of or resolving necrosis. They are thin-walled cysts with surrounding lung parenchyma **(Fig. 9)**. As the name suggests, they typically contain air and resolve with time spontaneously. However, when they occur in area of inflammation, fluid seepage may occur to produce air fluid levels; such lesions may take more time or may require drainage.
  - *Bronchopleural fistula*: This abnormal communication can be central or peripheral **(Fig. 10)**. Formation of bronchopleural fistula leads to air loculation in pleural space, pleural contents expelled in the form of sputum.
- Pericardial effusion is rarely seen.

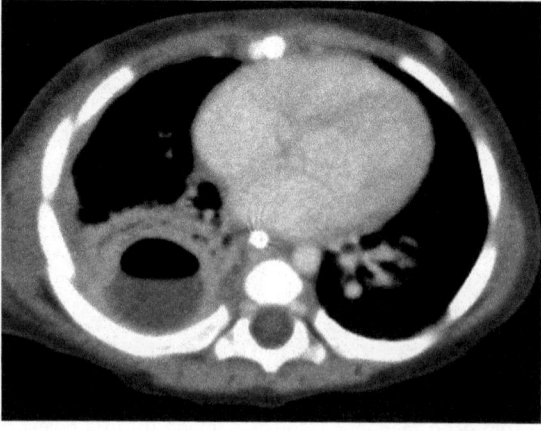

FIG. 8: Lung abscess. Axial contrast-enhanced computed tomography image in a 6-year-old girl showing an area of consolidation in right lower lobe with breakdown, air-fluid level, and thick peripheral enhancing walls.

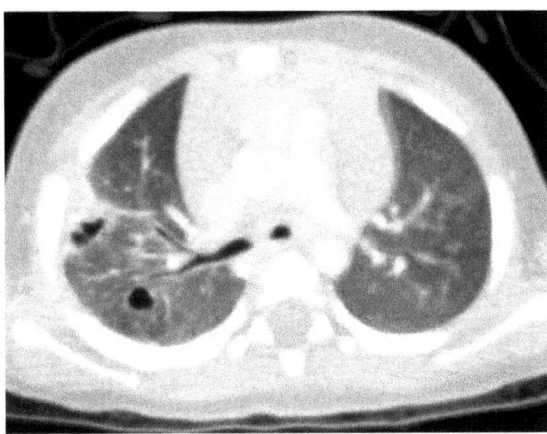

FIG. 9: Pneumatoceles. Axial contrast-enhanced computed tomography image in an 11-month-old boy following pneumonia showing small thin-walled air-filled lesions in the right lower lobe.

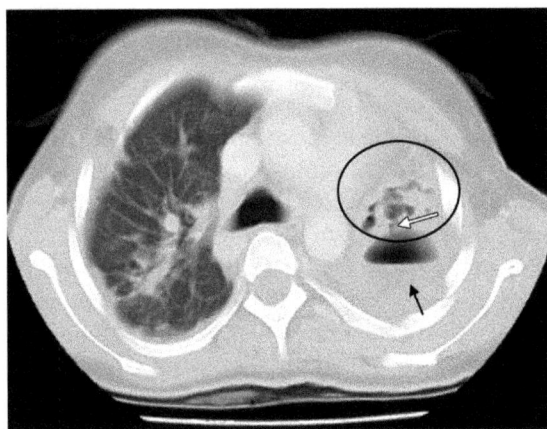

FIG. 10: Bronchopleural fistula. Axial contrast-enhanced computed tomography image in a 13-year-old girl showing destroyed left lung (circle) with irregularly dilated bronchi. One of the bronchus (white arrow) is communicating with the collection in the plural cavity (black arrow).

ROUND PNEUMONIA

Round pneumonia is a special entity generally accepted to be seen mostly in pediatric population up to the age of 8 years. It is usually seen in the age group of 3–5 years. As the name suggests, it appears as a spherical or rounded lesion on imaging.[7]

- *Clinical presentation*: Mild respiratory infectious prodrome followed by an acute febrile illness.

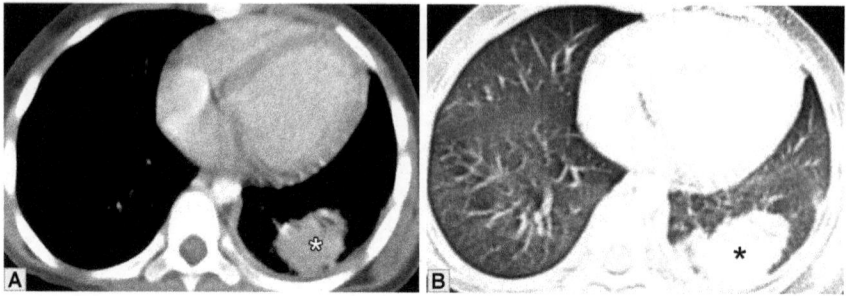

FIGS. 11A AND B: Round pneumonia (asterisk). (A) Mass like appearance; (B) lack of air bronchogram.

- *Pathology*:
  - In children, pathways of collateral ventilation namely pore of Kohn and channels of lambert are poorly developed.
  - Also, connective tissue septa are more closely apposed, and alveoli are smaller than adolescents and adults.
  - These factors are thought to have a role to play in producing a compact confluent area of pulmonary consolidation.
- *Imaging*:
  - It is mostly solitary.
  - More commonly seen in posterior and lower lobes. This is likely explained by the typical supine position and the effect of gravity on the bacteria laden fluid which passes to the most dependent bronchus and then to the periphery of the lung.
  - The size can range from 1–12 cm with a mean size of around 4 cm.
  - Two-thirds of cases show sharp margins while in adults' majority of these lesions show ill-defined lesions **(Figs. 11A and B)**.
  - Air bronchograms can often be seen within these lesions in children whereas they are rare in adults.
  - 95% of the lesions tend to undergo resolution while only small percentage of cases progress toward lobar pneumonia.
- *Differentials*: Bronchogenic cysts, loculated effusion, neuroblastoma, CPAM, etc.

Progressive Pneumonia

When the patient does not recover despite antibiotic therapy and instead worsens, it is called progressive pneumonia.

Fulminant Pneumonia

Progressive pneumonia where the conditions worsen over a short span of 24–48 hours is called fulminant pneumonia.

It is prudent to look for alternate causes and mimics of pneumonia in such situations.

Chronic Pneumonia

Pneumonia that does not resolve over a period of 1 month can be called chronic pneumonia/nonrevolving pneumonia.

Recurrent Pneumonia

Children with deficiencies in the local pulmonary or systemic host defenses or from underlying lung disorders that modify the lung defenses can have repeated episodes of pneumonia. It is usually defined as more than one episode of pneumonia in 12 months or more than three episodes in a lifetime.

The conditions leading to recurrent pneumonia can be broadly classified as following:
- Congenital malformations of upper or lower respiratory tract and cardiovascular system
- Recurrent aspirations
- Defects in clearance of airway secretions especially cystic fibrosis and ciliary abnormalities **(Figs. 12A to E)**
- Systemic and local immunity disorders
- Recurrent pneumonia limited to a specific lobe or segment can be caused by localized bronchial stricture or a congenital malformation **(Figs. 13A to D)**.

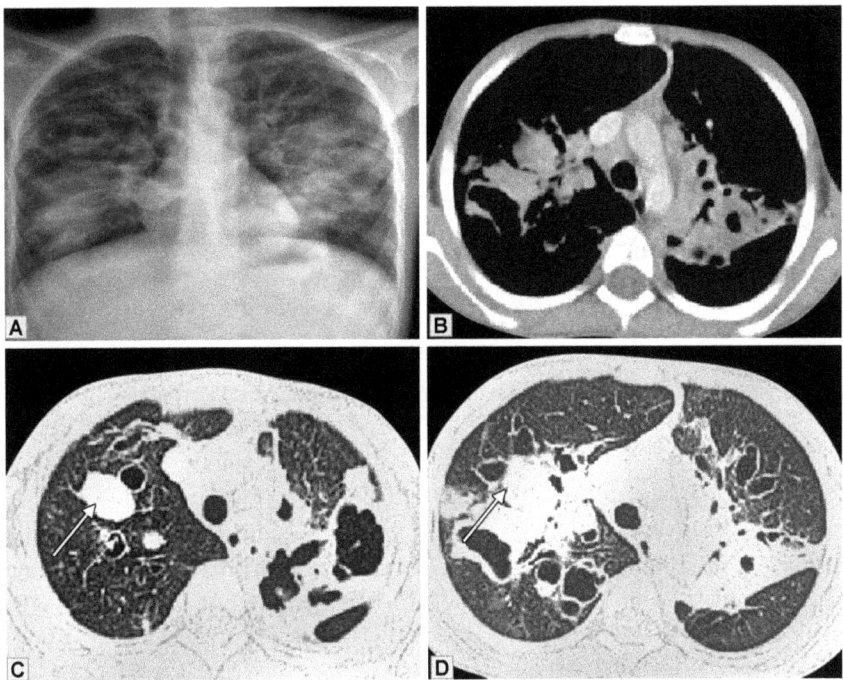

FIGS. 12A TO E: *Continued*

Continued

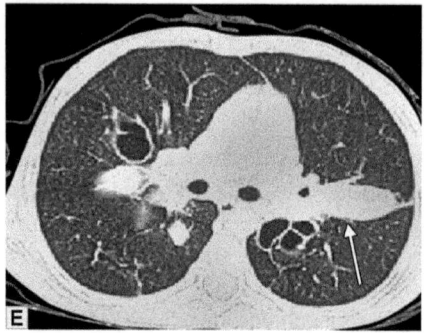

FIGS. 12A TO E: Nonresolving pneumonia in cystic fibrosis. (A) Bilateral hyperinflated lung fields, cystic bronchiectasis, elongated soft tissue shadows (bronchocele) in right lower lung zone, and consolidation in left middle lung zone. (B to E) Left lung upper lobe consolidation, bilateral central bronchiectasis, bronchocele (arrow).

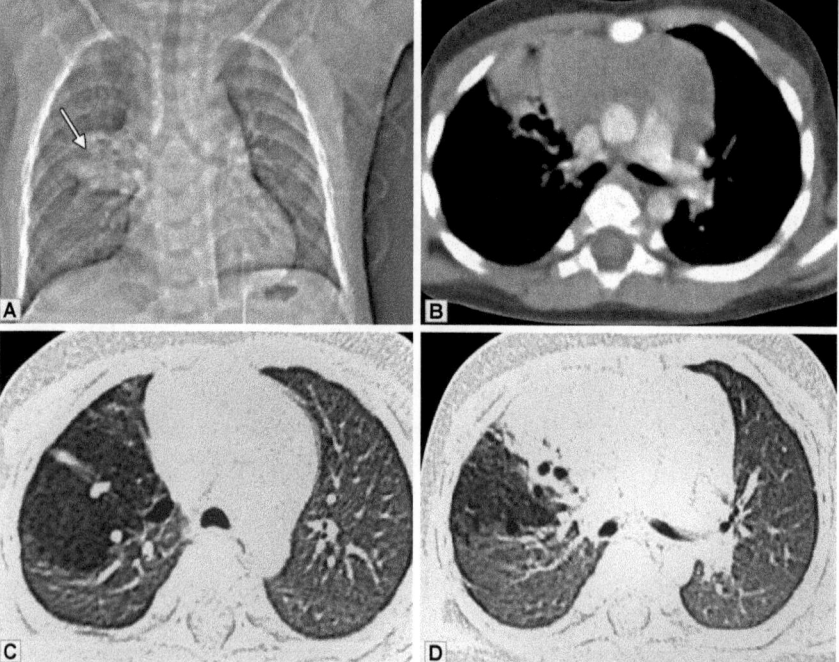

FIGS. 13A TO D: Nonresolving pneumonia due to segmental bronchial narrowing. (A) Right mid zone consolidation (arrow); (B) right upper lobe consolidation; (C and D) right upper lobe hyperlucency suggesting obstructive hyperinflation.

The predisposing condition can be identified in majority of cases and half of such cases were found to be due to aspiration syndrome. Immune disorders (including HIV infection), congenital heart disease, and asthma were the other common causes.[8,9]

Aspiration Syndrome

- In the pediatric group, aspiration occurs most frequently because of deglutition abnormality, congenital malformations, and gastroesophageal reflux.

- Any stasis resulting from narrowing of the esophageal lumen may lead to aspiration.[10]
- Usually, this does not occur in cases of acquired achalasia and stenosis, because children frequently adapt themselves to such conditions.
- Esophageal atresia usually is detected and surgically corrected before causing significant aspiration.
- Amongst those cases of compression by anomalous vessels, compression by double aortic arch is the one that most frequently causes symptoms.
- The diagnosis of H-type tracheoesophageal fistula may be late, as contrast-enhanced images cannot always easily demonstrate it.
- Chest radiography, sometimes supplemented by CT and esophageal gastroduodenal seriography (EGDS) are almost always enough to make the diagnosis in cases of aspiration syndrome.
- *Imaging*: Most frequent involvement of the posterior segments of the upper lobes and the upper segments of the lower lobes. This happens as aspiration occurs with the child in dorsal decubitus, like in most gastroesophageal reflux and vomiting episodes. In other situations, such as tracheoesophageal fistula and lack of motor coordination, other pulmonary segments may be affected **(Figs. 14A and B)**.
- Aspiration may result in atelectasis or pneumonia, the latter with or without atelectatic component. The absence of fever suggests pure atelectasis.
- *Lipoid pneumonia*: It is more rarely observed and is always iatrogenic. Lipoid pneumonia is not related to anatomical or functional anomalies. Aspiration occurs because of the use of mineral oil in the treatment of intestinal constipation or as an adjuvant in cases of intestinal subocclusion caused by *Ascaris lumbricoides*. The oil inhibits the cough reflex and ciliary motion, and silently reaches the alveoli. Because of the difficulty in removing the oil from the lungs, such pneumonias present a slow evolution pattern.

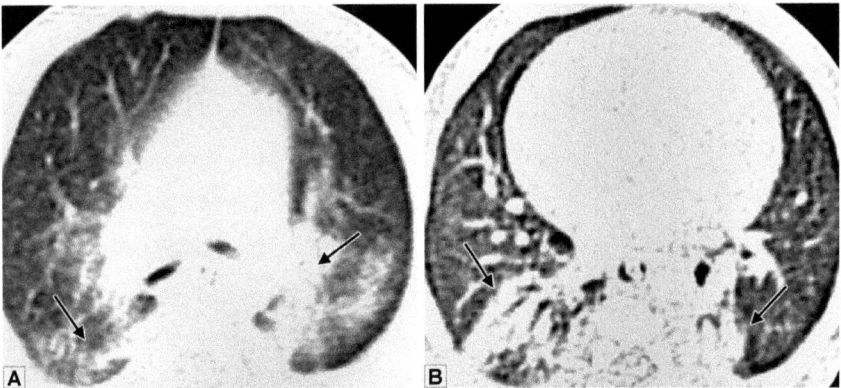

FIGS. 14A AND B: Recurrent pneumonia in a child with Down's syndrome with gastroesophageal reflux. Consolidation in bilateral lung dependent locations (arrows).

SECTION 3: Chest Infections

> **Other Related Chapters that can be Referred to:**
> ❏ Chapter 1: Chest Radiograph: Basics and Role
> ❏ Chapter 16: Bronchiectasis

■ REFERENCES

1. Koo HJ, Lim S, Choe J, Choi SH, Sung H, Do KH. Radiographic and CT features of viral pneumonia. Radiographics. 2018;38(3):719-39.
2. Foust AM, Phillips GS, Chu WC, Daltro P, Das KM, Garcia-Peña P, et al. International Expert Consensus Statement on Chest Imaging in Pediatric COVID-19 Patient Management: Imaging Findings, Imaging Study Reporting, and Imaging Study Recommendations. Radiol Cardiothorac Imaging. 2020;2(2):e200214.
3. O'Grady KAF, Torzillo PJ, Frawley K, Chang AB. The radiological diagnosis of pneumonia in children. Pneumonia. 2014;5(Suppl 1):38-51.
4. Pandey N, Mittal G, Agarwal N, Kakati B, Agarwal RK. Relationship between radiological findings with bacterial etiology of community acquired pneumonia in pediatric population. J Pure Appl Microbiol. 2021;15(4):2136-41.
5. Virkki R, Juven T, Rikalainen H, Svedström E, Mertsola J, Ruuskanen O. Differentiation of bacterial and viral pneumonia in children. Thorax. 2002;57(5):438-41.
6. de Benedictis FM, Kerem E, Chang AB, Colin AA, Zar HJ, Bush A. Complicated pneumonia in children. Lancet. 2020;396(10253):786-98.
7. Kim YW, Donnelly LF. Round pneumonia: Imaging findings in a large series of children. Pediatr Radiol. 2007;37(12):1235-40.
8. Lodha R, Puranik M, Natchu UC, Kabra SK. Recurrent pneumonia in children: clinical profile and underlying causes. Acta Paediatr. 2002;91(11):1170-3.
9. Owayed AF, Campbell DM, Wang EEL. Underlying causes of recurrent pneumonia in children. Arch Pediatr Adolesc Med. 2000;154:190-4.
10. de Oliveira GA, Pessanha LB, Guerra LF, Martins DL, Rondina RG, Silva JR. Aspiration pneumonia in children: an iconographic essay. Radiol Bras. 2015;48(6):391-5.

CHAPTER 8

Fungal Chest Infections

Ashu Seith Bhalla, Kana Ram Jat

- ❏ Classification of fungi
- ❏ Clinical features
- ❏ Aspergillosis
  - ➢ Invasive pulmonary aspergillosis
  - ➢ Chronic pulmonary aspergillosis
  - ➢ Allergic bronchopulmonary aspergillosis
- ❏ Other fungal infections
  - ➢ Mucormycosis
  - ➢ Pneumocystis pneumonia
  - ➢ Less common fungal infections

INTRODUCTION

- Fungal infections of the lung are being encountered increasingly due to the rising population of susceptible including children, especially the immunocompromised and transplant patients. However, these infections can occur in immunocompetent persons as well.
- The spectrum of immunocompromised hosts consists of those with overt immunodeficiency such as primary immunodeficiency diseases (PIDDs), human immunodeficiency virus (HIV), post bone marrow/organ transplantation, patients on chemotherapy, or receiving immunosuppressive drugs such as corticosteroids, uncontrolled diabetes mellitus (DM), cystic fibrosis, and postinfectious cavities.
- Fungi are ubiquitous organisms and lung involvement by these can be isolated or as a part of disseminated/systemic disease. Imaging findings of fungal infections can be variable according to host immune response and the implicated organism.

CLASSIFICATION OF FUNGI

- Fungi affecting respiratory tract may be classified as:
  - *Opportunist fungi*: These are ubiquitous organisms causing clinically significant disease only in a vulnerable host—*Aspergillus* species, *Mucorales* species (*Rhizopus, Mucor,* and *Rhizomucor*), *Candida, Fusarium, Cryptococcus,* and *Scedosporiosis*.
  - *Endemic fungi*: Found in only particular geographical region of the world—blastomycosis, histoplasmosis, and coccidioidomycosis.
- According to host immune status, there are different spectra of fungi which can cause pulmonary involvement. Also, some fungi are seen in both settings, i.e., in nonendemic regions these will be seen in immunocompromised individual mainly.

CLINICAL FEATURES

- Clinical presentation is nonspecific with fever, cough, chest pain, and hemoptysis.
- *When to clinically suspect pulmonary fungal infection:*
  - A patient with persistent pulmonary infiltrates and fever, not responding to typical antibacterial drugs, in susceptible population
  - A patient has some form of immune suppression
  - Associated skin, genitourinary, CNS, or bone involvement
  - Recent travel or exposure to endemic geographic regions

ASPERGILLOSIS

- Aspergillosis is the most common opportunistic fungal infection causing pulmonary infection.
- Pathogenic species include *A. fumigates, A. flavus, A. niger, A. terreus,* and *A. ustus*. These species are ubiquitous and only lead to disease in hosts who have immune functional defects or excessive immune response or have some structural lung disease which allows maturation of spores into tissue-invasive hyphae.
- The clinical presentation and imaging findings are not specific but are shared with other fungal infections.
- Various forms of *Aspergillus*-related lung disease include:
  - *Invasive pulmonary aspergillosis (IPA) (acute)*:
    - Angioinvasive
    - Airway invasive
  - *Chronic pulmonary aspergillosis (CPA)*:
    - Simple aspergilloma (SA)
    - Chronic cavitary pulmonary aspergillosis (CCPA)/chronic fibrosing pulmonary aspergillosis (CFPA)
    - Subacute invasive aspergillosis (SAIA)
    - *Aspergillus* nodule (AN)
  - Allergic bronchopulmonary aspergillosis (ABPA)

Invasive Pulmonary Aspergillosis
- *Aspergillus* is the most common invasive fungal infection in patients after hematopoietic stem cell transplantation (HSCT). It is more frequent in allogenic compared to autologous HSCT with highest incidence in mismatched-related donors.
- Aspergillus is also the most common cause of fungal lung infection in patients after solid organ transplant (SOT).
- IPA leads to damage of lung parenchyma and causes necrosis. IPA has been subdivided into angioinvasive and airway invasive aspergillosis forms.[1]
- The angioinvasive form predominantly involves the pulmonary artery branches, whereas the airway invasive form predominantly involves the bronchi and bronchioles.
- However, the two forms may coexist in the same patient, making it difficult to distinguish between the two types.

Angioinvasive Aspergillosis
- This is the most common form of IPA.
- Histologically, this form shows infiltration of lung tissue by fungus, with invasion of small arteries, vascular occlusion, and, often, infarction of involved lung.
- Serum galactomannan is positive in up to 80% patients with this form.[1]
- *Imaging*: High-resolution computed tomography (HRCT) chest should be performed early in the course of suspected IPA as most of the patients are not able to undergo tissue sampling for diagnosis.
- *If significant hemoptysis is present*:
  - Perform CT pulmonary angiography
  - Magnetic resonance imaging (MRI) may be done if CT is not feasible or for follow-up.
- *Chest radiographs*: The spectrum of findings include multiple, ill-defined 1–3 cm peripheral nodules, which coalesce over time.
  - Lobar or diffuse pulmonary consolidation is common, but less specific.
  - *"Air-crescent" sign*: It occurs because of cavitation in a nodule or mass (40%) **(Figs. 1A and B)**; usually indicates a good prognosis. It develops after several days after resolution of neutropenia. It is highly suggestive of IPA, however, has little impact on management.

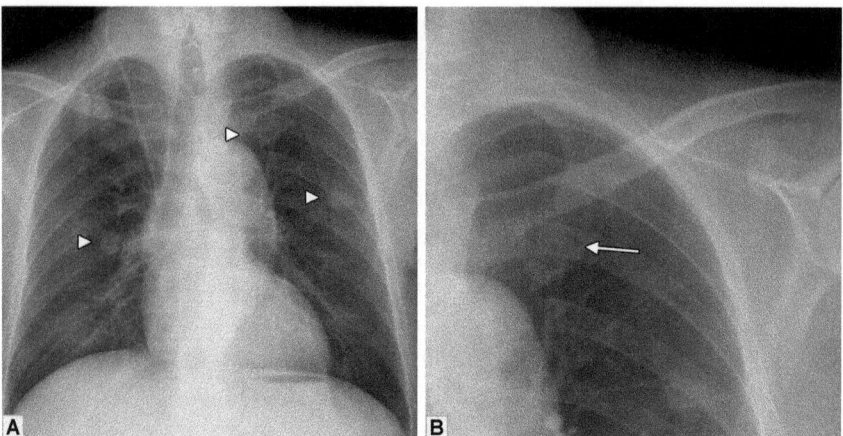

FIGS. 1A AND B: Chest radiographic signs of invasive pulmonary aspergillosis (IPA)— (A) multiple nodules (arrowheads) and (B) nodule with air crescent sign (arrow).

CT findings—multiple nodules which demonstrate:
- *CT halo sign*: Peripheral rim of ground-glass opacity (GGO) surrounding a focal dense parenchymal nodule **(Figs. 2A to F)**. It is nonspecific and has also been described in mucormycosis and granulomatous polyangiitis (GPA). However, in an appropriate clinical setting, it is highly suggestive of angioinvasive aspergillosis. It represents the central fungal nodule and surrounding area of coagulation necrosis or central infarct and surrounding hemorrhage.[2,3] It is seen in early stages of IPA. To be useful for IPA diagnosis, the CT scan must be performed early in the course of the disease. Most (75%) of the initial CT halo signs disappear within a week after IPA diagnosis.
- *Hypodense sign or internal low attenuation*:[1] Reported to be highly specific **(Figs. 2A to F)**, appears later than halo sign.
- *Reverse halo sign*: A central GGO surrounded by consolidation
- *"Air crescent sign"*: As the neutropenia improves, involves decrease in the ground-glass halo surrounding the nodule, followed by central hypodensity and subsequent cavitation giving the "air crescent sign".
- Pleural-based wedge-shaped areas of consolidation or alveolar consolidations **(Figs. 2A to F)**
- Masses (especially in SOT recipients)
- Pleural effusion is uncommon.
- Adenopathy is rare. Fissural, chest wall, or mediastinal invasion can also be seen.

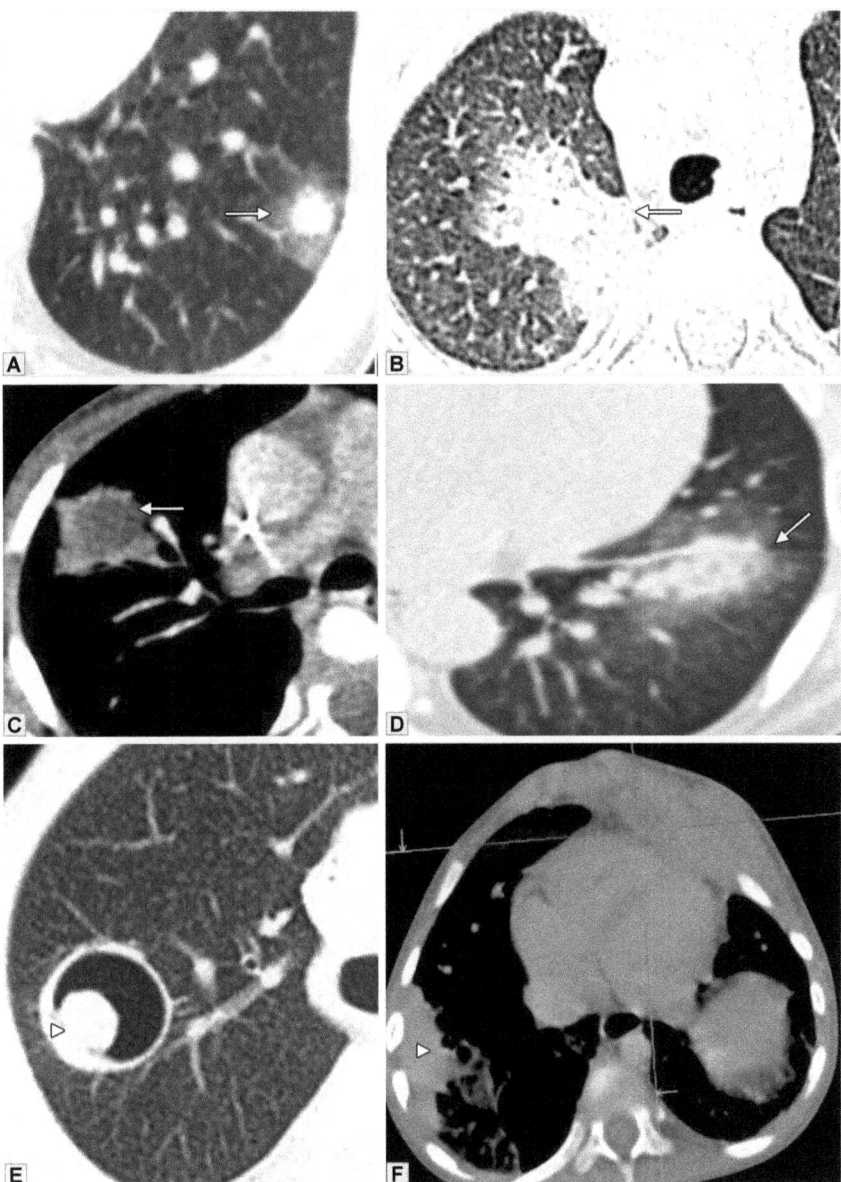

FIGS. 2A TO F: CT signs of invasive pulmonary aspergillosis (IPA)—(A) nodule with surrounding *ground-glass opacity;* (B) pleural-based areas of *consolidation* (arrow); (C) *Hypodense sign:* Appearance of central area of hypodensity (arrow) within the nodule/consolidation with surrounding enhancing wall; (D) consolidation with surrounding *ground-glass opacity* crossing across the fissure (arrow); (E) *crescent sign;* and (F) *chest wall* invasion (arrowheads).

MRI findings:
- MRI is complementary to CT in assessing the chest wall invasion in IPA,[1] however, early marrow changes can be assessed on MRI compared to CT.
- Postgadolinium rim enhancement giving a "target sign" and the "reverse target" on T2-weighted images (hyperintense center and hypointense rim) are strongly suggestive of IPA at a later stage of the disease.[1]
- MRI has a role in detection and follow-up of the IPA using rapid/short MRI protocols which can be acquired within a short-examination time to 2–12 minutes.[1-3]

Airway Invasive Aspergillosis

- Less common form (approximately 15% of cases)
- Serum galactomannan positive in up to 60% patients with this form[1]
- Bronchoalveolar lavage (BAL) is more likely to be positive for *Aspergillus* than in angioinvasive form.

CT findings include:
- Tracheal or bronchial wall thickening (tracheobronchitis) **(Figs. 3A and B)**
- Centrilobular nodules with tree in bud appearance in a patchy distribution
- Predominant peribronchial areas of consolidation or GGO mimicking bronchopneumonia **(Figs. 4A to C)**
- There are some differences in the laboratory and imaging pattern of IPA in clinical setting of neutropenic and non-neutropenic patients **(Table 1)**.[1]

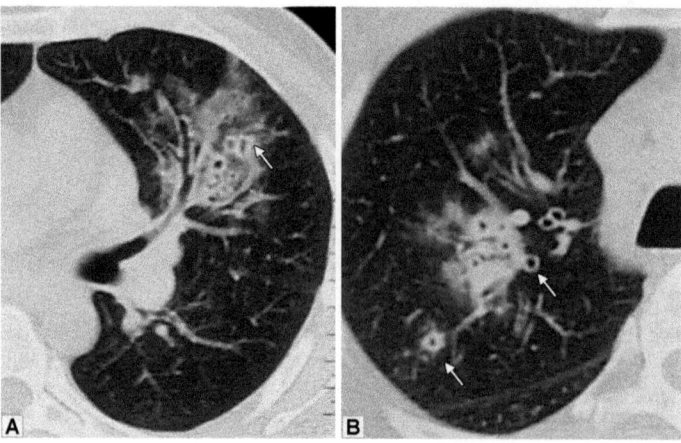

FIGS. 3A AND B: Airway invasive aspergillosis—(A) peribronchial consolidations and ground-glass opacity (GGO) and (B) bronchial wall thickening (arrows).

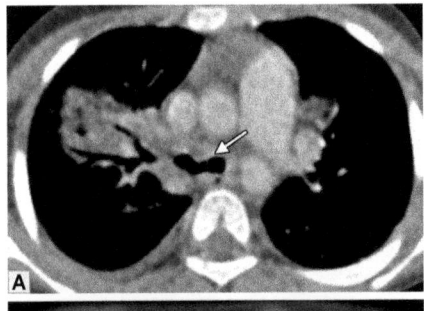
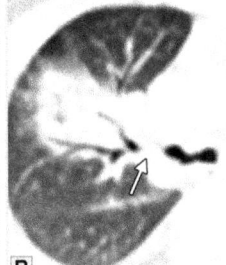
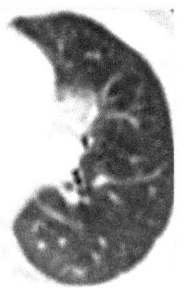
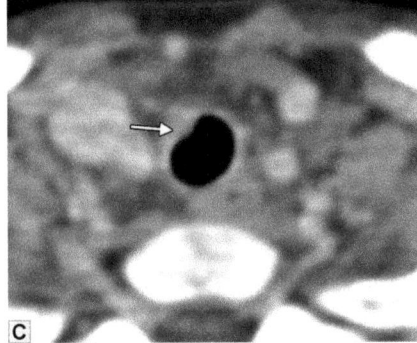

FIGS. 4A TO C: Airway invasive aspergillosis in a 10-year-boy.
(A) peribronchial consolidations with hypodense wall thickening of the anterior wall of carina (arrow);
(B) thickening of the right main bronchus causing irregularity and narrowing of the lumen (arrow); and
(C) focal eccentric wall thickening of the trachea (arrow).

TABLE 1: Difference in the clinical, laboratory, and CT imaging appearances of IPA in neutropenic and non-neutropenic patients.

	Neutropenic patients	Non-neutropenic patients
Susceptible population	Critically ill, ICU patients with neutropenia	Critically ill immunocompetent/immunosuppressed (other than neutropenia)
Pathology	Angioinvasion, hemorrhagic infarct, and coagulative necrosis	Airway invasive phase, pyogranulomatous reaction, followed by angioinvasion
Serum galactomannan	Elevated	Unreliable
CT findings	Nodules with halo, air crescent sign, hypodense sign, and peripheral wedge-shaped infarcts	Tracheobronchial wall thickening, centrilobular nodules with tree in bud opacities, consolidation, nodules, and GGO with peribronchial distribution

Chronic Pulmonary Aspergillosis

- Chronic pulmonary aspergillosis (CPA) is an umbrella term used to describe the diverse noninvasive/semi-invasive forms of aspergillosis.[1] CPA is an underrecognized entity and affects a large number of people with other underlying respiratory diseases. It is less common in children.
- Guidelines for the diagnosis and management of the entity and its diverse forms were formulated by a European Task Force and published in 2015.[5]

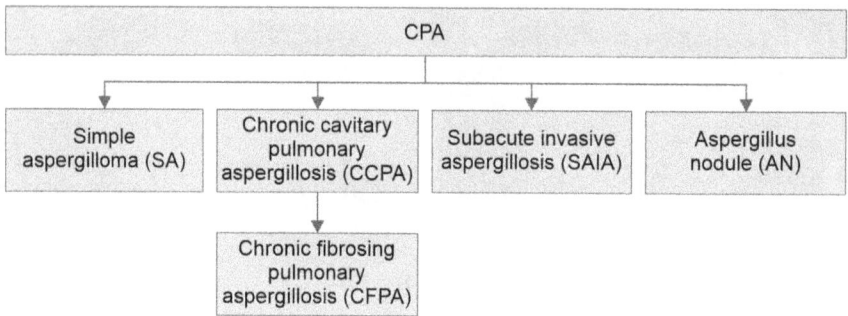

FLOWCHART 1: Subtypes of chronic pulmonary aspergillosis.

- CPA is further divided into several forms **(Flowchart 1)**. An overlap of the various forms is frequently seen.
- The diagnostic criteria are a combination of clinical, imaging, and laboratory findings.
- CPA develops in preexisting cavities or bronchiectasis but also itself leads to development of new cavities, enlargement of previous cavities, new nodules, and less frequently consolidation.
- CT angiography (CTA) may reveal enlarged bronchial arteries, nonbronchial systemic collaterals, or even pseudoaneurysms.
- There is paucity of literature pertaining to this entity in children.
- Common in patients with sequelae to prior tuberculosis (TB), nontuberculous mycobacterial (NTM) infection, or ABPA. Less common causes include sarcoidosis (fibrocavitary stage), chronic cavities of hydatid cyst, or cystic interstitial lung diseases.

Simple Aspergilloma

- While aspergilloma may be seen in most of the other forms of CPA, "SA" refers to presence of a fungal ball in a single cavity.
- The term "aspergilloma" refers to a "fungal ball" which comprises fungal hyphae and the surrounding extracellular matrix.
- In this form, there are no systemic symptoms, no progression, and usually very few or no serological or microbiological evidence of aspergillus species.
- These patients may present with hemoptysis.
- The characteristic sign described on chest radiograph and CT is the "Monod sign" adjacent to the mycetoma. It was earlier known as "air crescent sign"**(Figs. 5A and B)**. "Monod sign" is preferred here to differentiate it from the air crescent sign in IPA.
- On CT, SA appears as low density, nonenhancing contents within a cavity **(Figs. 5A and B)**.
- On MRI, the aspergilloma is hypointense on T2-weighted images and iso to hypointense on T1-weighted images.
- An aspergilloma can develop in pulmonary cavities in a dilated bronchus (as in cystic fibrosis) or even in the pleural cavity.

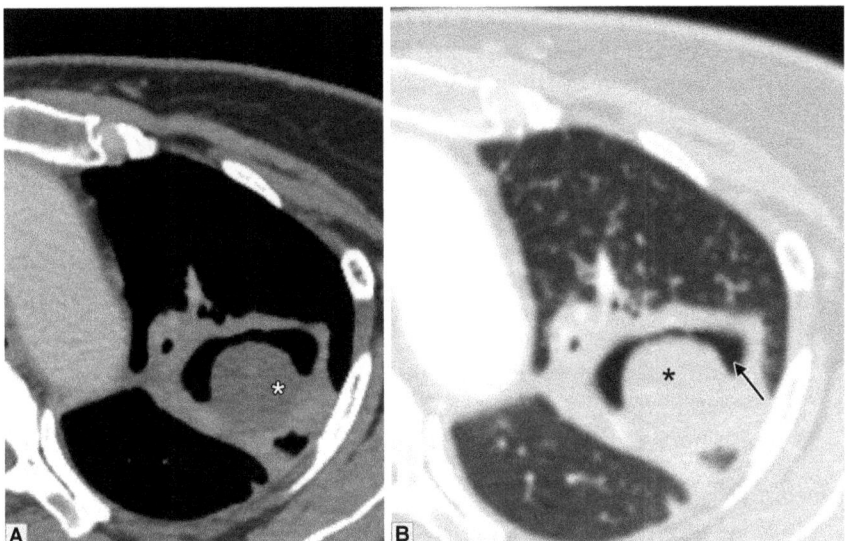

FIGS. 5A AND B: Simple aspergilloma—(A) intracavitary low-attenuation soft tissue (asterisk) and (B) peripheral incomplete rim or air density (arrow).

Subacute Invasive Aspergillosis

- *Synonyms/previous terminology*: Chronic necrotizing aspergillosis/semi-invasive aspergillosis (SAIA) occurs in debilitated or mildly immunocompromised patients.
- While the clinical and radiological features are similar to CCPA, SAIA shows more rapid progression. Also, serological and/or microbiological evidence of aspergillus species is more likely to be seen in this form.
- On imaging besides nodules and cavitation, consolidation with necrosis and "abscesses" may be seen.

Aspergillus Nodule

- This is an uncommon form of CPA. Presenting as noncavitating nodules.
- The imaging appearance of this form is indistinguishable from other infective/malignant causes of nodules. Larger lesions may also show central necrosis; however, invasion is not seen.

Allergic Bronchopulmonary Aspergillosis

Allergic bronchopulmonary aspergillosis is a dysregulated immune response to *Aspergillus fumigatus* conidia which is seen in patients of bronchial asthma or cystic fibrosis.

Clinical Manifestations

The most frequent presentation is of poorly controlled asthma. Respiratory symptoms include shortness of breath, expectoration, wheeze, or hemoptysis.

Diagnostic criteria (Several criteria exist. According to consensus guideline recommended by International Working Group of ABPA complicating asthma formed by the International Society for Human and Animal Mycology) in 2013:[6]
- *Predisposing conditions*: Bronchial asthma and cystic fibrosis
- *Obligatory criteria*:
    - Raised serum immunoglobulin E (IgE) levels against *Aspergillus fumigatus* (>0.35 KUA/L) or positive aspergillus skin test (AST)
    - Elevated serum IgE (total) levels > 1,000 IU/μL
- *Other criteria (two out of three should be present)*:
    1. Positive S. IgG antibodies against *A. fumigatus*
    2. Imaging findings c/w ABPS (bronchiectasis is no longer a part of essential criteria)
    3. Peripheral eosinophilia >500 cells/μL

Imaging

- Imaging findings in ABPA show a "remitting-relapsing" course, and have classically been described as "fleeting shadows".
- During the acute phase, areas of consolidations and mucus-filled dilated bronchi are seen. In the intercurrent phase, bronchiectasis and bronchial wall thickening are present. Mucus plugging due to inspissated secretions may be present even during remissions.

Chest radiograph:
- May not show any abnormality in up to half of the cases
- Findings during acute phase include consolidation, bronchoceles seen as "toothpaste" or "gloved finger" opacities **(Fig. 6)** or areas of atelectasis.
- After remission, residual changes include tram-track opacities, ring shadows, hyperinflation, and areas of emphysema.

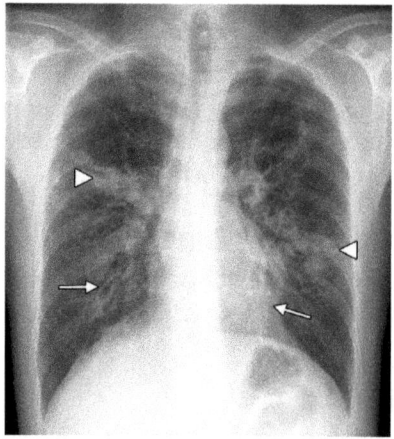

FIG. 6: CXR in ABPA—central bronchiectasis (arrowheads) and bronchocele/finger-in-glove opacities (arrows).
(ABPA: allergic bronchopulmonary aspergillosis; CXR: chest X-ray)

Computed tomography:
- Bronchiectasis is the most frequent finding on CT. While the distribution is classically described as central (involving inner two-thirds of the lungs), it has been shown that bronchiectasis extends to the periphery of the lungs in up to 40% of the patients.
- Morphology of bronchiectasis is cylindrical in less severe forms while it may be varicose/cystic in severe disease **(Figs. 7A to C)**.
- Another characteristic finding of ABPA is the presence of high-attenuation mucus (HAM) within the dilated bronchi on NCCT **(Figs. 7A to C)**. The high density is due to desiccated secretions and presence of iron, manganese, and calcium salts.
- Other findings seen due to mucus impactions are centrilobular nodules including tree-in-bud opacities.
- Consolidation is a less frequent finding and when confined to single lobe simulates infectious pneumonia. Collapse may also be seen.
- Parenchymal fibrosis, even cavities or bullae may develop. Pleural thickening and pneumothorax are also described.
- Aspergilloma can develop within the dilated bronchi.

Magnetic resonance imaging: The mucus plugs within the dilated bronchi usually demonstrate high signal on T1WI and low T2 signal intensity, referred to as "inverted mucoid impaction signal" (IMIS) sign **(Figs. 8A and B)**.

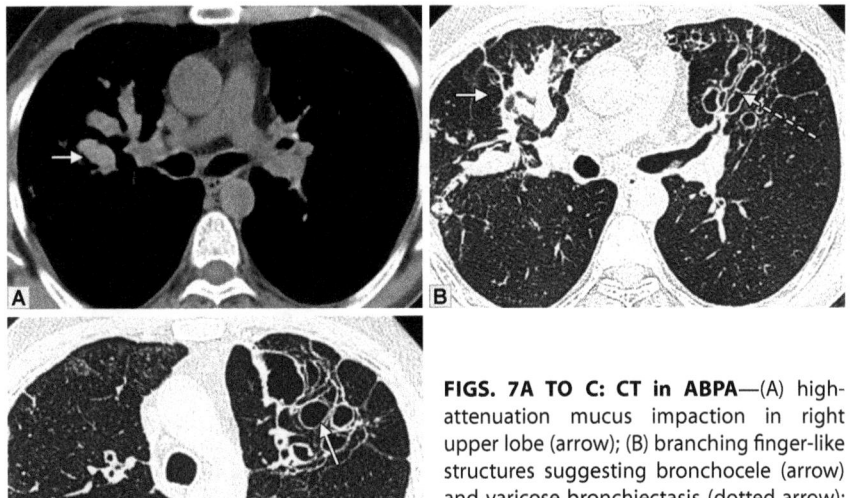

FIGS. 7A TO C: CT in ABPA—(A) high-attenuation mucus impaction in right upper lobe (arrow); (B) branching finger-like structures suggesting bronchocele (arrow) and varicose bronchiectasis (dotted arrow); and (C) higher section showing cystic bronchiectasis (arrow).
(ABPA: allergic bronchopulmonary aspergillosis; CT: computed tomography)

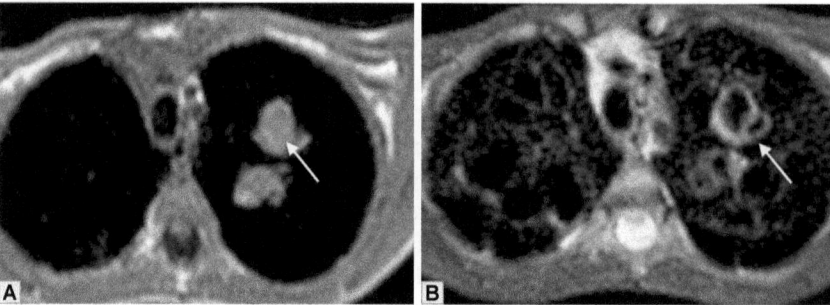

FIGS. 8A AND B: MRI in ABPA in a 16-year-girl. *Inverted mucus impaction signal sign.* (A) T1W image: High signal intensity tubular structures in LUL (arrow) and (B) T2W image: Hypointense signal (arrow).
(ABPA: allergic bronchopulmonary aspergillosis; MRI: magnetic resonance imaging)

Staging of Allergic Bronchopulmonary Aspergillosis

- *Clinical*: There are seven clinical stages of ABPA (zero to six) based on symptoms, radiology, IgE levels, requirement of steroids, and complications (cor pulmonale).[7] Details of the staging are beyond the scope of this chapter.
- *Radiological classification (based on HRCT)*: There are four subcategories of ABPA based on imaging. All the categories should satisfy basic diagnostic criteria of ABPA. The imaging findings are as follows:
  1. ABPA-S (serological ABPA): Normal HRCT
  2. ABPA-B: ABPA with bronchiectasis
  3. ABPA-HAM: ABPA showing high-attenuation mucus along with bronchiectasis
  4. ABPA-CPF (ABPA-chronic pleuropulmonary fibrosis): ABPA showing at least two radiological features of fibrosis without mucus impaction or HAM

■ OTHER FUNGAL INFECTIONS

The other important fungi include *Mucor* species, *Cryptococcus neoformans, Histoplasma capsulatum, Pneumocystis Jirovecii, Candida albicans, Blastomyces dermatitidis, Coccidioides immitis, Paracoccidioides brasiliensis, Fusarium solani, Trichophyton* species, *Microsporum* species, *Scedosporium* species.

Mucormycosis

- *Organism*: Mucormycosis is an angioinvasive infection caused by filamentous fungi which include *Rhizopus, Mucor,* and *Lichtheimia.*
- *Pathology*: These are angioinvasive, and cause early and rapidly progressive tissue necrosis and subsequent thrombosis.

- *Clinical scenarios*: The immunocompromised hosts including those with uncontrolled DM, solid organ or bone marrow transplant, PIDDs [e.g., chronic granulomatous disease (CGD)], or on immunosuppressive drugs, are more susceptible for acquiring these infections. It is the second most common and most severe opportunistic fungal infection in transplant recipients after *Aspergillus*. Amongst SOTs, disseminated disease most frequent in liver transplant (up to 55%). Reported mortality in disseminated disease is up to 90%.
- *Clinical presentation*: It presents more frequently disseminated form including rhinosinocerebral and cutaneous manifestations. Patients present with nonspecific respiratory symptoms with or without fever and pleuritic chest pain. Infection can rapidly progress with development of hemoptysis and rhinocerebral symptoms.
- *Imaging findings*: Chest radiograph/CT findings:
  - Areas of wedge-shaped/mass-like consolidation[4]
  - Solitary or multiple nodules or masses frequently with cavitation
  - Unilateral or bilateral pleural effusions (20%)
  - Unilateral or bilateral hilar and mediastinal lymphadenopathy (10%)
  - A "reversed halo sign"/bird's nest sign—reversed halo sign appears as a central GGO surrounded by denser consolidation **(Figs. 9 and 10)**. Presence of irregular and intersecting areas of stranding or irregular lines within the area of GGO is described as the bird's nest sign. It is a strong indicator of mucormycosis versus IPA.

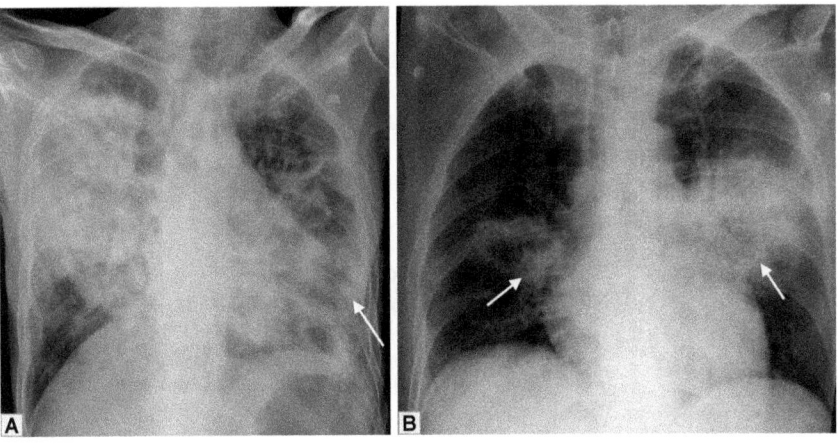

FIGS. 9A AND B: CXR in mucormycosis. Multifocal large consolidations transgressing fissures—(A) consolidation with central lucency (arrow) and (B) multifocal consolidation with central ground-glass opacity (GGO) (arrows).

- Consolidations directly crossing the fissures or invasion of the chest wall and pulmonary arteries are more common with mucormycosis than IPA.[4]
  - Pulmonary arterial pseudoaneurysms **(Figs. 10A to C)** may also be seen.
- Imaging findings of mucormycosis can be unusual/aggressive in appearance in immunodeficiency. In children with primary cell-mediated immunodeficiency such as CGD, mucormycosis may present as mass-like consolidation, and contiguous chest wall or vertebral involvement **(Figs. 11A to D)**.[8]
  - When to suspect pulmonary mucormycosis over IPA is summarized in **Table 2**.

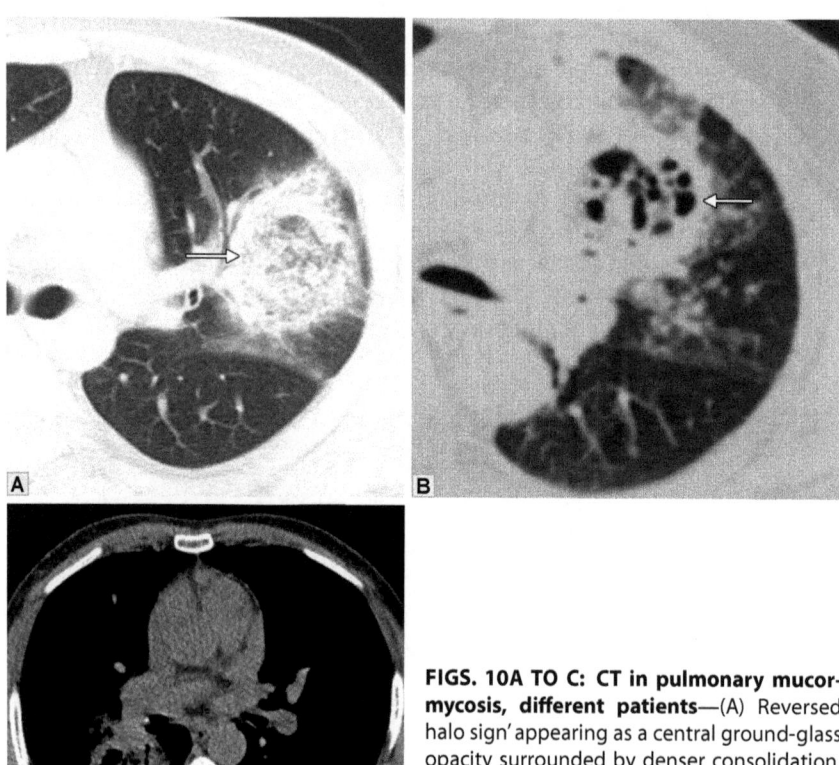

FIGS. 10A TO C: CT in pulmonary mucormycosis, different patients—(A) Reversed halo sign' appearing as a central ground-glass opacity surrounded by denser consolidation. (B) Central irregular and intersecting strands or irregular lines giving an appearance of "bird's nest" sign. (C) "Bird's nest" sign on mediastinal window.

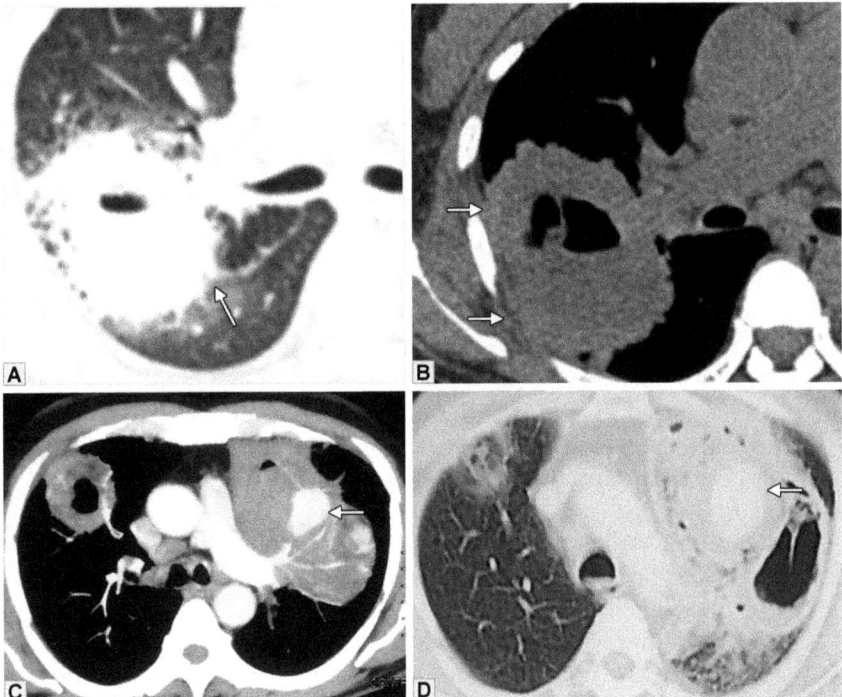

FIGS. 11A TO D: Complications of pulmonary mucormycosis. Two patients A and B. *Patient A*: Mass-like consolidation with cavitation seen in right upper lobe, invading the fissure, and involving the adjacent lower lobe (arrow in A). Chest wall invasion also seen. The consolidation was also found adherent to adjacent rib at surgery (B). *Patient B*: Multiple large areas of consolidation and cavities in both lungs (C and D). Contrast-filled outpouching (arrow) s/o pseudoaneurysm arising from segmental pulmonary artery branch within the areas of consolidation.

TABLE 2: When to suspect mucormycosis over aspergillosis.[1-4]	
Imaging findings favoring Mucormycosis	Imaging findings favoring invasive Aspergillosis
Concomitant sinusitis	Clusters of centrilobular nodules
Voriconazole prophylaxis	Peribronchial consolidations
Presence of multiple (≥10) nodules	Bronchial wall thickening
Reversed halo sign/Bird's nest sign	
Pleural effusion	

Pneumocystis Pneumonia

- *Organism*: *Pneumocystis jirovecii* is a yeast-like fungal microorganism.
- *Pathology*: Pathologically, pneumocystis pneumonia (PCP) is characterized by foamy, intra-alveolar exudates. Cavitation, vascular invasion, vasculitis, and even noncaseating, calcified granulomas are some atypical pathological patterns reported.
- *Clinical scenarios*: It forms the most common acquired immunodeficiency syndrome (AIDS), defining illness, and affects the patient when CD4 levels < 100 cells/mm^3.
- *Clinical presentation*: The presentation in an immunocompromised host other than AIDS is usually acute and manifested by an abrupt onset of fever, dry cough, dyspnea, respiratory insufficiency, and hypoxemia. In HIV infected individuals, the most common manifestations of PCP are subacute onset of progressive dyspnea, fever, nonproductive cough, and chest discomfort that worsens within days to weeks.
- *Imaging findings*:
  - On chest radiograph, it may present as diffuse bilateral airspace opacities or fine reticulonodular opacities or ill-defined hazy GGOs or consolidation.
  - HRCT findings are summarized in the **Box 1**.
  - Ground-glass opacities are by far the most common finding **(Figs. 12A and B)**.
  - Patients may develop extensive bilateral consolidations in more severe forms.

BOX 1 | HRCT findings in pneumocystis pneumonia in the order of frequency.

Common imaging patterns:
- Patchy or diffuse, symmetric bilateral ground-glass opacity (GGO)
- Perihilar, central, or upper lobe predominance
- Distinct "mosaic" pattern due to areas of normal lung intervening between areas of GGOs
- Thin or thick-walled cysts, irregular cavities
- Pneumothorax
- Consolidation
- Reticulation and septal thickening (resolving disease)

Uncommon imaging patterns:
- Bronchiectasis or bronchiolectasis
- Small nodules, centrilobular, or diffuse
- Large nodules or masses
- Pleural effusions
- Lymphadenopathy

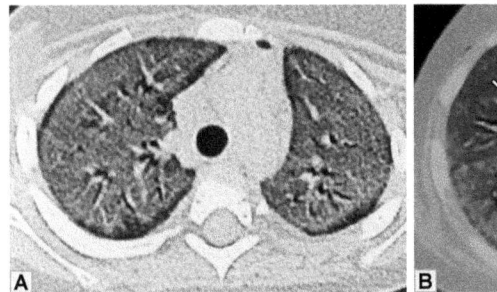
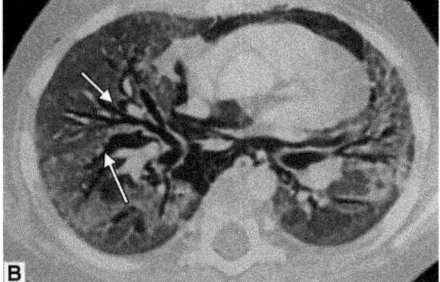

FIGS. 12A AND B: Pneumocystis pneumonia—(A) diffuse ground-glass opacity (GGO) with peripheral subpleural sparing and (B) pulmonary interstitial emphysema (arrows in B).

- Presence of smooth interlobular septal thickening and intralobular linear opacities superimposed on the GGOs resulting in a "crazy-paving" pattern suggests resolving phase of infection.
- *Cystic changes in PCP*:
  - Cystic changes are seen in 20–35% of patients of *Pneumocystis jirovecii* pneumonia (PJ)P who have AIDS **(Figs. 13A and B)**, while these cysts are uncommon in non-AIDS immunocompromised patients.
  - Cysts are variable in appearance being thick or thin walled. Complex cysts, cysts occurring in clusters, and cysts with an irregular shape are also seen.
  - Upper lobe predominance is common.
  - Due to rupture of the cysts, there is a high incidence of pneumothoraces.
  - After therapy, these cysts/cavities eventually regress, resulting either in complete disappearance, residual nodules or masses, or both.
- *Stages of disease*: **Table 3** clubs the imaging patterns according to the phases of PCP infection.

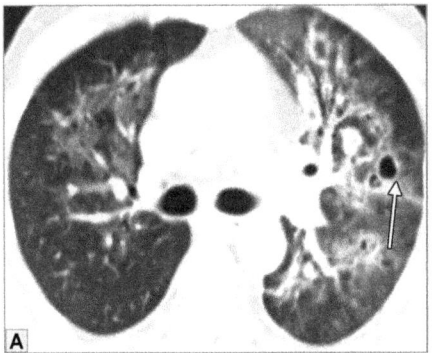
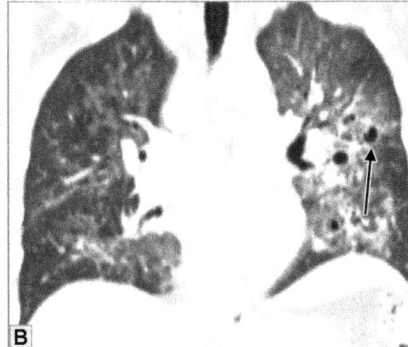

FIGS. 13A AND B: Cyst in PCP—(A) bilateral central GGO and reticulations and (B) thin-walled cysts (arrows).

TABLE 3: HRCT and pathological findings according to the phases of PCP infection.

Stage of PCP	HRCT findings pathological findings
Acute phase	• Scattered areas of ground-glass • Intra-alveolar exudates as well opacity as mild thickening of the airspace consolidation alveolar septa
Resolving or subacute	*Interstitial abnormalities*: • Thickened interlobular and • Reticular opacities intralobular septa • Organization of intra-alveolar • Crazy paving exudates
Chronic	• Diffuse interstitial fibrosis • Fibrosis • Honeycombing • Giant cell and granulomatous • Mild, peripheral bronchiectasis reaction

Less Common Fungal Infections

Clinical and imaging features of other less common fungi are discussed in **Table 4**.

TABLE 4: Clinicoradiologic spectrum of other less common fungal infections.

Fungi	Source	Population affected by it	Imaging features

Cryptococcus neoformans	Soil containing pigeon droppings	Transplant recipients (SOT more than HSCT), HIV, steroid use	• Solitary or multiple small well-defined subpleural nodules with upper and mid zone predominance; in a clustered nodular pattern, cavitation is present in 10–40%:[6]
			  ○ Focal areas of consolidation
			  ○ Concomitant CNS lesions

Candida albicans **(Figs. 14A and B)**		HSCT, lung, liver transplants, and other immunocompromised state	Nodules with surrounding ground glass opacities, consolidation, diffuse ground glass opacities, and diffuse random/miliary nodules

Continued

Continued

Fungi	Source	Population affected by it	Imaging features
Fusarium solani	Soil and plant	HSCT and lung transplant	Airspace/interstitial opacities, nodules with or without halo sign, pulmonary infarction, sinusitis
Histoplasma capsulatum	Endemic fungus in Asia, Africa, South America, parts of north America Caves harboring bats	HSCT and lung transplant, HIV infection	• Acute pulmonary histoplasmosis (nonspecific findings with acute consolidation, nodules, and lymphadenopathy) • Disseminated form (miliary random pulmonary nodules) • Chronic cavitary pulmonary histoplasmosis (thick-walled cavities with extensive fibrosis) • Mediastinal fibrosis
Coccidioides immitis and C. posadasii	Endemic in regions of ports of Mexico (northern) and southwestern region of United States (also known as Valley fever)	SOT, within first year	• Acute—multilobar consolidations, resolve at one area and appear at new locations-known as "phantom consolidations" • Chronic—fibrocavitary disease in lungs, chronic osteomyelitis, and meningitis • Disseminated—miliary nodules and lymphadeno-pathy associated with skin, bone, and brain lesions
Blastomyces dermatitidis	Endemic in central and southeastern United States and southern Canada		• Acute form—consolidation/nodule, overwhelming infection with adult respiratory distress syndrome • Chronic form—mass-like lesions that look like lung cancer or upper lobe cavitary lesions. Lymphadenopathy is seen less commonly than histoplasmosis
Phaeohypho-mycosis (Figs. 15A to D)	Black fungi in soil or marshland	Neutropenia, HSCT, HIV, SOT, and malignancy	Skin and subcutaneous tissue infection, CNS involvement, and cavitary lung nodules

(CNS: central nervous system; HIV: human immunodeficiency virus; HSCT: hematopoietic stem cell transplantation; SOT: solid organ transplantation)

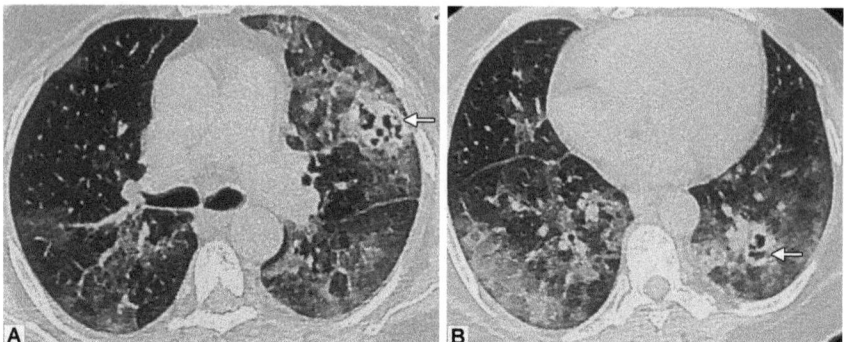

FIGS. 14A AND B: Disseminated candidiasis with pulmonary involvement. (A) Cavitating nodule with surrounding ground-glass opacities (arrow) and (B) in addition, multifocal areas of ground-glass opacity (GGOs) involving both lungs.

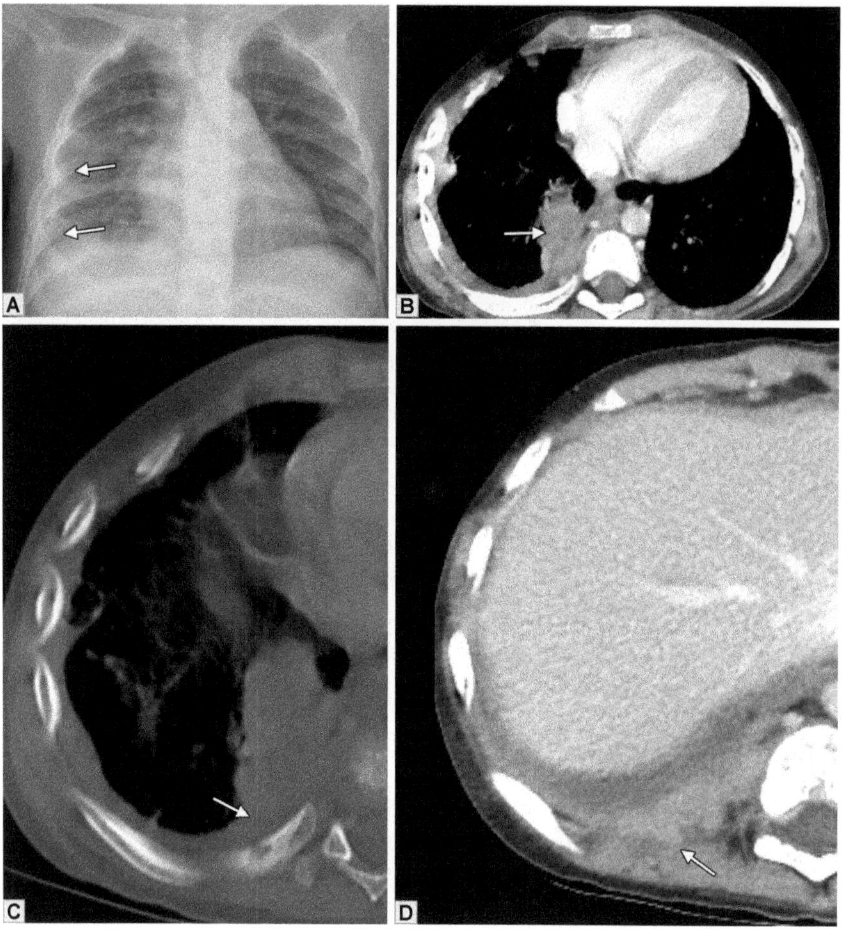

FIGS. 15A TO D: Phaeohyphomycosis. (A) CXR and (B to D) CT axial images—(A) peripheral pleural based nodules (arrows in A and B); adjacent rib sclerosis and lytic lesion (arrow in C); and pleural thickening (arrow in D).

CONCLUSION

Fungi are ubiquitous in the environment; the clinical features are largely governed by the immune status of the patient.

Other Related Chapters that can be Referred to:
- Chapter 10: Chest Infections in Immunocompromised Host
- Chapter 16: Bronchiectasis

REFERENCES

1. Garg A, Bhalla AS, Naranje P, Vyas S, Garg M. Decoding the Guidelines of Invasive Pulmonary Aspergillosis in Critical Care Setting: Imaging Perspective. Indian J Radiol Imaging. 2023;33(3):382-91.
2. Wahba H, Truong MT, Lei X, Kontoyiannis DP, Marom EM. Reversed halo sign in invasive pulmonary fungal infections. Clin Infect Dis. 2008;46(11):1733-7.
3. Chamilos G, Marom EM, Lewis RE, Lionakis MS, Kontoyiannis DP. Predictors of pulmonary zygomycosis versus invasive pulmonary aspergillosis in patients with cancer. Clin Infect Dis. 2005;41(1):60-6.
4. Jung J, Kim MY, Lee HJ, Park YS, Lee SO, Choi SH, et al. Comparison of computed tomographic findings in pulmonary mucormycosis and invasive pulmonary aspergillosis. Clin Microbiol Infect. 2015;21(7):684.e11-8.
5. Patterson TF, Thompson GR, Denning DW, Fishman JA, Hadley S, Herbrecht R, et al. Practice Guidelines for the Diagnosis and Management of Aspergillosis: 2016 Update by the Infectious Diseases Society of America. Clin Infect Dis. 2016;63(4):e1-e60.
6. Agarwal R, Chakrabarti A, Shah A, Gupta D, Meis JF, Guleria R, et al. Allergic bronchopulmonary aspergillosis: review of literature and proposal of new diagnostic and classification criteria. Clin Exp Allergy. 2013;43(8):850-73.
7. Blum U, Windfuhr M, Buitrago-Tellez C, Sigmund G, Herbst EW, Langer M. Invasive pulmonary aspergillosis. MRI, CT, and plain radiographic findings and their contribution for early diagnosis. Chest. 1994;106(4):1156-61.
8. Jana M, Sinha P, Garg P, Naranje P, Kabra SK, Bhalla AS. Imaging findings in chronic granulomatous disease (CGD). Indian J Pediatr. 2022.

CHAPTER 9

Chest Tuberculosis

Taruna Yadav, Sushil K Kabra

- ❑ Imaging modalities
  - ➢ Chest radiograph
  - ➢ Ultrasonography
  - ➢ Computed tomography
  - ➢ Magnetic resonance imaging
  - ➢ ^{18}F-fluorodeoxyglucose PET-CT
- ❑ Choice of modality
- ❑ Imaging findings
  - ➢ Pulmonary TB
  - ➢ Extrapulmonary TB
- ❑ Signs of activity
- ❑ Specific situations
  - ➢ Tuberculosis in HIV
  - ➢ Immune reconstitution inflammatory syndrome
  - ➢ Tuberculosis in primary immunodeficiency disorders
  - ➢ Drug-resistant TB
  - ➢ Congenital TB

■ INTRODUCTION

- Tuberculosis (TB) continues to be a public health challenge with an estimate of about 10 million affected across the world. Children and young adolescents aged under 15 years represent about 11% of all TB cases globally.[1] In India, about 342,000 incident cases of pediatric TB are estimated to occur every year accounting for 31% of the global burden and 13% of the overall TB burden in the country.
- In the chest, TB involves the lungs [pulmonary TB (PTB)] and multiple extrapulmonary sites [extrapulmonary TB (EPTB)]. EPTB sites in the chest include—lymph nodes, pleura, pericardium, and chest wall. Airway involvement can occur in both PTB and EPTB.
- The types of manifestations a patient develops are largely dependent on their inherent immunity. Based on this, the classification is into forms such as primary pulmonary complex (PPC), progressive pulmonary lesion (PPL), or reactivation TB. In this chapter, the discussion will proceed site-wise.

- Multimodality imaging is paramount in the diagnosis and follow-up of thoracic TB in children. Nonspecific clinical symptoms, paucibacillary nature of pediatric PTB, and long time taken in microbiological investigations with less sensitivity make the use of appropriate imaging mandatory for early diagnosis for starting of treatment.
- Primary TB may be asymptomatic in children with complete healing. Late childhood or adolescent presentation may be due to active TB (due to reinfection or reactivation) or complications resulting from fibrotic sequelae of previous infection (superadded bacterial infection or cavitary aspergilloma). So, differentiation of active versus inactive disease is essential to prevent further cases of TB and avoid potential risks of antitubercular treatment in children with inactive disease.

IMAGING MODALITIES

Role of various imaging modalities is discussed below.

Chest Radiograph

- In a child with suspected thoracic TB, chest radiograph (CXR) is the first modality despite its low sensitivity (approximately 67%) of detection as compared to more sensitive cross-sectional imaging modalities (CT/MRI).
- It serves as an initial screening modality. Frontal CXR is most commonly used. Lateral CXR may be used in few cases to confirm the presence of hilar or subcarinal lymphadenopathy **(Figs. 1A and B)**.
- CXR may suffice in those patients with history of contact, compatible clinical features, and characteristic or suggestive imaging **(Figs. 1A and B)**.

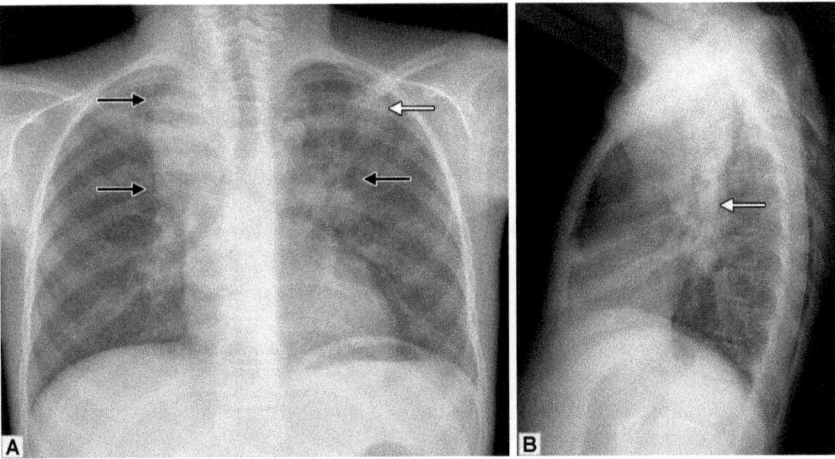

FIGS. 1A AND B: Suggestive chest radiographs in pulmonary tuberculosis. Bilateral hilar and paratracheal lymphadenopathy (black arrows in A) with lung involvement (white arrow in A). Doughnut sign (white arrow in B).

Ultrasonography

- Chest ultrasonography is increasingly being used for the evaluation of pleura, mediastinal lymphadenopathy, and lung involvement. Ultrasonographic window for lung and mediastinum evaluation in pediatric chest is excellent due to the absence of costal cartilage calcifications, thin chest wall with less subcutaneous fat, and presence of thymus in young children.
- In children, a combination of ultrasound and CXR increases the diagnostic efficiency for thoracic TB. Point-of-care ultrasound (POCUS) at bedside is gaining widespread popularity in emergency and critical care settings. Interim response assessment of therapy can be done at multiple time points due to lesser cost and absence of radiation in USG. Differentiation between minimal pleural effusion and residual pleural thickening is also feasible. Costochondral junction or rib TB can also be followed up on USG. USG findings/technique of various compartments are described subsequently.

Computed Tomography

- Although CT involves ionizing radiation, with newer radiation dose reduction techniques such as iterative reconstruction, CT doses are reducing over time (see Chapter 3). Faster acquisition can allow for imaging of the whole chest in a single breath hold reducing motion artifacts. Increasing availability and excellent sensitivity of CT make it the imaging modality of choice in all complex cases with TB. Indications for CT chest are listed in **Box 1**.
- For a thorough baseline evaluation of all compartments of the thorax and accurate differentiation of active from healed infection, an initial contrast-enhanced CT is advised. During follow-up, noncontrast CT with HRCT reconstruction in cases of parenchymal disease or MRI in cases of nodal and pleural disease can be used.

BOX 1 | **Indication of CT chest in pediatric tuberculosis.**

- Normal/equivocal chest radiograph—to detect radiographically occult nodal, parenchymal, pleural tuberculosis with a strong clinical suspicion of tuberculosis
- To differentiate between latent/healed/active pulmonary tuberculosis in indeterminate cases
- For evaluation of complications of TB—tracheobronchial compression + lobar collapse, bronchiectasis, and bronchopleural fistula
- Differentiation of tubercular from nontubercular infections in complex cases/ immunosuppressed host
- Preprocedural/presurgical evaluation—before diagnostic/therapeutic bronchoscopy or evaluation of bronchopleural fistula, before VATS decortication

(CT: computed tomography; TB: tuberculosis; VATS: video-assisted thoracic surgery)

Magnetic Resonance Imaging

- With the advent of newer developments in MRI with faster, breath-hold, and motion-corrected sequences, MRI is increasingly being used in the follow-up of patients requiring prolonged treatment particularly multidrug-resistant TB (MDR-TB) as a radiation-free modality.[1] Interim treatment response assessment with MRI is a viable option to avoid radiation with good contrast resolution **(Fig. 2)**.
- MRI has good sensitivity for the evaluation of PTB and EPTB, particularly for the evaluation of parenchymal cavitation, mediastinal lymph nodal disease, pleural effusion, in the diagnosis and response assessment in children.[2] Contrast-enhanced MRI is not mandatory for nodal evaluation; however, it increases the conspicuity of necrosis and is helpful in accurate assessment of disease activity.

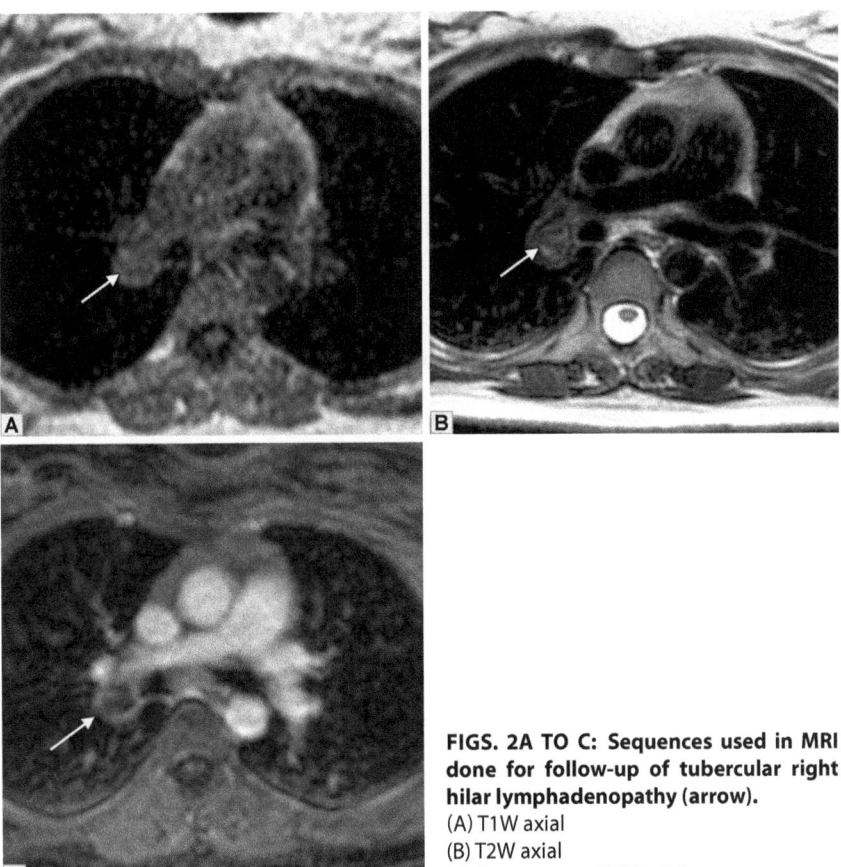

FIGS. 2A TO C: Sequences used in MRI done for follow-up of tubercular right hilar lymphadenopathy (arrow).
(A) T1W axial
(B) T2W axial
(C) Post contrast T1W axial

^{18}F-Fluorodeoxyglucose PET-CT

Higher radiation dose, higher cost, less availability of ^{18}F-fluorodeoxyglucose positron emission tomography computed tomography (^{18}F-FDG PET-CT) make it a less valuable imaging modality in the management of TB despite its high sensitivity.

■ CHOICE OF MODALITY

The CXR alone can suffice in case of highly suggestive symptoms. CT and USG can be used as additional investigation in case of equivocal diagnosis or complications.

■ IMAGING FINDINGS

Pulmonary TB

Chest Radiograph

- Highly suggestive CXR findings include miliary shadows, hilar or mediastinal adenopathy, or fibrocavitary chronic parenchymal lesions.[2] In cases of nonspecific CXR findings such as consolidations, in-homogenous shadows, or bronchopneumonia, etc., a repeat CXR after a course of antibiotics should be performed, followed by microbiological tests.
- Chest radiography was identified by the guideline development group (GDG) of the WHO as a critical tool to evaluate the severity of intrathoracic disease. As indicated under the recommendation remarks, nonsevere intrathoracic or PTB disease refers to—intrathoracic lymph node TB without airway obstruction, uncomplicated TB pleural effusion or paucibacillary, noncavitary disease confined to one lobe of the lungs and without a miliary pattern **(Figs. 3A and B)**. Extensive or advanced disease in children under 15 years of age is usually defined by the presence of cavities or bilateral disease on CXR **(Figs. 4A to D)**.[3]
- Common sites of involvement are the right middle and lower lobe in primary TB in children. Patterns of involvement are shown in **Table 1** and **Figures 5A and B**.

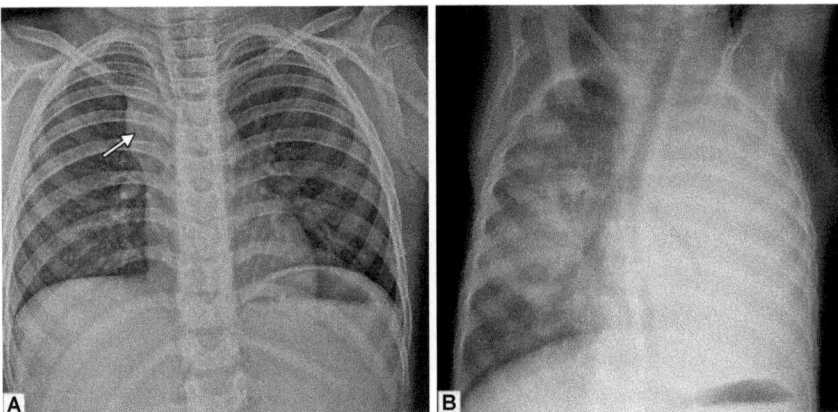

FIGS. 3A AND B: Nonsevere and severe disease on chest radiograph. Right paratracheal lymphadenopathy alone (A). Bilateral consolidation and left opaque hemithorax (B).

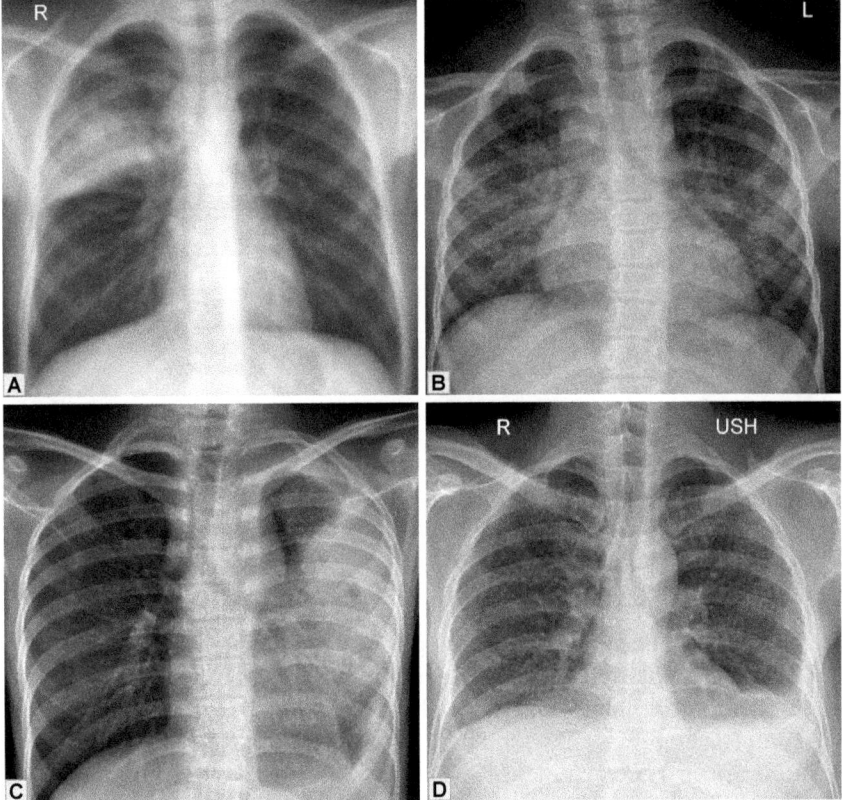

FIGS. 4A TO D: Patterns on CXR, active disease. Primary disease: right paratracheal LN and right upper lobar consolidation (A). Progressive primary disease (B and C). Miliary tuberculosis with left pleural effusion (D).
(CXR: chest radiograph; LN: lymph node)

TABLE 1: Lung parenchymal findings on chest radiograph.		
Presentation	**Lobar involvement**	**Radiographic manifestation**
Primary tuberculosis	Middle and lower lobe of right lung more than left lung	• Focal or multifocal consolidation + cavitation • Multiple clustered nodules • Miliary pattern
Progressive primary disease	More than one lung segment, even entire lobe	• Lobar consolidation • Miliary spread • Bronchopneumonia pattern
Post-primary tuberculosis	Upper lobe more than lower lobe	• Consolidation with cavitation • Centrilobular nodules may be with tree in bud pattern
Sequelae of previous infection	Upper lobe more than lower lobe	• Fibrosis • Bronchiectasis • Paracicatricial emphysema

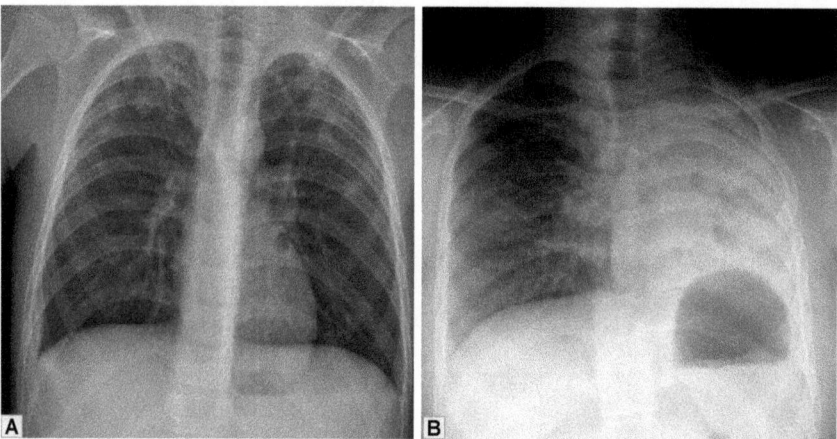

FIGS. 5A AND B: Patterns on CXR, tubercular sequelae. Bilateral upper lobar fibrosis (A). Destroyed left lung with bronchiectasis (B).

Ultrasonography

- It has not gained acceptance as a primary modality for lung. It can help when CT is not available, or patient is unable to undergo CT.
- Evaluation of lung parenchymal abnormalities on USG requires a complete zone-wise assessment.
- USG can only detect pleural-based consolidations as overlying air leads to absence of an acoustic window in rest of the nonpleural-based nodules/consolidations. Lung assessment by USG also has an initial learning curve.

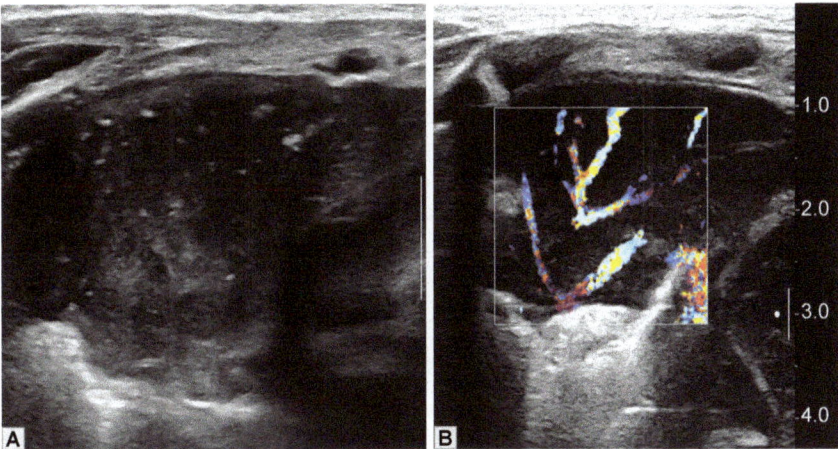

FIGS. 6A AND B: Ultrasound in consolidation. Gray scale (A) and Doppler (B) images. Hepatization (A) and preserved internal vascularity (B).

- Consolidations and collapse are seen as hypoechoic areas with and without air bronchograms. Evolution of consolidation with resolution or development of cavitation/lung abscess can be detected by USG **(Figs. 6A and B)**.

Computed Tomography
- *Consolidation* with or without cavitation is the hallmark of pulmonary involvement. Consolidation can be unifocal or multifocal **(Figs. 7A and B)**. Collapse of lung segments secondary to bronchial compression by nodes can also be seen. On CT, consolidation is seen as an area of increased density obscuring the vessels; however, on contrast-enhanced computed tomography (CECT), the normal pulmonary vessels are seen in the consolidated lung.

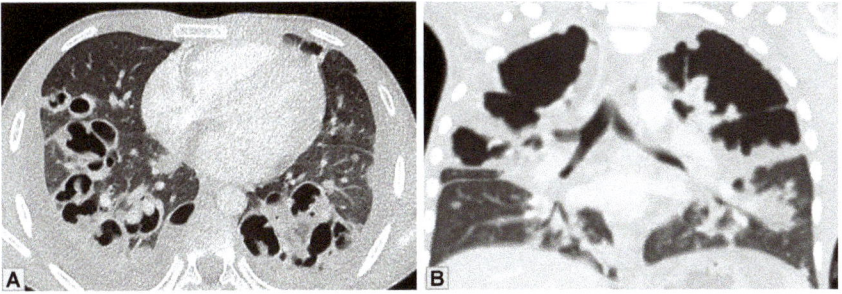

FIGS. 7A AND B: Consolidation in CT. Extensive upper lobar consolidation with internal necrosis and cavitation.

- *Nodules* of all types are encountered in TB—large nodules, small nodules (centrilobular, random, and perilymphatic) and micronodules (miliary) **(Figs. 8A to C)**. Among these, centrilobular nodules (CLNs) are the most frequent and perilymphatic distribution is the least frequent.
  - Tree-in-bud opacities are a type centrilobular nodules (2-4 mm) appearing as sharply marginated linear branching opacities.
  - Perilymphatic nodules (PLNs) are distributed along the bronchovascular bundles and subpleural region. They are infrequent in TB, but these have been recently reported including the "galaxy sign" which is considered typical of sarcoidosis. However, this appearance is infrequent in TB and the presence of PLN still favors sarcoidosis.
  - Miliary nodules are 1-3-mm well-defined nodules, having bilateral random distribution, which develop due to hematogenous spread of the infection. These may be associated with septal thickening.

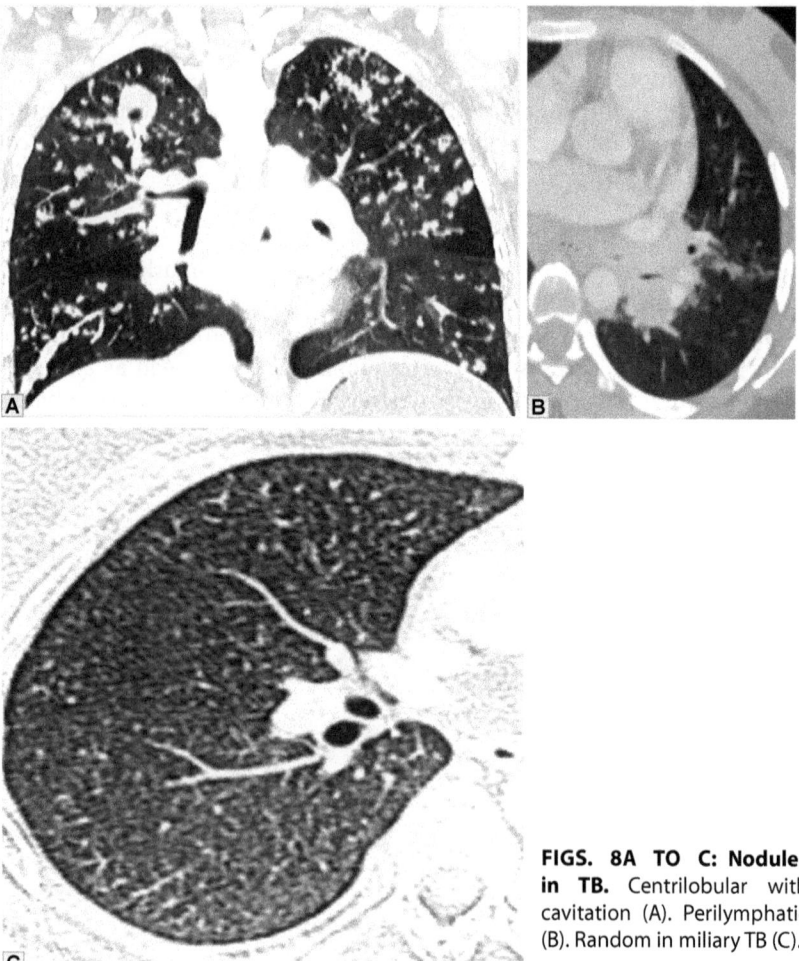

FIGS. 8A TO C: Nodules in TB. Centrilobular with cavitation (A). Perilymphatic (B). Random in miliary TB (C).
(TB: tuberculosis)

CHAPTER 9: Chest Tuberculosis

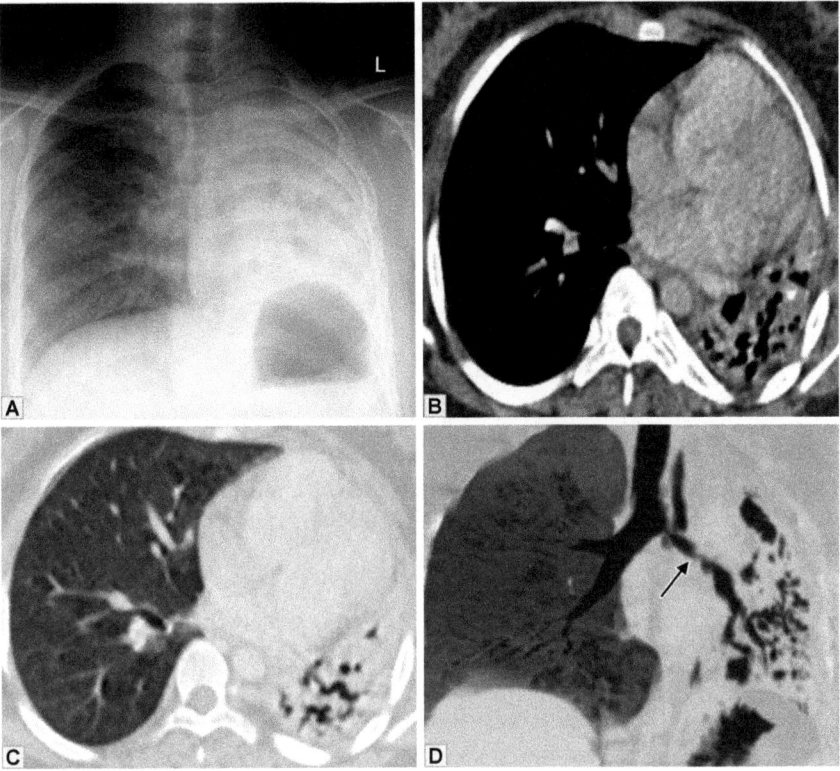

FIGS. 9A TO D: Sequelae of TB. CXR (A), axial CECT (B and C), Coronal MinIP (D) images. Opaque left hemithorax with ipsilateral mediastinal shift (A). Destroyed left lung with bronchiectasis (B and C). Irregularity and stricture left main bronchus (arrow in D).
(CECT: contrast-enhanced computed tomography; CXR: chest radiograph; MinIP: minimum intensity projection; TB: tuberculosis)

- *Larger nodules* (1–4 cm) can occur due to coalescence of smaller nodules. These have irregular margins and are surrounded by satellite nodules. Peribronchial distribution suggests active disease.
- Sequelae can be seen in the form of fibrosis and paracicatricial emphysema. Traction bronchiectasis can be seen in the affected areas. Cavities may persist, and can be colonized by *Aspergillus* (**Figs. 9A to D**).

Magnetic Resonance Imaging

- MRI is not a primary modality but can detect most changes, e.g., if MRI is done for nodes.
- With the advent of newer sequences with less motion sensitivity and related artifact, evaluating tubercular parenchymal changes has become possible using MRI. Consolidation, cavities, and larger nodules are well detected on T2W MRI. MRI lacks the sensitivity of CT in detecting smaller nodules.

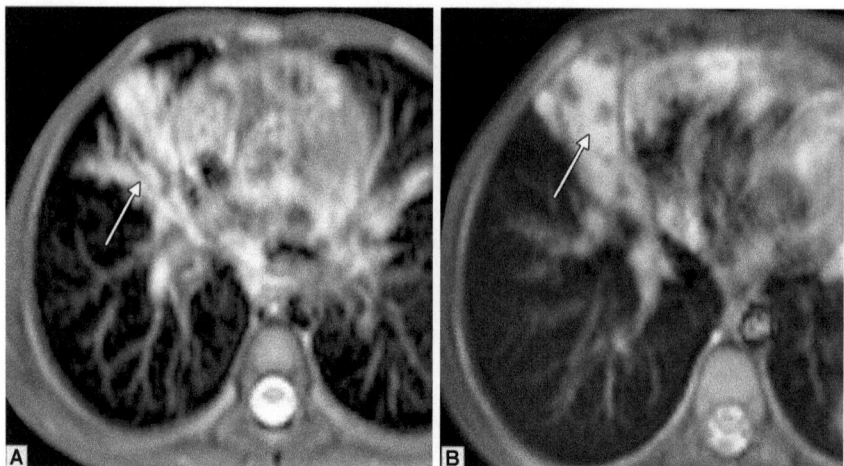

FIGS. 10A AND B: MRI in tubercular consolidation T2W fat-suppressed axial images. Consolidation in right middle lobe (arrow in A), seen as hyperintense structure. Areas of cavitation (arrow in B).

- Consolidation is seen as T2W hyperintense areas with variable diffusion restriction **(Figs. 10A and B)**.
- Nodules are detected as T2W hyperintense lesions, and are difficult to detect on T1W images.

Extrapulmonary TB

Lymphadenopathy

Chest Radiograph

- Mediastinal lymphadenopathy is more common in children than adults and may be the sole radiographic pattern of primary tubercular infection. Mediastinal lymphadenopathy can occur alone or in combination with cervical lymphadenitis (most common site of nodal involvement) and/or enlargement of axillary, abdominal lymph nodes.
- Signs of lymphadenopathy on plain radiographs **(Figs. 11A to C)** are enlisted in **Box 2**.[4]

Ultrasonography

- Mediastinal lymph nodes can be assessed by USG. Different USG probes (linear-parasternal approach, endocavitary/convex/microconvex—suprasternal approach), most commonly in combination, are used for the mediastinal assessment **(Figs. 12A and B)**. Only paratracheal, prevascular, subcarinal nodes can be adequately assessed with USG with limited use for lower and posterior mediastinal lymph nodes due to poor window. It requires operator's familiarity with the modality and an initial learning curve due to limited parasternal and suprasternal window. Technique is also described in Chapter 2.

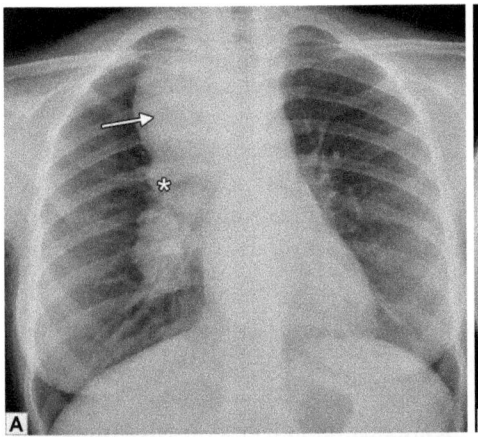
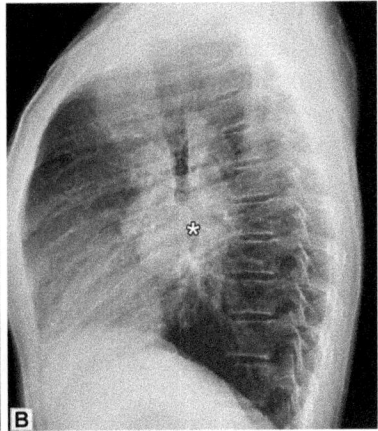
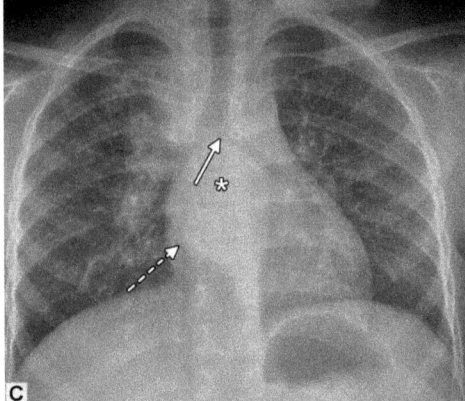

FIGS. 11A TO C: Signs of LN on CXR. PA (A) and lateral (B) radiograph; PA radiograph of another patient (C). Right paratracheal (arrow in A) LN seen as widened right paratracheal stripe. Right hilar LN, seen as doughnut sign (asterisk on A and B). Subcarinal LN (asterisk in C), causing widened carinal angle (arrow); and displacement of azygoesophageal line (dashed arrow).
(CXR: chest radiograph; LN: lymph node)

BOX 2 | CXR signs of lymphadenopathy.

PA radiograph:
- Widening of right paratracheal stripe (right paratracheal LN)
- Widened carinal angle (subcarinal LN)
- Displacement of azygoesophageal line (subcarinal LN)
- Hilar enlargement (hilar LN)
- Left-sided superior mediastinal widening (prevascular LN)

Lateral radiograph:
- "Doughnut sign" in hilar lymph nodes (mass-like lobulated shadow posteroinferior to bronchus intermedius)
- Loss of retrosternal lucency (prevascular LN)

(CXR: chest radiograph; LN: lymph node; PA: posteroanterior)

- In an expert operator's hands, USG can be more sensitive than CXR for mediastinal nodal assessment.
- In addition, screening of the neck for cervical lymph nodes and abdomen for periportal/retroperitoneal lymph nodes, hepatosplenomegaly/liver, or splenic granulomas may support the diagnosis of disseminated TB. Tubercular lymph nodes are hypoechoic, oval to round in shape with or without internal anechoic necrotic areas. On healing, lymph nodes show decrease in size, disappearance of necrotic areas, and foci of calcifications with shadowing.

Contrast-enhanced Computed Tomography
- Right paratracheal, hilar, and subcarinal are the most common sites affected. On CT, nodes show central necrosis, ghost-like, heterogeneous **(Figs. 13A to F)**, or even homogeneous enhancement. Obscuration of perinodal fat and conglomeration are signs of activity. Calcification may be seen initially and increases with treatment.
- Reappearance or perinodal fat is one of the earliest signs of response.
- With treatment, the nodes become more homogeneous with reduction of necrosis. Increase in calcification is also seen.
- Residual nodes post completion of treatment are seen in up to a third of the patients. This would represent nonresponse to therapy, but some persistent nodes do not always represent active disease.

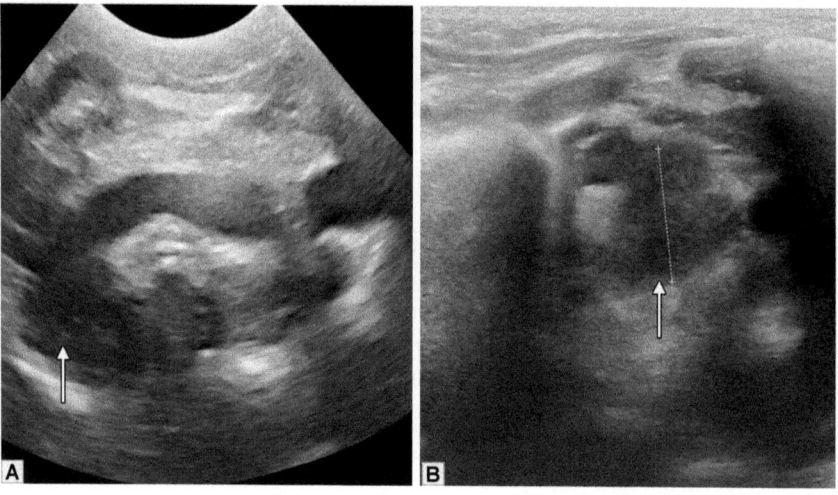

FIGS. 12A AND B: Ultrasound in lymphadenopathy. Suprasternal US with curvilinear sector probe (A). Right parasternal US with linear transducer (B). Enlarged right paratracheal lymph node (arrow).

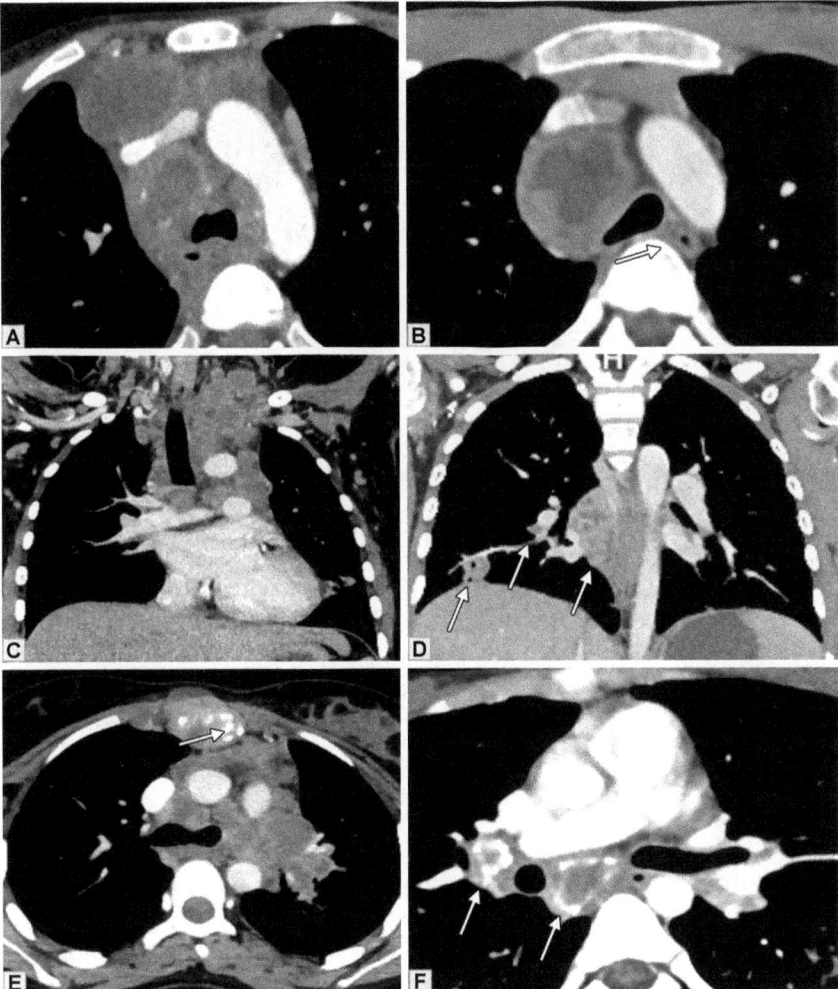

FIGS. 13A TO F: CT in intrathoracic lymphadenopathy in 6 different patients (A to E) with thoracic tuberculosis. (A) Multiple necrotic mediastinal lymph nodes causing mild SVC and tracheal compression. (B) Large right paratracheal lymph node with peripheral rim enhancement causing significant tracheal compression (arrow). (C) Bulky necrotic mediastinal nodes in coronal image. (D) Ghon's complex—arrows [subpleural parenchymal focus (Ghon's focus) along with enlarged necrotic draining right hilar and subcarinal lymph nodes]. (E) Mediastinal nodes along with sternal lytic lesion (white arrow) caused by tuberculosis. (F) Peripherally calcified necrotic lymph nodes (arrows) in partially healed tuberculosis during treatment.

Magnetic Resonance Imaging

- On MRI, tubercular lymph nodes (LNs) may show variable signal on imaging **(Figs. 14A to D)**. The characteristic necrotic node is seen as peripheral rim enhancement with a central core which is T2W hyperintense.[5] Other possible appearances include T2 homogeneously

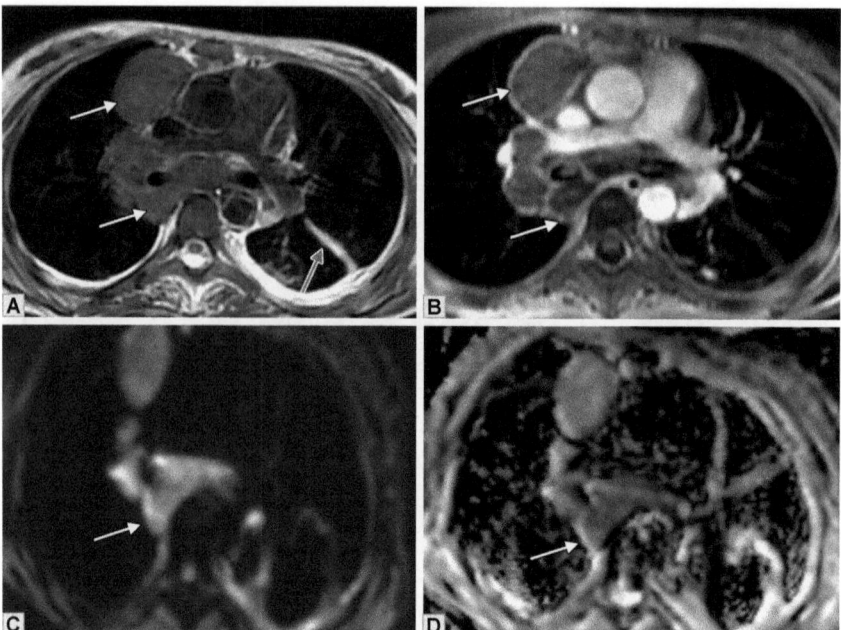

FIGS. 14A TO D: Contrast-enhanced MRI in tubercular lymphadenopathy. Axial T2-weighted (A), postcontrast T1-weighted image (B), DWI (C), and ADC map (D). Multiple enlarged T2 hypointense right paratracheal, right hilar, and subcarinal lymph nodes (arrows in A). Peripheral enhancement with central nonenhancing areas (B). Mild left pleural effusion (gray arrow in A). Mild diffusion restriction in the subcarinal node (arrow in C and D). Facilitated diffusion in right paratracheal nodes (C and D).

hyperintense with homogenous contrast enhancement, T2 hyperintense with thin rim of T2 hypointense SI, and heterogenous hyperintense with minimal or no enhancement. The T1 and T2 signal ratio, when compared to the multifidus muscle, tends to decrease with treatment.[6]

Pleural Involvement

- Pleural effusion in TB can be free flowing or loculated, and is seen on CXR with an opacity along the costophrenic angles progressing medially with meniscus sign **(Figs. 15A to D)**.
- Slowly over time, pleural effusion gets loculated with thickening of visceral and parietal pleura (also see Chapter 26).
- Loculations in the effusion and chronic changes with volume loss suggest empyema. It is hard to differentiate between pleural thickening and small pleural fluid in chronic cases on radiograph.
- With healing calcification and increase in pleural thickening, volume loss sets in.
- Evaluation of the stage of empyema is similar to that in other organisms causing infected pleural fluid collections (IPFCs). It is discussed in Chapter 26.

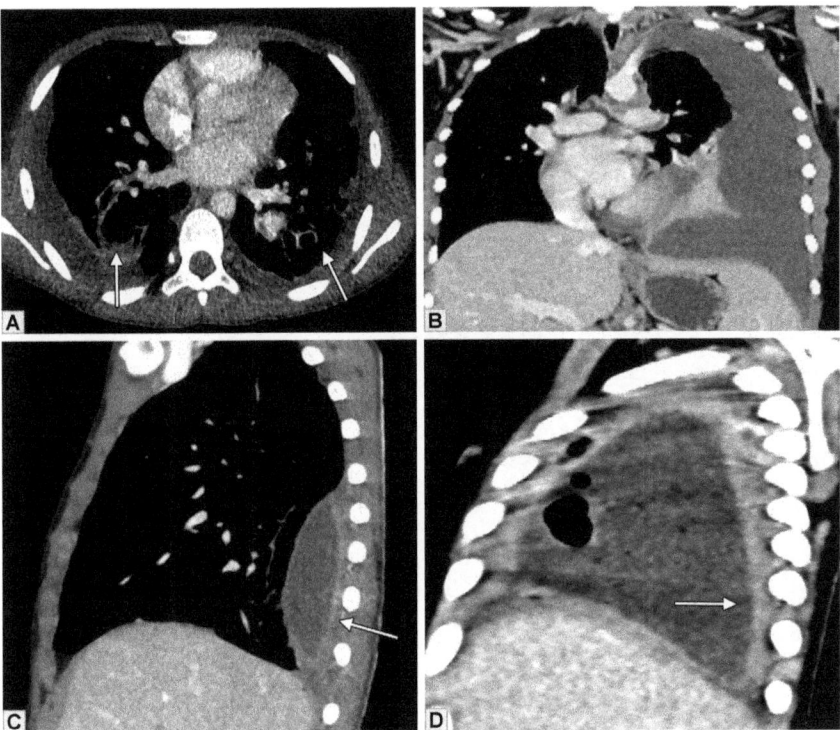

FIGS. 15A TO D: Multiple modes of presentations of pleural tuberculosis. Bilateral cavitary lesions (arrows in A) in lungs with bilateral pleural effusion (A). Left pleural effusion (B). (C and D) A 13-year-old boy. Loculated empyema with thick peripherally enhancing wall (arrow in C). Thick enhancing pleural peel (arrow in D).

Chest Wall Involvement
- Chest wall involvement can present with extrapleural involvement ribs or vertebral erosions which may be detected on CXR. CT is a superior modality to visualize subtle bone destruction **(Figs. 16A to C)**. It can present with a cold abscess with endophytic and exophytic components.
- Osteomyelitis of chest wall bones is seen including sternum, ribs, or vertebrae.
- Bone destruction with abscess/collection showing peripheral enhancement is present.
- USG is useful in superficial part involvement, while MRI is for spinal TB.
- MRI is superior to CT in the detection of epidural component and marrow changes.

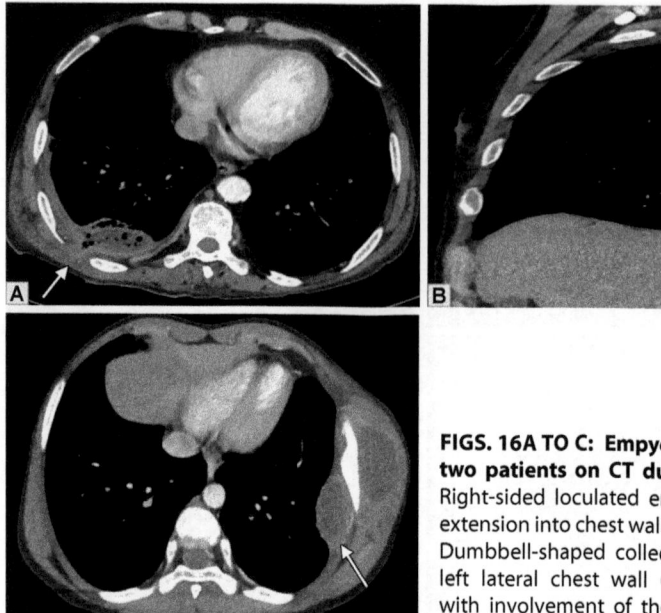

FIGS. 16A TO C: Empyema necessitans in two patients on CT due to tuberculosis. Right-sided loculated empyema with early extension into chest wall (arrows in A and B). Dumbbell-shaped collection is seen along left lateral chest wall (arrow in C) along with involvement of the adjacent rib with sclerosis and periosteal reaction.

Large Airway Involvement

- Trachea and major bronchi may be involved in multiple different ways primarily with associated wall thickening (smooth or irregular), endoluminal mass or ulceration, or as peribronchial soft tissue thickening leading to narrowing of lumen trachea or bronchi.
- Enlarged necrotic nodes may also erode into bronchus.
- Damage to the bronchial wall and parenchymal destruction will result in bronchiectasis after healing **(Figs. 17A and B)**.

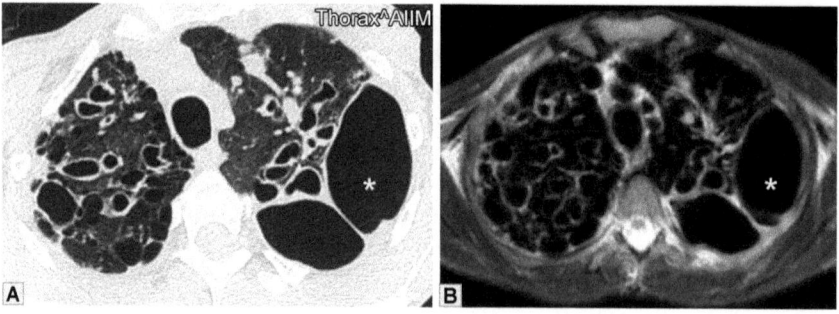

FIGS. 17A AND B: Post-tubercular bronchiectasis. Axial contrast-enhanced computed tomography (A), and axial T2W MR (B) images. Cystic and varicoid bronchiectasis. Thin-walled cavities (asterisk).

- Peripheral small airways are also filled with inflammatory exudates resulting in "tree in bud" opacities.
- Sometimes an entire lung parenchymal can be destroyed due to TB.

SIGNS OF ACTIVITY

Differentiation of residual active disease from sequelae can be challenging in post-treatment settings. Salient points are given below:
- *Parenchyma*:
  - *Active*: Thick-walled cavities, consolidation, and centrilobular nodules
  - *Inactive*: Thin-walled cavities, fibrotic bands, and well-defined nodules
- *Nodes*:
  - *Active*: Node enhancement (rim or inhomogeneous), conglomeration, and obscuration of perinodal fat. Active nodes can also be occasionally homogeneous.
  - *Inactive*: Homogeneous, discrete, and reappearance of perinodal fat.

SPECIFIC SITUATIONS

Tuberculosis in HIV

- Radiological findings of TB in patients with HIV can be atypical.
- In *HIV-associated PTB*, the imaging manifestations are dependent on the level of immunosuppression at the time of overt disease. HIV-seropositive patients with a CD4 T lymphocyte count < $200/mm^3$ have prominent mediastinal/hilar lymphadenopathy while cavitation is less common. Cavitation is seen in those with higher CD4 counts. In severe immunosuppression, miliary or disseminated disease is common.

Immune Reconstitution Inflammatory Syndrome

- Immune reconstitution inflammatory syndrome (IRIS) is a delayed and vigorous immune reaction to subclinical TB infection in acquired immune deficiency syndrome (AIDS) patients when antiretroviral therapy is started.[7] Recently, IRIS has also been reported in non-HIV patients.
- Paradoxical worsening of the pulmonary disease is seen after initiation of therapy.
- *Imaging findings*: Worsening of lymphadenopathy/extrapleural disease and pulmonary consolidations and/or nodules or other extrapleural sites occurs.

Tuberculosis in Primary Immunodeficiency Disorders

- Children with deficient cell-mediated immunity (T cell immunodeficiency) or phagocytic disorders (e.g., chronic granulomatous disease) are prone to infection with TB.
- The imaging findings can be atypical (also see Chapter 10).

Drug-resistant TB

- Drug-resistant TB (DR-TB) is a major public health problem due to spread of drug-resistant organisms. It is associated with high mortality consequent to ineffectiveness of therapy.
- The diagnosis of DR-TB is based on the demonstration of drug resistance on culture sensitivity.
- *Imaging findings*:
  - These are similar to drug-sensitive TB, except that multiple cavities with signs of chronicity, i.e., bronchiectasis/calcified granulomas are more common in MDR-TB **(Figs. 18A to D)**.
  - A strong correlation between imaging findings and the mode of acquisition of drug-resistance has been demonstrated:
    - In primary drug resistance, i.e., without anti-TB therapy or a therapy of <1 month, noncavitary consolidation, pleural effusion, and a primary TB pattern of disease are more common.
    - In secondary drug resistance, i.e., developing after therapy of longer than 1 month, cavitary consolidations and a reactivation pattern of the disease usually seen.

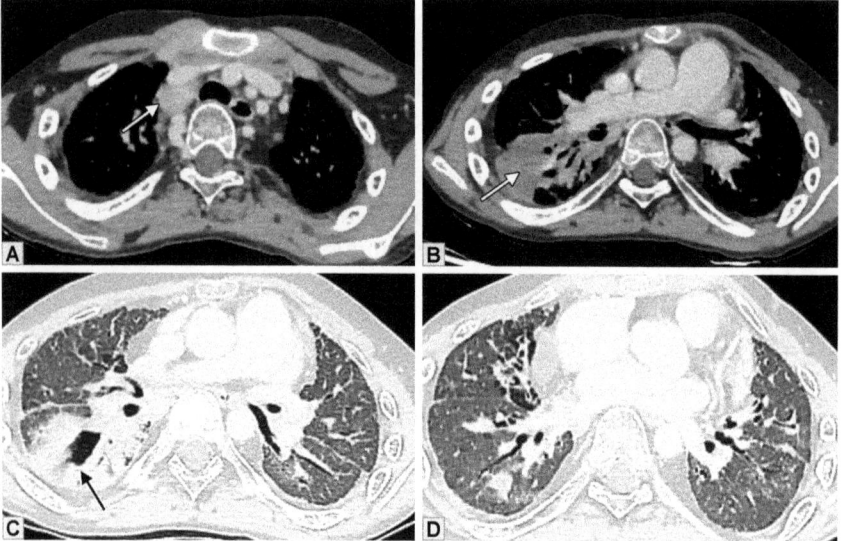

FIG. 18A TO D: Drug resistant TB in a 10-year-boy with fibrotic ILD. (A) Enlarged right paratracheal lymphadenopathy (arrow). (B and C) Right lower lobe superior segment consolidation with cavitation (arrow). (D) Peribronchial fibrosis.

Congenital TB
- Congenital TB presents in neonates or infants, and has a high mortality. A diagnosis of congenital TB can only be made if both the tuberculous nature of the lesion, and antenatal origin of the infection can be proven.[6]
- *Routes of infection*: Acquired by aspiration of infected amniotic fluid during passage through birth canal wherein lungs are affected first, or by ingestion where gastrointestinal (GI) tract is affected, or through transplacental route where liver is affected initially.
- *Imaging findings depend upon mode of acquisition*:[8]
  - Miliary or interstitial pattern is seen in hematogenous spread, while patchy bronchopneumonia or diffuse air space disease develops in infections acquired due to aspiration of infected material.
  - In addition, multiple pulmonary nodules or cysts which show peripheral rim enhancement on CT, or hilar and mediastinal adenopathy may also be present.

CONCLUSION

Due to nonspecific symptoms of PTB and EPTB, a full understanding and pattern recognition of imaging presentations of the various forms of the disease and disease activity is essential for early detection, timely management, and to prevent further spread of this potentially fatal but treatable infection in the community.

Other Related Chapters that can be Referred to:
- Chapter 10: Chest Infections in Immunocompromised Host
- Chapter 26: Pleural Disorders: Imaging

REFERENCES

1. Pillay T, Andronikou S, Zar HJ. Chest imaging in paediatric pulmonary TB. Paediatr Respir Rev. 2020;36:65-72
2. Singh V, Parakh A. What is new in the management of childhood tuberculosis in 2020? Indian Pediatrics. 2020;57:1172-6.
3. Concepcion NDP, Laya BF, Andronikou S, Daltro PAN, Sanchez MO, Uy JAU, et al. Standardized radiographic interpretation of thoracic tuberculosis in children. Pediatr Radiol. 2017;47(10):1237-48.
4. Bhalla AS, Goyal A, Guleria R, Gupta AK. Chest tuberculosis: Radiological review and imaging recommendations. Indian J Radiol Imaging. 2015;25(3):213-25.
5. George A, Andronikou S, Pillay T, Goussard P, Zar HJ. Intrathoracic tuberculous lymphadenopathy in children: a guide to chest radiography. Pediatr Radiol. 2017;47(10):1277-82.
6. Singh R, Naranje P, Bhalla AS, Pandey S. Magnetic resonance imaging in response assessment of mediastinal tuberculous lymphadenopathy: Going beyond size. Lung India. 2021;38(5):431-7.
7. Walker NF, Stek C, Wasserman S, Wilkinson RJ, Meintjes G. The tuberculosis-associated immune reconstitution inflammatory syndrome: recent advances in clinical and pathogenesis research. Curr Opin HIV AIDS. 2018;13(6):512-21.
8. Neyaz Z, Gadodia A, Gamanagatti S, Sarthi M. Imaging findings of congenital tuberculosis in three infants. Singapore Med J. 2008;49(2):e42-6.

CHAPTER 10

Chest Infections in Immunocompromised Host

Manisha Jana, Nitin Dhochak

- ❑ Primary immunodeficiency disorders (PIDs)
- ❑ Classification of PIDs
- ❑ Infections in immunodeficiency
- ❑ Noninfectious complications
- ❑ Specific primary immunodeficiency disorders
  - ➢ Predominantly humoral (B-cell) disorders
  - ➢ Cellular and combined (T-cell and B-cell) disorders
  - ➢ Phagocytic disorders (disorders of granulocyte, monocyte, and macrophages)
  - ➢ Complement deficiencies
  - ➢ Miscellaneous
- ❑ Secondary causes of immunodeficiency
  - ➢ Human immunodeficiency virus infection
- ❑ Approach on imaging

■ INTRODUCTION

- The term, immunocompromised hosts, refers to patients with a diminished immune function which may be inherited (primary immune deficiency disorders) or acquired. There are diverse etiologies of acquired diminution of immunity, including patients on immunosuppression for organ transplants (solid or hematopoietic), diabetes, acquired immunodeficiency syndrome (AIDS), or steroid therapy.
- These patients suffer from recurrent infections which can involve multiple systems including lung, gastrointestinal tract (GIT), skin, head, and neck. Besides infections, impaired immunity also results in other manifestations which include autoimmune disorders and certain malignancies. Pulmonary manifestations further include interstitial lung diseases (ILDs).[1-3]
- Imaging is an important component of monitoring and surveillance of patients with primary immunodeficiency disorder (PID). In addition, a diagnosis of PID and hence appropriate evaluation can be suggested in those with recurrent lower respiratory tract infection (LRTIs), aggressive infections, and lower lobe bronchiectasis.

- Chest radiographs with restricted use of CT form the imaging armamentarium. Low-dose CT technique can be employed. MR chest should be considered in those requiring frequent imaging.

PRIMARY IMMUNODEFICIENCY DISORDERS (PIDs)

The term, PIDs, refers to disorders wherein genetic defects result in impairment of immunity.[4] While incidence of individual entities is rare, when assessed together, the reported prevalence is about 1–4 per 1,000 (accessed on 22/4/2022, *uptodate.com*). Several of these result from mutation in a single gene. However, several different mutations may result in a clinically similar phenotype. The term "inborn errors of immunity (IEI)" is also employed.

The clinical manifestations in PIDs are often multisystem, and several are associated with characteristic abnormalities such as cardiac or skeletal anomalies. Thorax, particularly the lungs, is frequently affected in PIDs.

CLASSIFICATION OF PIDS

- The classification system followed by most centers is the one given by International Union of Immunological Societies (IUIS), wherein there are 10 categories.[5] Common causes are enlisted in **Table 1**.
- The other less common categories include autoinflammatory diseases, complement deficiencies, bone marrow failure, and phenocopies of PIDs. Phenocopies refer to disorders that can mimic IEI.
- A simpler way to comprehend PIDs and associated complications is to consider two broad categories—those of adaptive and innate immunity **(Table 2)**. Adaptive immunity refers to T-cell, and B-cell-mediated, or combined immunodeficiencies. Innate immunodeficiency refers to a deficiency of immune response which is mediated by neutrophil and complements. Innate immune system is fast and nonspecific.

TABLE 1: Common causes of primary immunodeficiency disorders.

Cellular and humoral immunodeficiency	Severe combined immunodeficiency
Antibody deficiency	• Common variable immunodeficiency • Agammaglobulinemia (X-linked or autosomal recessive) • Hyper-IgM • Selective IgA deficiency
Syndromic combined immunodeficiencies	• Hyper-IgE • Wiskott–Aldrich syndrome
Immune dysregulatory diseases	Chediak–Higashi syndrome
Phagocytic disorders	• Chronic granulomatous disease • Leukocyte adhesion defect

TABLE 2: Disorders of adaptive and innate immunity.	
Disorders of adaptive immunity	**Disorders of innate immunity**
T-cell IDs (usually part of combined, not isolated) *B-cell IDs:* • Common variable immunodeficiency • X-linked agammaglobulinemia • Hyper-IgM syndrome *Combined IDs:* • Severe combined immunodeficiency syndrome • DiGeorge syndrome • Hyper-IgE syndrome • Ataxia telangiectasia • Wiskott–Aldrich syndrome	• Phagocytic disorders • Complement deficiency disorders

(ID: immunodeficiency)

- The discussion in this chapter is based on pulmonary complications and their imaging patterns, and subsequently, a brief discussion of specific entities. Only the more common PIDs will be discussed.

■ INFECTIONS IN IMMUNODEFICIENCY

- The site and causative organism for various infections in immunocompromised host depend on the type of immunodeficiency. This is described in **Table 3**.

TABLE 3: Causative organisms in various immunodeficiency disorders.		
Category	**Site of infection**	**Causative organism**
Humoral (B-cell) immunodeficiency	Respiratory tract, GIT, skin infections, meningitis, and sepsis	*Pneumococcus* **(Figs. 1A and B)**, *Haemophilus, Staphylococcus aureus, Meningococcus,* and *Pseudomonas*
Combined T- and B-cell immunodeficiency	Systemic viral infections, GIT	Viruses (especially RSV and EBV), *Pneumocystis, Toxoplasma, Cryptosporidium,* nontubercular mycobacteria
Phagocytic disorders	Respiratory tract, liver abscess, lung abscess, GIT, and urinary tract	*Candida, Nocardia* **(Figs. 2A to D)**, *Aspergillus, Staphylococcus, Pseudomonas,* nontubercular mycobacteria
Complement deficiency	Meningitis, systemic bacterial infections	*Neisseria, Haemophilus, Streptococci, CMV,* and *HSV*

(CMV: *Cytomegalovirus*; EBV: Epstein–Barr virus; GIT: gastrointestinal tract; HSV: herpes simplex virus; RSV: respiratory syncytial virus)

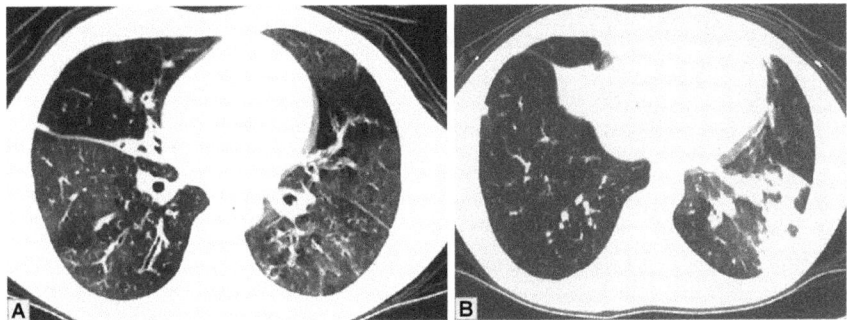

FIGS. 1A AND B: Acquired immunodeficiency after splenectomy, presenting with recurrent pneumococcal pneumonia. Diffuse central bronchiectasis. RML collapse and left lower lobe consolidation.
(RML: right middle lo be)

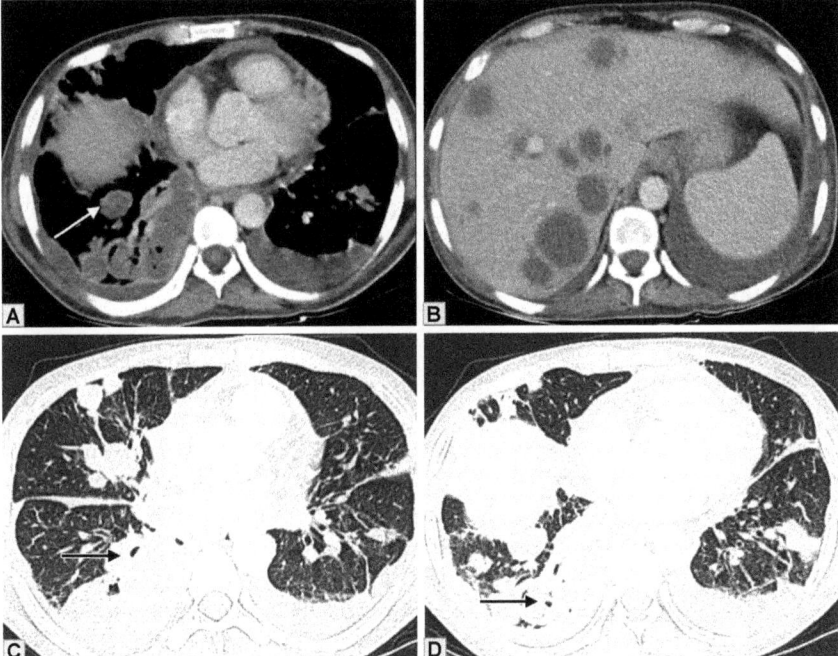

FIGS. 2A TO D: Secondary cellular and combined immunodeficiency in a patient of nephrotic syndrome with long-term corticosteroid treatment. Disseminated nocardia infection. Low attenuation lung nodules (arrow) and pleural effusion (A). Multiple hepatic abscesses (B). Multiple lung nodules, few showing cavitation (arrows in C and D).

- In children living with HIV (CLHIV), the risk of developing pulmonary infections complications is related to the decrease in CD4 cell count in addition to the other risk factors. **Table 4** summarizes the pulmonary infections in relation to the CD4 cell count.

TABLE 4: Pulmonary infections in HIV related to CD4 cell count.

CD4 cell count (cells/mm^3)	Infections
<50	• Cytomegalovirus pneumonia • Disseminated fungal infections • Disseminated mycobacterial infections (tubercular/nontubercular)
50–100	• Nocardia pneumonia • *Mycobacterium avium* complex • *Histoplasma capsulatum* • *Coccidioides* species • *Blastomyces* species • *Invasive aspergillus* • *Toxoplasma gondii*
100–200	• *Rhodococcus equi* • Mycobacterial tuberculosis (primary pattern) • Pneumocystis pneumonia
200–400	• Recurrent bacterial infections • Mycobacterial tuberculosis (reactivation pattern)
400–500	Bacterial infections
Any CD4 cell count	Bacterial pneumonia

NONINFECTIOUS COMPLICATIONS

- Noninfectious complications of PIDs are described in **Table 5**, and complications in acquired immunodeficiency (HIV) in **Table 6**.
- Interstitial lung disease in the background of common variable immunodeficiency (CVID) can be of various types. Commoner are organizing pneumonia, lymphocytic interstitial pneumonia (LIP), and *granulomatous lymphocytic ILD (GL-ILD)*. GL-ILD is an unusual complication of CVID. It shows a mixed restrictive and obstructive pattern on pulmonary function test. On imaging, it manifests as consolidation, septal thickening, nodule (GGO/solid) having a peribronchial distribution and lower lobe predominance. It is usually associated with lymphadenopathy and splenomegaly, and has a poor prognosis.
- *Kaposi's sarcoma* is classically associated with CD4 cell count of <200; however, few reports suggest its occurrence in CD4 cell count of >300 also. Common imaging findings include poorly defined lung nodules, peribronchovascular consolidation with flame-shaped hilar radiation, ground-glass opacities, interlobular septal thickening, and fissural nodules.

TABLE 5: Noninfectious complications in primary immunodeficiency disorders.

CVID	- Sarcoid-like lymphadenopathy - ILD
	NHL: - Incidence increased (approximately 7%) - Usually extranodal
IgA deficiency	- Autoimmune thrombocytopenic purpura - Autoimmune hemolytic anemia - Juvenile rheumatoid arthritis and thyroiditis
Hyper-IgE syndrome	- Osteopenia, easy fracturability - Aneurysms
SCID	ILD (ADA-deficient variety of SCID): Pulmonary alveolar proteinosis pattern
Wiskott–Aldrich syndrome	- Lymphoma, myeloproliferative disorders - Kaposi's sarcoma - Necrotizing vasculitis and aneurysm formation
Ataxia telangiectasia	- Cerebellar degeneration - Radiation sensitivity
Chronic granulomatous disease	- Lymphadenopathy - Antral fistula - Esophagitis and esophageal strictures - GI strictures
Hyper-IgM syndrome	- Autoimmune disorders (arthritis, inflammatory bowel disease) - Susceptibility to hepatobiliary neoplasms

(ADA: adenosine deaminase; CVID: common variable immunodeficiency; GI: gastrointestinal; Ig: immunoglobulin; ILD: interstitial lung disease; NHL: non-Hodgkin's lymphoma; SCID: severe combined immunodeficiency)

TABLE 6: Noninfectious complications associated with HIV.

Hodgkin's lymphoma	- Associated with Epstein–Barr virus infection - Risk is highest with CD4 count between 225 and 249 cells/mL[9]
Kaposi's sarcoma	- Most common AIDS-defining malignancy - Associated with HHV-8, also known as Kaposi sarcoma-associated herpes virus
Multicentric Castleman's disease	- Also associated with HHV-8 - CD4 count is usually >200 cell/mL
Primary effusion lymphoma	- Rare complication associated with HHV-8 - B-cell NHL presenting as effusion with no solid pleural masses - Poor prognosis
Pulmonary artery hypertension	- Prevalence in HIV-infected patients is approximately 25 times higher than the non-HIV infected - Increased chance at counts <200 cells/mL
Diffuse infiltrative lymphocytosis syndrome	Manifests as a Sjögren-like disease causing bilateral parotitis, lymph nodal enlargement, and involvement of lungs, nervous system, liver, kidneys, and digestive tract

(HHV-8: human herpes virus 8; HIV: human immunodeficiency virus; NHL: non-Hodgkin's lymphoma)

- *Multicentric Castleman's disease* is a lymphoproliferative disorder which clinically presents with recurrent fever, malaise, and weight loss. The imaging features include hilar, mediastinal and axillary enhancing lymph node enlargement, ill-defined centrilobular nodules, peribronchovascular thickening, ground-glass opacities, and consolidation.
- *Diffuse infiltrative lymphocytosis syndrome* is a rare multisystem syndrome seen in HIV-infected patients resulting from CD8+ cell proliferation and infiltration into various organs. Various manifestations of this syndrome are as follows:
- *Lymphocytic interstitial pneumonia*:
  - LIP is part of lymphocytosis syndrome associated with Epstein–Barr virus (EBV).
  - It is commoner in HIV-infected children than adults and is AIDS-defining illness in the former.
  - It is usually seen at near-normal CD4 cell counts.
  - Patients respond to initiation of antiretroviral therapy (ART) alone.
  - Imaging features include ill-defined centrilobular and subpleural nodules, ground-glass opacities, basal reticulations, interlobular septal thickening, and thin-walled cysts **(Figs. 3A to C)**.

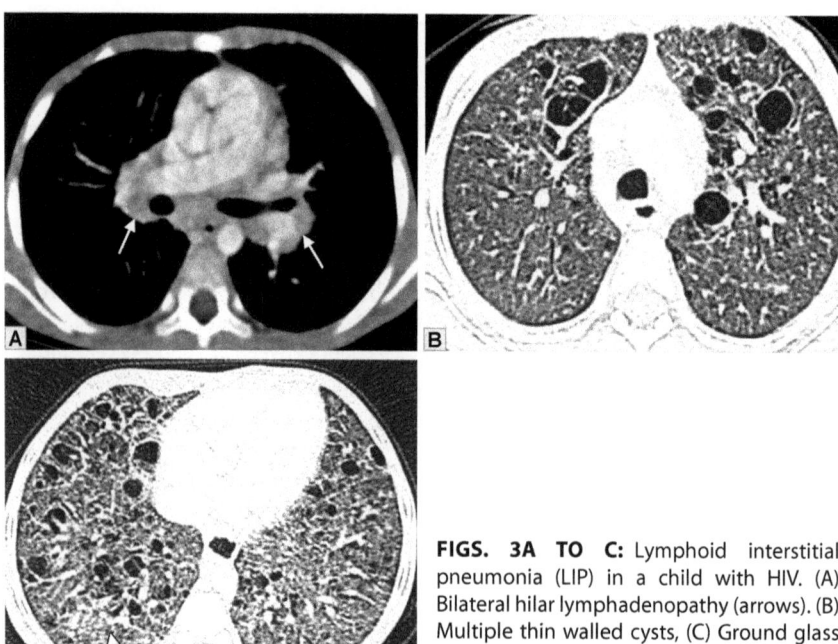

FIGS. 3A TO C: Lymphoid interstitial pneumonia (LIP) in a child with HIV. (A) Bilateral hilar lymphadenopathy (arrows). (B) Multiple thin walled cysts, (C) Ground glass opacity, cysts and perilymphatic nodules (arrow).

- *Multilocular thymic cysts (MTC)*:
  - Also part of lymphocytosis syndrome
  - Usually benign, rarely undergo malignant transformation
  - On imaging, they present as anterior mediastinal multilocular cystic mass which may show areas of soft tissue attenuation on CT.
- *Follicular bronchiolitis (FB)*:
  - Reactive condition characterized pathologically by lymphoid follicles confined to the peribronchial region
  - Seen in both children and adults with HIV positivity
  - Usually resolve with highly active ART
  - It may mimic chronic obstructive pulmonary disease (COPD) clinically
  - Imaging features include centrilobular and peribronchial nodules with or without peribronchial thickening and occasional GGO.

■ SPECIFIC PRIMARY IMMUNODEFICIENCY DISORDERS

Predominantly Humoral (B-cell) Disorders

These are the most common PIDs comprising about 70% of these disorders:[6]

- These defects result in impaired antibody production and are a heterogeneous group comprising several disorders.
- Host response to bacterial infection requires the combined action of antibodies, complement system, and phagocytes.
- A defect in any of these three components will lead to recurrent pyogenic infections especially with encapsulated bacteria.

In the primary forms, affected children present with recurrent otitis media, sinusitis, pneumonia or even meningitis or septicemia.

Common Variable Immunodeficiency (Figs. 4A to C)

- In CVID, there are absent or very low circulating antibodies, but B cell number is normal.
- All major classes of antibodies are affected
- On occurrence of stimulation, B cells respond and proliferate in number but are unable to further differentiate and produce antibodies.
- Age of presentation is variable (early childhood to adulthood) and both sexes may be affected.
- Patients present with recurrent sinopulmonary infections, meningoencephalitis in late childhood or adulthood.
- Splenomegaly and lymphadenopathy, lymphoid hyperplasia of the gastrointestinal tract (GIT), and generalized lymphoproliferative disorders are also seen.
- Patients are prone to develop interstitial lung disease (ILD), bronchiectasis, and lymphoreticular malignancies.
- Granulomatous lymphocytic ILD (GLILD) is a diffuse lung disease seen in up to 15% patients of the CVID.

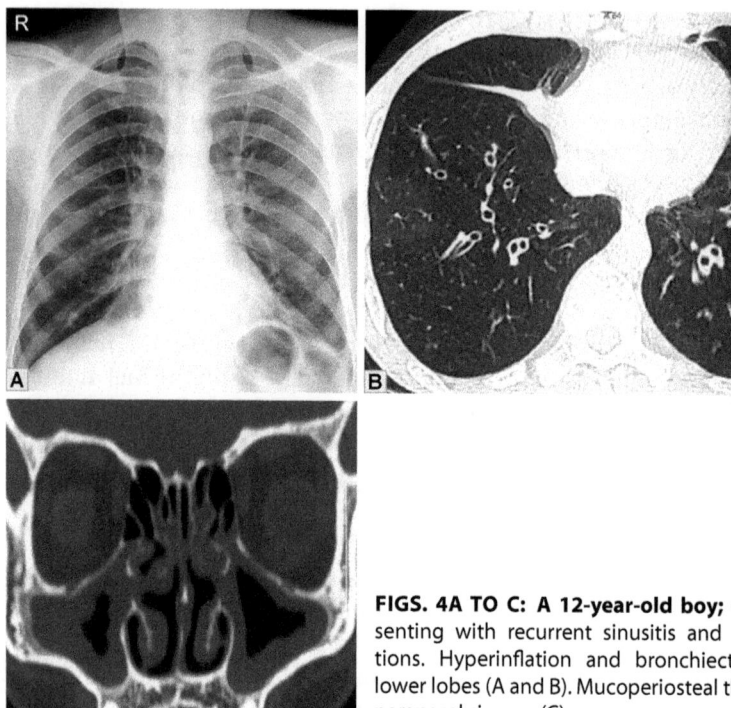

FIGS. 4A TO C: A 12-year-old boy; CVID representing with recurrent sinusitis and chest infections. Hyperinflation and bronchiectasis in the lower lobes (A and B). Mucoperiosteal thickening of paranasal sinuses (C).
(CVID: common variable immunodeficiency)

X-linked Agammaglobulinemia

(*Synonym:* Bruton's agammaglobulinemia)
- Less common than IgA deficiency or CVID
- Absent circulating antibodies, markedly reduced number of circulating mature B cells
- During the first 6–9 months of life, maternal IgG antibodies protect the infant from infections.
- Patients present in late infancy or early childhood with recurrent sinopulmonary infections, enteroviral meningoencephalitis, and intestinal giardiasis.
- *Imaging*: Middle and lower lobe bronchiectasis, typically small adenoids (and other lymphoid tissues)
- The comparison between two major humoral immunodeficiencies—CVID and X-linked agammaglobulinemia is presented in **Table 7**.

IgA Deficiency

- Most common primary immunodeficiency disorder
- Frequent in Caucasian populations
- Varied spectrum, with several affected children being asymptomatic

CHAPTER 10: Chest Infections in Immunocompromised Host

TABLE 7: Comparison between CVID and X-linked agammaglobulinemia.

	CVID	X-linked agammaglobulinemia
Age of onset	Variable, early childhood to adulthood	Early childhood
Defect	• Low levels of circulating antibodies • B cells normal	Low levels of mature B cells and plasma cells
T cell functions	Abnormal in up to 60% patients	Normal
Infections	Recurrent sinopulmonary infections	Similar, but chronic meningo-encephalitis more common
Imaging	• Pneumonia • Atelectasis • Bronchial wall thickening • Bronchiectasis • Normal or increased lymphoid tissue—lymphadenopathy • Splenomegaly	*Similar:* • Bronchiectasis in lower and middle lobes • Lymphoid tissues (e.g., adenoids, tonsil) small or absent • No splenomegaly • Meningitis or encephalitis
Autoimmune disorders and malignancies	• Autoimmune disorders seen in up to 20% patients • Lymphoreticular malignancies	Increased malignancy risk
Treatment	Intravenous immunoglobulin replacement	Similar

(CVID: common variable immunodeficiency)

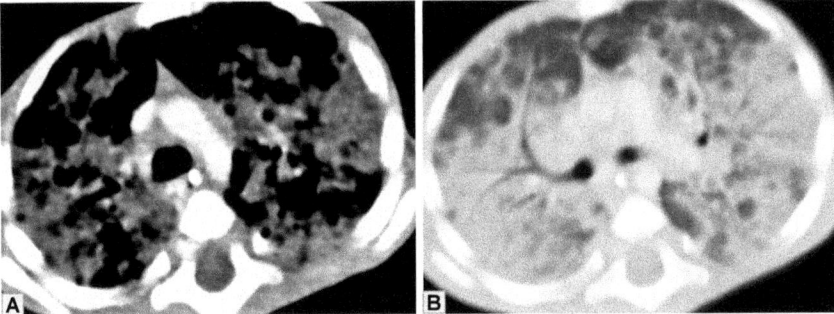

FIGS. 5A AND B: IgA deficiency. Areas of consolidation in both lungs (A). Septal thickening in both upper lobes (B).

- Affected individuals are prone to respiratory and GIT infections, allergy, autoimmune disorders, and also malignancies.
- Imaging findings are mostly related to the recurrent pyogenic infections **(Figs. 5A and B)**.
- Treatment is mostly supportive.

Hyper-IgM Syndrome
- This primary immunodeficiency disease is associated with diminished levels of IgG with normal or increased circulating IgM levels.
- This may be X-linked or non-X-linked.
- Similar to other disorders of this group, recurrent pyogenic infections are seen.

Cellular and Combined (T-cell and B-cell) Disorders
- Disorders of cellular immunodeficiency should be suspected in those with severe/recurrent viral infections. These disorders also result in fungal infections (cutaneous/systemic), parasitic infections, acid-fast bacilli, and *Pneumocystis jirovecii* infections.
- T-cell disorders nearly always have associated poor humoral immunity, as antibody production is dependent on T cells.
- Immunization with live vaccines (e.g., BCG) should be avoided in the severe forms.
- These babies are also prone to graft-versus-host reaction to blood transfusions.

DiGeorge Syndrome
(*Synonym*: Thymic aplasia or hypoplasia)
- Failure of development of the third and fourth pharyngeal pouches results in absent/hypoplastic thymus with dysmorphic facies.
- Tetany (resulting from lack of the parathyroid) and congenital defects of the heart and great vessels are also present.
- Associated with congenital cardiovascular anomalies (conotruncal abnormalities, tetralogy of Fallot, interrupted aortic arch, double aortic arch, and right-sided aortic arch), gastrointestinal, renal anomalies, and cognitive delay.
- *Chest radiograph*: Narrow superior mediastinum, findings due to the aortic anomalies (e.g., right-sided aortic arch) and cardiac anomalies **(Figs. 6A and B)**.
- *Computed tomography (CT)*: Variable severity—hypoplasia or aplasia of thymus **(Figs. 7A and B)**.
- Treatment is mostly supportive, those with the severe complete form may require BMT.

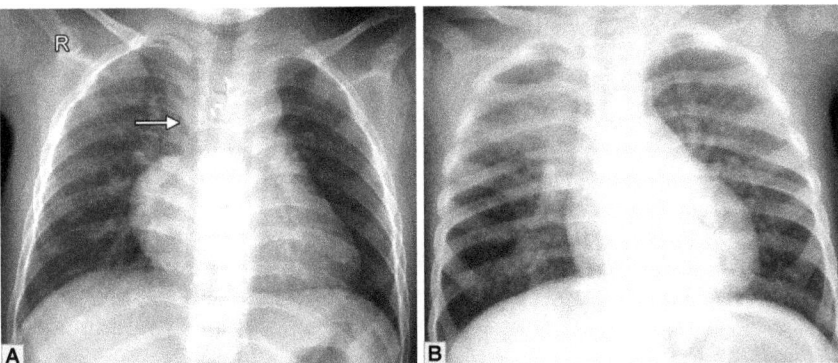

FIGS. 6A AND B: Radiographic findings in thymic hypoplasia and aplasia. Thymic aplasia (A) in an infant: Narrow cardiac pedicle (arrow). Associated cardiac anomalies suggested by surgical clips. Thymic hypoplasia (B) in 10-month-old infant: Narrow cardiac pedicle and absent thymic shadow on radiograph (B).

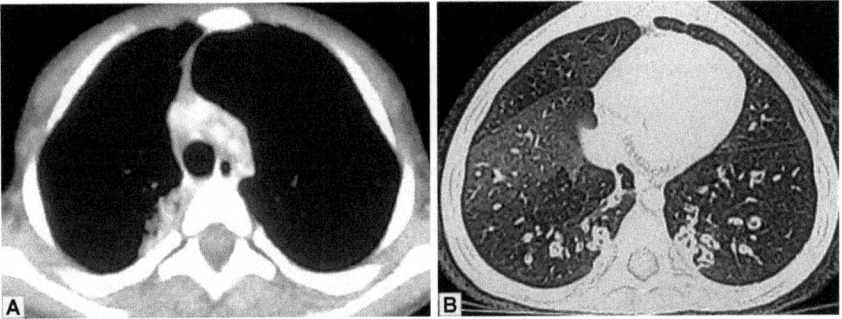

FIGS. 7A AND B: Imaging findings in thymic hypoplasia/aplasia. Thymic hypoplasia in 10-month-old infant. Very small thymus (A). Bronchiectasis of both lower lobes secondary to recurrent infection and aspiration (B).

Severe Combined Immunodeficiency

- Severe combined immunodeficiency (SCID) is a group of disorders characterized by absent T cell and B cell function [natural killer (NK) cells may also be affected].
- Presents in infancy, with male infants being more frequently affected.
- Typical presentation is with failure to thrive, chronic diarrhea, rashes, pneumonia, oral thrush, and sepsis since early infancy.
- *Adenosine deaminase (ADA) deficiency subtype*: Characteristic skeletal imaging findings with flared anterior costochondral junctions, metaphyseal cupping, squaring of scapular tip, and "bone in bone" appearance of vertebral bodies.
- *Chest imaging*: Recurrent or severe pneumonia [usual organisms include *Pneumocystis jirovecii*, respiratory syncytial virus (RSV), cytomegalovirus (CMV), and bacteria]

- Thymic shadow is absent.
- *Treatment*: Bone marrow transplant (BMT)

Partial Combined Immunodeficiency Syndromes

These include multiple entities such as Wiskott–Aldrich syndrome, ataxia telangiectasia, and cartilage-hair hypoplasia.

Wiskott–Aldrich syndrome:
- X-linked recessive disorder which comprises the triad—eczema, thrombocytopenia (small defective platelets), and recurrent infections
- Complications include massive bleed, infection, and lymphoreticular malignancy.

Ataxia telangiectasia:
- Characterized by ataxia, cutaneous and conjunctival telangiectasia, oculomotor apraxia, and partial immunodeficiency **(Figs. 8A to D)**
- The patients are prone to develop lymphoma, T-cell leukemias, and breast and ovarian cancers.

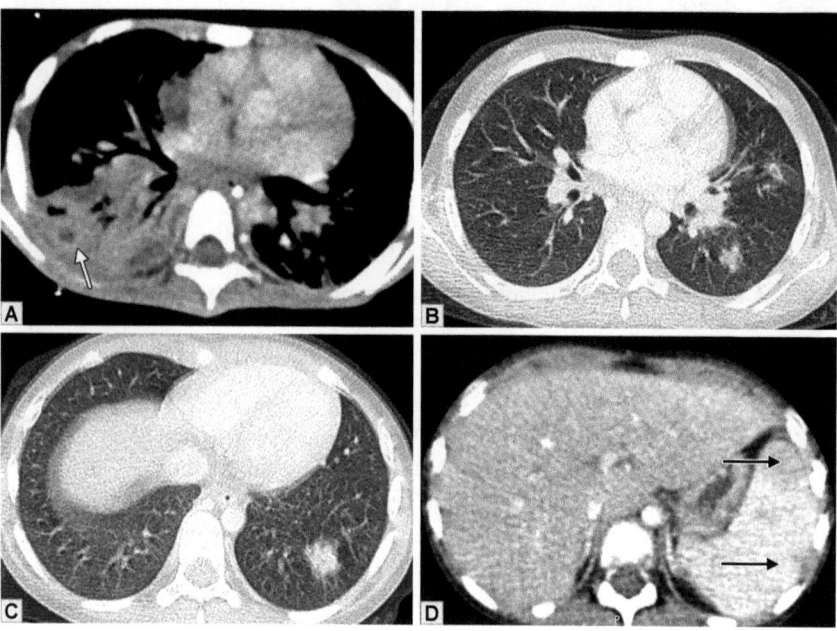

FIGS. 8A TO D: Ataxia telangiectasia, presenting with staphylococcal infection. Axial soft tissue (A), lung window (B and C), and contrast-enhanced computed tomography abdomen (D). Right lower lobe consolidation with central liquefaction (arrow in A). Multifocal nodules (B and C). Multiple peripheral splenic infarcts (arrows in D).

Phagocytic Disorders (Disorders of Granulocyte, Monocyte, and Macrophages)
Chronic Granulomatous Disease
- Presents in infancy
- Pulmonary infection commonly caused by *Staphylococcus, Aspergillus, Burkholderia, Nocardia* (**Figs. 9A to D**).
- Common infections may present with unusual imaging appearances.
- Aspergillus infection in CGD can present with multilobar consolidation, nodules, and conglomerate necrotic mediastinal lymphadenopathy.
- Lymphadenopathy, hepatic and splenic granuloma formation, antral stricture, duodenal fold thickening, and enteric fistulas.[7]
- Mucormycosis in CGD can have a locally aggressive mass-like appearance and adjacent bone/chest wall infiltration.[8]

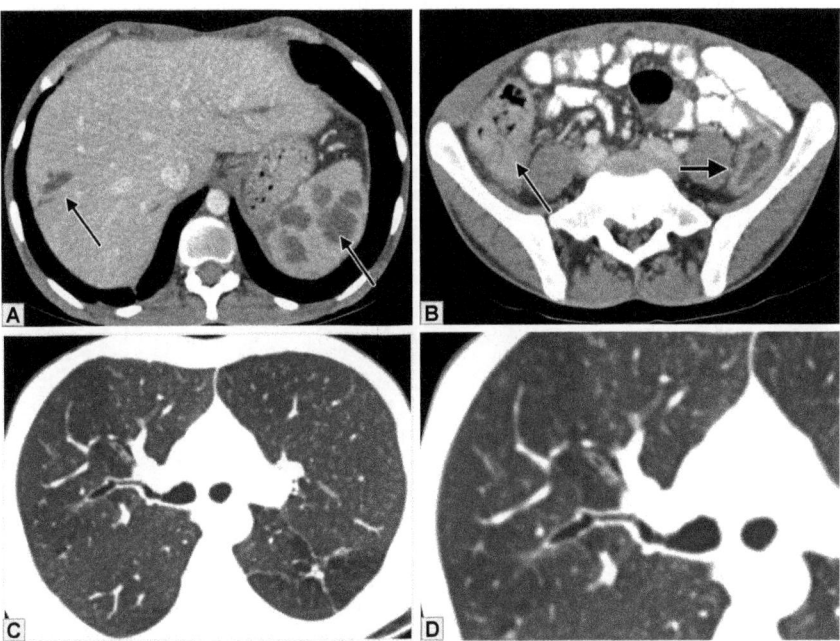

FIGS. 9A TO D: Chronic granulomatous disease. Resolving hepatic abscess (arrows in A). Multiple splenic abscesses. Enlarged retroperitoneal lymph nodes (not shown). Wall thickening of cecum (thin arrow in B) and descending colon (thick arrow in B). Bronchiectasis and air trapping secondary to recurrent chest infections (C and D).

Leukocyte Adhesion Defect
- It presents in infancy with delayed separation of umbilical cord, umbilical cord and skin infections.
- Group of phagocytic disorders where there is a defect in transport of leukocytes from blood vessels to the site of injury.
- The most common type is caused by defect in *integrin-b* gene.
- Marked neutrophilic leukocytosis and absence of pus are indicators of this disorder.
- Common causative organisms include *Staphylococcus*, *Pseudomonas*, *Klebsiella*, various fungi, and *Acinetobacter* (**Figs. 10A to D**).

Cyclical Neutropenia
- It is a rare autosomal dominant disorder presenting with cyclical neutropenia (every 14–35 days).
- It usually presents in the 1st year of life.
- Clostridial sepsis leading to intestinal ulceration and bleeding is a life-threatening complication.

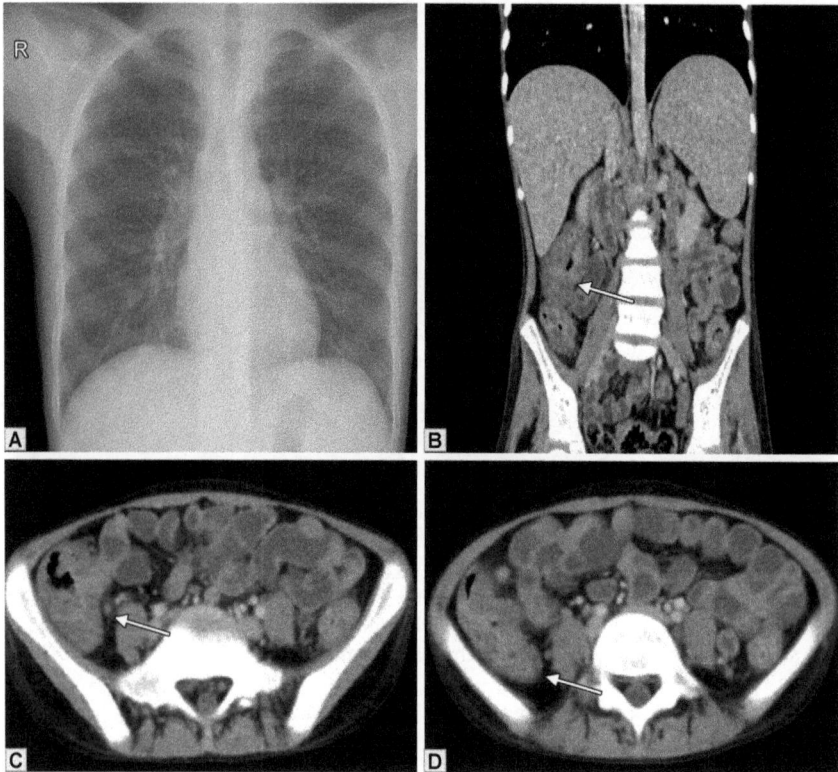

FIGS. 10A TO D: Leukocyte adhesion defect in a 10-year-old boy, with suspected tuberculosis. Chest radiograph (A), coronal (B) and axial CECT abdomen (C and D). Bilateral lower zone early bronchiectasis (A). Mural thickening of IC junction and cecum (arrows in B to D).

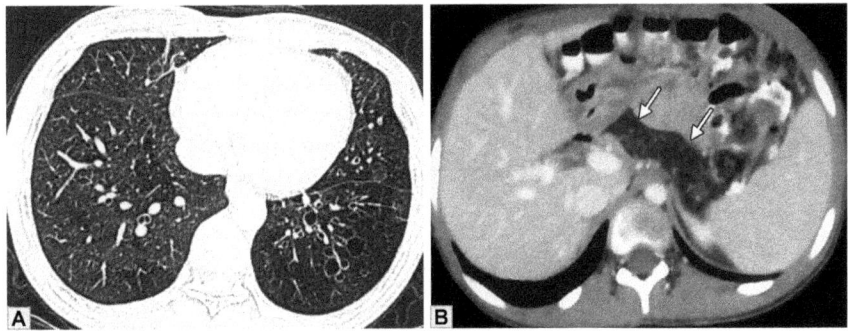

FIGS. 11A AND B: Shwachman diamond syndrome with episodes of neutropenia. Bilateral lower lobe bronchiectasis (A). Fatty replacement of pancreas, without any calcification (arrows in B) (B). Sweat chloride test was negative, ruling out cystic fibrosis.

Shwachman–Diamond Syndrome
- It is a rare inherited disorder that mimics cyclical neutropenia, but usually associated with dysmorphic facies and skeletal abnormality.
- Neutropenia and bone marrow failure
- Pancreas shows fatty atrophy **(Figs. 11A and B)**.

Complement Deficiencies
- These are the most rare form of PIDDs.
- Different forms show variable severity.
- Complement factor 1-4 deficiencies have more frequent pyogenic infections, while those with complement factor 5-9 deficiencies are prone to *Nocardia* infection.

Miscellaneous
- *Hyper-IgE syndrome* is a form of PIDD presenting in infancy with recurrent staphylococcal infections and increased serum IgE levels **(Figs. 12A to C)**.

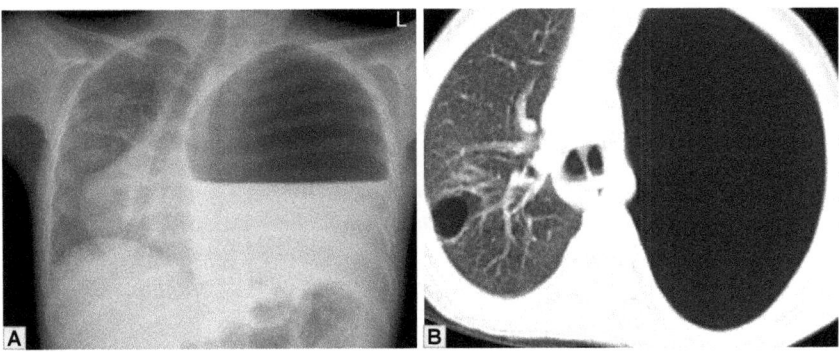

FIGS. 12A TO C: *Continued*

Continued

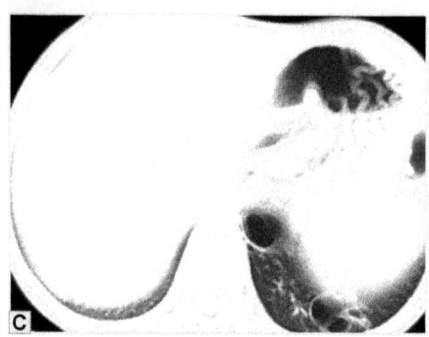

FIGS. 12A TO C: A 10-year-old boy with hyper-IgE syndrome. Recurrent staphylococcal pneumonia. Large pneumatocele with air fluid level in left lung (A). Large left upper lobe pneumatocele and multiple other variable sized pneumatoceles in both lungs (B and C).

- Imaging findings are of recurrent pneumonia with multiple, often persistent pneumatoceles.
- Osteopenia is also seen. Coarse facial features, retained primary teeth, are other clinical associations.

Mendelian Susceptibility to Mycobacterial Diseases
- Mendelian susceptibility to mycobacterial diseases (MSMD) is a group of rare genetic disorders characterized by susceptibility of the individual to mycobacterial pathogens.
- The genotype is heterogeneous; and till date, approximately 19 genes in the interaction between T cell/NK cell and phagocytes have been implicated in this disorder. The most severe of them are caused by interferon-gamma receptor 1 and 2 deficiency **(Figs. 13A to E)**.
- The clinical presentation also varies—from presenting at neonatal/early infancy period with accelerated BCG response (BCGosis) to recurrent infections with various mycobacteria during infancy, early childhood, or adolescence.[9]
- In addition to mycobacterium tuberculosis and nontubercular mycobacteria, these patients are prone to infection by several other microorganisms such as *Salmonella typhi*, other *Salmonella* species, *Burkholderia*, *Listeria*, *Leishmania donovani*, *Cryptococcus*, *Histoplasma capsulatum*, and *Coccidioidomycoses*. The infection causing organism in MSMD patients varies depending upon the local prevalence of diseases.
- The causative organism sometimes can provide a clue to the underlying immune defect genotype. For example, mycobacterial infection with CMV infection suggests complete autosomal recessive variant of interferon-gamma (IFN-γ) receptor R1/R2 defect, or complete STAT-1 defect.
- Presentation can be with multiorgan involvement.
- Multifocal tubercular osteomyelitis can also be seen in IFN-γσ receptor deficiency
- In selected subtypes, IFN can be helpful. Hematopoietic stem cell transplantation (HSCT) is the management of choice.

CHAPTER 10: Chest Infections in Immunocompromised Host

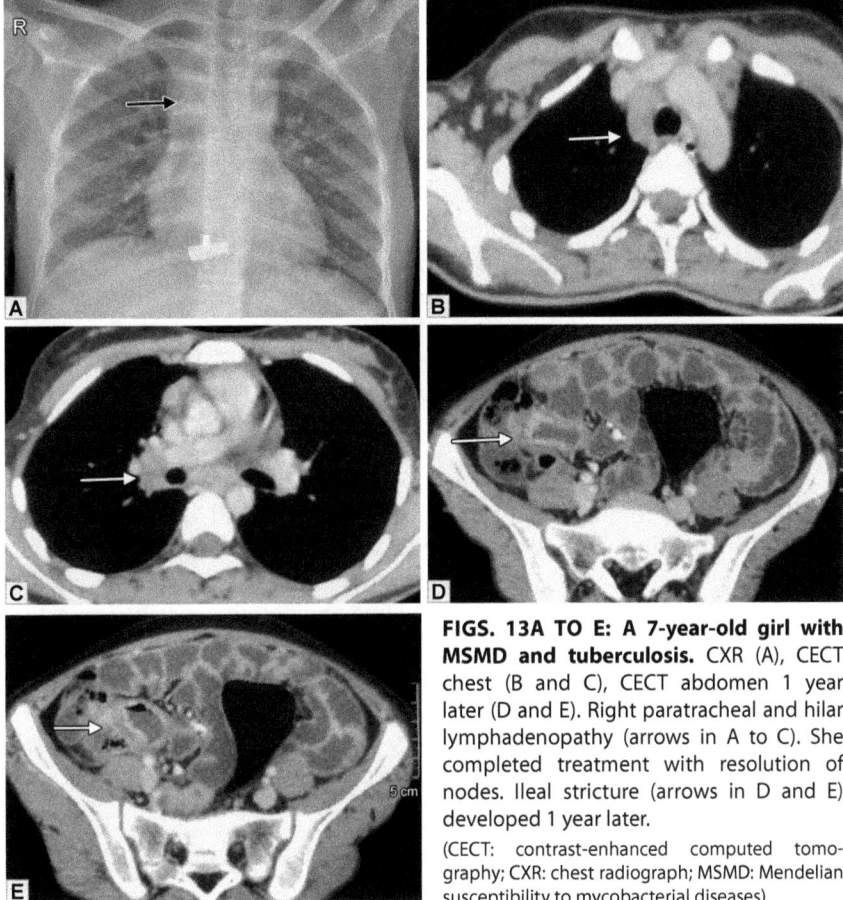

FIGS. 13A TO E: A 7-year-old girl with MSMD and tuberculosis. CXR (A), CECT chest (B and C), CECT abdomen 1 year later (D and E). Right paratracheal and hilar lymphadenopathy (arrows in A to C). She completed treatment with resolution of nodes. Ileal stricture (arrows in D and E) developed 1 year later.
(CECT: contrast-enhanced computed tomography; CXR: chest radiograph; MSMD: Mendelian susceptibility to mycobacterial diseases)

■ SECONDARY CAUSES OF IMMUNODEFICIENCY

Various secondary causes can cause immunodeficiency, by affecting different components of the immune system. The infectious and noninfectious complications of HIV will be discussed in this chapter.

Human Immunodeficiency Virus Infection
- Human immunodeficiency virus (HIV) and acquired immunodeficiency syndrome (AIDS) are modern pandemics first identified >40 years ago.
- There are multiple direct and indirect manifestations of the disease with significant morbidity and mortality.
- The clinical scenario has changed with the introduction of effective ART, with more lasting and chronic complications compared to pre-ART era, when HIV-related deaths were more numerous.

- There is a similar change in the incidence of classic AIDS-defining illnesses. However, the non-AIDS-defining illnesses continue to cause morbidity in these patients with respiratory disease being one of the most common.[1]

The spectrum of HIV-related pulmonary involvement may be categorized based on the following:
- *AIDS-defining diseases*: Among the exhaustive list of AIDS-defining illnesses, recurrent pneumonias, *Pneumocystis jirovecii* pneumonia, Kaposi sarcoma, mycobacterial infections, LIP, or pulmonary lymphoid hyperplasia complex is important respiratory condition that will be discussed subsequently [Centre for Disease Control and Prevention (CDC)].[2]
- *Pulmonary complications*—which may be infectious or noninfectious.[3]

APPROACH ON IMAGING

- The imaging findings in immunodeficiency depend on the causative organism, and are listed in **Table 8**. While there is significant overlap in imaging findings of various causative organisms as well as various subgroups of PIDD, sometimes a few imaging pointers may be indicative of a specific organism.
- Additionally, sometimes there may be some specific imaging markers, which can be crucial in narrowing the differential diagnosis **(Table 9)**. Both extrapulmonary and pulmonary imaging findings guide the nature of further investigations/sampling **(Figs. 14A to D)**.

TABLE 8: Pattern-based approach in identifying causative organism in PIDD.	
Radiologic pattern	Causative organism
Lobar consolidation	Bacterial infection
Multifocal consolidation	Bacterial, invasive fungal
Consolidation crossing the fissures	Invasive fungal
"Mass-like" consolidation	Invasive fungal (mucor and *Aspergillus*)
Necrotic lymphadenopathy and conglomeration	Invasive fungal and TB
Contiguous chest wall invasion	Invasive fungal and TB
(PIDD: primary immunodeficiency disease; TB: tuberculosis)	

CHAPTER 10: Chest Infections in Immunocompromised Host

TABLE 9: Imaging clues toward different PIDDs.

Thoracic findings	Type of PIDDs
Absent/small thymic shadow	• DiGeorge syndrome • SCID • Partial combined immunodeficiency syndromes
Bronchiectasis	CVID
Persistent/expanding pneumatoceles	Hyper-IgE syndrome
Diffuse alveolar hemorrhage (DAH)	Wiskott–Aldrich syndrome
Empyema/IPFCs	Hyper-IgE syndrome
Associated findings	
Skeletal abnormalities: • Flared anterior end of rib • Metaphyseal cupping • Vertebral "bone within bone" appearance • Squared scapular tip	SCID (ADA deficiency subtype)
Osteopenia	Hyper-IgE syndrome
Aortic arch anomalies	DiGeorge syndrome
Cardiac defects	DiGeorge syndrome
Short-limb dwarfism, metaphyseal dysplasia	Cartilage hair hypoplasia
Liver and splenic abscess, abdominal adenopathy	Chronic granulomatous disorder
Gastric antral narrowing and duodenal fold thickening	Chronic granulomatous disorder
Ureteral/urethral strictures, UB wall thickening, and renal infections	Chronic granulomatous disorder
Osteomyelitis	Chronic granulomatous disorder
Splenomegaly, tonsillar/adenoid enlargement	• CVID • X-linked agammaglobulinemia

(ADA: adenosine deaminase; CVID: common variable immunodeficiency; IPFC: infected pleural fluid collection; PIDD: primary immunodeficiency disease; SCID: severe combined immunodeficiency)

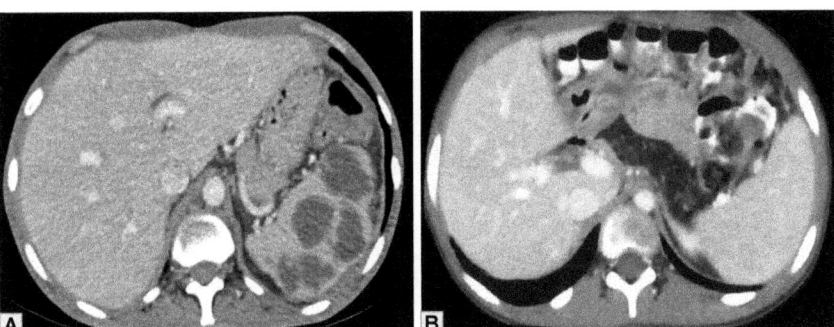

FIGS. 14A TO D: *Continued*

Continued

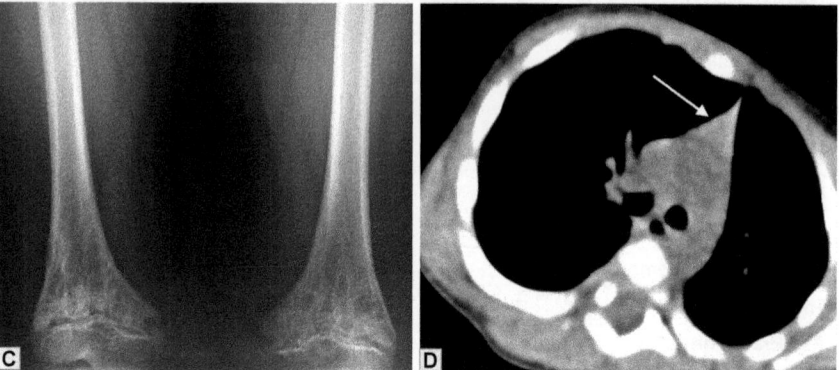

FIGS. 14A TO D: Imaging pointers in various immunodeficiencies. Deep organ (splenic) abscesses in chronic granulomatous disorder (A). Pancreatic fatty atrophy in Shwachman–Diamond syndrome (B). Metaphyseal chondrodysplasia in cartilage hair hypoplasia (C). Small thymic shadow in thymic hypoplasia (arrow in D).

Other Related Chapters that can be Referred to:
- Chapter 8: Fungal Chest Infections
- Chapter 16: Bronchiectasis

REFERENCES

1. Reda SM, ElGhoneimy DH, Afifi HM. Clinical predictors of primary immunodeficiency diseases in children. Allergy Asthma Immunol Res. 2013;5(2):88-95.
2. Ahuja J, Kanne JP. Thoracic infections in immunocompromised patients. Radiol Clin N Am. 2014;52:121-36.
3. Oh YW, Effmann EL, Godwin JD. Pulmonary infections in immunocompromised hosts: the importance of correlating the conventional radiologic appearance with the clinical setting. Radiology. 2000;217(3):647-56.
4. Jeffrey Modell Foundation. National Primary Immunodeficiency Resource Center. [online] Available from http://www.info4pi.org. [Last accessed August, 2018].
5. Bousfiha AA, Moundir A, Tangye SG, Picard C, Jeddane L, Al-Herz W, et al. The 2022 Update of IUIS Phenotypical Classification for Human Inborn Errors of Immunity. J Clin Immunol. 2022;42(7):1508-20.
6. Yin EZ, Frush DP, Donnelly LF, Buckley RH. Primary immunodeficiency disorders in pediatric patients: clinical features and imaging findings. Am J Roentgenol. 2001;176:1541-52.
7. Sherwani P, Bhalla AS, Jana M, Naranje P, Kabra SK, Gupta AK, et al. Thoracic manifestations of primary immunodeficiency disorders. Indian J Pediatr. 2020;87(10):846-9.
8. Jana M, Sinha P, Garg P, Naranje P, Kabra SK, Bhalla AS. Imaging Findings in Chronic Granulomatous Disease (CGD). Indian J Pediatr. 2022 Dec 1. doi: 10.1007/s12098-022-04350-6. Epub ahead of print. PMID: 36454508.
9. Errami A, El Baghdadi J, Ailal F, Zaki-Dizaji M, Aghdam KR, Mortaz E, et al. Mendelian susceptibility to mycobacterial disease: an overview. Egypt J Med Hum Genet. 2023;247 (2023).

SECTION 4

Diffuse Lung Diseases and Miscellaneous

CHAPTER 11: Diffuse Lung Diseases: Part 1
CHAPTER 12: Diffuse Lung Diseases: Part 2
CHAPTER 13: Pulmonary Complications in Congenital Heart Diseases

CHAPTER 11

Diffuse Lung Diseases: Part 1

Deeksha Bhalla, Priyanka Naranje

- ❏ Pattern-based approach in infants
  - ➢ Diffuse lung diseases with increased lung volume
  - ➢ Diffuse lung disease with decreased-lung volume
  - ➢ Diffuse lung disease with normal lung volume
- ❏ Pattern-based approach to classification in older children
  - ➢ Ground-glass opacity-dominant pattern
  - ➢ Cyst-dominant diffuse lung disease
  - ➢ Nodule-dominant diffuse lung disease
  - ➢ Reticular pattern (septal thickening)-dominant diffuse lung disease

■ INTRODUCTION

Among pediatric diffuse lung disease (DLD), childhood interstitial lung disease (chILD) forms a vast and heterogeneous spectrum that differs considerably from that in adults. They often affect parts of the pulmonary lobule other than the interstitium. It is also of note to mention that the entities encountered in infancy are a unique set of developmental disorders, and thus a separate classification for these has been proposed by the American Thoracic Society in 2013.[1] A pattern-based approach to childhood ILD is beneficial to narrow differential diagnosis, since it is often difficult to pinpoint an exact etiological diagnosis.

■ PATTERN-BASED APPROACH IN INFANTS

This section will discuss the approach to radiological classification of ILDs in infants, as proposed by Liang et al.[2] A stepwise approach is to be followed as described below:
1. The first step is to classify lung volume as low, normal, or high.

2. Hyperinflated lungs will show more than six anterior ribs above the diaphragm and flattened domes on radiographs. On CT, there will be reduced attenuation of the lungs with/without focal areas of air trapping and increased anteroposterior (AP) diameter of chest.
3. DLDs presenting with hyperinflated lungs include *Filamin A (FLNA)* mutation and neuroendocrine cell hyperplasia of infancy (NEHI).
4. Low-lung volume may be symmetric or asymmetric. There is persistent raised diaphragmatic dome above the 5th anterior rib in two or more radiographs. The X-ray attenuation may be high or low. When asymmetric, there may be compensatory hyperinflation of the contralateral lung, ipsilateral small pulmonary artery.
5. DLDs presenting with low-lung volume are far more common, including the group of surfactant dysfunction disorders and pulmonary hypoplasia, which may be primary or secondary to chest wall, diaphragmatic, or abdominal defects.
6. DLDs with normal/variable lung volume are trisomy 21, bronchopulmonary dysplasia, NKX-2 mutation, and pulmonary interstitial glycogenolysis (PIG).

Further classification is discussed under the following headings:

Diffuse Lung Diseases with Increased Lung Volume

The proposed algorithm for DLDs with hyperinflated lungs/increased lung volume is depicted in **Flowchart 1 and Figure 1**.

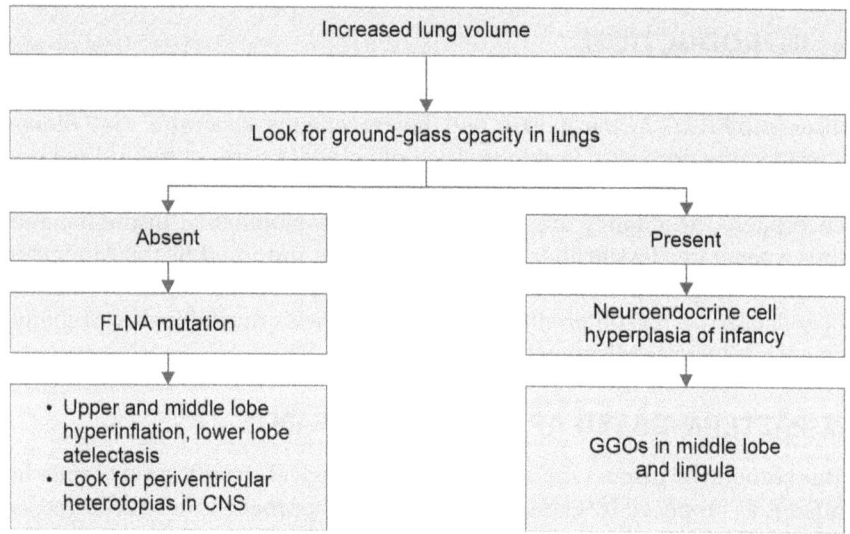

FLOWCHART 1: Approach to DLD with hyperinflated lungs.
(DLD: diffuse lung disease; FLNA: filamin A; CNS: central nervous system; GGO: ground-glass opacity)

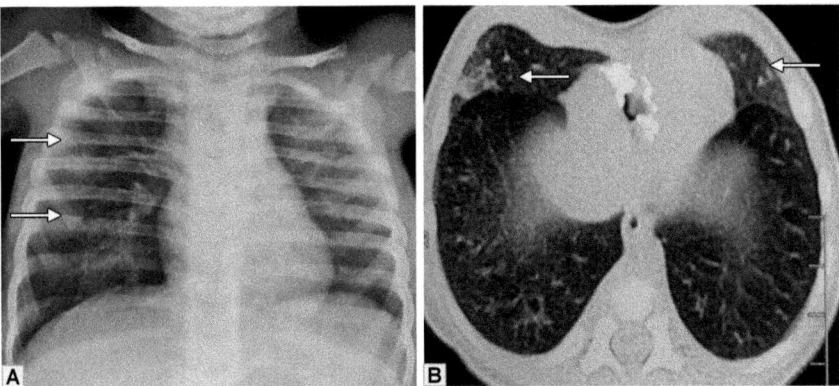

FIGS. 1A AND B: DLD with hyperinflated lungs. *Neuroendocrine cell hyperplasia of infancy.* (A) Frontal chest radiograph shows hyperinflated lungs with asymmetric involvement (right>left) (arrows). (B) Axial HRCT shows a pectus excavatum deformity as ground-glass opacity (GGO) in the right middle lobe and lingula (arrows) with sparing of the lower lobes. This is neuroendocrine cell hyperplasia of infancy.
(DLD: diffuse lung disease; HRCT: high-resolution computed tomography)

Diffuse Lung Disease with Decreased-lung Volume

The proposed algorithm for DLDs with decreased lung volume is depicted in **Flowchart 2 and Figure 2.**

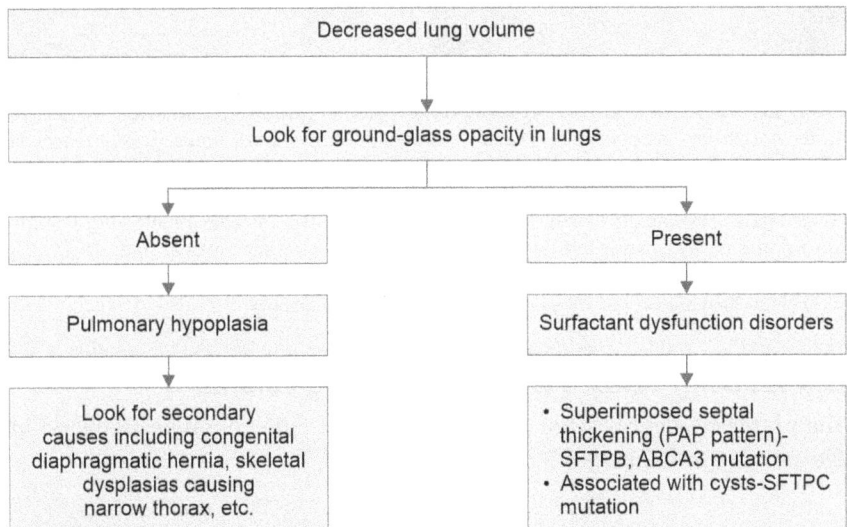

FLOWCHART 2: Approach to DLD with low-lung volume.
(DLD: diffuse lung disease; PAP: pulmonary alveolar proteinosis; SFTPB: surfactant protein B; ABCA3: ATP-binding cassette transporter A3; SFTPC: surfactant protein C)

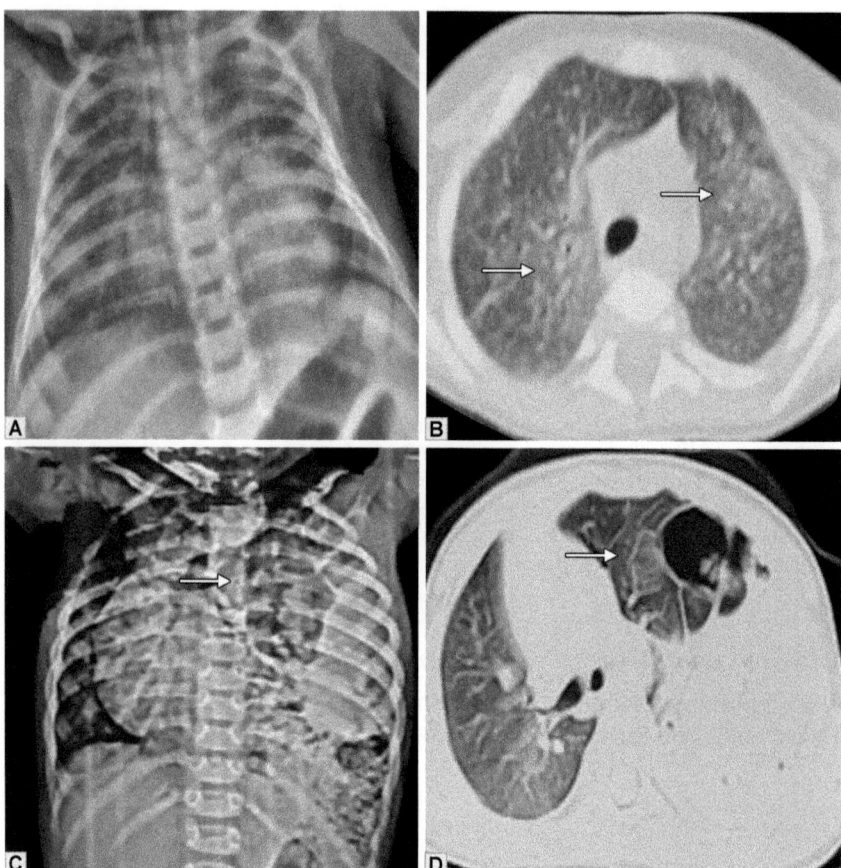

FIGS. 2A TO D: DLD with decreased-lung volume (different patients). (A and B) *Surfactant protein deficiency.* (A) Frontal radiograph shows small lungs (barely reach till anterior end of 5th rib) with a diffuse haze. (B) HRCT shows multiple areas of ground-glass opacity (GGO) in both upper lobes (arrows). (C and D) *Pulmonary hypoplasia secondary to congenital diaphragmatic hernia.* (C) Frontal radiograph shows reduced left lung volume (arrow) and partly opaque left hemithorax with contralateral mediastinal shift. (D) On CT, there is herniation of bowel loops into the left hemithorax with a small left lung (arrow).
(DLD: diffuse lung disease; HRCT: high-resolution computed tomography)

Diffuse Lung Disease with Normal Lung Volume

The proposed algorithm for DLDs with normal lung volume is depicted in **Flowchart 3 and Figure 3**.

CHAPTER 11: Diffuse Lung Diseases: Part 1

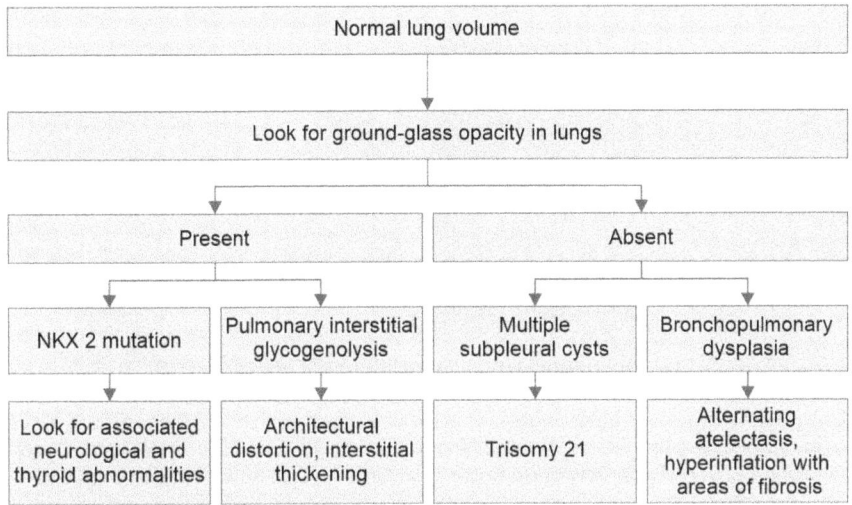

FLOWCHART 3: Approach to DLD with normal lung volume.
(DLD: diffuse lung disease)

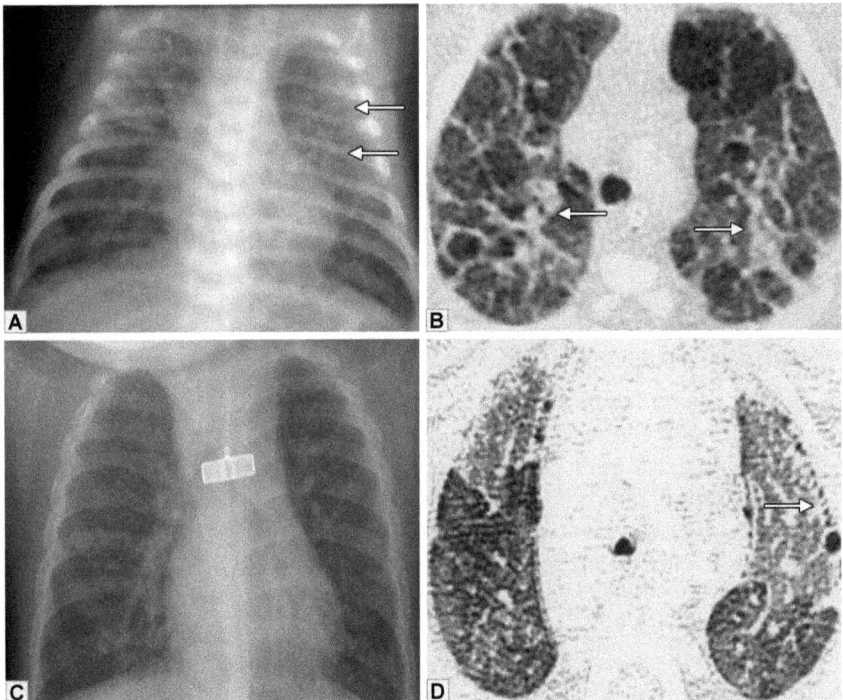

FIGS. 3A TO F: *Continued*

Continued

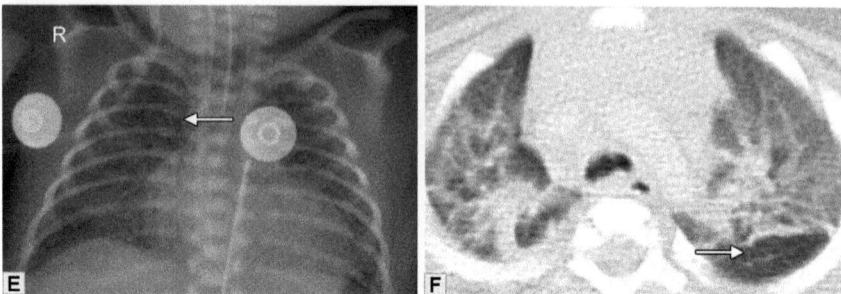

FIGS. 3A TO F: DLD with normal lung volume (different patients). (A and B) *Pulmonary interstitial glycogenolysis.* (A) On the frontal chest radiograph, anterior ends of 6 ribs are seen, which suggests normal lung volume. Multiple reticular opacities are seen in both lungs (arrows). (B) Axial CT shows symmetric interstitial thickening. (C and D) *Trisomy 21.* (C) Frontal radiograph in a child with Down's syndrome shows normal lung volume. (D) Small subpleural cysts are seen on the axial CT (arrow). (E and F) *Bronchopulmonary dysplasia.* (E) Radiograph shows normal lung volume with granular lungs and "ropy" opacities in the right upper lobe (arrows). (F) HRCT shows areas of fibrosis and atelectasis alternating with hyperinflation (arrow).
(DLD: diffuse lung disease; HRCT: high-resolution computed tomography)

■ PATTERN-BASED APPROACH TO CLASSIFICATION IN OLDER CHILDREN

Imaging patterns in older children show some overlap with those seen in adults, though etiologies differ. A stepwise approach must be followed in these patients as well, in which the initial step must be to recognize the predominant abnormality in the lung. This may be GGO, nodules, cysts, or fibrosis.

Further classification is discussed under the following headings.

Ground-glass Opacity-dominant Pattern

- When predominant GGO is identified on HRCT, a crucial factor in classifying etiology is the clinical course, whether presentation and evolution have been acute or chronic. In case of acute presentation and rapid deterioration, pulmonary edema, hemorrhage, and acute respiratory distress syndromes (ARDS) must be considered.[3,4]
- While in case of chronic progressive disease, or waxing and waning course, the cellular NSIP, desquamative interstitial pneumonia (DIP), or alveolar hemorrhage patterns may be identified.
- The pulmonary alveolar proteinosis (PAP) pattern, which refers to GGO with superimposed septal thickening or "crazy paving", is also encountered frequently.

The pattern-based approach to GGO dominant DLD is summarized in **Flowchart 4 and Figure 4**.

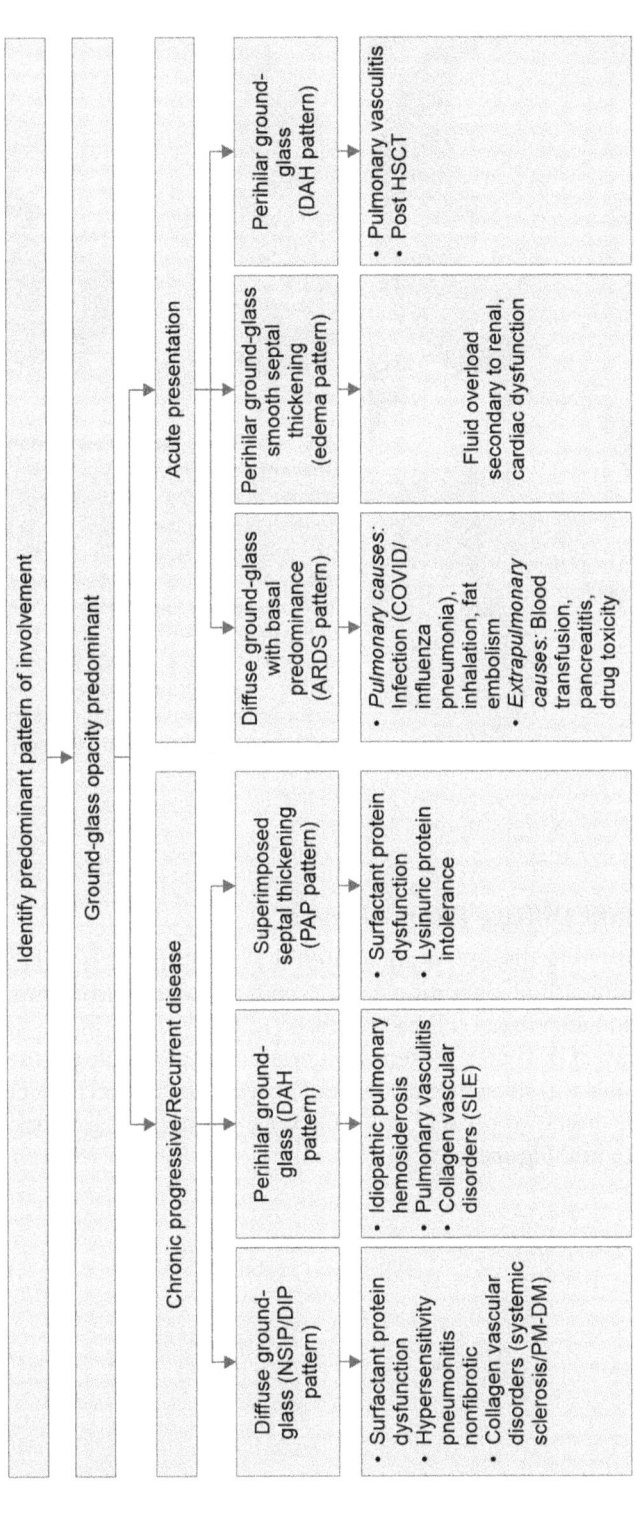

FLOWCHART 4: Approach to GGO-predominant lung disease in children.
(GGO: ground-glass opacity; HSCT: hematopoietic stem cell transplantation; NSIP: nonspecific interstitial pneumonia; DIP: desquamative interstitial pneumonia; DAH: diffuse alveolar hemorrhage; SLE: systemic lupus erythematosus; PAP: pulmonary alveolar proteinosis)

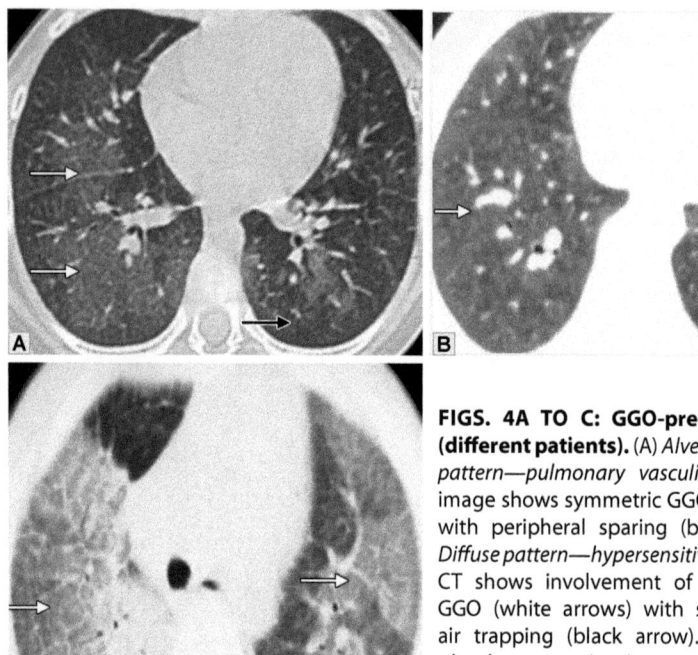

FIGS. 4A TO C: GGO-predominant DLD (different patients). (A) *Alveolar hemorrhage pattern—pulmonary vasculitis*: HRCT axial image shows symmetric GGO (white arrows) with peripheral sparing (black arrow). (B) *Diffuse pattern—hypersensitivity pneumonitis*: CT shows involvement of both lungs by GGO (white arrows) with spared areas of air trapping (black arrow). (C) *Pulmonary alveolar proteinosis pattern—surfactant protein dysfunction.* GGO with superimposed septal thickening (white arrows) in GM-CSF receptor deficiency.

(DLD: diffuse lung disease; GGO: ground-glass opacity; HRCT: high-resolution computed tomography; GM-CSF: granulocyte-macrophage colony-stimulating factor)

Cyst-dominant Diffuse Lung Disease

- When cystic lung disease is encountered in children, it is usually the lymphoid interstitial pneumonia (LIP) pattern or in association with multisystem Langerhans cell histiocytosis (LCH).
- Earlier stages of LCH may present with predominant nodules in the lung. These nodules will subsequently undergo cavitation to form lung cysts.
  The pattern-based approach to cystic lung disease is summarized in **Flowchart 5 and Figure 5**.

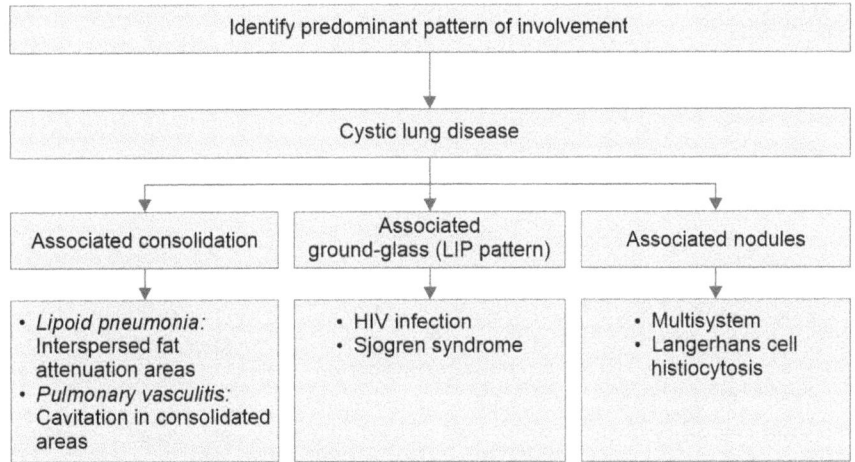

FLOWCHART 5: Approach to cystic lung disease in children.
(LIP: lymphoid interstitial pneumonia; HIV: human immunodeficiency virus)

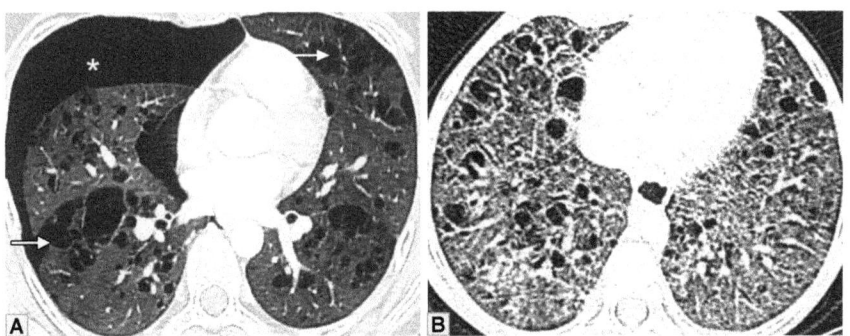

FIGS. 5A AND B: Cystic DLD (different patients). (A) *Langerhans cell histiocytosis.* Axial HRCT shows multiple variable sized lung cysts in both lungs with relative sparing of posterior lungs and right pneumothorax (*). (B) *Lymphocytic interstitial pneumonia (HIV infection).* Diffuse involvement (no zonal predilection) of the lungs is seen with uniform sized cysts and ground-glass opacity.

Nodule-dominant Diffuse Lung Disease

- When a predominant nodular pattern is identified, the distribution of the nodules must be characterized.
- Centrilobular nodules are seen in the terminal bronchioles of the secondary pulmonary lobule, while perilymphatic nodules follow the interstitium along bronchovascular bundles. Random nodules do not respect either of these distributions.

  The pattern-based approach to nodule-dominant DLD is summarized in **Flowchart 6 and Figure 6.**

SECTION 4: Diffuse Lung Diseases and Miscellaneous

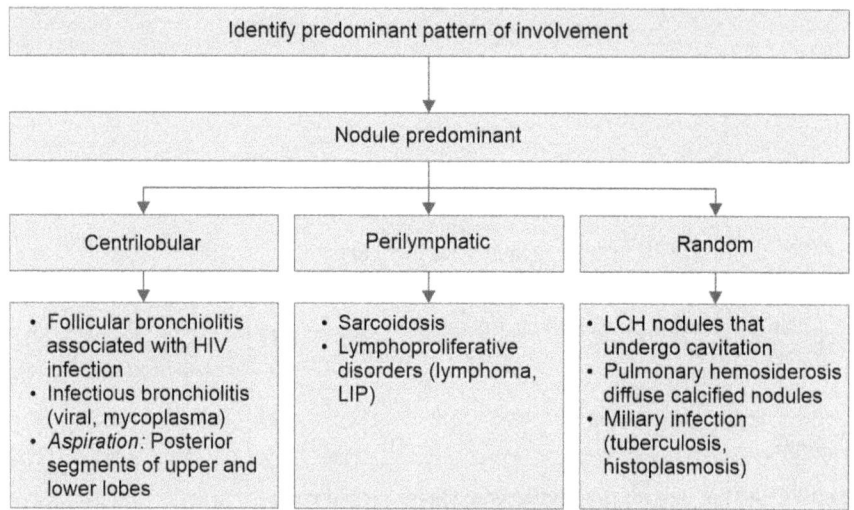

FLOWCHART 6: Approach to nodular lung disease in children.
(HIV: human immunodeficiency virus; LCH: Langerhans cell histiocytosis)

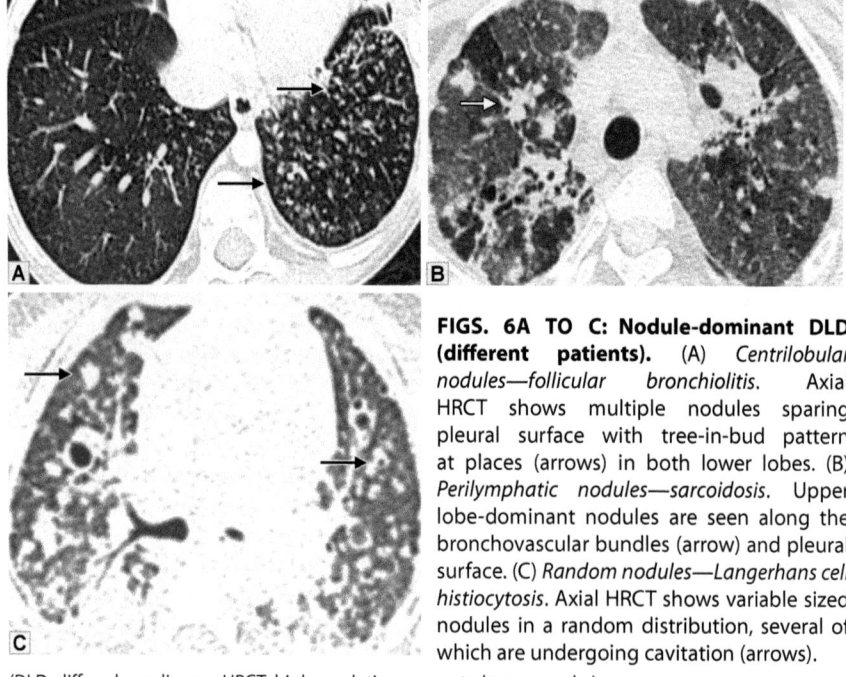

FIGS. 6A TO C: Nodule-dominant DLD (different patients). (A) *Centrilobular nodules—follicular bronchiolitis.* Axial HRCT shows multiple nodules sparing pleural surface with tree-in-bud pattern at places (arrows) in both lower lobes. (B) *Perilymphatic nodules—sarcoidosis.* Upper lobe-dominant nodules are seen along the bronchovascular bundles (arrow) and pleural surface. (C) *Random nodules—Langerhans cell histiocytosis.* Axial HRCT shows variable sized nodules in a random distribution, several of which are undergoing cavitation (arrows).

(DLD: diffuse lung disease; HRCT: high-resolution computed tomography)

Reticular Pattern (Septal Thickening)-dominant Diffuse Lung Disease

- The first point of differentiation must be between fibrotic septal thickening or infiltrative septal thickening (due to fluid or cells infiltrating the interstitium).
- Among infiltrative causes, in children, congenital vascular anomalies such as pulmonary veno-occlusive disease or lymphatic obstruction secondary to malignancy such as leukemia are foremost causes of infiltrative septal thickening.
- Fibrotic lung disease is characterized by irregular septal thickening, volume loss, and architectural distortion.
- An important difference is that usual interstitial pneumonia (UIP), the dominant pattern seen in adults, is not encountered in children.
- Fibrotic ILD patterns can be categorized as subpleural fibrosis (SPF) or airway centric fibrosis (ACF).[5]
- Subpleural fibrosis resembles the fibrotic nonspecific interstitial pneumonia (NSIP) picture seen in adults, with fibrotic strands and architectural distortion seen at the periphery of the lung.
- Airway-centric fibrosis involves the axial interstitium, with peribronchovascular fibrosis and traction bronchiectasis.
  The pattern-based approach to nodule-dominant DLD and fibrotic lung disease is summarized in **Flowchart 7 and Figure 7**.

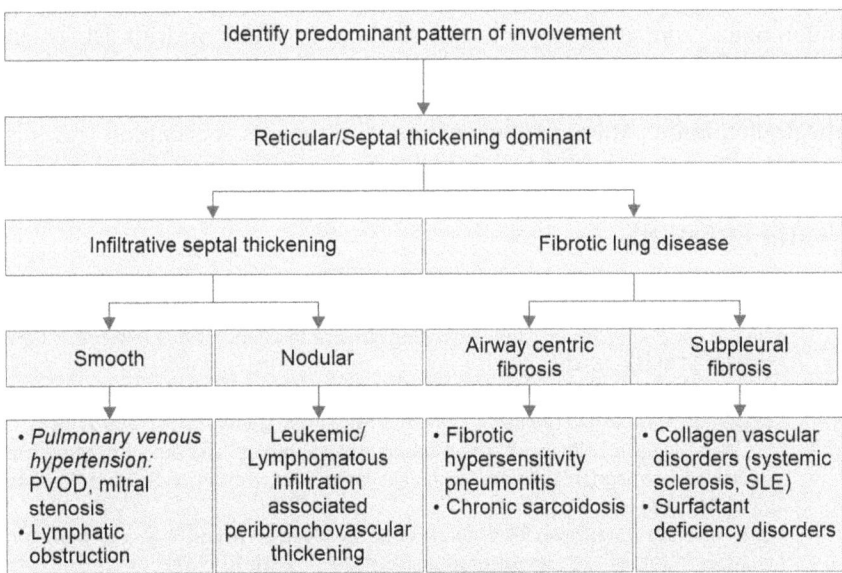

FLOWCHART 7: Pattern-based approach to reticular pattern on HRCT in children.
(HRCT: high-resolution computed tomography; PVOD: pulmonary veno-occlusive disease; SLE: systemic lupus erythematosus)

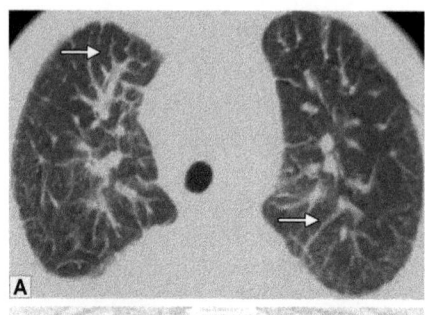
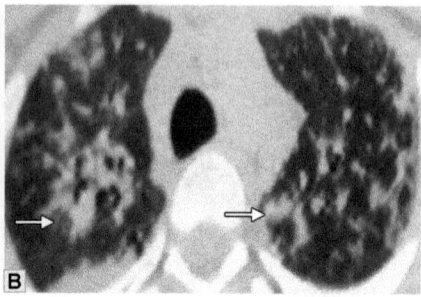
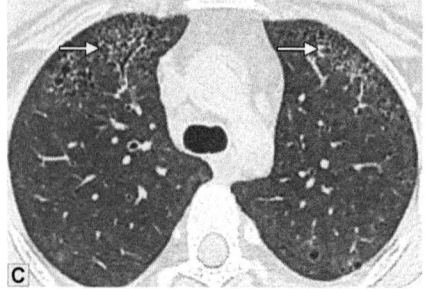

FIGS. 7A TO C: Reticular-dominant DLD. (A) *Infiltrative septal thickening—lymphatic obstruction.* Axial HRCT shows smooth symmetric septal thickening (arrows). (B) *Fibrotic lung disease—airway centric.* Coarse, irregular reticular opacities are seen in central distribution (arrows) in a child with fibrosis secondary to presumed hypersensitivity. (C) *Fibrotic lung disease—subpleural.* HRCT shows irregular septal thickening in peripheral distribution (arrows) in a child with systemic sclerosis ILD.
(DLD: diffuse lung disease; HRCT: high-resolution computed tomography; ILD: interstitial lung disease)

CONCLUSION

It is essential to follow a pattern-based approach to narrow imaging differentials and guide meaningful workup in children with DLDs. In infants, the first step is recognizing lung volume, followed by determining presence of GGO in lungs. In older children, the first step is categorizing the predominant pattern of involvement; and then its distribution which is usually sufficient to reach a set of diagnoses.

REFERENCES

1. Kurland G, Deterding RR, Hagood JS, Young LR, Brody AS, Castile RG, et al. An official American Thoracic Society clinical practice guideline: classification, evaluation, and management of childhood interstitial lung disease in infancy. Am J Respir Crit Care Med. 2013;188(3):376-394.
2. Liang T, Vargas SO, Lee EY. Childhood Interstitial (diffuse) lung disease: Pattern recognition approach to diagnosis in infants. Am J Roentgenol. 2019;212(5):958-967.
3. Qi Y, Wang L, Qian L, Zhang X. The etiology, clinical profile, and outcome of diffuse alveolar hemorrhage in children: a ten-year single-center experience. Transl Pediatr. 2021;10(11):2921-8.
4. Fan K, McArthur J, Morrison RR, Ghafoor S. Diffuse alveolar hemorrhage after pediatric hematopoietic stem cell transplantation. Front Oncol. 2020;10:1757.
5. Bhalla D, Jana M, Naranje P, Bhalla AS, Kabra SK. Fibrosing interstitial lung disease in children: An HRCT-based analysis. Indian J Pediatr. 2023;90(2):153-9.

CHAPTER 12

Diffuse Lung Diseases: Part 2

Deeksha Bhalla, Manisha Jana

- ❏ Childhood interstitial lung disease entities more prevalent in infancy
  - ➢ Diffuse developmental disorders
  - ➢ Growth abnormalities
  - ➢ Surfactant dysfunction disorders
  - ➢ Specific conditions of unknown or poorly understood etiology
- ❏ Disorders not specific to infancy
  - ➢ Disorders of normal host
  - ➢ Disorders related to systemic disease processes
  - ➢ Disorders of immunocompromised host
  - ➢ Miscellaneous

INTRODUCTION

- The reported prevalence of childhood interstitial lung disease (chILD) varies considerably across institutes, from 0.13 to 16.2 per 100,000 children per year.[1] There is a relative lack of understanding about this entity contributed in part by its low prevalence as well as by the complex multitude of specific etiologies that differ from adults.
- In the practice guideline proposed by American Thoracic Society, in children presenting with symptoms of diffuse lung disease, exclusion of common etiologies such as infection, aspiration, and congenital heart disease must be carried out at the first step.[2] Once this is done, a "chILD syndrome" is diagnosed, which is then classified by a multidisciplinary team (MDT) based on etiopathogenesis. This classification system is detailed below **(Box 1)**. The imaging pattern-based approach is described in Chapter 11. This chapter briefly discusses specific entities with emphasis on how the radiologist can contribute to the MDT.

> **BOX 1** **Classification of childhood diffuse lung disease (DLD).**
>
> A. *Disorders more prevalent in infancy:*
> - *Diffuse developmental disorders:*
>   - Acinar dysplasia
>   - Alveolar dysplasia
>   - Alveolar capillary dysplasia with misalignment of pulmonary veins
> - *Growth abnormalities:*
>   - Congenital alveolar dysplasia
>   - Bronchopulmonary dysplasia
>   - Chromosomal abnormalities
> - *Surfactant dysfunction disorders:*
>   - *SPFTB* mutations
>   - *SPFTC* mutations
>   - *ABCA3* mutations
>   - *NKX2.1* mutations
> - *Specific conditions of undefined etiology:*
>   - Neuroendocrine cell hyperplasia of infancy
>   - Pulmonary interstitial glycogenolysis
>
> B. *Disorders not specific to infancy:*
> - *Disorders of normal host—infectious/postinfectious processes:*
>   - Exposure related—hypersensitivity pneumonitis
>   - Aspiration pneumonia
>   - Eosinophilic pneumonias
> - *Disorders related to systemic disease processes:*
>   - Immune-related disorders
>   - Storage disorders
>   - Sarcoidosis
>   - Langerhans cell histiocytosis
>   - Malignant infiltrates
> - *Disorders of immunocompromised host:*
>   - Opportunistic infections
>   - Obliterative bronchiolitis
>   - Follicular bronchiolitis/lymphocytic interstitial pneumonia
> - *Disorders masquerading as interstitial lung disease:*
>   - Arterial hypertensive vasculopathy
>   - Veno-occlusive disease
>   - Lymphatic disorders
> - *Unclassified*: Nondiagnostic biopsies, end-stage disease, etc.

■ CHILDHOOD INTERSTITIAL LUNG DISEASE ENTITIES MORE PREVALENT IN INFANCY

Diffuse Developmental Disorders

- Present with respiratory failure at birth or in first few hours of life.[3,4]
- Include acinar dysplasia, alveolar dysplasia, and alveolar capillary dysplasia with misalignment of pulmonary veins (ACD-MPV). The latter is associated with pulmonary lymphangiectasia as well as multiple gastrointestinal and genitourinary abnormalities.
- No characteristic radiologic appearance or diffuse airspace opacification is seen. Air leaks (pneumothorax or pneumomediastinum) may be associated.

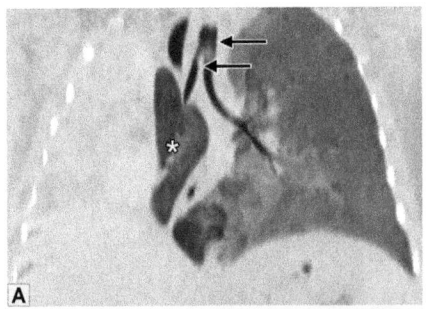
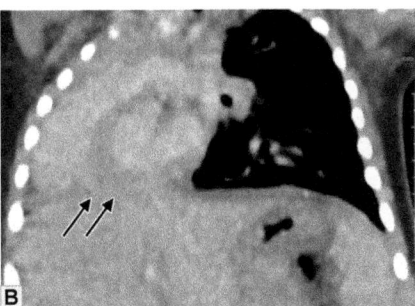
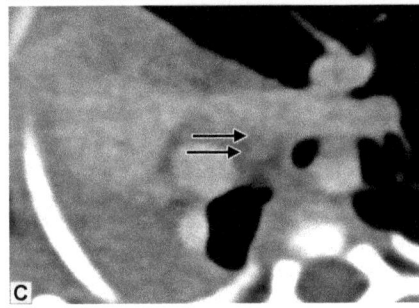

FIGS. 1A TO C: Pulmonary hypoplasia. A 3-month-old boy with respiratory distress since birth. (A) Hypoplastic right lung (*) with an abnormally oriented high-riding carina (arrows). (B) Ipsilateral mediastinal shift seen with normal diaphragm (arrows). (C) Rudimentary right pulmonary artery (arrows) compared to the much larger caliber of left pulmonary artery.

Growth Abnormalities

Pulmonary Hypoplasia

- May be primary, but more commonly secondary to lesions in the thorax that limits space for lung growth.
- The most common cause is congenital diaphragmatic hernia, others include severe oligohydramnios and skeletal dysplasias causing narrow thorax.
- The affected lung is uniformly small in volume with no ground glass opacities **(Figs. 1A to C)**.

Chronic Neonatal Lung Disease (Bronchopulmonary Dysplasia)

- "Classic" bronchopulmonary dysplasia (BPD) is seen in infants exposed to high-oxygen pressures during neonatal period as part of treatment for hyaline membrane disease.
- The radiographic appearance is that of variable lung volume with coarse reticular opacities. CT better depicts areas of hyperinflated lung and cystic lucencies alternating with fibrosis and atelectasis **(Figs. 2A to C)**. Bronchial wall thickening may be seen.
- "New" form of BPD has emerged due to increased survival of extremely premature infants (24–26 weeks). Histological features correspond to the gestational age of the child at delivery.
- The imaging findings are subtle, with less pronounced fibrosis and airway involvement.[5]

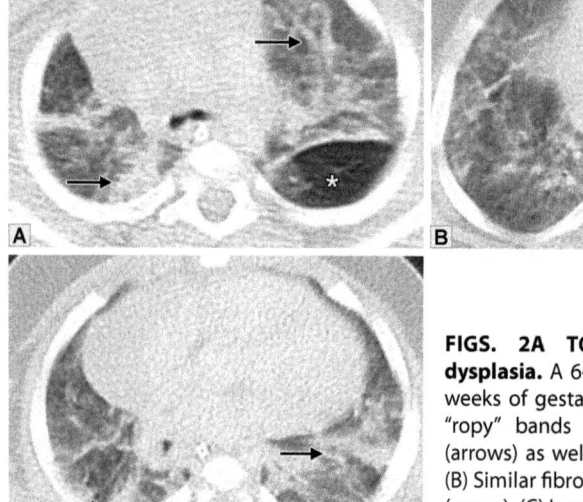

FIGS. 2A TO C: Bronchopulmonary dysplasia. A 6-month-old boy born at 25 weeks of gestation. (A) Upper lobes show "ropy" bands and atelectatic segments (arrows) as well as areas of hyperinflation. (B) Similar fibrotic bands in the lower lobes (arrow). (C) Increasing atelectasis is present in dependent segments (arrows) due to prolonged ventilation.

Chromosomal Abnormalities
- Trisomy 21 presents with multiple subpleural cysts. In a CT series of children with Down's syndrome, anteromedial segments of the lung were involved in 100% cases[6] **(Figs. 3A to C)**.
- Filamin A (FLNA) mutation causes hyperinflation of upper and middle lobes, with varying degrees of lower lobe atelectasis. Coarse septal thickening may be associated.
- There are associated gray matter heterotopias, vascular aneurysms, and connective tissue disorders (hyperextensibility).

Surfactant Dysfunction Disorders
- These are groups of uncommon disorders that result from mutations in surfactant proteins.
- Presentation and imaging features vary based on the specific protein involved **(Table 1; Figs. 4 and 5)**.

CHAPTER 12: Diffuse Lung Diseases: Part 2

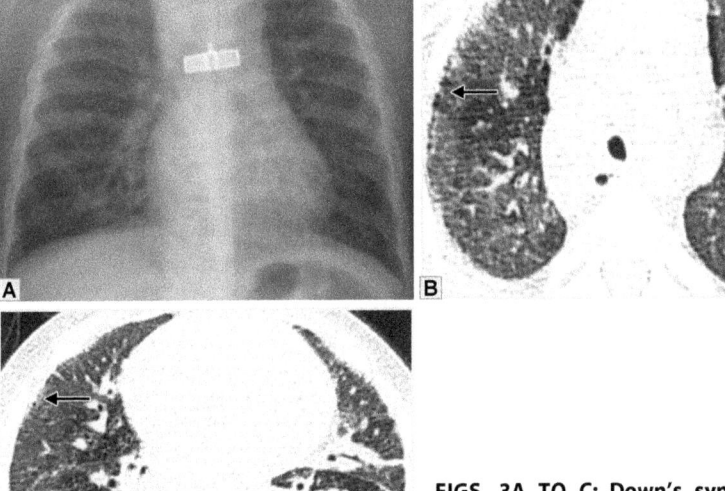

FIGS. 3A TO C: Down's syndrome. (A) Frontal radiograph, normal appearing lungs with maintained lung volume. (B and C) Multiple small subpleural cysts are seen (arrows), more numerous in upper lobes.

TABLE 1: Surfactant protein deficiency causing interstitial lung disease in children.

Surfactant protein	Presentation	Radiological pattern
Surfactant protein B (SFTPB)	• AR inheritance • Early infancy—respiratory distress • Usually fatal	PAP
Surfactant protein C (SFTPC)	• AD/de novo mutation • Older infants, children, and adults	• Ground–glass opacity (93%) and cysts (40%)[7] • Patterns • NSIP, DIP, and CPI
ATP-binding cassette A (ABCA3)	Infants, older children, and young adults—severity less than SFTPB mutations[8]	NSIP, DIP, and CPI
NK2 homeobox 1 (NKX2-1)—Encodes thyroid transcription factor 1 (TTF-1)	Brain, thyroid, lung syndrome—choreoathetosis, congenital hypothyroidism, neonatal respiratory distress/recurrent infections[9]	Ground–glass opacity, interstitial thickening
Granulocyte macrophage colony-stimulating factor (GM-CSF) receptor mutation	Older children—progressive dyspnea[10]	PAP (should be suspected when SFTPB or ABCA3 mutation not demonstrated with this pattern)

(AR: autosomal recessive; AD: autosomal dominant; PAP: pulmonary alveolar proteinosis; NSIP: nonspecific interstitial pneumonitis; DIP: desquamative interstitial pneumonia; CPI: chronic pneumonitis of infancy)

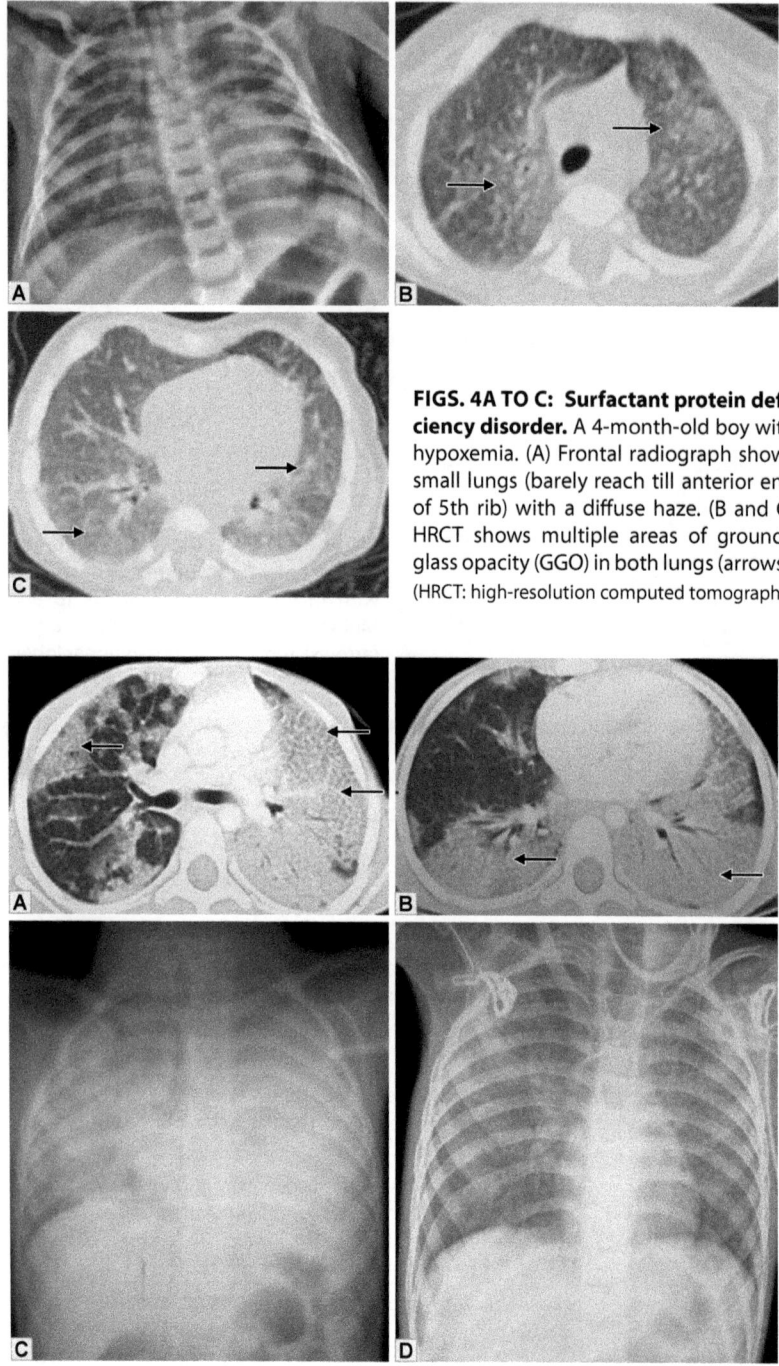

FIGS. 4A TO C: Surfactant protein deficiency disorder. A 4-month-old boy with hypoxemia. (A) Frontal radiograph shows small lungs (barely reach till anterior end of 5th rib) with a diffuse haze. (B and C) HRCT shows multiple areas of ground–glass opacity (GGO) in both lungs (arrows).
(HRCT: high-resolution computed tomography)

FIGS. 5A TO D: GM-CSF receptor mutation. A 3-month-old term infant with respiratory distress. (A and B) CT done in April 2021 shows GGO in both lungs (left > right) with superimposed septal thickening (arrows). (C and D) Serial radiographs from March (C) and June (D) 2021 show progressive clearing of the lungs with supportive therapy.
(GGO: ground–glass opacity; GM-CSF: granulocyte macrophage colony-stimulating factor)

Specific Conditions of Unknown or Poorly Understood Etiology

Neuroendocrine Cell Hyperplasia of Infancy

- Neuroendocrine cell hyperplasia of infancy (NEHI) refers to an increased number of neuroendocrine cells within the "neuroepithelial bodies" in the airway epithelium.
- Term infants who present with tachypnea, hypoxia, crackles, and retractions; not responding to steroids or bronchodilators.
- Patchy ground-glass opacity, with distribution in right middle lobe and lingula is the most common CT finding, followed by mosaic attenuation with air trapping. This CT pattern of NEHI has been reported to be 100% specific[11] **(Figs. 6A to C)**.
- Routine histopathology is seldom diagnostic, immunostaining for bombesin is necessary for pathologic confirmation which is not part of routine evaluation. Therefore, CT must suggest the diagnosis to guide pathological evaluation.

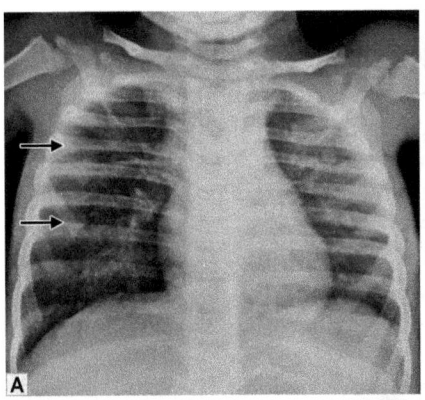
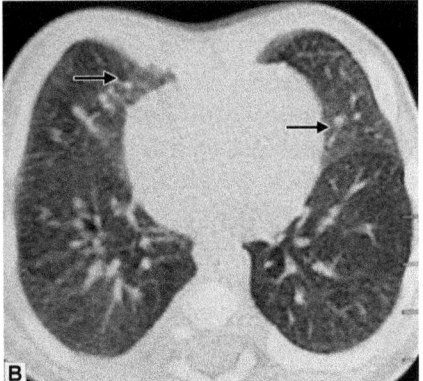
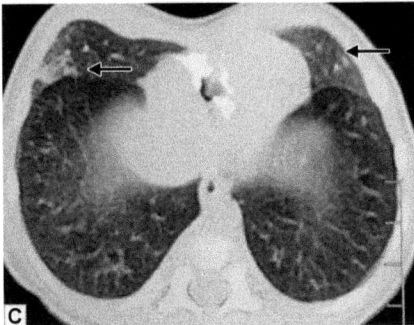

FIGS. 6A TO C: Neuroendocrine cell hyperplasia of infancy. A 40-day-old girl child with persistent tachypnea and hypoxemia. (A) Frontal chest radiograph shows asymmetric hyperinflated lungs (right > left) (arrows). (B and C) Axial HRCT shows pectus excavatum deformity, causing asymmetric appearance on radiographs, as well as GGO in the right middle lobe and lingula (arrows) with sparing of the lower lobes.
(GGO: ground–glass opacity; HRCT: high-resolution computed tomography)

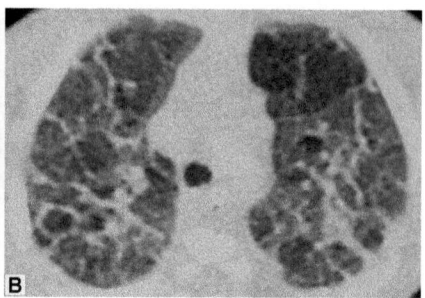
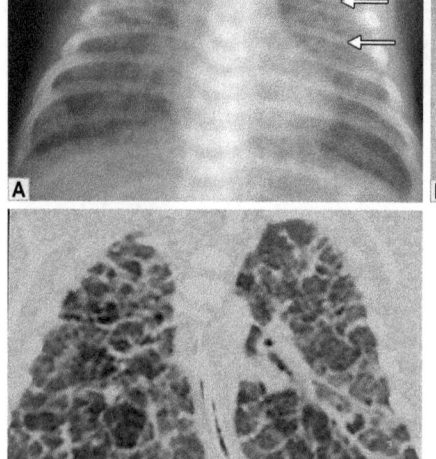

FIGS. 7A TO C: Pulmonary interstitial glycogenolysis. A 45-day-old boy with respiratory distress and hypoxemia. (A) Frontal radiograph, normal lung volume (anterior ends of 6 ribs seen). Multiple reticular opacities in both lungs (arrows). (B and C) CT shows extensive symmetric interstitial thickening, with no zonal predilection.

Pulmonary Interstitial Glycogenolysis

- Pulmonary interstitial glycogenolysis (PIG) may be primary or secondary (associated with pulmonary hypoplasia, adjoining congenital lung abnormalities such as cysts or bronchopulmonary dysplasia).
- This entity is characterized by mesenchymal cell proliferation in the alveolar walls, which may be reactive.
- Presentation often at birth or during neonatal period.
- Good prognosis with improvement over time.
- Nonspecific imaging features may show overlap with lung growth disorders.
- Combination of interstitial thickening, architectural distortion, ground-glass opacity and air trapping[12] (**Figs. 7A to C**).

■ DISORDERS NOT SPECIFIC TO INFANCY

Disorders of Normal Host

Bronchiolitis Obliterans

- It refers to severe, fixed obstruction at the level of the small airways. It may be secondary to a variety of processes, including infections (adenovirus), hematopoietic stem cell or lung transplant (secondary to graft versus host disease), connective tissue disease, drugs, and toxins.
- The presenting symptoms are tachypnea, dyspnea, and wheeze, with a mean age at onset of 7.5 months as found by Lino et al.[13]
- Chest radiographs demonstrate hyperinflation and may show peribronchial thickening (**Figs. 8A to D**).
- On CT, mosaic attenuation is the striking feature which may be accompanied by bronchial wall thickening or bronchial dilatation (**Figs. 9A to C**).

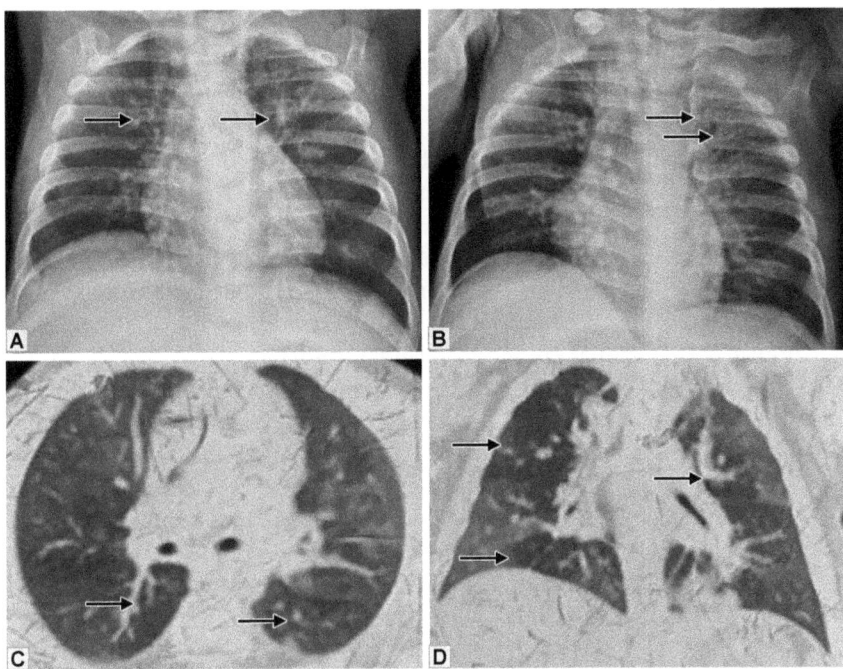

FIGS. 8A TO D: Postinfectious bronchiolitis obliterans. A 10-month-old boy with recurrent episodes of pneumonia since birth. (A) Radiograph done in April 2023 shows hyperinflated lungs with peribronchial thickening in upper zones (arrows). (B) Follow-up radiograph done in May reveals a superadded patch of consolidation (arrows). (C and D) Mosaic attenuation in both lungs with areas of air trapping (arrows), suggestive of postinfectious bronchiolitis obliterans.

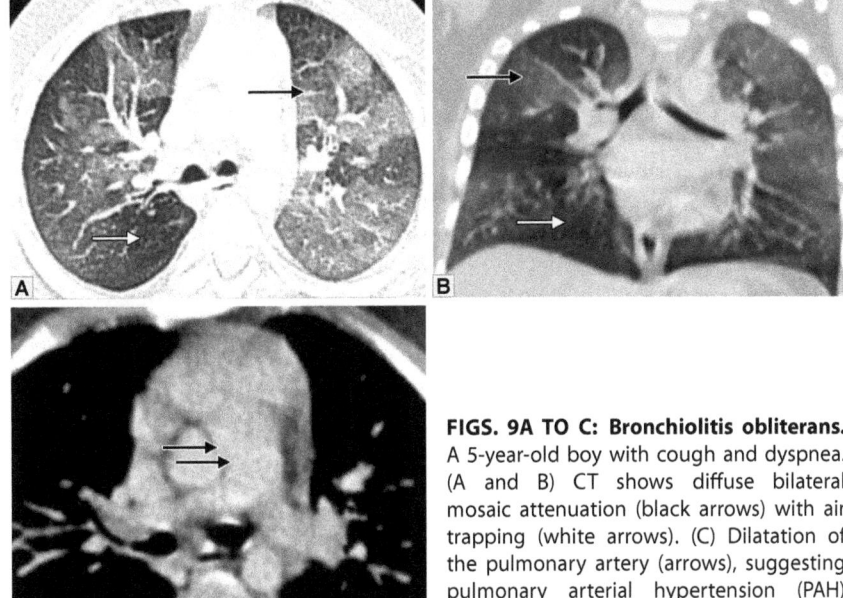

FIGS. 9A TO C: Bronchiolitis obliterans. A 5-year-old boy with cough and dyspnea. (A and B) CT shows diffuse bilateral mosaic attenuation (black arrows) with air trapping (white arrows). (C) Dilatation of the pulmonary artery (arrows), suggesting pulmonary arterial hypertension (PAH) secondary to the lung changes.

Hypersensitivity Pneumonitis

- Similar to adults, hypersensitivity pneumonitis (HP) in children is related to environmental exposure to antigens.
- Common exposures in children are often related to bird or fungal antigens, unlike occupational exposure in adults.
- Classic presentation is with dyspnea, cough, wheeze, and mid-inspiratory rales.
- The "typical" nonfibrotic presentation is with parenchymal abnormality in the form of GGO and mosaic attenuation; and small airway abnormality in the form of centrilobular nodules and air trapping. The abnormality is diffuse, with no zonal predilection **(Figs. 10A to C)**.
- The "typical" fibrotic form, on the other hand, presents with traction bronchiectasis, reticulations, and architectural distortion in mid lung zones with sparing of lower lungs **(Figs. 11A to D)**. The "three density" pattern with alternating areas of air trapping, GGO, and normal lung is also characteristic. Peribronchovascular fibrosis and upper lung zone predominance are also compatible with HP.[14]
- Bronchoalveolar lavage (BAL) shows lymphocytosis, with increased CD8+ cells and a low CD4+/CD8+ ratio.

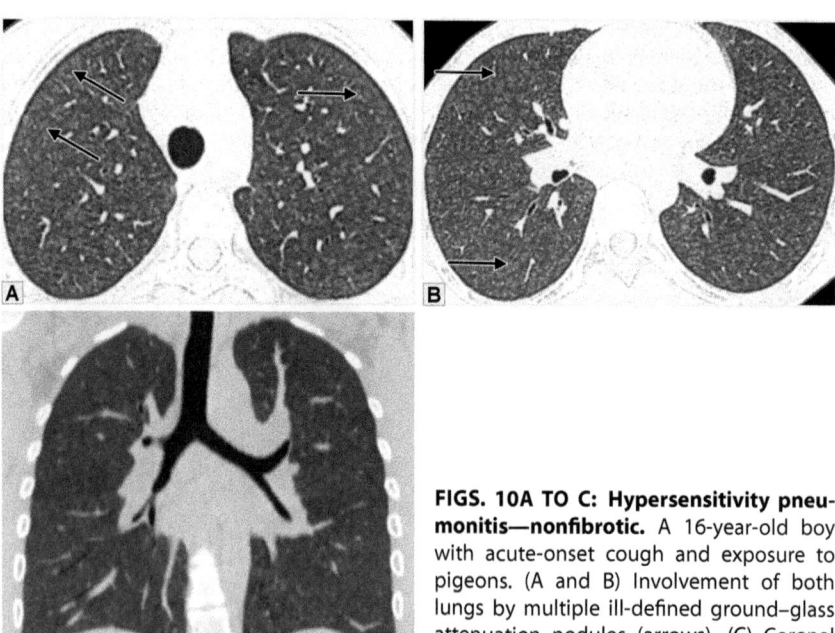

FIGS. 10A TO C: Hypersensitivity pneumonitis—nonfibrotic. A 16-year-old boy with acute-onset cough and exposure to pigeons. (A and B) Involvement of both lungs by multiple ill-defined ground–glass attenuation nodules (arrows). (C) Coronal CT demonstrates the diffuse ground–glass haze without an apicobasal gradient.

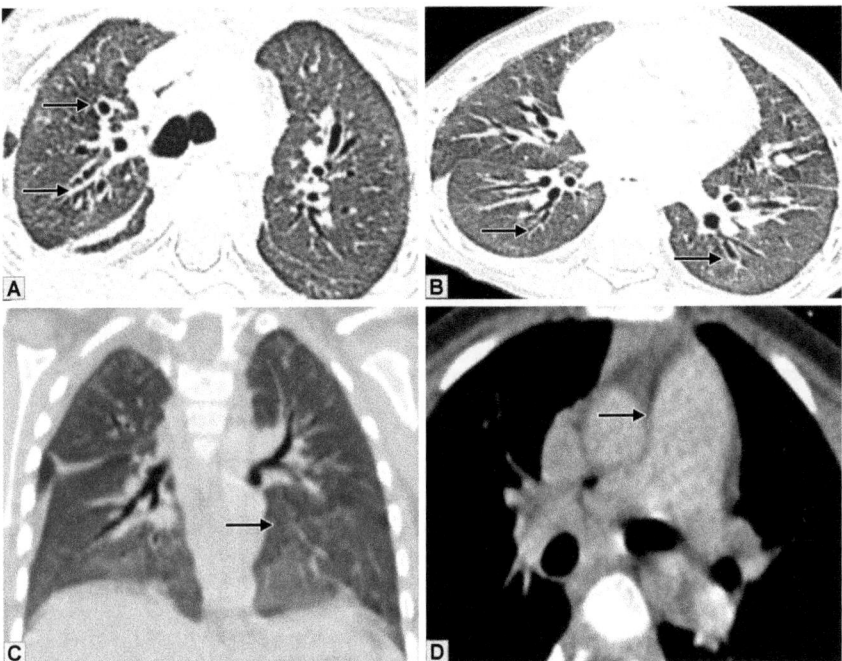

FIGS. 11A TO D: Hypersensitivity pneumonitis—fibrotic. (A) Ground–glass attenuation in the upper lobes with traction bronchiectasis (arrows). (B and C) Peribronchovascular fibrosis in the parahilar regions of lower lobes with traction bronchiectasis (arrows in B) and mosaic attenuation (arrow in C). (D) Pulmonary arterial dilatation is also noted secondary to lung fibrosis.

Exogenous Lipoid Pneumonia

- In adults, it is related to aspiration of mineral oils as an occupational hazard. In children, this is often related to cultural practices involving nasal oil application for cleansing or oral administration as a laxative.
- It presents with cough, dyspnea, tachypnea, and rarely even with fever or hemoptysis.
- Diagnosis is made by demonstration of lipid-laden macrophages in BAL or lung biopsy.
- The radiographic picture is of airspace opacification. Expansile pneumonia may be seen in the right upper lobe.
- On CT, there are dependent consolidations and GGO, which progress to diffuse involvement in severe disease[15] **(Figs. 12A to C)**. Right upper lobe involvement has also been frequently reported. Fat attenuation in areas of consolidation may be seen in lipoid pneumonia **(Figs. 13A to C)**.

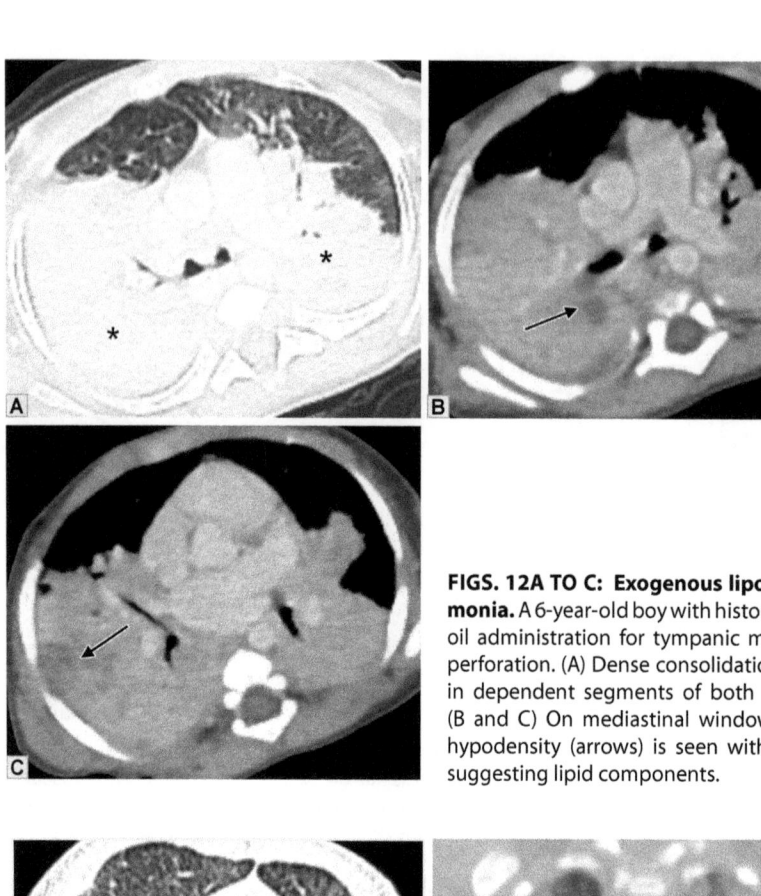

FIGS. 12A TO C: Exogenous lipoid pneumonia. A 6-year-old boy with history of aural oil administration for tympanic membrane perforation. (A) Dense consolidation is seen in dependent segments of both lungs (*). (B and C) On mediastinal window, central hypodensity (arrows) is seen within these, suggesting lipid components.

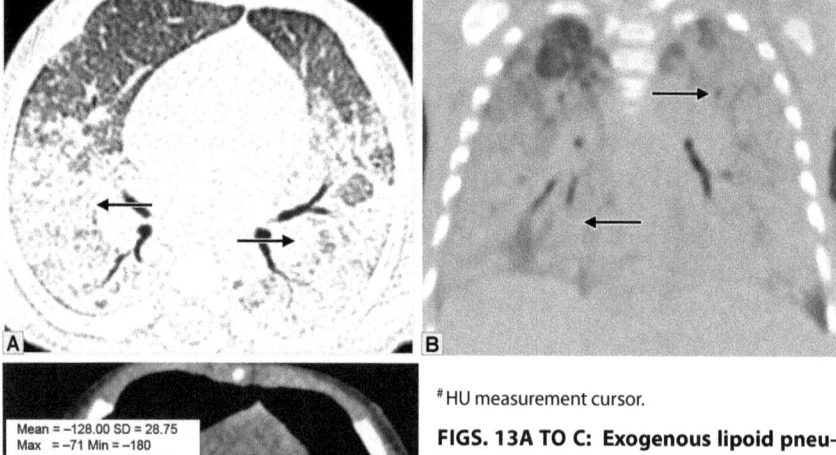

#HU measurement cursor.

FIGS. 13A TO C: Exogenous lipoid pneumonia. A 7-year-old boy with cough and fast breathing. (A) Dependent consolidation seen in both lungs (arrows) with interspersed GGO. (B) On the coronal section, extensive involvement of posterior lungs is seen (arrows). (C) On mediastinal window, there are multiple fat attenuation areas (−128 HU) within the consolidation.

(GGO: ground-glass opacity)

Eosinophilic Pneumonias

- Infiltration of the lung parenchyma (both alveoli and interstitial space) by eosinophils.
- Demonstration of eosinophilia on BAL (>20–25%) is sufficient for diagnosis, biopsy is usually not necessary. Peripheral blood eosinophilia may be associated.[16]
- The various forms are detailed in **Table 2**.

TABLE 2: Clinical features, pathophysiology, and imaging findings of pulmonary disorders with eosinophilia.

	Presentation	Etiopathogenesis	Imaging features
• Primary • Acute eosinophilic pneumonia	• Recent smoke or irritant exposure • Respiratory distress with hypoxia	Idiopathic	• GGO, dense consolidation in random distribution with pleural effusion • Dramatic response to steroids
Chronic eosinophilic pneumonia	Progressive symptoms, initially cough followed by systemic symptoms	• Idiopathic • T-cell abnormalities described in some adult studies	• Peripheral ground glass and consolidation (negative picture of pulmonary edema) • Response to steroids • May evolves into lung fibrosis
Hyper-eosinophilic syndrome	Multisystem involvement including skin, lung, cardiac involvement, and myeloproliferative disorder. New-onset asthma may be seen	• May be idiopathic, reactive (lymphoid variant) or primary (neoplastic) • Blood and tissue hypereosinophilia	• Nonspecific • Patchy GGO/consolidation
Parasitic Loeffler syndrome	Transient (7–10 days) cough and wheeze	Hypersensitivity reaction to migration of larvae through lung to intestine	Migratory pulmonary infiltrates in peripheral location
Visceral larva migrans	More pronounced than Loeffler with other organ involvement (liver, heart, and retina)	Larvae of *Toxocara* species that are trapped in their lifecycle	Similar features
Tropical pulmonary eosinophilia (TPE)	• Cough (paroxysmal and nocturnal) • Dyspnea, weakness, and weight loss	Hypersensitivity reaction to microfilaria (*Wuchereria* and *Brugia*) antigens in pulmonary vasculature	Reticulonodular pattern in mid to lower zones, miliary mottling, bronchiectasis **(Figs. 14A and B)**

(GGO: ground–glass opacity)

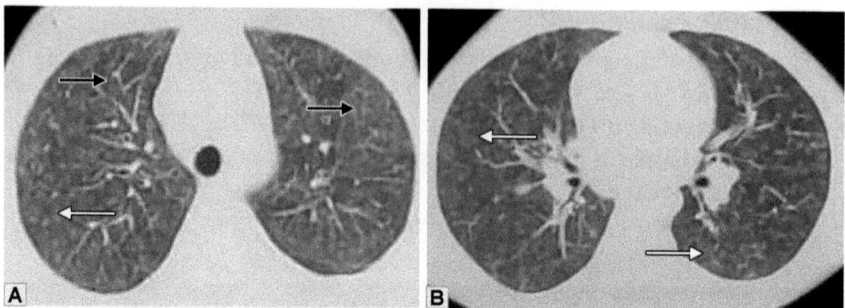

FIGS. 14A AND B: Tropical pulmonary eosinophilia. A 15-year-old girl who was a resident of Bihar, with acute-onset dyspnea and eosinophilia. Multiple tiny nodules scattered throughout both lungs with ground–glass attenuation (white arrows). Few areas of septal thickening are also noted (black arrows).

Idiopathic Pulmonary Hemosiderosis
- Recurrent episodic pulmonary hemorrhage causing hemoptysis and iron deficiency anemia. Symptoms have a waxing and waning course.
- Usually in children under 10 years; both sex equally affected.
- Unclear etiology, autoimmune theory, and sensitivity to cow milk protein proposed.
- In the acute phase, CT findings of diffuse alveolar hemorrhage are seen with central GGO and consolidation, which typically resolve in 2 weeks **(Figs. 15A to D)**. Hemosiderin-laden macrophages are found in alveoli on biopsy.
- In chronic disease, interstitial thickening and fibrosis are noted **(Figs. 16A to C)**. Interstitial hemosiderin deposition with interlobular septal thickening seen on pathology.

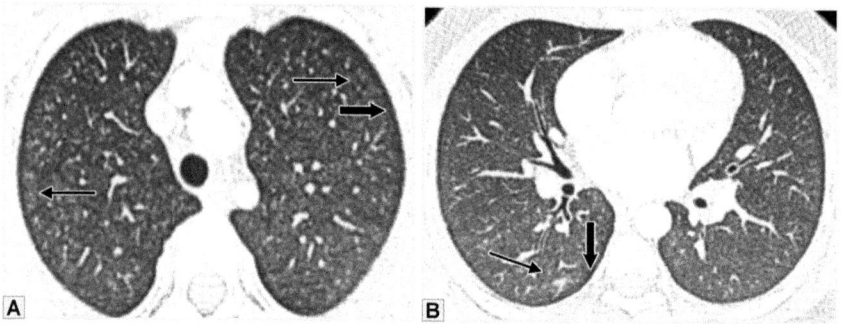

FIGS. 15A TO D: *Continued*

Continued

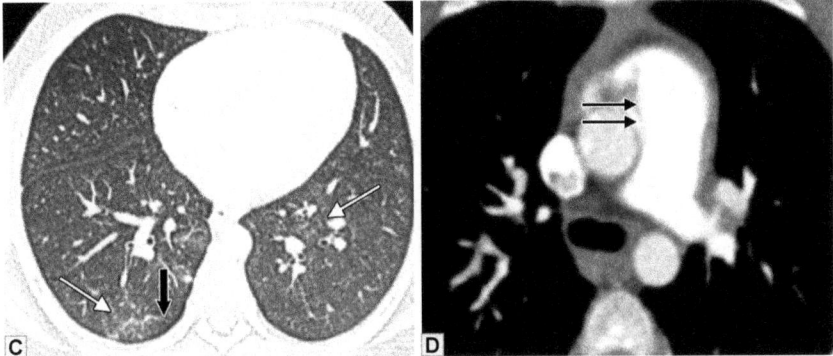

FIGS. 15A TO D: Idiopathic pulmonary hemosiderosis. A 9-year-old boy with recurrent pulmonary hemorrhage. (A to C) Axial lung window sections show ill-defined nodules (black arrows) as well as GGO and septal thickening (white arrows), with immediate subpleural sparing (solid arrows). (D) PAH is also noted (arrows) secondary to the repeated hemorrhage. (GGO: ground–glass opacity; PAH: pulmonary arterial hypertension)

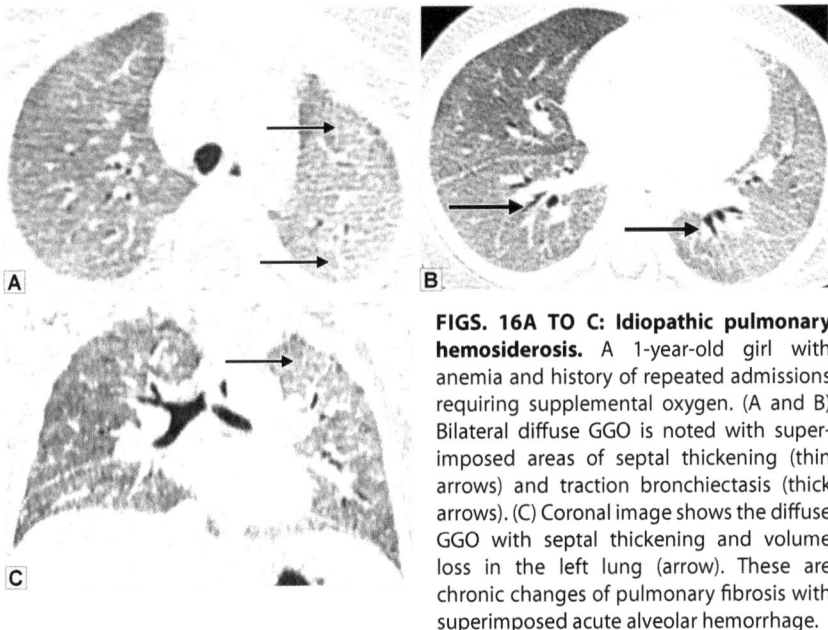

FIGS. 16A TO C: Idiopathic pulmonary hemosiderosis. A 1-year-old girl with anemia and history of repeated admissions requiring supplemental oxygen. (A and B) Bilateral diffuse GGO is noted with super-imposed areas of septal thickening (thin arrows) and traction bronchiectasis (thick arrows). (C) Coronal image shows the diffuse GGO with septal thickening and volume loss in the left lung (arrow). These are chronic changes of pulmonary fibrosis with superimposed acute alveolar hemorrhage.

Disorders Related to Systemic Disease Processes

Storage Disorders

The lung parenchymal changes in lysosomal storage disorders[17] are summarized in **Flowchart 1**. Illustrative cases are shown in **Figures 17 and 18**.

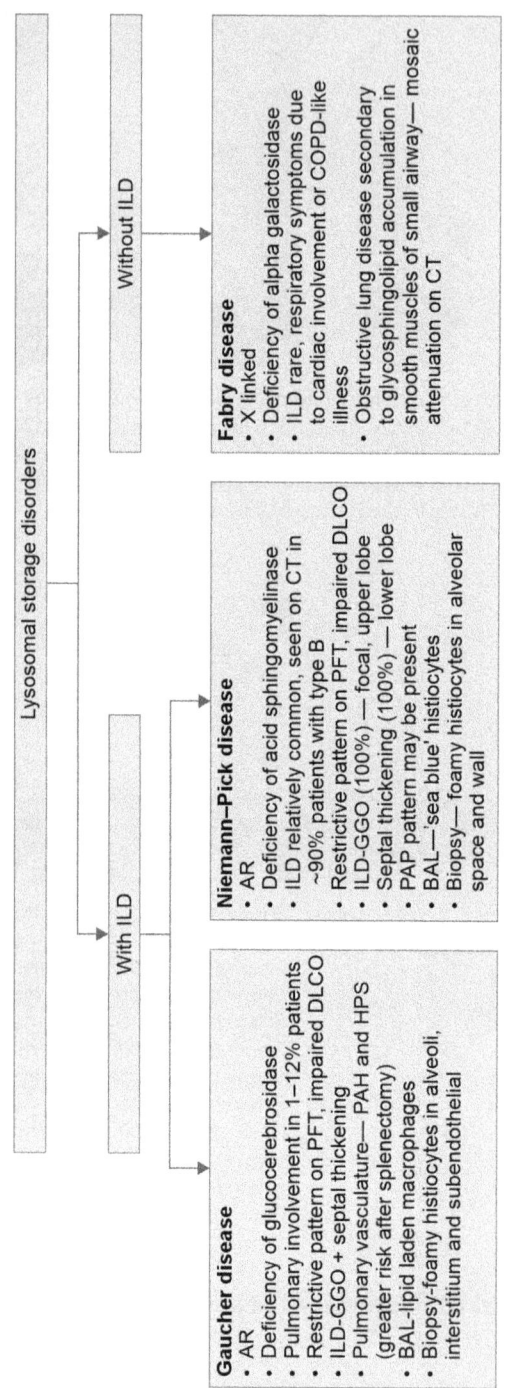

FLOWCHART 1: Summary of lung involvement in lysosomal storage disorders.

(AR: autosomal recessive; PFT: pulmonary function tests; DLCO: diffusing capacity of lungs for carbon monoxide; GGO: ground–glass opacity; PAH: pulmonary arterial hypertension; HPS: hepatopulmonary syndrome; PAP: pulmonary alveolar proteinosis; COPD: chronic obstructive pulmonary disease)

CHAPTER 12: Diffuse Lung Diseases: Part 2

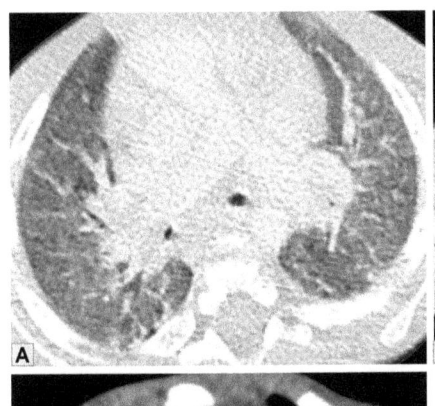
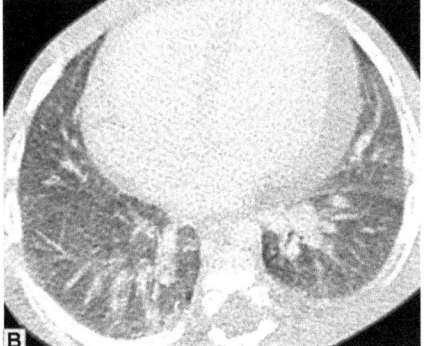
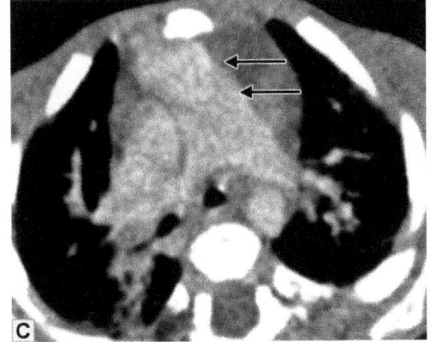

FIGS. 17A TO C: Gaucher's disease (GD). A 1-year-old boy with diagnosed GD and dyspnea. (A and B) Diffuse, symmetric GGO present in both lungs. (C) Significant dilatation of the pulmonary artery seen suggesting PAH (arrows).

(GGO: ground–glass opacity; PAH: pulmonary arterial hypertension)

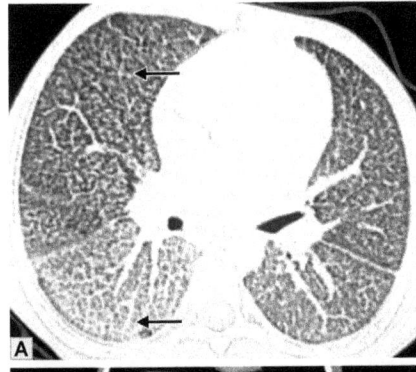
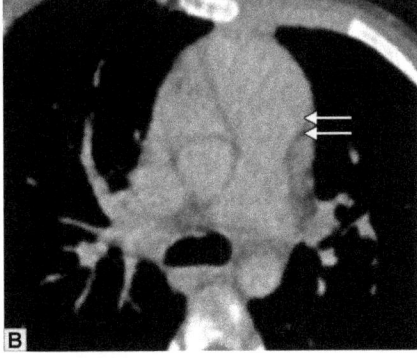
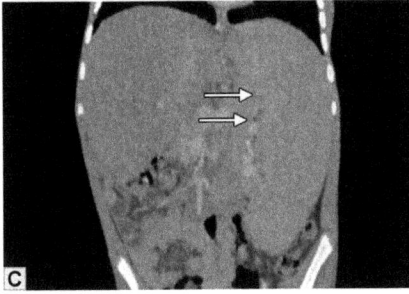

FIGS. 18A TO C: Storage disorder with lung involvement. A 9-year-old boy with hepatosplenomegaly and anemia. (A) Diffuse GGO with superimposed septal thickening (arrows) in both lungs. (B) PA dilatation is also noted (arrows). (C) Moderate splenomegaly (arrows) in the abdomen.

(GGO: ground–glass opacity; PA: pulmonary artery)

Immune Disorders

Pulmonary hemorrhage syndromes:
- Mostly associated with capillaritis
- Can be seen in multiple syndromes including vasculitides such as microscopic polyangiitis, granulomatosis with polyangiitis (Wegener's granulomatosis), Goodpasture's syndrome as well as collagen vascular disorders (CVD) including systemic lupus erythematosus (SLE), progressive systemic sclerosis (PSS), and polymyositis–dermatomyositis (PM-DM).
- Positive serum antineutrophil cytoplasmic antibodies (ANCAs) are diagnostic; however, lung biopsy may be required in their absence to demonstrate capillaritis.
- Patients present with dyspnea accompanied by episodic hemoptysis and anemia.
- Bilateral symmetric GGO with parahilar predominance is observed **(Figs. 19 and 20)**. Multifocal fluffy or nodular GGO may also be seen in the acute phase.

Nonhemorrhagic disease:
- Interstitial lung disease is commonly associated with CVD. The pattern of involvement differs according to the underlying etiology. These are summarized in **Table 3**.
- Early findings are often nonspecific and include GGO and septal thickening, while advanced disease often shows nonspecific interstitial pneumonitis (NSIP) pattern, with lower lobe predominant GGO, septal thickening, traction bronchiectasis and honeycombing **(Figs. 21 and 22)**.

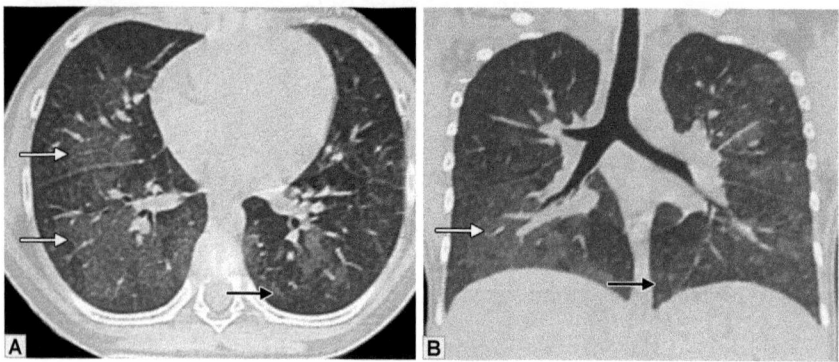

FIGS. 19A AND B: Pulmonary hemorrhage due to vasculitis. A 7-year-old girl with celiac disease. Bilateral GGO (white arrows) in parahilar distribution is noted with sparing of subpleural lung zones (black arrows).

(GGO: ground-glass opacity)

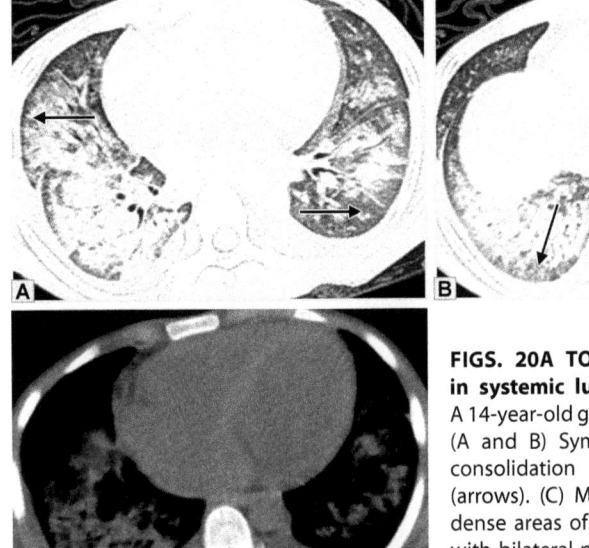

FIGS. 20A TO C: Alveolar hemorrhage in systemic lupus erythematosus (SLE). A 14-year-old girl with acute-onset dyspnea. (A and B) Symmetric parahilar GGO and consolidation with subpleural sparing (arrows). (C) Mediastinal window showing dense areas of consolidation (white arrow) with bilateral pleural effusion secondary to pleuritis in SLE.
(GGO: ground–glass opacity)

TABLE 3: Imaging patterns of ILD in connective tissue disorders.	
Collagen vascular disorder	ILD pattern
Systemic sclerosis	NSIP, interstitial fibrosis, and pulmonary artery hypertension
Polymyositis–dermatomyositis	NSIP and organizing pneumonia
Juvenile idiopathic arthritis	LIP and chronic bronchiolitis
Sjogren syndrome	LIP and chronic bronchiolitis
(ILD: interstitial lung disease; LIP: lymphocytic interstitial pneumonitis; NSIP: nonspecific interstitial pneumonitis)	

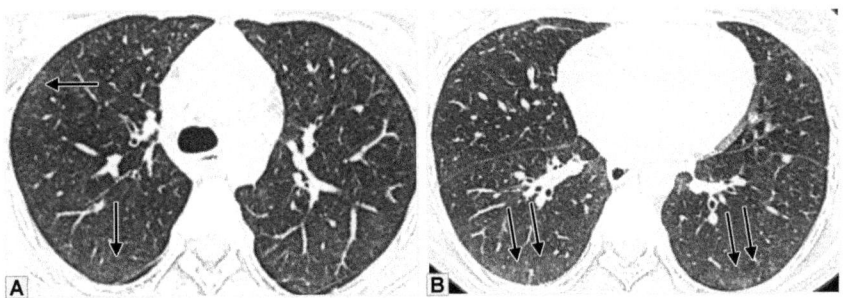

FIGS. 21A TO C: *Continued*

Continued

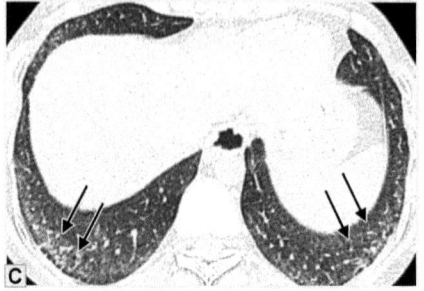

FIGS. 21A TO C: Early ILD in limited systemic sclerosis. A 15-year-old with no pulmonary symptoms. Both lungs show peripheral subpleural GGO (arrows), with a distinct apicobasal gradient.

(GGO: ground–glass opacity; ILD: interstitial lung disease)

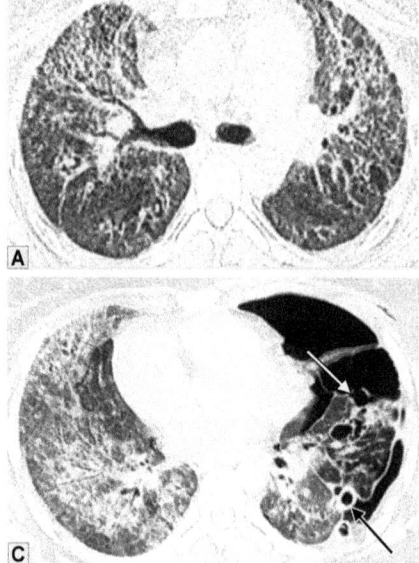
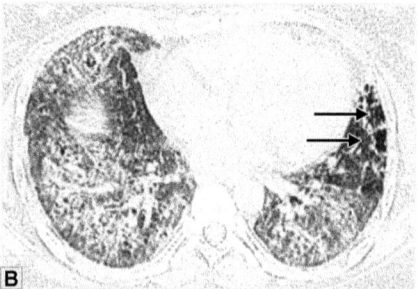

FIGS. 22A TO C: Nonspecific interstitial pneumonitis secondary to surfactant deficiency. An 18-year-old girl with progressive dyspnea. (A) Extensive subpleural reticulation and interlobular septal thickening is noted. (B) Small subpleural cysts are also seen (arrows). (C) HRCT taken 2 weeks after the previous study due to exacerbation of symptoms reveals moderate left pneumothorax due to rupture of one of the subpleural cysts (white arrow). A drainage tube had been placed (black arrow).

(HRCT: high-resolution computed tomography)

Granulomatosis with polyangiitis (GPA):
- Formerly known as Wegener's granulomatosis. It is a T-cell-mediated disorder that affects kidney as well as respiratory tract (both upper and lower).
- Necrotizing vasculitis as well as pulmonary parenchymal inflammation is present. c-ANCA is positive in up to 85% patients with active disease.

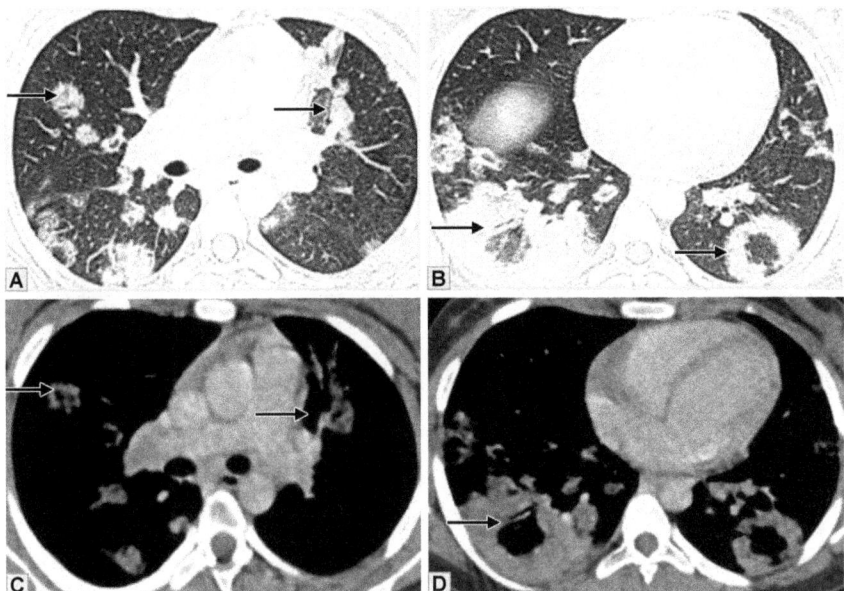

FIGS. 23A TO D: Granulomatosis with polyangiitis. A 13-year-old girl with hemoptysis. Multiple nodules with central ground–glass attenuation (arrows) in the mid lungs (A and C). Similar larger masses are seen in lower lungs (B and D).

- Multifocal variable sized (2 mm to several centimeters) pulmonary nodules are seen on CT. Larger nodules often undergo cavitation **(Figs. 23A to D)**.
- Pulmonary consolidation representing infarct or hemorrhage is also seen.

Langerhans cell histiocytosis:
- In children, multisystem (MS) involvement is seen affecting bones, liver, skin, spleen, central nervous system (CNS), and lung. Pulmonary involvement is seen in 20–50% children with MS-LCH.[18]
- Unlike adults, isolated pulmonary involvement is rare in children. There is no association with smoking.
- Radiographs show a reticulonodular pattern in early disease. On CT, multiple nodules are observed which undergo cavitation to form thin-walled lung cysts of bizarre shapes.
- Pneumothorax is a frequent and recurrent complication in these children due to rupture of cysts **(Figs. 24A to E)**.
- The upper lobe predominance observed in adults is not seen in children, but characteristic sparing of lung base as well as costophrenic angles is observed **(Figs. 25A to C)**.
- Bronchoalveolar lavage shows CD1a-positive cells, but with low sensitivity. The role of lung biopsy remains unclear.

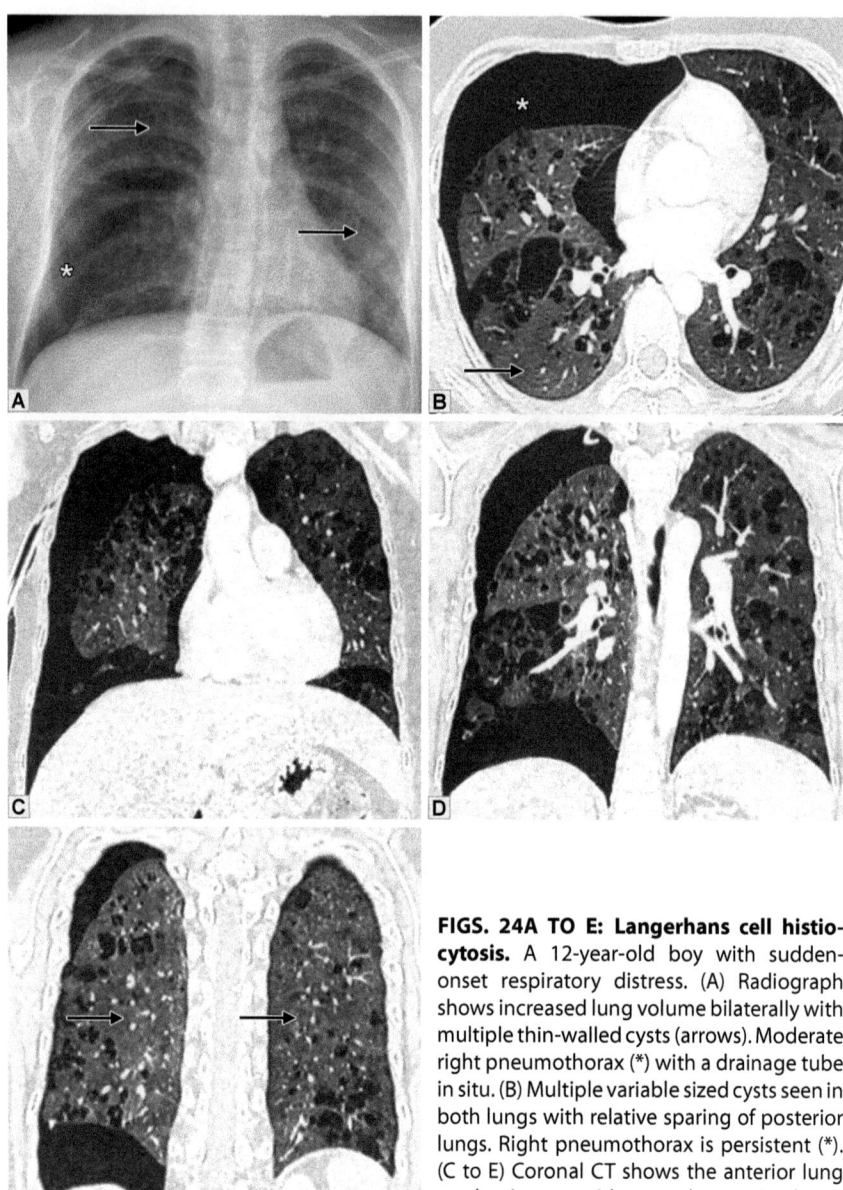

FIGS. 24A TO E: Langerhans cell histiocytosis. A 12-year-old boy with sudden-onset respiratory distress. (A) Radiograph shows increased lung volume bilaterally with multiple thin-walled cysts (arrows). Moderate right pneumothorax (*) with a drainage tube in situ. (B) Multiple variable sized cysts seen in both lungs with relative sparing of posterior lungs. Right pneumothorax is persistent (*). (C to E) Coronal CT shows the anterior lung predominance with spared posterior lungs (arrows).

CHAPTER 12: Diffuse Lung Diseases: Part 2

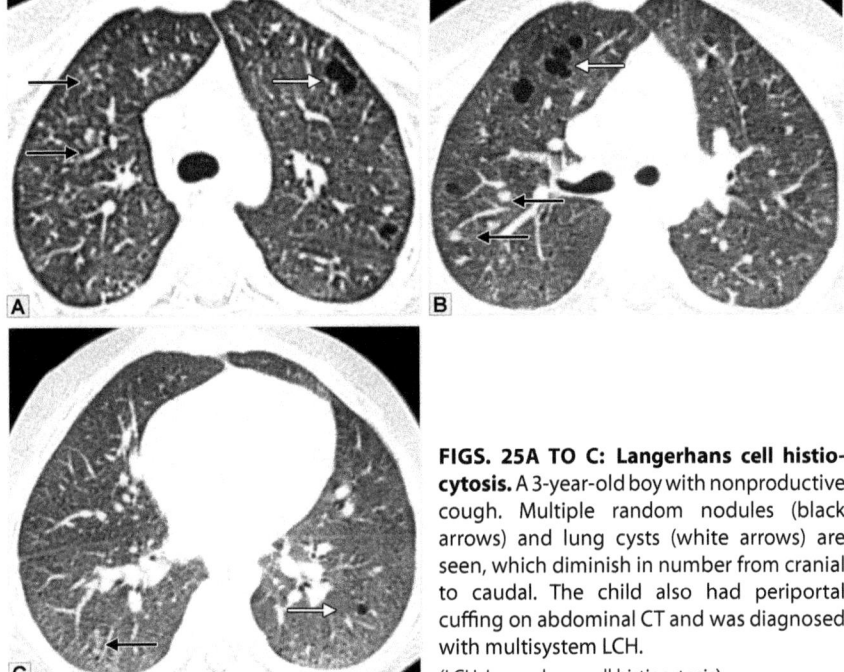

FIGS. 25A TO C: Langerhans cell histiocytosis. A 3-year-old boy with nonproductive cough. Multiple random nodules (black arrows) and lung cysts (white arrows) are seen, which diminish in number from cranial to caudal. The child also had periportal cuffing on abdominal CT and was diagnosed with multisystem LCH.
(LCH: Langerhans cell histiocytosis)

Sarcoidosis:
- There are two forms of childhood sarcoidosis. In children <5 years, a classical triad of arthritis, uveitis, and skin rash is seen without pulmonary involvement.
- The other form is seen in older children (adolescents) who present with multisystem involvement resembling adults, including pulmonary, nodal, ocular, joint (arthritis), and cutaneous (erythema nodosum). Hepatic and splenic involvement may also be seen.
- Classical stages of thoracic sarcoidosis have been described, which are isolated lymphadenopathy, combined nodal and parenchymal involvement, isolated parenchymal involvement, and pulmonary fibrosis.
- Small nodules in perilymphatic distribution are characteristic, with coalescence of these to form consolidation.
- In advanced stages, upper-lobe and airway-centric fibrosis with traction bronchiectasis and architectural distortion is noted.
- Good response to steroids is usually seen in early disease, but up to ~25% patients have high-risk disease that shows relentless progression to pulmonary fibrosis.[19]

Disorders of Immunocompromised Host
Lymphocytic Interstitial Pneumonitis/Follicular Bronchiolitis
- These represent a continuum of lymphocytic infiltrative disorders. Follicular bronchiolitis (FB) is a localized disease, while lymphocytic interstitial pneumonitis (LIP) has diffuse involvement.
- In children, these are most often associated with human immunodeficiency virus (HIV) infection and acquired immunodeficiency syndrome (AIDS). Up to ~40% of children with AIDS reported to develop LIP.[20]
- Other associations include Sjogren syndrome and congenital immunodeficiencies such as common variable immunodeficiency (CVID).
- Follicular bronchiolitis shows multiple centrilobular tree-in-bud nodules **(Figs. 26A and B)**, while LIP shows a combination of GGO in peripheral lung and nodules. Peribronchovascular cysts are also associated **(Figs. 27A to D)**.

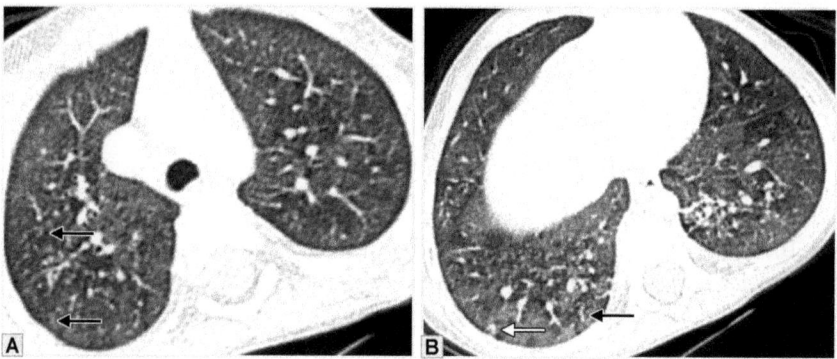

FIGS. 26A AND B: Follicular bronchiolitis. A 2-year-old boy with wheezing. Small centrilobular nodules (black arrows) are seen, with some of these showing "tree-in-bud" appearance (white arrow). Mosaic attenuation is also noted in both lungs, suggesting small-airway involvement.

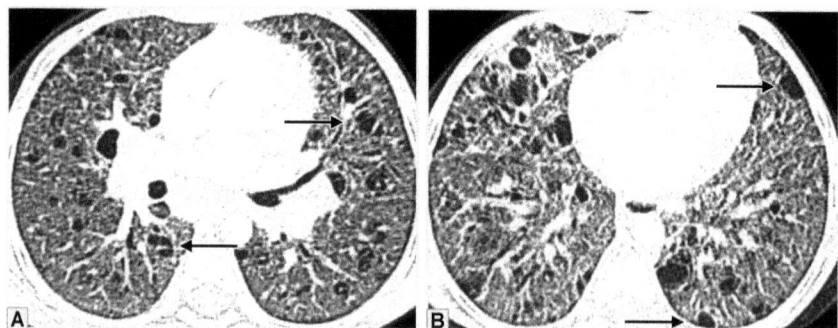

FIGS. 27A TO D: *Continued*

Continued

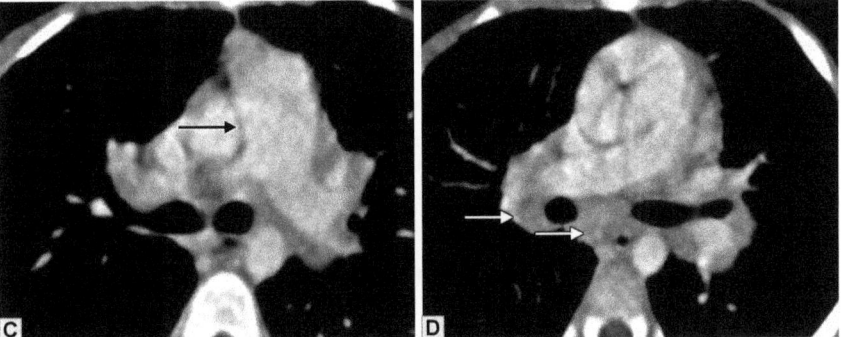

FIGS. 27A TO D: Lymphocytic interstitial pneumonitis. A 6-year-old boy with HIV-positive status. (A and B) Diffuse ground–glass haze in both lungs, with multiple small cysts seen distributed along bronchovascular bundles and in subpleural location (arrows). (C) Pulmonary artery dilatation is present (arrow). (D) Multiple enlarged lymph nodes are also seen in the bilateral hila and the subcarinal location (arrows).

Miscellaneous

Pulmonary Alveolar Microlithiasis

- This is a rare condition seen in both children and adults, with female predominance. It is inherited as an autosomal recessive disorder.
- Deposition of calcium phosphate microliths in alveoli.
- Patients are often asymptomatic till late in the disease course, family screening is essential in a diagnosed patient.[21]
- On radiographs, coalescent high-density nodules that obscure heart borders and alveoli are characteristic, though a diffuse "sand-like" haze is more commonly seen in children.
- On CT, GGO is found representing microscopic calcification with superimposed calcific nodules representing macroscopic deposits.
- "Black pleura" sign is described on radiographs as a strip of peripheral lucency underlying the ribs, which corresponds to tiny subpleural cysts on CT. The cysts represent early pulmonary fibrosis.

■ REFERENCES

1. Hime NJ, Zurynski Y, Fitzgerald D, Selvadurai H, Phu A, Deverell M, et al. Childhood interstitial lung disease: A systematic review. Pediatr Pulmonol. 2015;50(12):1383-92.
2. Kurland G, Deterding RR, Hagood JS, Young LR, Brody AS, Castile RG, et al. An official American Thoracic Society clinical practice guideline: classification, evaluation, and management of childhood interstitial lung disease in infancy. Am J Respir Crit Care Med. 2013;188(3):376-94.
3. Ferraro VA, Zanconato S, Zamunaro A, Carraro S. Children's Interstitial and Diffuse Lung Diseases (ChILD) in 2020. Child Basel Switz. 2020;7(12):280.
4. Semple TR, Ashworth MT, Owens CM. Interstitial Lung Disease in Children Made Easier…Well, Almost. Radiogr Rev Publ Radiol Soc N Am Inc. 2017;37(6):1679-703.

5. Liang T, Vargas SO, Lee EY. Childhood Interstitial (Diffuse) Lung Disease: Pattern Recognition Approach to Diagnosis in Infants. AJR Am J Roentgenol. 2019;212(5):958-67.
6. Biko DM, Schwartz M, Anupindi SA, Altes TA. Subpleural lung cysts in Down syndrome: prevalence and association with coexisting diagnoses. Pediatr Radiol. 2008;38(3):280-4.
7. Mechri M, Epaud R, Emond S, Coulomb A, Jaubert F, Tarrant A, et al. Surfactant protein C gene (SFTPC) mutation-associated lung disease: high-resolution computed tomography (HRCT) findings and its relation to histological analysis. Pediatr Pulmonol. 2010;45(10):1021-9.
8. Bullard JE, Wert SE, Whitsett JA, Dean M, Nogee LM. ABCA3 mutations associated with pediatric interstitial lung disease. Am J Respir Crit Care Med. 2005;172(8):1026-31.
9. Carré A, Szinnai G, Castanet M, Sura-Trueba S, Tron E, Broutin-L'Hermite I, et al. Five new TTF1/NKX2.1 mutations in brain-lung-thyroid syndrome: rescue by PAX8 synergism in one case. Hum Mol Genet. 2009;18(12):2266-76.
10. Suzuki T, Sakagami T, Young LR, Carey BC, Wood RE, Luisetti M, et al. Hereditary pulmonary alveolar proteinosis: pathogenesis, presentation, diagnosis, and therapy. Am J Respir Crit Care Med. 2010;182(10):1292-304.
11. Brody AS, Guillerman RP, Hay TC, Wagner BD, Young LR, Deutsch GH, et al. Neuroendocrine cell hyperplasia of infancy: diagnosis with high-resolution CT. AJR Am J Roentgenol. 2010;194(1):238-44.
12. Castillo M, Vade A, Lim-Dunham JE, Masuda E, Massarani-Wafai R. Pulmonary interstitial glycogenosis in the setting of lung growth abnormality: radiographic and pathologic correlation. Pediatr Radiol. 2010;40(9):1562-5.
13. Lino CA, Batista AKM, Soares MAD, de Freitas AE, Gomes LC, M Filho JH, et al. Bronchiolitis obliterans: clinical and radiological profile of children followed-up in a reference outpatient clinic. Rev Paul Pediatr. 2013;31(1):10-6.
14. Raghu G, Remy-Jardin M, Ryerson CJ, Myers JL, Kreuter M, Vasakova M, et al. Diagnosis of hypersensitivity pneumonitis in adults. An Official ATS/JRS/ALAT Clinical Practice Guideline. Am J Respir Crit Care Med. 2020;202(3):e36-69.
15. Marangu D, Gray D, Vanker A, Zampoli M. Exogenous lipoid pneumonia in children: A systematic review. Paediatr Respir Rev. 2020;33:45-51.
16. Giovannini-Chami L, Blanc S, Hadchouel A, Baruchel A, Boukari R, Dubus JC, et al. Eosinophilic pneumonias in children: A review of the epidemiology, diagnosis, and treatment. Pediatr Pulmonol. 2016;51(2):203-16.
17. Borie R, Crestani B, Guyard A, Lidove O. Interstitial lung disease in lysosomal storage disorders. Eur Respir Rev. 2021;30(160):200363.
18. Sharma S, Dey P. Childhood pulmonary Langerhans cell histiocytosis in broncho-alveolar lavage: A case report along with review of literature. Diagn Cytopathol. 2016;44(12):1102-6.
19. Chiu B, Chan J, Das S, Alshamma Z, Sergi C. Pediatric Sarcoidosis: A Review with Emphasis on Early Onset and High-risk Sarcoidosis and Diagnostic Challenges. Diagn Basel Switz. 2019;9(4):160.
20. Becciolini V, Gudinchet F, Cheseaux JJ, Schnyder P. Lymphocytic interstitial pneumonia in children with AIDS: high-resolution CT findings. Eur Radiol. 2001;11(6):1015-20.
21. Helbich TH, Wojnarovsky C, Wunderbaldinger P, Heinz-Peer G, Eichler I, Herold CJ. Pulmonary alveolar microlithiasis in children: radiographic and high-resolution CT findings. AJR Am J Roentgenol. 1997;168(1):63-5.

CHAPTER 13

Pulmonary Complications in Congenital Heart Diseases

Anisha Garg, Amarinder S Malhi

- ❑ Complications involving airways
  - ➢ Airway compression
  - ➢ Tracheobronchomalacia
  - ➢ Tracheal stenosis
  - ➢ Abnormal bronchial branching pattern
  - ➢ Plastic bronchitis
- ❑ Complications involving lung parenchyma
  - ➢ Infection
  - ➢ Atelectatic and emphysematous changes
  - ➢ Pulmonary edema
  - ➢ Pulmonary hemorrhage
- ❑ Complications involving pulmonary vasculature
  - ➢ Altered pulmonary blood flow
  - ➢ Hemoptysis—major aorto-pulmonary collateral arteries
  - ➢ Pulmonary arteriovenous malformations
  - ➢ Venovenous collaterals
  - ➢ Thromboembolic complications
- ❑ Complications involving pleura and thoracic cage
- ❑ Complications related to cardiac surgery

■ INTRODUCTION

- Cardiac and respiratory systems lie in close proximity to each other and show developmental and functional interdependence. Lungs and heart experience similar genetic and perinatal insults. Their disorders also present with overlapping symptoms adding to the diagnostic dilemma.
- Moreover, cardiac interventions in congenital heart diseases (CHDs) can lead to pulmonary complications including infections. Likewise, lung disorders can adversely affect the management and even preclude surgeries for congenital cardiac diseases. Therefore, it is imperative to identify and understand respiratory comorbidities in CHD patients for comprehensive patient care.
- The intrathoracic complications of CHDs are discussed compartment wise.

COMPLICATIONS INVOLVING AIRWAYS

Airway complications present with an obstructive pattern of lung dysfunction and include the following **(Table 1)**.

Airway Compression

- Airway compression is common in CHDs due to cardiac and pulmonary artery enlargement or vascular malposition. Children are more likely to be symptomatic because of their smaller, more collapsible airways. Large left-to-right shunts as seen in ventricular septal defect (VSD), patent ductus arteriosus (PDA), and truncus arteriosus lead to pulmonary overcirculation which dilates the central pulmonary vessels and enlarges the left atrial and overall heart size. Pulmonary stenosis and rare cases of tetralogy of Fallot (TOF) with dysplastic regurgitant pulmonary valve are also associated with enlarged pulmonary arteries. In these cases, the left main bronchus is most susceptible to obstruction as it gets pinched between the left atrium and left pulmonary artery causing left lower lobe atelectasis **(Figs. 1A to C)**.

TABLE 1: Airway complications.[3]		
	Imaging	Association/cause
Airway compression	Tracheal narrowing, surface indentation, and displacement	Vascular ring, slings, cardiomegaly, and dilated pulmonary arteries
Tracheobroncho-malacia (TBM)	• 50% AP diameter reduction of trachea in expiration • Invagination of posterior tracheal membrane (frown sign)	• Tracheoesophageal fistula, prolonged intubation • Vascular and nonvascular compression
Complete tracheal rings	Rounded narrow trachea with fixed diameter	Pulmonary artery sling
Subglottic stenosis	Hourglass narrowing	Prolonged intubation
Airway branching anomalies	• Tracheal bronchus, bridging bronchus • Horseshoe lung • Isomerism • Double right sidedness* • Double left sidedness*	• Pulmonary sling • Scimitar syndrome • Heterotaxy
Plastic bronchitis	Airway casts larger than mucus plugs, no bronchiectasis or air trapping	Cavopulmonary anastomosis
Primary ciliary dysfunction	Middle/lower lobe bronchiectasis, mucus plugging, and sinusitis	Dextrocardia and heterotaxy

Double right sidedness: Bilateral eparterial bronchi and three lobes of lungs.
Double left sidedness: Bilateral hyparterial bronchi and two lobes of lungs.

CHAPTER 13: Pulmonary Complications in Congenital Heart Diseases

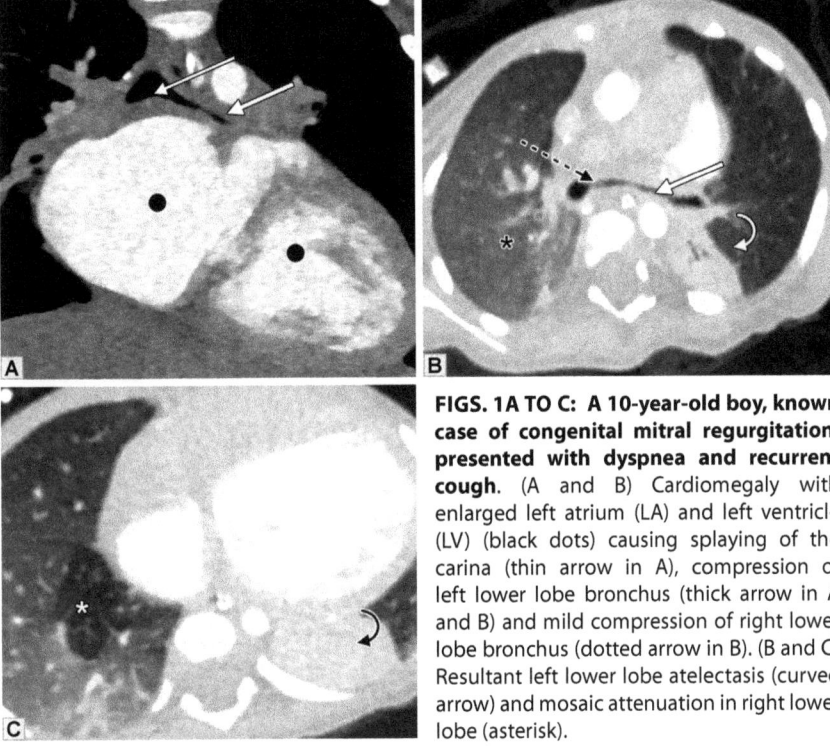

FIGS. 1A TO C: A 10-year-old boy, known case of congenital mitral regurgitation, presented with dyspnea and recurrent cough. (A and B) Cardiomegaly with enlarged left atrium (LA) and left ventricle (LV) (black dots) causing splaying of the carina (thin arrow in A), compression of left lower lobe bronchus (thick arrow in A and B) and mild compression of right lower lobe bronchus (dotted arrow in B). (B and C) Resultant left lower lobe atelectasis (curved arrow) and mosaic attenuation in right lower lobe (asterisk).

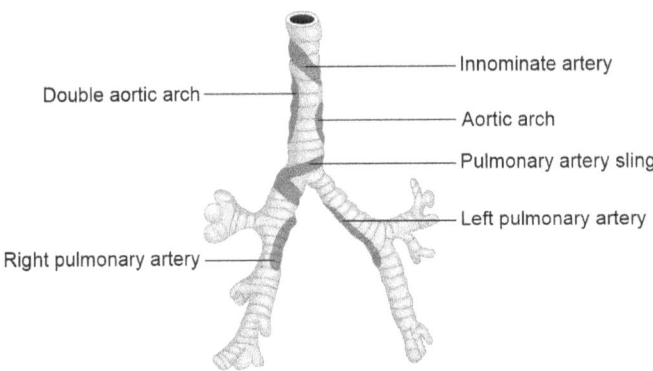

FIG. 2: Sites of vascular compression on trachea.

- Vascular rings can completely or incompletely encircle the trachea and esophagus with narrowing of their lumen **(Fig. 2)**. Double aortic arch and right aortic arch with aberrant left subclavian artery are two of the most common symptomatic vascular rings. The latter forms a loose ring completed by PDA or ligamentum arteriosum. Pulmonary artery sling is an aberrant left pulmonary artery arising from right pulmonary artery. Its unusual course between the trachea and esophagus causes compression of the distal trachea and right main bronchus with right lung hyperinflation.

- The extrinsic vascular or nonvascular compression on trachea ultimately leads to degeneration of tracheal cartilage or tracheomalacia which exacerbates the airway obstruction. Computed tomography angiography (CTA) can diagnose and assess the degree of tracheal narrowing.[1]

Tracheobronchomalacia

- Tracheobronchomalacia (TBM) refers to softening of the tracheal and/or bronchial cartilaginous rings with subsequent inward collapse of the posterior tracheal membrane. This causes luminal narrowing especially during expiration. Primary TBM occurs due to intrinsic cartilage deficiency or in association with tracheoesophageal fistula (TEF) which occurs concurrently in many CHDs. Secondary causes include vascular and nonvascular indentation and prolonged intubation. It is critical to diagnose this condition preoperatively as it can result in poor postoperative outcomes.
- Children present with barky cough, stridor, and recurrent respiratory tract infections. A reduction of >50% anteroposterior diameter between inspiratory and expiratory CT with invagination of posterior tracheal membrane (frown sign) is diagnostic.

Tracheal Stenosis

- Complete tracheal rings cause a circumferential reduction in tracheal lumen which appears as a narrow-rounded fixed caliber trachea **(Figs. 3A to D)**. The long-segment stenosis along with a low-positioned carina at T6–7 vertebral level gives the appearance of a T-shaped trachea. The frequent association of pulmonary artery sling with complete tracheal rings in about two-thirds of the cases has been labeled as the ring–sling complex. Other components of this complex are blind ending right upper lobe bronchus, bridging right bronchus arising from the left bronchus and right lung hypoplasia or air trapping.

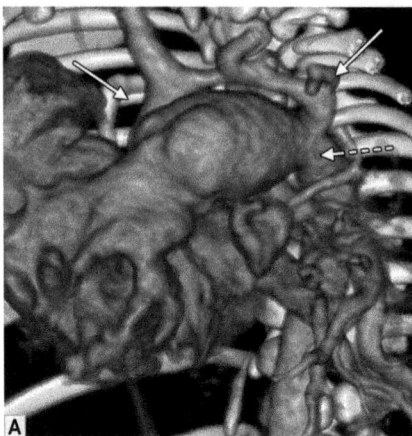
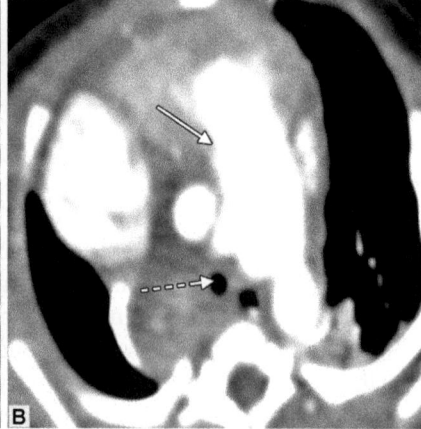

FIGS. 3A TO D: *Continued*

Continued

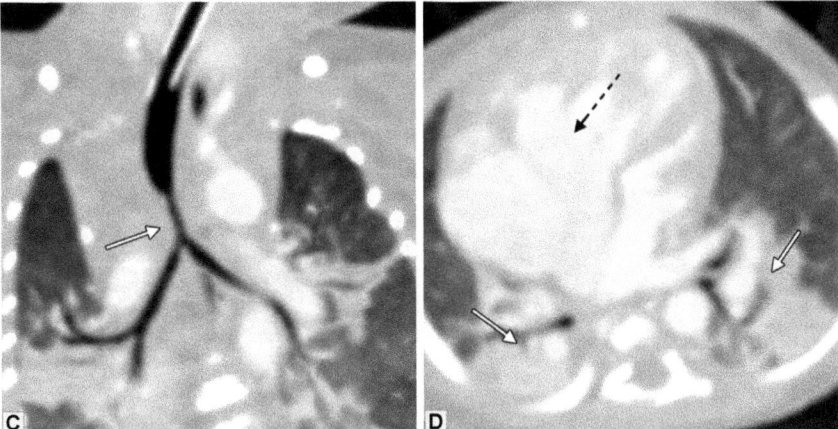

FIGS. 3A TO D: 10-year-old girl with multiple congenital anomalies and stridor. (A) Volume rendered (VRT) image of CT angiography: Preductal type of coarctation of aorta with narrowing of the arch from the level of brachiocephalic artery up to the left subclavian artery (arrows). Descending aorta is supplied by the PDA (dotted arrow). (B) Dilated main pulmonary artery (MPA) (arrow) suggestive of PAH. Trachea (dotted arrow) is narrow and rounded due to complete cartilaginous rings. (C) Resultant stenosis of trachea (arrow) just proximal to carina with narrow bronchi. (D) Bilateral lower lobe aspiration pneumonitis (arrows). Also note dilated right atrium (RA) and right ventricle (RV) due to PAH (dotted arrow).

- Subglottic stenosis commonly occurs in these patients due to prolonged intubation, especially in a postoperative setting. The mucosal edema and ischemia at the site of cuff of the endotracheal tube produces an hourglass narrowing with subsequent fibrosis.

Abnormal Bronchial Branching Pattern

- Displaced or supernumerary bronchi are rarely associated with CHDs and present with recurrent pneumonia and hemoptysis. Tracheal bronchus arises from the right wall of trachea within 2 cm of carina and may be the sole or accessory supply of right upper lobe. A low-positioned endotracheal tube may block its origin with right upper lobe atelectasis. The bronchial anomalies associated with pulmonary artery sling have been described above. In heterotaxy syndromes, mirror image bronchial anatomy occurs consisting of either bilateral right-sided or left-sided bronchi or corresponding mirror image lung lobulation **(Figs. 4 and 5)**. Right isomerism is especially notorious for its association with complex cyanotic CHDs.
- Scimitar syndrome may have a peculiar finding of horseshoe lung which is a tongue-like extension of right lung across the midline and behind the heart merging with the left lung. Bronchial agenesis is rare and more common on the left side. It is generally accompanied by pulmonary artery and lobar agenesis with resultant ipsilateral volume loss and tracheomediastinal shift **(Figs. 6A to D)**.

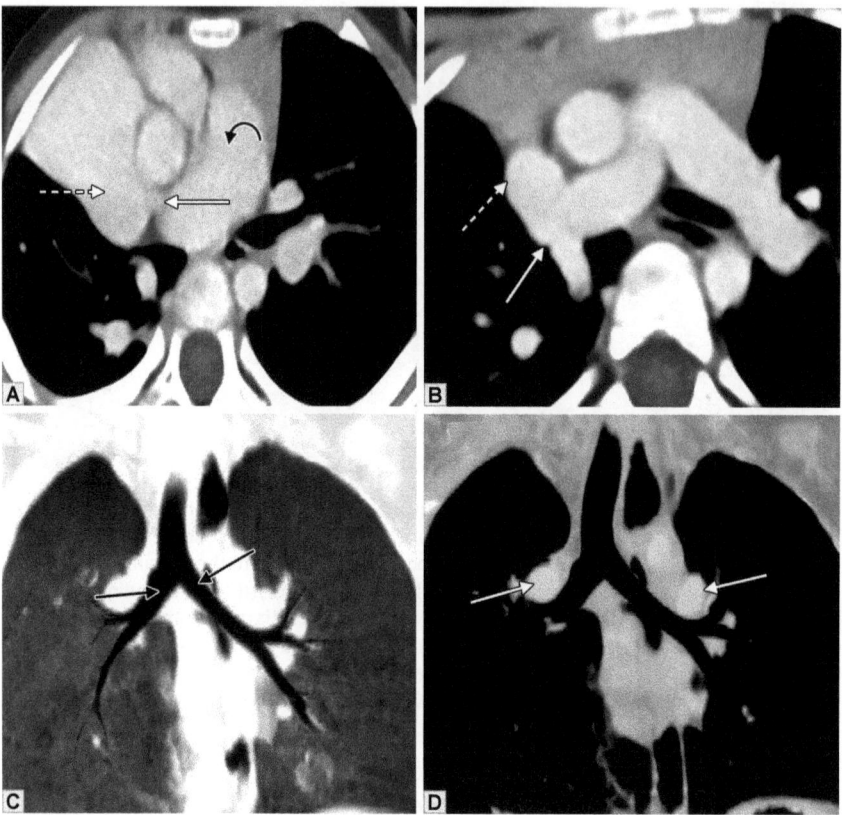

FIGS. 4A TO D: A 3-year-old girl, 45 XY karyotype, suspected case of CHD. (A) Small atrial septal defect (ASD) (arrow) with normally positioned but dilated RA (dotted arrow). Left atrium (LA) (curved arrow) and ventricular situs is normal (not shown). (B) Right superior pulmonary vein (arrow) draining into superior vena cava (dotted arrow): Supracardiac partial anomalous pulmonary venous return. (C) Coronal Minip: Bilateral left-sided bronchi (arrows) with hyparterial position (arrows in D). Left-sided bronchial situs with normal atrial situs suggestive of situs ambiguous.

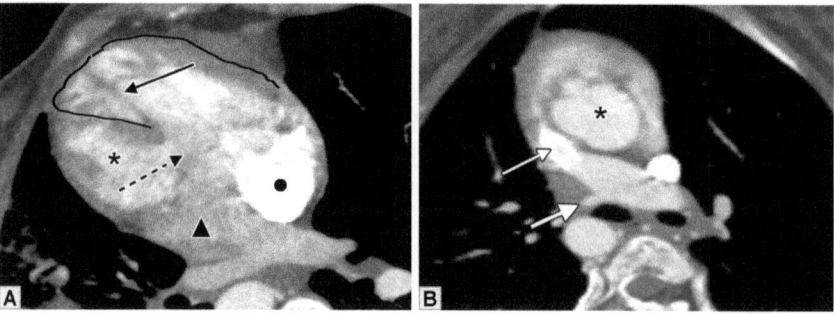

FIGS. 5A TO F: *Continued*

CHAPTER 13: Pulmonary Complications in Congenital Heart Diseases

Continued

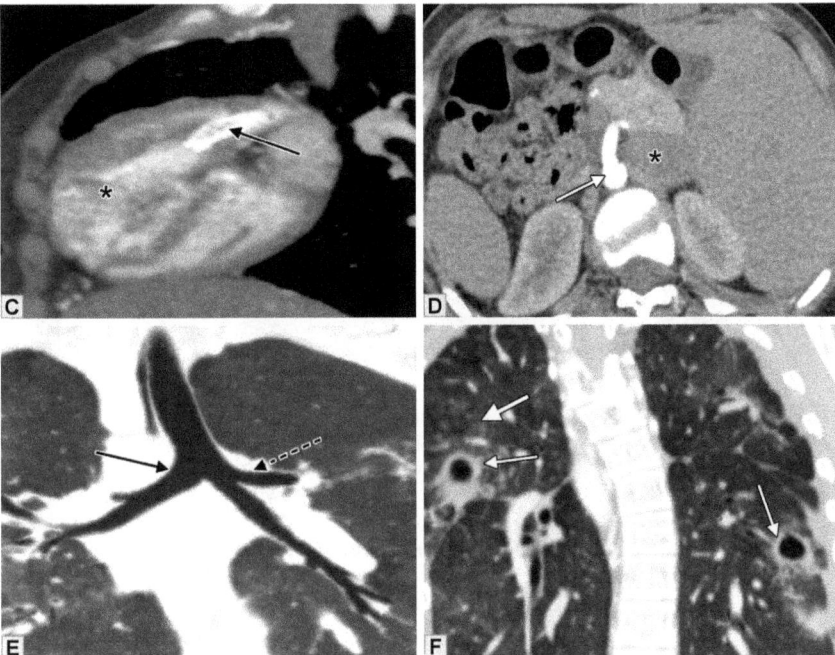

FIGS. 5A TO F: 15-year-old girl with high grade fever and dyspnea. (A) Morphological RV (outlined in black) with moderator band (arrow) and RA (black dot) on left side. LV (asterisk) and LA (arrowhead) are on right side. Basal VSD is noted (dotted arrow): Cardiac situs inversus. (B) Ascending aorta (asterisk) anterior and to left of MPA (thin arrow): L-TGA. MPA shows right ventricular outflow tract (RVOT) stenosis with stent in situ (arrow). RPA is hypoplastic (thick arrow). (C) Both MPA (arrow) and ascending aorta (not shown) arise from anteriorly placed RV (asterisk): Double outlet right ventricle (DORV). (D) Liver and IVC (asterisk) on left and spleen and aorta (arrow) on right: Abdominal situs inversus. (E) Morphological left bronchus on right (dotted arrow) and morphological right bronchus (arrow) on left. (F) Multiple cavities (thin arrows) and nodules (thick arrow) in both lungs likely due to septic emboli. Final diagnosis: Situs inversus with DORV, L TGA, VSD, hypoplastic RVOT and RPA with infection.

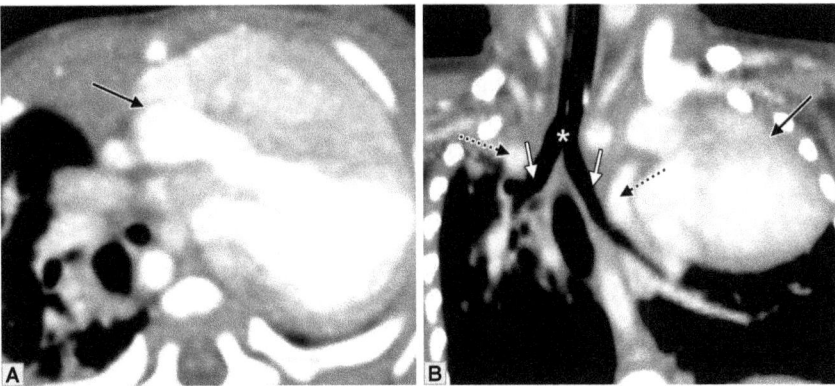

FIGS. 6A TO D: *Continued*

Continued

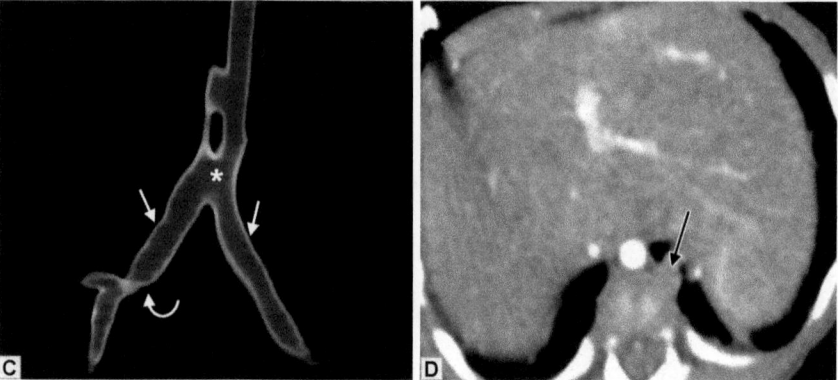

FIGS. 6A TO D: CT angiography of a patient with recurrent cough. (A and B) Heart is rotated with upward deviation to left side due to left upper lobe agenesis (black arrows). Bilateral hyparterial bronchi noted below pulmonary arteries (dotted arrows in B). (C) Volume-rendered technique (VRT) image of tracheobronchial tree shows bilateral lower lobe bronchi (short arrows) arising from carina (asterisk) with stenosis of the distal portion of right lower lobe bronchus (curved arrow). Bilateral upper lobe bronchi are not seen—agenesis. Same anatomy is also depicted in (B). (D) Midline liver and hemiazygos continuation of inferior vena cava (IVC) (arrow).

Plastic Bronchitis

Chronic central venous hypertension is an inherent complication in patients of Fontan surgery. This may cause increased fluid seepage through the peribronchial lymphatics which forms casts within the bronchial lumen. On CT scan, they appear as partial or complete filling defects with atelectasis, ground-glass opacities (GGOs), and consolidation in downstream lung parenchyma. Notably, there is no bronchiectasis/air trapping. Patients present with wheezing, dyspnea, and expectoration of pearly white casts. Bronchoscopic extraction of casts leads to rapid resolution of symptoms.

■ COMPLICATIONS INVOLVING LUNG PARENCHYMA

Altered pulmonary hemodynamics result in varying degrees of lung hypoplasia and a restrictive lung physiology in half of the patients of CHD. Their ability to compensate for acute parenchymal insults both in pre- and postoperative settings is thus limited **(Table 2)**.

CHAPTER 13: Pulmonary Complications in Congenital Heart Diseases

TABLE 2: Parenchymal complications.[3]

	Imaging	Association/cause
Infection	Lobar or peribronchial consolidation	Bacterial
	Dense nodules, Halo sign	Angioinvasive aspergillus
	Peribronchial soft tissue and centrilobular nodules	Airway invasive aspergillus
	Peribronchial thickening, patchy air trapping, and subsegmental atelectasis	Respiratory syncytial virus
	Random nodules with ground-glass opacity (GGOs) and central cavitation	Septic emboli
Atelectasis and emphysematous changes	Mosaic attenuation	Vascular compression, pulmonary edema, mucus plugging, and aspiration
Pulmonary edema	Septal thickening, GGOs, pleural and pericardial effusions, and consolidation	Hypoplastic left heart syndrome, total anomalous pulmonary venous return, cor triatriatum, large left-to-right shunt, left ventricular failure, ARDS and reperfusion injuries following surgery for tetralogy of Fallot
Pulmonary lymphatic perfusion syndrome	Septal thickening, pleural and pericardial chylous effusion, mediastinal edema, and enlarged nodes	Hypoplastic left heart syndrome, total anomalous pulmonary venous return
Pulmonary hemorrhage	GGOs, consolidation	Eisenmenger's, bleeding diathesis

Infection

- Pulmonary infections are the most frequent noncardiac complications. Among them, respiratory syncytial virus (RSV) has been found to be the foremost infection in children < 2 years.[2] It presents as bronchiolitis causing peribronchial thickening, patchy air trapping, and subsegmental atelectasis. Surgeries performed during the active phase of RSV infection are associated with higher incidence of pulmonary hypertension.
- Bacterial infections give rise to lobar or peribronchial segmental consolidation. Dense nodules surrounded by GGOs and associated with wedge-shaped infarct like consolidation and herald serious infections like angioinvasive aspergillosis. On the other hand, airway invasive aspergillosis generally causes peribronchial consolidation, centrilobular nodules, and tree-in-bud opacities. Septal thickening with interspersed GGOs suggests atypical infections such as mycoplasma **(Figs. 7 and 8)**.

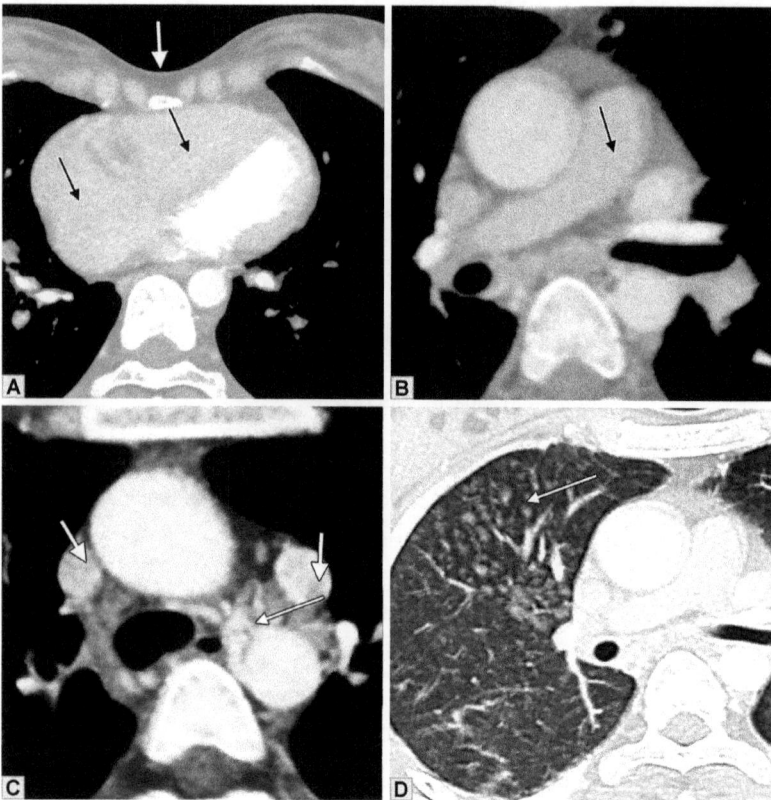

FIGS. 7A TO D: CT bronchial angiogram of a 22-year-old female with fever and hemoptysis. Echo findings suspicious for tetralogy of Fallot (TOF) physiology. (A) Dilated right atrium (RA) and right ventricle (RV) (arrows). Note pectus excavatum. (B) Relatively small main pulmonary artery (MPA) (arrow). (C) Multiple mediastinal collaterals arising from common and right bronchial (thin arrow). Duplicated superior vena cava (SVC) (thick arrows). (D) Centrilobular nodules in segmental distribution in right middle lobe (RML) (arrow) suggest superimposed infection.

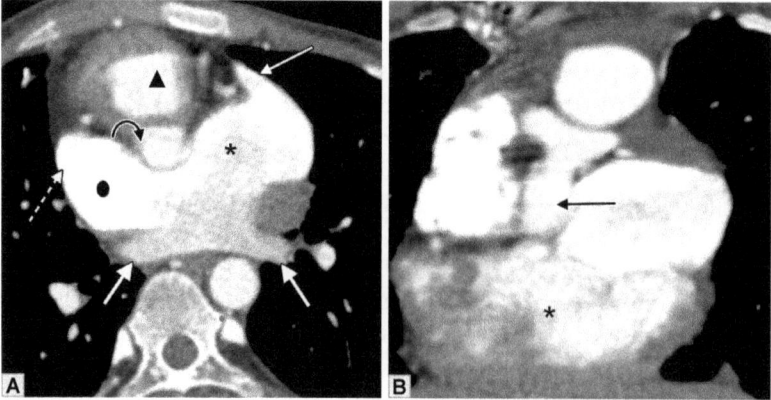

FIGS. 8A TO D: *Continued*

Continued

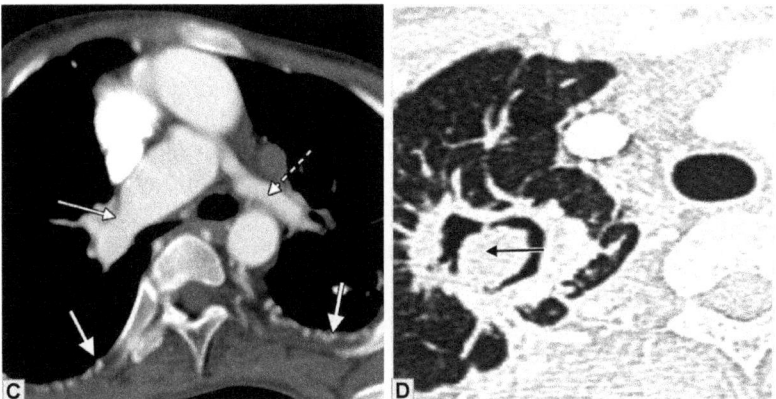

FIGS. 8A TO D: CT bronchial angiogram of a patient with single ventricle physiology. (A) Left atrium (LA) (asterisk) with LA appendage (thin arrow) and draining pulmonary veins (thick arrows). Right atrium (RA) (black dot) with broad RA appendage (dotted arrow). Interatrial septum not seen suggestive of atrial septal defect (ASD). Ascending aorta (arrowhead) is anterior and right of the narrow caliber main pulmonary artery (MPA) (curved arrow) suggests D-transposition of great arteries (D-TGA). (B) Ascending aorta (not shown) and narrow caliber MPA (arrow) arising from the single ventricle (asterisk). (C) Dilated right pulmonary artery (RPA) (thin arrow) and hypoplastic left pulmonary artery (LPA) (dotted arrow). Also note multiple major aortopulmonary collateral arteries (MAPCAs) (thick arrows). (D) Thick-walled cavity with soft tissue within in right upper lobe (arrow)—aspergilloma in old TB cavity.

- In the postoperative period, patients of CHDs face a heightened susceptibility to infections. Nosocomial and ventilator-associated pneumonias are the primary lung infections, the usual isolates being *Pseudomonas* and *Klebsiella* followed by *Candida*. Surgical site infections such as sternal osteomyelitis, mediastinal and pleural collections, infection of the prosthetic grafts, and endocarditis affecting the prosthetic valves are also prevalent. Furthermore, these infections can extend to the lungs, manifesting as septic pulmonary emboli. They appear as multiple ill-defined nodules surrounded by GGOs that often cavitate **(Figs. 5A to F)**.[3]

Atelectatic and Emphysematous Changes

Obstruction of both large and small airways can arise from various factors such as extrinsic pressure from vascular structures, pulmonary edema, mucus plugging, and aspiration particularly in postoperative patients. A mosaic pattern of lung attenuation with patchy atelectasis is seen, especially in neonates **(Figs. 1A to C)**.[2]

Pulmonary Edema

- On CT scans, pulmonary edema appears as peribronchial and septal thickening with interspersed GGOs and consolidation in a perihilar and dependent distribution. It arises from the disruption of starling forces, which is linked to abnormal cardiac function and postoperative complications. Left ventricular failure, large volume left-to-right shunts, and left atrial venous hypertension such as in cor triatriatum, hypoplastic left heart syndrome (HLHS), and total anomalous pulmonary venous return (TAPVR) can lead to fluid accumulation in the lung interstitium, decreasing the lung compliance.
- Pulmonary lymphatic perfusion syndrome occurs due to high central venous pressures causing distension of pulmonary lymphatics (lymphangiectasia) and leakage of lymph. The constellation of findings consisting of pulmonary edema, chylous pleural and pericardial effusions, mediastinal edema, lymphadenopathy, and plastic bronchitis is a clue to diagnosis **(Figs. 9A to D)**. Magnetic resonance and conventional lymphangiography can localize the site of lymphatic leakage and serve as a guide for percutaneous embolization.[3]
- Furthermore, postoperative acute respiratory distress syndrome (ARDS) and reperfusion-hyperperfusion injuries following corrective procedures for TOF, pulmonary atresia, and univentricular physiology can result in altered capillary permeability and pulmonary edema.

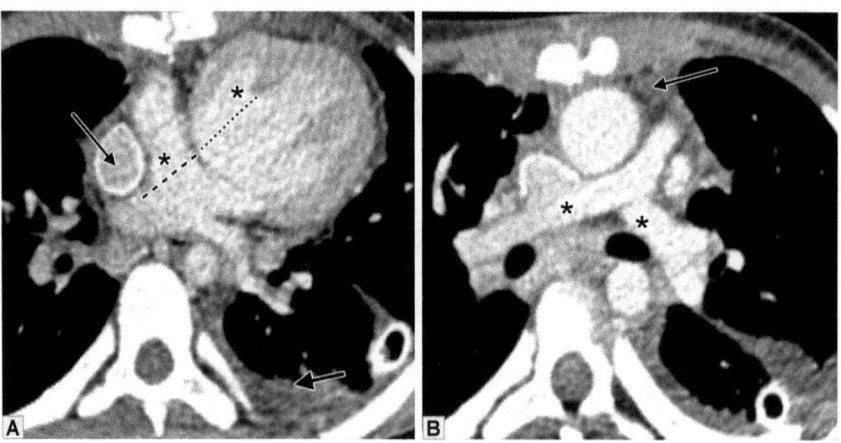

FIGS. 9A TO D: *Continued*

Continued

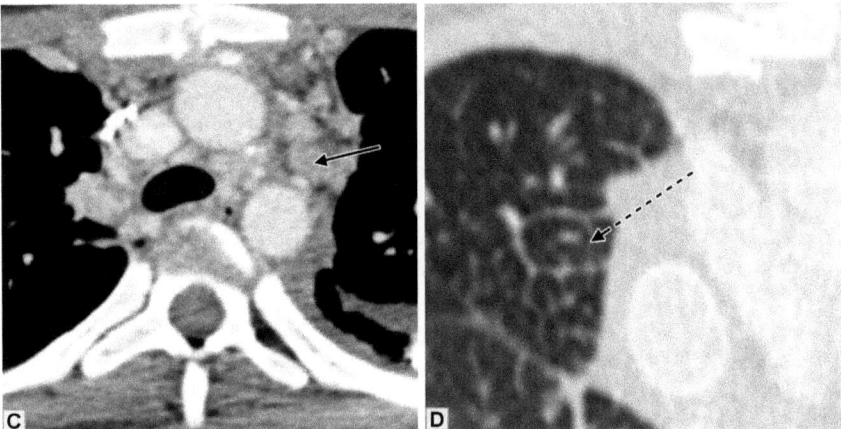

FIGS. 9A TO D: A 18-years-old boy, postoperative of Fontan procedure, presented with dyspnea. (A) Small RA and RV due to tricuspid atresia with atrial septal defect (ASD) and ventricular septal defect (VSD) (dotted lines). Extracardiac Fontan shunt (thin arrow), left pleural effusion (thick arrow). (B) Small pulmonary arteries (asterisks). Mild mediastinal edema (arrow). (C) Multiple small mediastinal nodes (arrow). (D) Zoomed lung window image: Septal thickening in right middle lobe (RML) (dotted arrow). This constellation of findings suggests lymphatic hyperperfusion syndrome.

Pulmonary Hemorrhage

Pulmonary hemorrhage is an infrequent phenomenon. It is encountered in cases of CHD complicated by Eisenmenger's syndrome especially when accompanied by both clotting and bleeding diathesis with life-threatening consequences. Radiologically, it mimics pulmonary infection and edema. Rapid clearing in 3-4 days, lack of dependent gradient and history of hemoptysis with significant drop in hemoglobin levels are helpful differentiating features.[2]

■ COMPLICATIONS INVOLVING PULMONARY VASCULATURE

Apart from central vascular anomalies, peripheral pulmonary blood vessels can also develop pathologies that lead to respiratory symptoms **(Table 3)**.

SECTION 4: Diffuse Lung Diseases and Miscellaneous

TABLE 3: Pulmonary vascular complications.[3]

	Imaging	Association/cause
Increased pulmonary blood flow	Pulmonary artery hypertension—dilated central pulmonary arteries with peripheral pruning, mosaic perfusion, centrilobular GGOs, and neovascular proliferation	Left-to-right shunt, complex CHD with unobstructed pulmonary outflow tract such as atrioventricular septal defect and truncus arteriosus
Decreased pulmonary blood flow	Small pulmonary arteries pulmonary artery stenosis, and pulmonary oligemia	TOF, pulmonary atresia, tricuspid atresia with pulmonary stenosis, and transposition of great arteries with pulmonary stenosis
Hemoptysis	Major aortopulmonary collateral arteries	TOF, pulmonary atresia, tricuspid atresia with pulmonary stenosis, and transposition of great arteries with pulmonary stenosis
PAVM	Dilated pulmonary artery and vein with a tangle of vessels, adjoining GGOs	Cavopulmonary anastomosis
Venovenous collaterals	Large-dilated veins from upper extremities to pulmonary veins	Cavopulmonary anastomosis
Pulmonary thromboembolism	Filling defects in pulmonary arteries	Cavopulmonary anastomosis and Eisenmenger's syndrome
Paradoxical embolism	Cerebral abscess and cerebral infarct	Intracardiac shunts, pulmonary AVMs, and venovenous collaterals

(AVM: arteriovenous malformation; CHD: congenital heart diseases; GGO: ground-glass opacity; TOF: tetralogy of Fallot)

Altered Pulmonary Blood Flow

- Increased pulmonary blood flow occurs in large left-to-right shunts leading to reflex pulmonary artery vasoconstriction and vascular remodeling and development of *pulmonary artery hypertension (PAH)* **(Figs. 10A to C)**. There is right ventricular dysfunction and eventually, reversal of left-to-right shunt known as Eisenmenger's syndrome. The reversal of shunt relieves the pressure on right heart but causes increased cyanosis, erythrocytosis, and risk of thromboembolic complications. Imaging studies reveal dilated central pulmonary arteries with peripheral pruning. Associated mosaic perfusion, centrilobular GGOs, and neovascular proliferation in the form of subpleural beading (Sheehan's vessels) are seen.
- On the other hand, decreased pulmonary blood flow in cases of TOF, pulmonary atresia, and tricuspid atresia with pulmonary stenosis may be responsible for reduced lung volumes and oversimplification of alveolar architecture. There are symptoms of diffuse lung disease, severe enough to cause PAH.

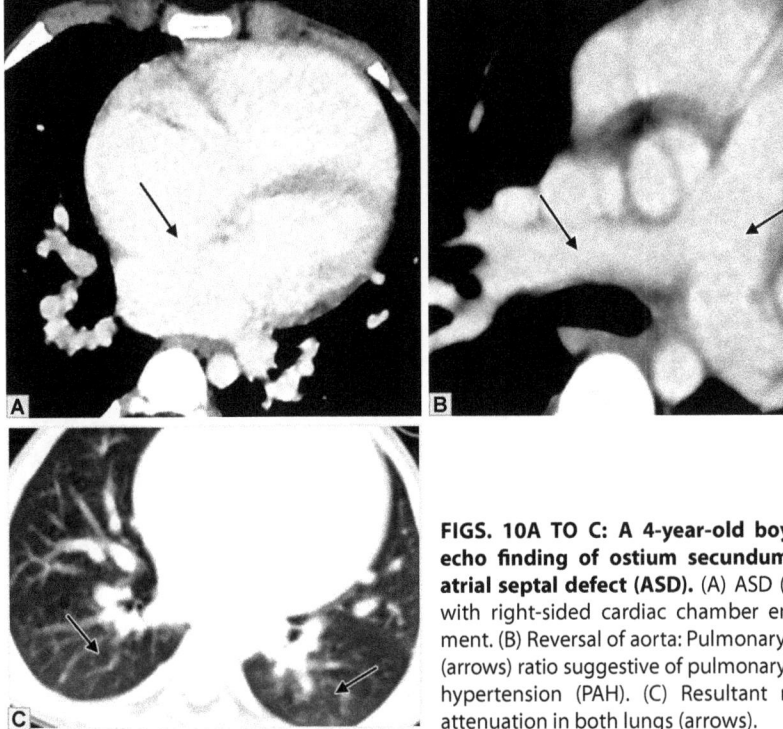

FIGS. 10A TO C: A 4-year-old boy with echo finding of ostium secundum type atrial septal defect **(ASD).** (A) ASD (arrow) with right-sided cardiac chamber enlargement. (B) Reversal of aorta: Pulmonary artery (arrows) ratio suggestive of pulmonary artery hypertension (PAH). (C) Resultant mosaic attenuation in both lungs (arrows).

Hemoptysis—Major Aortopulmonary Collateral Arteries

- In CHDs with severely compromised pulmonary blood flow such as TOF and pulmonary atresia, lung perfusion is maintained either via PDA or major aortopulmonary collateral arteries (MAPCAs) **(Figs. 8A to D)**. MAPCAs are persistent fetal segmental arteries that arise from bronchial arteries, aorta, and its first order branches like subclavian artery and connect to the pulmonary vasculature.
- The MAPCAs may be essential or nonessential. Essential MAPCAs are the sole supply to a pulmonary segment whereas nonessential ones occur in addition to the segmental pulmonary artery causing lung hyperperfusion. Large MAPCAs can develop segmental PAH and subsequently result in pulmonary hemorrhage and hemoptysis. They can be treated with unifocalization, ligation, or coil embolization.

Pulmonary Arteriovenous Malformations

Pulmonary arteriovenous malformations (PAVMs) are a unique manifestation of the altered hemodynamics in patients who have undergone cavopulmonary anastomosis for univentricular heart physiology **(Figs. 11A to E)**. They are postulated to arise as a result of exclusion of hepatic antiangiogenic factors from the pulmonary circulation and hence are more common on

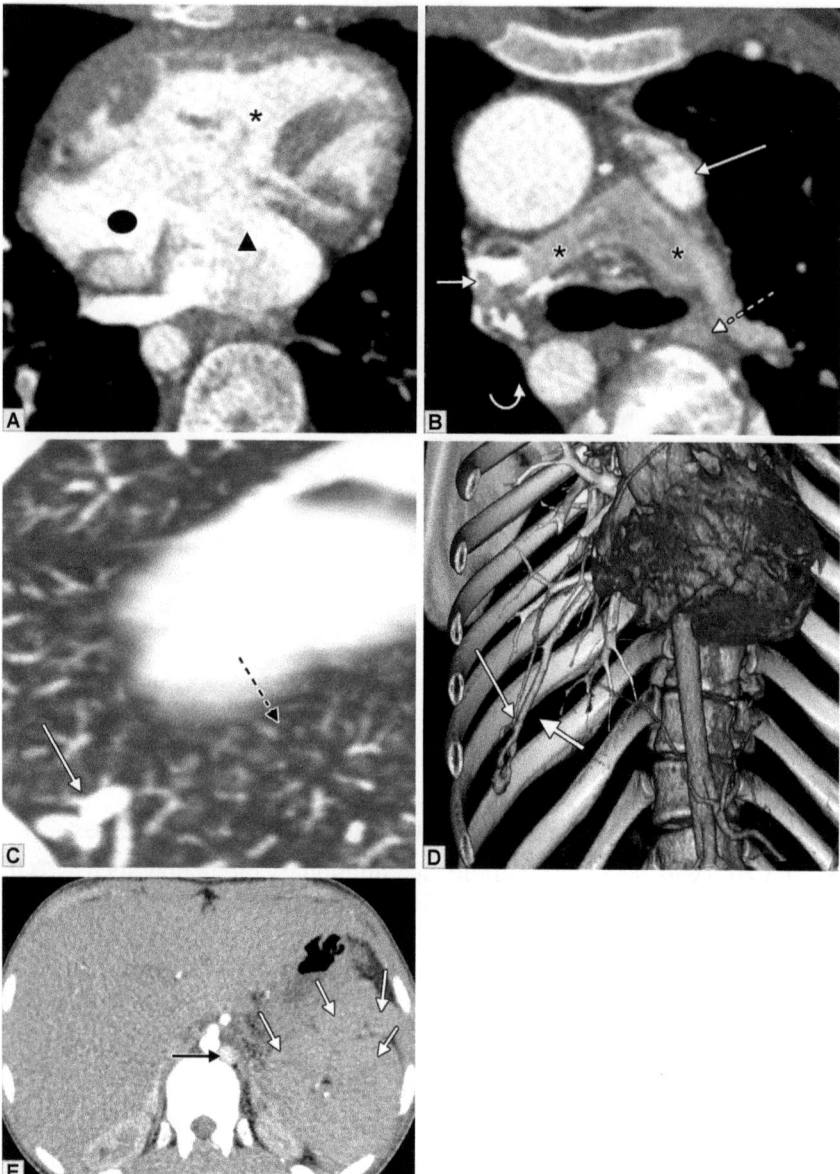

FIGS. 11A TO E: CT angiogram of a patient operated for univentricular physiology (Kawashima procedure). (A) Single ventricle (asterisk) with both right atrium (RA) (circle) and left atrium (LA) (arrowhead) draining into it. (B) Small caliber pulmonary arteries (asterisks). Blood from both superior vena cava (SVC) (arrows) and hemiazygos continuation of inferior vena cava (IVC) (dotted arrow) redirected to pulmonary circulation causing heterogeneous opacification. Also note right-sided descending aorta (curved arrow). (C) Zoomed maximum intensity projection (MIP) image of right lower lobe: Pulmonary arteriovenous malformation (PAVM) (arrow) and few ground-glass nodules (dotted arrow) due to aspirated blood. (D) Volume-rendered technique (VRT) image of the same region shows PAVM with feeding artery (thin arrow) and draining vein (thick arrow). (E) Polysplenia (arrows) and hemiazygos continuation of IVC (black arrow) suggestive of left isomerism.

the side opposite the inferior vena cava (IVC) drainage. Glenn procedure (superior cavopulmonary anastomosis) has greater incidence of PAVMs than Fontan operation (bicaval anastomosis). CT pulmonary angiography (CTPA) depicts a tangle of vessels in periphery of the lung with one or more dilated pulmonary arteries and veins extending up to it. Surrounding GGOs, indicative of microvascular telangiectasia may be seen. A feeding artery size > 3 mm and symptomatic PAVMs are indications for embolization.

Venovenous Collaterals

Systemic–pulmonary venovenous collaterals (VVCs) are a manifestation of the raised central venous pressures in Fontan circulation and participate in right-to-left shunting. They descend from the region of upper extremities into the left side of mediastinum and drain into pulmonary veins or left atrium.

Thromboembolic Complications

In Fontan circulation, the cavopulmonary blood flow is passive and nonpulsatile due to exclusion of the right ventricular pump. Hence, there is increased susceptibility to systemic venous thrombosis and pulmonary embolism. Similarly, in Eisenmenger's syndrome, pulmonary arteries are dilated with sluggish blood flow. Combined with chronic cyanosis, erythrocytosis, and hypercoagulability, this leads to increased incidence of thrombosis. Furthermore, patients with CHD are predisposed to paradoxical embolism due to systemic–pulmonary communications including intracardiac shunts and PAVMs.[4,5]

■ COMPLICATIONS INVOLVING PLEURA AND THORACIC CAGE

Pleural effusion can occur as a consequence of infection, cardiac failure, chylothorax, or direct trauma to thoracic duct during surgery **(Table 4 and Figs. 9A to D)**.

Deformities of thoracic cage such as pectus excavatum, scoliosis, and skeletal dysplasias such as Ellis–van Creveld and short rib polydactyly syndromes can be associated with CHDs **(Table 4)**. Pectus excavatum causes compression of the right ventricle and lungs leading to ventricular dysfunction and restrictive lung disease **(Figs. 7A to D)**.

TABLE 4: Pleural and thoracic complications.[3]		
	Imaging	Association/cause
Pleural effusion		Infection, cardiac failure, chylothorax, and trauma to thoracic duct
Pectus excavatum	Decrease AP diameter of thorax (Haller index > 2)	Idiopathic

TABLE 5: Surgical complications.[3]		
	Imaging	Association/cause
Post transplant lymphoproliferative disorders (PTLD)	Parenchymal nodules and mass-like consolidation, lymphadenopathy	Epstein–Barr virus
Pleuroparenchymal fibroelastosis (PPFE)	Apical pleural thickening, subpleural fibroatelectatic changes	Idiopathic
Injury	Chylothorax, diaphragmatic palsy, vocal cord palsy, and subglottic stenosis	Injury to thoracic duct, phrenic nerve, and recurrent laryngeal nerve prolonged Intubation

COMPLICATIONS RELATED TO CARDIAC SURGERY (TABLE 5)

Infections, atelectasis, congestive cardiac failure, and pulmonary edema are frequent in the postoperative period. Cardiac interventions can be complicated by injuries to mediastinal structures leading to chylothorax, diaphragmatic palsy, recurrent laryngeal nerve palsy, and subglottic stenosis. Fontan procedure is associated with lymphatic hyperperfusion syndrome **(Figs. 9A to D)**. Posttransplant lymphoproliferative disorder (PTLD) occurs within 10 years after cardiac transplantation and presents as nodules and mass-like consolidations with mediastinal lymphadenopathy. Pleuropulmonary fibroelastosis (PPFE), though mostly seen after bone marrow transplantation, has been reported to occur postcardiac transplantation. It presents as apical pleural thickening with subpleural fibrotic changes. Contrary to adults where it presents insidiously, affected children show a rapid relentless progression.[3]

CONCLUSION

The intricate relationship between the cardiac and respiratory systems underscores the importance of recognizing and addressing respiratory comorbidities in CHD cases. This holistic approach to patient care is essential for achieving better outcomes and ensuring effective management of both systems.

Other Related Chapters that can be Referred to:
- Chapter 18: Pulmonary Artery Imaging
- Chapter 19: Pulmonary Veins Imaging
- Chapter 20: Lymphatic Anomalies: Imaging and Interventions

REFERENCES

1. Newman B. Airway abnormalities associated with congenital heart disease. Pediatr Radiol. 2022;52(10):1849-61.
2. Healy F, Hanna BD, Zinman R. Pulmonary complications of congenital heart disease. Paediatr Respir Rev. 2012;13(1):10-5.
3. Rapp JB, White AM, Otero HJ, Biko DM. Computed tomography of the airways and lungs in congenital heart disease. Pediatr Radiol. 2022;52(13):2529-37.
4. Saremi FE. Cardiac CT and MR for adult congenital heart disease. In: Saremi F (Ed) Cardiac CT and MR for Adult Congenital Heart Disease. New York, NY: Springer; 2013.
5. King WG, Schowengerdt KO. Pulmonary Disease Associated with Congenital Heart Disease. In: Wilmott RW, Deterding R, Li A, Ratjen F, Sly P, Zar HJ (Eds). Kendig's Disorders of the Respiratory Tract in Children, 9th edition. Phliadelphia: Elsevier; 2019. pp. 615-25.

SECTION 5

Airway Imaging

CHAPTER 14: Upper Airway Imaging
CHAPTER 15: Central Airway Imaging
CHAPTER 16: Bronchiectasis
CHAPTER 17: Small Airway Diseases

CHAPTER 14

Upper Airway Imaging

Smita Manchanda, Ankita Aggarwal

- ❏ Classification
- ❏ Etiological approach
  - ➤ Congenital
  - ➤ Infective
- ➤ Vascular malformations
- ➤ Masses/Lymphoid enlargement
- ➤ Miscellaneous

INTRODUCTION

- Upper airway refers to part of respiratory tract extending from anterior nares to upper trachea (up to the thoracic inlet).
  The imaging modalities include plain radiographs, ultrasound (USG), and contrast-enhanced computed tomography (CECT).
- Plain radiographs are especially useful in the emergency setting including suspected foreign body (FB) and infective conditions. USG is a portable, easily available, radiation-free imaging modality with the added advantage of dynamic evaluation of the airway without sedation. A good acoustic window is available in the pediatric age group because of thin musculature and unossified cartilages. The normal anatomy of the airway on radiograph and USG is shown in **Figures 1 and 2**, respectively.

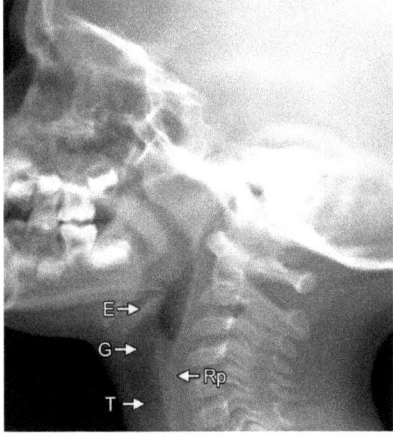

FIG. 1: Normal anatomy on lateral radiograph of the neck showing: epiglottis (E), glottis (G), trachea (T), prevertebral/retropharyngeal space (Rp).

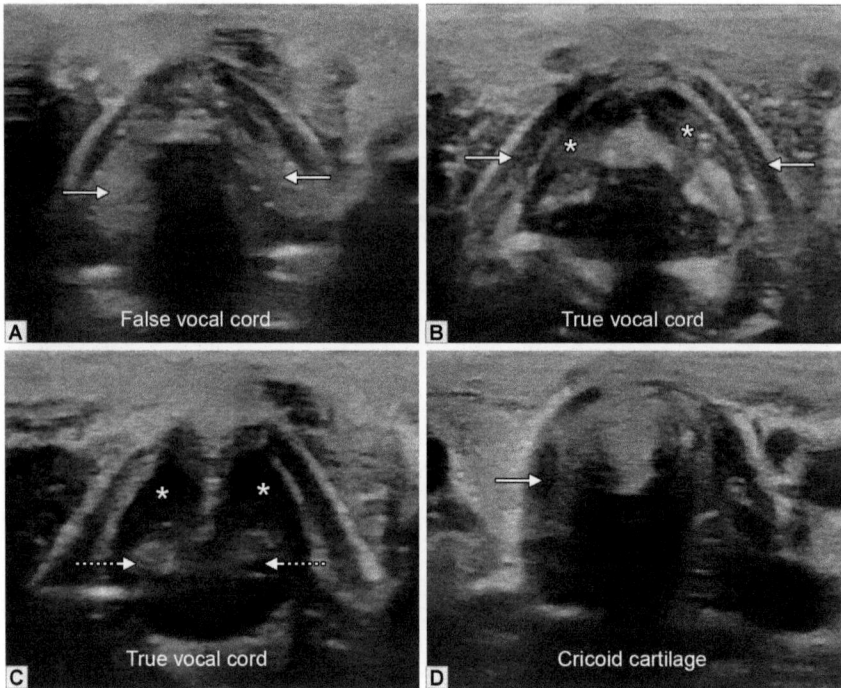

FIGS. 2A TO D: Normal USG of the larynx. (A) level of false vocal cords (arrows). (B) True vocal cords in abduction (asterisks) during normal respiration. Thyroid cartilage (arrows). (C) True vocal cords (asterisks) in adduction during phonation. Arytenoid cartilage marked as dotted arrows. (D) A complete ring of cricoid cartilage (arrow).

CECT has a role in delineating the extent of disease especially tumors and space infections. MRI is used as problem solving especially in cases of vascular malformations and tumors.

CLASSIFICATION

The abnormalities of upper airway can be classified under the following headings:
- *Based on compartment*:
  - Intrinsic/mural abnormalities
  - Extrinsic compression
  - Intraluminal obstruction

- *Based on etiology*:
  - Congenital
  - Infective
  - Vascular malformations
  - Masses/neoplastic
  - *Miscellaneous*: Foreign body and iatrogenic strictures

ETIOLOGICAL APPROACH

The etiological approach to upper airway abnormalities is followed in this chapter as detailed below.

Congenital

The congenital causes of upper airway obstruction can be at the level of nasopharynx, oropharynx, or larynx.

Nasopharynx

The causes of nasopharyngeal airway obstruction include choanal atresia, pyriform aperture stenosis, frontonasal dysplasia, encephalocele, and midface hypoplasia/craniofacial syndromes (detailed discussion of these entities is beyond the scope of this chapter).

Oropharynx

Cleft lip, cleft palate, pharyngeal hypotonia, micrognathia, retrognathia, macroglossia, and glossoptosis are causes of obstruction at the level of oropharynx (detailed discussion of these entities is beyond the scope of this chapter).

Larynx

The characteristic symptom of upper-airway obstruction is stridor which can be inspiratory, expiratory, or biphasic. Inspiratory stridor is due to an obstruction above the glottis, expiratory stridor because of airway obstruction in the lower trachea, and biphasic stridor is associated with a glottic or subglottic lesion. The common causes of laryngeal anomalies include laryngomalacia, vocal-cord paralysis, laryngeal web, cleft, subglottic stenosis, and hemangioma. The key clinical and imaging features are summarized in **Table 1**[1-3] and illustrated in **Figures 3 to 7**.

TABLE 1: Key clinical and imaging features of congenital causes of laryngeal airway obstruction.

Disease	Site/etiology	Clinical	Imaging
Laryngomalacia (most common congenital laryngeal anomaly)	• Shortened aryepiglottic folds • Prolapse of the cuneiform and corniculate cartilages over the laryngeal inlet • Immaturity of neuromuscular control/cartilaginous structures	• Presentation usually 2 weeks after birth • Inspiratory stridor especially in supine position/agitated child	• Usually does not undergo imaging • *Chest radiograph:* Aspiration can cause recurrent pulmonary infections
Vocal cord paralysis (second most common)	Vocal cords *Bilateral:* Idiopathic or CNS cause (Arnold–Chiari, spinal dysraphism)	*Bilateral VC palsy:* Airway emergency with a near-normal phonation and a high-pitched inspiratory stridor	• *USG:* Immobile vocal cords • *Chest radiograph:* Aspiration can cause recurrent pulmonary infections
• Congenital subglottic stenosis • 2 types: Membranous/cartilaginous **(Figs. 3A and B)**	• Diameter < 4 mm of the cricoid region in a full-term infant • <3 mm in a premature infant • Incomplete recanalization of the laryngotracheal tube during the 3rd month of gestation	Biphasic stridor, dyspnea, and labored breathing	*Lateral and AP radiographs:* Narrowing at level of subglottis
Laryngeal web[3] **(Figs. 4A and B)**	• Webs are typically in the anterior portion of the glottis and may have a subglottic extension • Lack of complete separation of connective tissue of vocal folds • Most common associated anomaly is subglottic stenosis	Dysphonia at birth and/or respiratory distress	• *CT:* Delineates the craniocaudal extent of the web and its thickness • Congenital lateral pharyngeal diverticula may also be seen in association. Unilateral, cystic/air-filled structures connected to the tonsillar fossa or the pyriform sinus
Vallecular cyst **(Figs. 5A and B)**	• Fluid filled cyst in supraglottic location • May be associated with laryngocele **(Figs. 6A and B)**	Inspiratory stridor, feeding difficulties, and undernutrition	*USG:* Well-defined anechoic lesion in the supraglottis
Subglottic hemangioma **(Figs. 7A and B)**	• Hemangioma at the level of subglottis • Benign, congenital vascular tumor	Respiratory distress, biphasic stridor along with difficulty in feeding	• *USG Doppler:* Echogenic lesion with increased vascularity in the subglottis • *CT/MRI:* Extent of lesion (neck/mediastinum)

(VC: vocal cord)

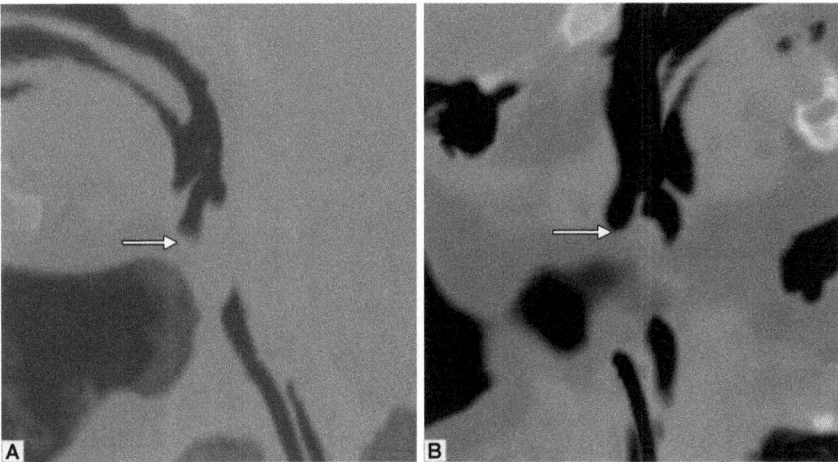

FIGS. 3A AND B: Congenital subglottic stenosis. (A) Sagittal minimum intensity projection image. (B) Coronal minimum intensity image. (A and B) Abrupt termination of the upper airway (arrows) at the level of hypopharynx.

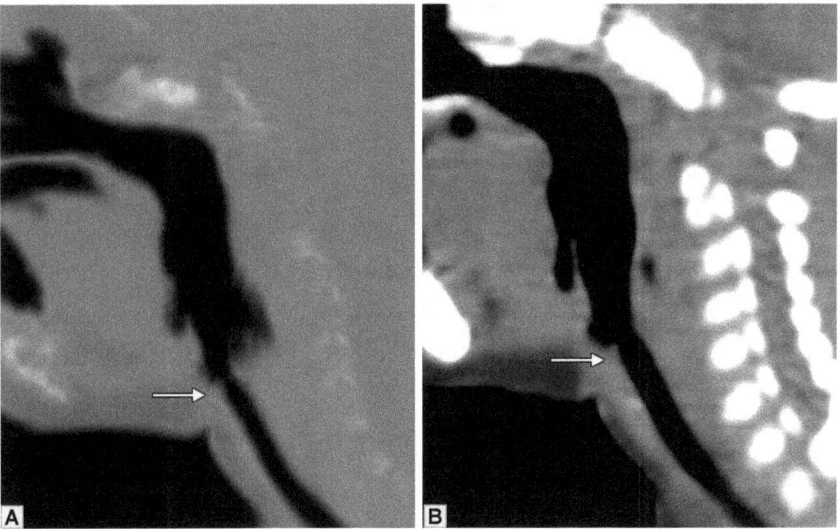

FIGS. 4A AND B: Laryngeal web. CECT sagittal images of the neck. A thin partial membrane (arrows) along the anterior larynx causing minimal compromise of the airway.
(CECT: contrast-enhanced computed tomography)

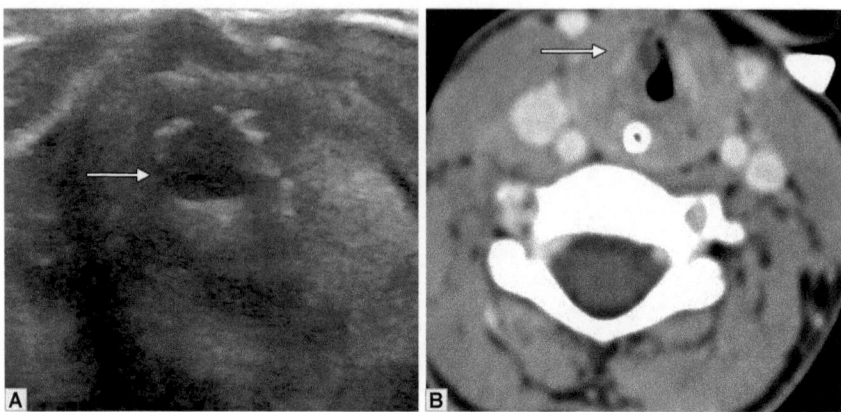

FIGS. 5A AND B: Congenital laryngeal cyst. (A) USG image. (B) CECT image. (A and B) Thin-walled fluid-filled, nonenhancing, cystic lesion (arrows) seen on the right side of the laryngeal ventricle.
(USG: ultrasound; CECT: contrast-enhanced computed tomography)

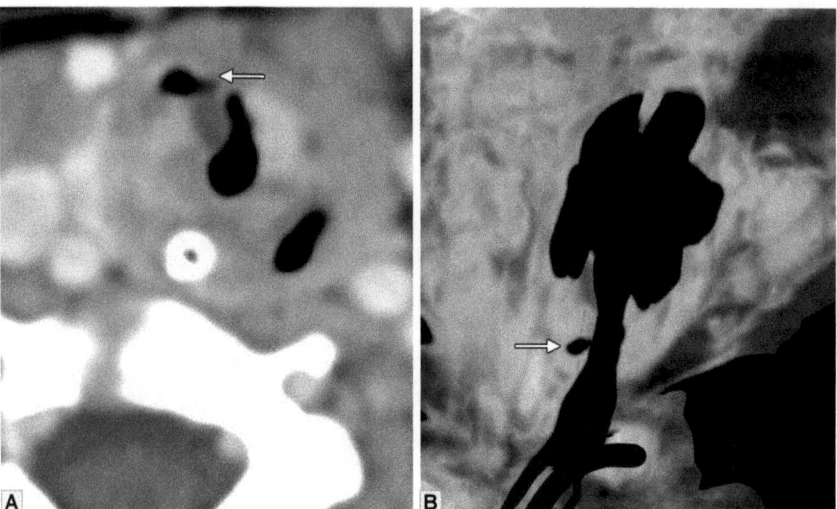

FIGS. 6A AND B: External laryngocele. (A) CECT images. (B) Minimum intensity projection image. (A and B) Well-defined thin-walled air-filled lesion (arrows) in the right paraglottic region which is communicating with the laryngeal ventricle.
(CECT: contrast-enhanced computed tomography)

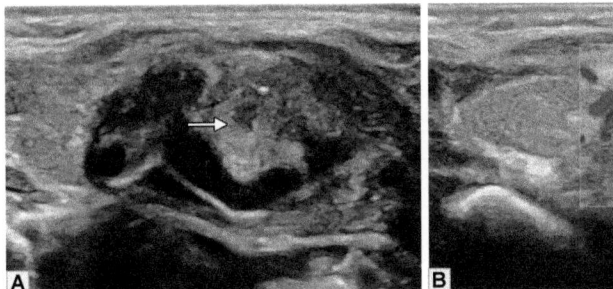
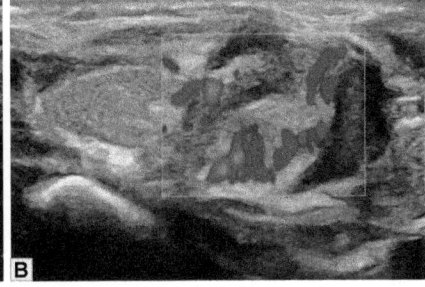

FIGS. 7A AND B: Subglottic hemangioma. (A) Sagittal oblique USG image. (B) Color Doppler. (A) Homogenous hyperechoic mass (arrow) in the subglottis. (B) Marked vascularity seen within the lesion.

Infective

- Upper airway infections in children involve the pharynx or sinonasal tract with fever, cough, rhinorrhea, and similar mild symptoms. However, involvement of airway and adjoining sites such as epiglottis (epiglottitis), larynx (laryngitis), or trachea (tracheitis) can result in emergent situation. These children present with change of voice or hoarseness and respiratory distress, besides cough. Adjoining collections in peritonsillar and retropharynx affect the airway by secondary compression.[4,5]
- The key clinical and imaging features of these entities have been summarized in **Table 2**[4,5] and illustrated in **Figures 8 to 11**.

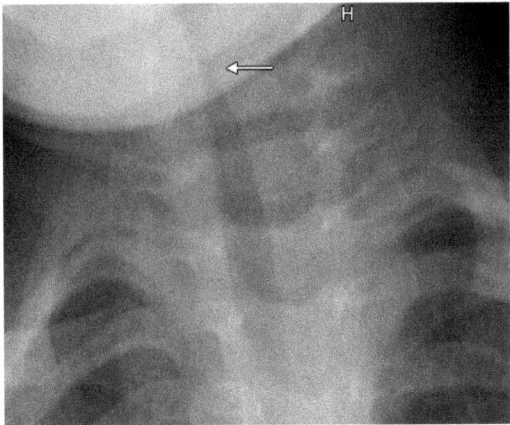

FIG. 8: Steeple sign. Frontal radiograph of the neck depicts tapering of the upper trachea (arrow), similar to the church steeple, hence called steeple sign. This is a classic finding in a case of croup (laryngotracheobronchitis).

TABLE 2: Key clinical and imaging features of upper airway infections in children.

Disease	Sites	Organism	Clinical	Imaging (radiographs in most infections, CT is not performed/indicated)
Laryngotracheobronchitis (Croup) (Fig. 8)	• Larynx • Trachea • Bronchi	Viral (parainfluenza virus I, II, or III)	Age: 6 months to 6 years "Barking" type cough	• AP: Subglottis swelling results in "steeple sign" • Lateral: Hyperinflation of hypopharynx
Supraglottitis (epiglottitis)	Epiglottis and aryepiglottic folds	Haemophilus influenzae type B bacteria, viruses ±	Age: 2–4 years Fever and triad of drooling, dysphagia, and distress	• Lateral: Thumbprint sign of swollen epiglottis and aryepiglottic folds
Tracheitis	Trachea	Bacterial (primary or super added)	Age: 6 months to 14 years Fever, stridor, and respiratory distress	Lateral: Irregular tracheal margin
Retropharyngeal abscess (Figs. 9A to D)	Retropharyngeal space	Bacterial (group A beta-hemolytic streptococci. Staphylococcus aureus)	Age: 6 months to 6 years Fever, tender unilateral lymphadenopathy, dysphonia ("hot potato" voice) neck pain, neck stiffness	• Lateral: Widening of retropharyngeal space • CT: Rim-enhancing collection in retropharyngeal space
Acute tonsillitis and peritonsillar abscess (Quinsy) (Fig. 10)	Adjacent to palatine tonsil between capsule and pharyngeal muscles	Bacterial polymicrobial	Age: >10 years Severe unilateral soreness of throat, muffled voice, and trismus	• CT: Tonsillar enlargement • Inflammation/collection in peritonsillar region
Ludwig's angina (Figs. 11A and B)	Inflammation and cellulitis of the submandibular and sublingual spaces	Bacterial polymicrobial	Mean age 9 years Fever, pain, and a bull neck appearance	• USG: Hypoechoic collections • CECT: Reveals extent of inflammation and rim-enhancing collections

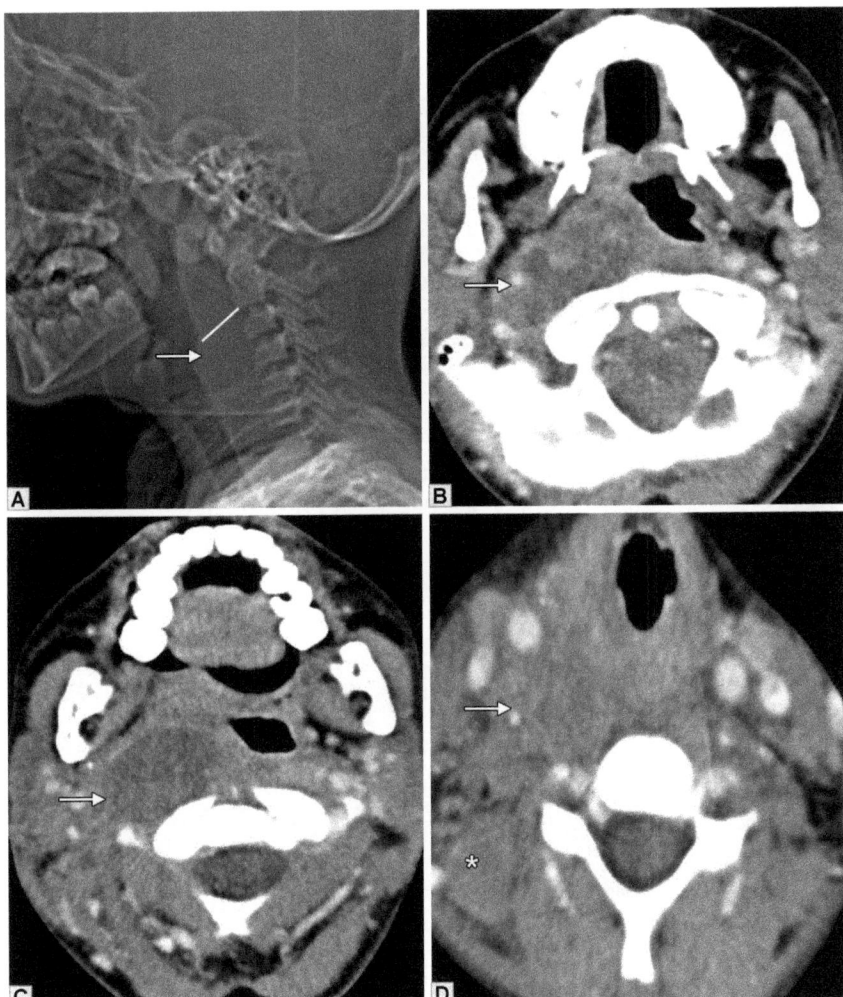

FIGS. 9A TO D: Retropharyngeal abscess. (A) CT scanogram. (B to D) CECT axial images at level of maxilla (B), mandible (C), oropharynx (D). (A) Widening of the prevertebral space (white line). (B to D) A hypoenhancing collection (arrows) in right parapharyngeal and prevertebral space causing mass effect and narrowing of the airway. Right posterior cervical lymph nodes (asterisk).
(CECT: contrast-enhanced computed tomography)

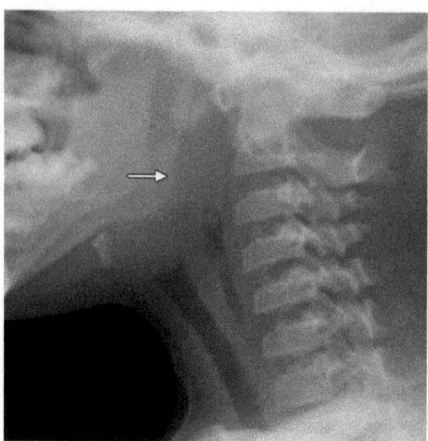

FIG. 10: Acute tonsillitis and adenoiditis. Lateral radiograph of the neck shows a large soft tissue mass (arrow) epicentered in oropharynx and hypopharynx causing obliteration of the airway.

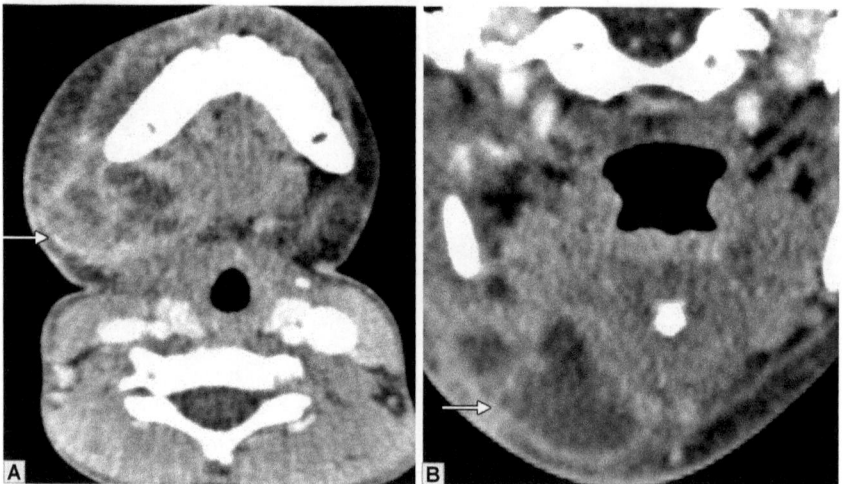

FIGS. 11A AND B: Ludwig's angina. CECT images of the neck. Thick multilocular peripherally enhancing collection (arrows) in right submandibular and sublingual space.
(CECT: contrast-enhanced computed tomography)

Retropharyngeal abscess:
- A space infection which can cause extrinsic compression of the airway and is potentially life threatening.
- The retropharyngeal space (RPS) is located posterior to the pharynx (nasopharynx, oropharynx, and hypopharynx), larynx, and trachea and extends cranially up to the skull base and caudally to the mediastinum at the level of carina. In close proximity of the RPS are the danger space and the prevertebral space.

- In children, an upper respiratory tract infection spreads to the retropharyngeal lymph nodes which suppurate and lead to abscess formation.
- Complications of RPA include airway compression, spread of inflammation to adjacent structures, necrotizing fasciitis, and abscess rupture with resultant aspiration of purulent material. Mediastinal spread of the disease can cause mediastinitis, pericarditis, pleuritis, and empyema. Lateral spread can cause internal jugular vein thrombosis and carotid artery pseudoaneurysms. Posterior spread can lead to osteomyelitis and vertebral subluxation.
- *Imaging:*[4,5] Lateral soft-tissue neck radiography reveals widening of the soft tissues in the RPS. A prevertebral space thickness of <6 mm at C3 level is considered normal in children and <6 mm at C2 and <22 mm at C6 vertebral level is normal in adults. Any widening is considered pathological and needs urgent clinical evaluation and management. FB or gas in the RPS can also be well visualized and should alert the radiologist for possible abscess formation. CECT shows the entire extent of the abscess and any complications.

Vascular Malformations

- Large low-flow vascular malformations in the head and neck region (**Figs. 12 and 13**) can be multicompartmental and can extend into the parapharyngeal and retropharyngeal spaces and cause extrinsic airway narrowing.
- These are usually multicystic transpatial lesions, with occasional hemorrhage and fluid levels because of prior hemorrhage or infection. Phleboliths can be seen as hyperdense foci on CT and small areas of signal void on MRI.[6]

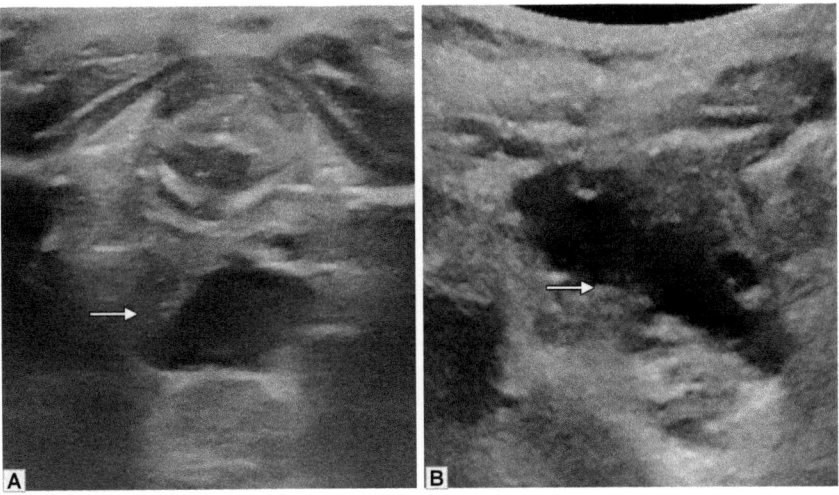

FIGS. 12A TO D: *Continued*

Continued

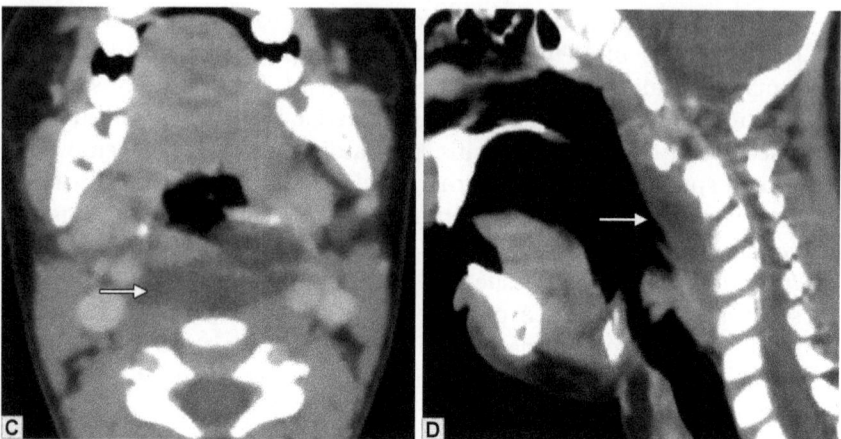

FIGS. 12A TO D: Low-flow vascular malformation. (A and B) USG images. (C and D) CECT images. (A and B) Septated cystic lesion (arrows) in the postcricoid and retropharyngeal space. (C and D) A lobulated, septated, fluid attenuation lesion (arrows) in the retropharyngeal space with no significant contrast enhancement.
(CECT: contrast-enhanced computed tomography)

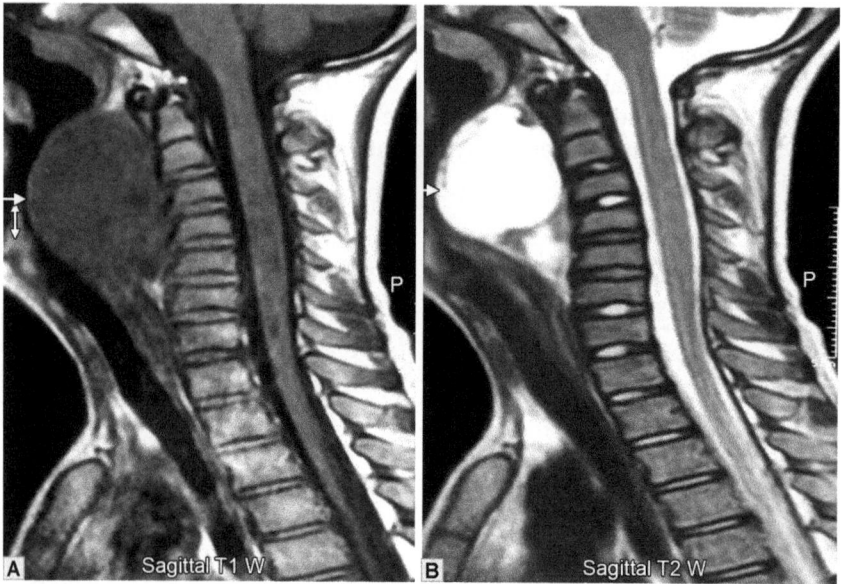

FIGS. 13A TO C: *Continued*

Continued

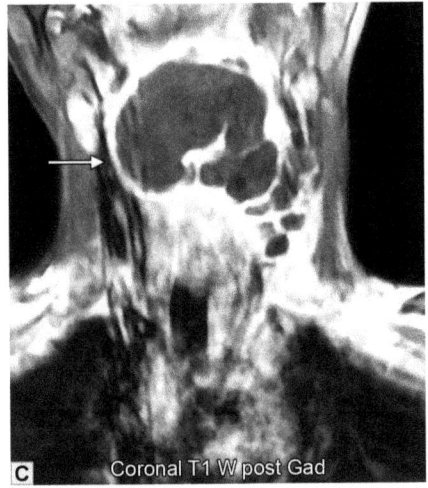

FIGS. 13A TO C: Retropharyngeal lymphatic malformation. (A) Sagittal T1W image, (B) sagittal T2W image, and (C) PG T1W image. (A) A lobulated T1W hypointense mass (arrow) in the retropharyngeal region. (B) Multilocular T2W hyperintense cystic lesion (arrow) with few thick septa within. (C) The cystic lesion shows thick enhancement of the periphery and septa. It is seen to cause marked compromise of the airway (arrow) and is extending from C2-C7 vertebral level.

Masses/Lymphoid Enlargement

Lymphoidal Enlargement/Waldeyer's Ring

- *Waldeyer's ring* is a ring of lymphoidal tissue in the nasopharynx and oropharynx.
- It is composed of four tonsillar structures, namely, palatine tonsil, adenoids, lateral wall of oropharynx, and lingual tonsils at the base of the tongue. They act as the first line of defense against any microbe that enters via the aerodigestive tract. They are common site of involvement in Hodgkin lymphoma in pediatric and young adult population.[7] Atypical infections including fungal infections like *Entomophthoromycosis* can present with diffuse circumferential inflammatory soft-tissue thickening along the Waldeyer ring, nasopharynx, oropharynx, and larynx and thickened soft tissues of face and neck with cervical lymphadenopathy.
- *Adenoid hypertrophy* is a frequent cause of nasal obstruction in pediatric age group. It is the lymphoidal soft tissue proliferation along the posterosuperior wall and roof of the nasopharynx. They enlarge in the age of 3-7 years after which they regress in size. They become pathological when they cause severe compromise of the airway, recurrent sinusitis, or chronic otitis media.
  - Lateral radiograph of the neck is done at the end of inspiration with neck in slight extension so as to negate the effect of soft tissue elevation during swallowing or respiration which can narrow the nasopharynx.
  - *Three measurements can be done*: Adenoid–nasopharynx ratio (A/N), the adenoid thickness, and the linear distance between antrum and the adenoid tissue.[8] A/N ratio is the most common method to assess for airway narrowing **(Fig. 14)**. This is measured from the straight part of the basiocciput to the maximum convexity of the adenoid (A) to the distance between basiocciput to hard palate (N).

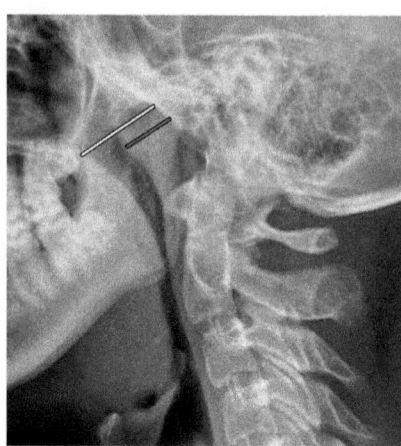

FIG. 14: Adenoid hypertrophy. Lateral radiograph of the neck shows soft tissue opacity in the region of nasopharynx consistent with adenoid hypertrophy. The black line depicts the adenoid size (A) and white line depicts the nasopharyngeal airway (N). In this case, the A/N ratio is 0.65.

- In the neonatal age group, congenital goiter and infantile hemangioma can significantly narrow the airway and cause respiratory distress. Diffuse and homogeneous enlargement of the thyroid gland is seen in cases of *congenital goiter* with narrowing of the adjacent airway. *Infantile hemangiomas* are lobulated, well-defined lesions with increased echogenicity, and arterial flow on color Doppler. *Subglottic hemangioma* is a common cause of neonatal respiratory distress and obstruction at subglottic level. Respiratory distress and biphasic stridor along with difficulty in feeding are the classical presentation during the proliferative phase of the hemangioma. USG Doppler typically reveals an echogenic lesion with increased vascularity in the subglottis.
- *Tumors*: The common tumors in the pediatric age group which can be multicompartmental and cause significant airway narrowing include teratomas, lymphoma, neuroblastoma **(Figs. 15A and B)**, rhabdomyosarcoma, Ewing's family of tumors **(Figs. 16A and B)**, and plexiform neurofibromas.

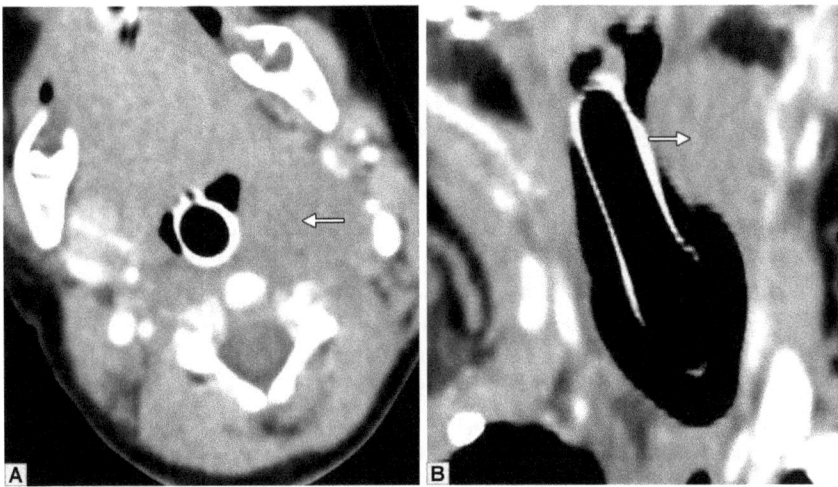

FIGS. 15A AND B: Left parapharyngeal space neuroblastoma. CECT images of the neck. A relatively well-defined homogeneous mass (arrows) in left parapharyngeal space, indenting and causing mild narrowing of the airway anteromedially and displacement of carotid vessels posterolaterally.
(CECT: contrast-enhanced computed tomography)

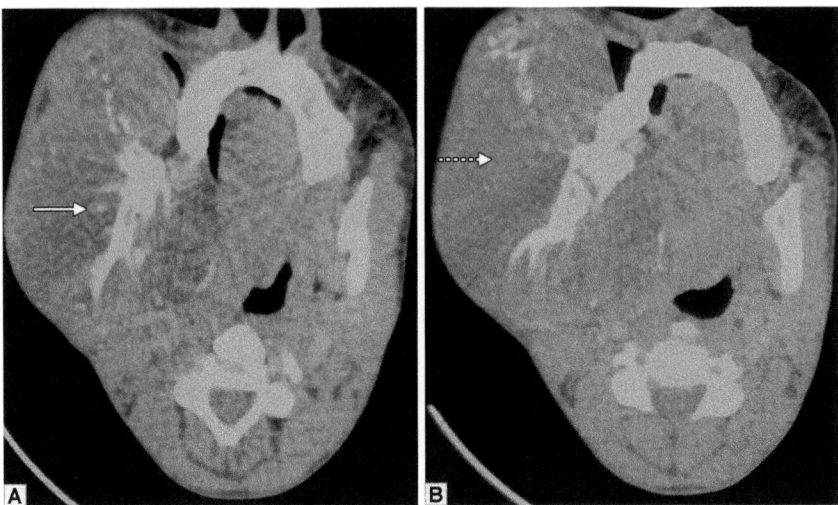

FIGS. 16A AND B: Ewing's sarcoma. CECT axial images. Lytic destruction of the right hemimandible with spiculated periosteal reaction (arrow), associated with a large soft tissue component (dotted arrow) extending to the intraoral, oropharyngeal, and right parapharyngeal space causing mass effect and luminal compromise of the airway.
(CECT: contrast-enhanced computed tomography)

Miscellaneous

Foreign Body

- Upper airway FB aspiration/inhalation results in an emergent presentation, this is unlike FBs in the bronchi which can have acute or chronic presentation.[6]
- Imaging is indicated to localize the FB.
- Initially a chest radiograph of chest is performed (inspiratory + expiratory/ lateral decubitus). For suspected upper airway FB, frontal and lateral neck radiographs are to be done [STN (soft tissue neck)—AP/lateral].
- The sites of impaction in upper airway include larynx or trachea.
- Further, upper esophageal FBs can also present with airway symptoms due to compromise. The acute of impaction is at the level of cricoid cartilage, and rarely these can erode at the trachea. These can lead to superadded infection and abscess formation **(Figs. 17A to D)**.

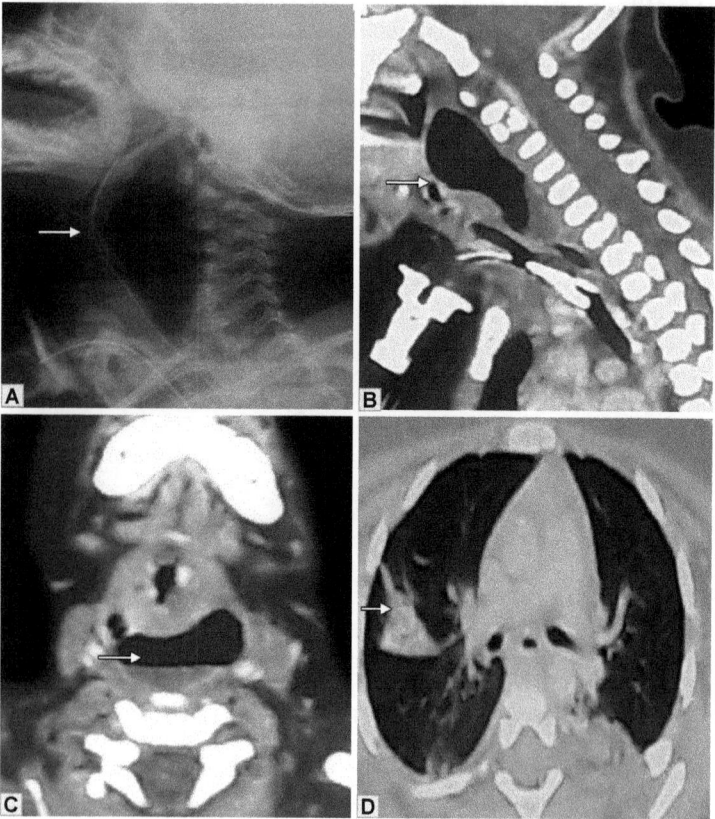

FIGS. 17A TO D: Prevertebral/retropharyngeal abscess post foreign body impaction. (A) Lateral radiograph of the neck, (B and C) CECT neck images, and (D) CECT chest axial lung window. (A) Widening of the prevertebral space with presence of large pocket of air (arrow) causing airway luminal compromise. (B and C) Large prevertebral abscess with air–fluid level (arrows) causing near complete occlusion of the airway with distal tracheostomy tube in situ. (D) Consolidation in right lung (arrow).
(CECT: contrast-enhanced computed tomography)

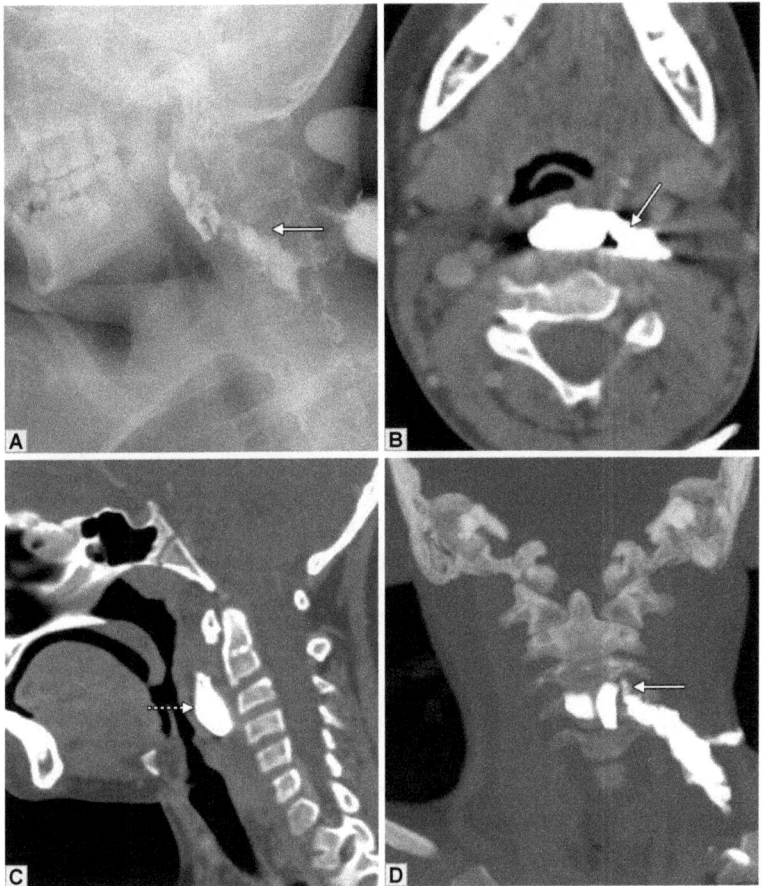

FIGS. 18A TO D: Retropharyngeal abscess and fistula formation post foreign body penetration (wooden stick) in the neck. (A) Conventional fistulogram, (B and C) CT sinogram images, and (D) maximum intensity projection image (MIP). (A to D) A thick irregular fistula (arrows) is seen extending from left lateral side of the lower neck, superiorly and medially and terminating in a retropharyngeal collection (dotted arrow).

- Fistula formation can occur along the site of penetration **(Figs. 18A to D)**.
- If the radiographs do not reveal an FB, and the patient is symptomatic and/or clinical suspicion of aspiration is high noncontrast computed tomography (NCCT) of neck and chest is performed.
- Normal imaging does not exclude an FB.

Iatrogenic/accidental Strictures and Fistulae

- Prolonged endotracheal intubation may lead to tracheal stenosis and subglottic stenosis **(Figs. 19A and B)**.
- Stricture more likely with cuffed endotracheal tube with higher cuff pressure (>30 mm Hg) and prolonged intubation time leading to wall ischemia and fibrosis.

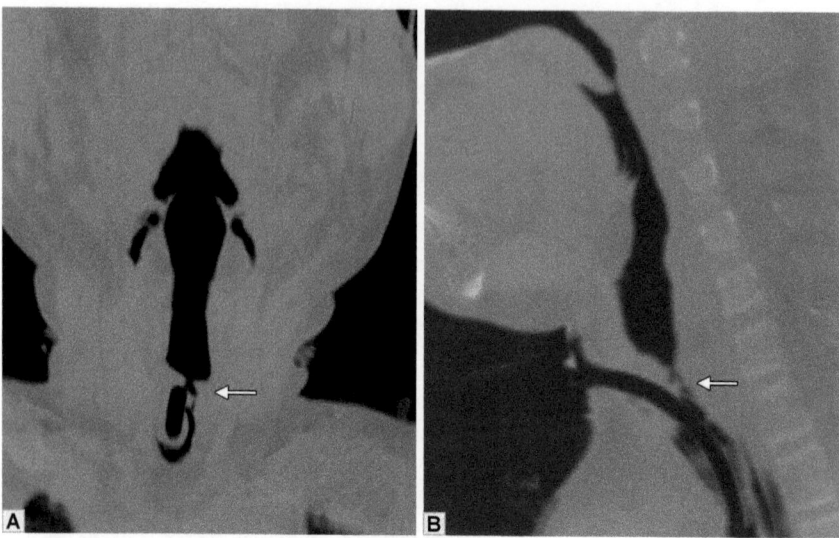

FIGS. 19A AND B: Postintubation subglottic stenosis. (A) CECT coronal image (B) minimal intensity projection images. (A and B) Near complete occlusion of the subglottic airway (arrows) with distal tracheostomy in situ.
(CECT: contrast-enhanced computed tomography)

- Clinically presents with inspiratory stridor or monophasic expiratory wheeze on exertion.
- Imaging helpful in detecting extension of stricture.
- Treatment modalities include rigid bronchoscopy with balloon dilation, stenting, or surgery.
- Corrosive poisoning can damage the mucosa and lead to ulcerations **(Fig. 20)**. Healing may lead to fibrosis and stenosis.

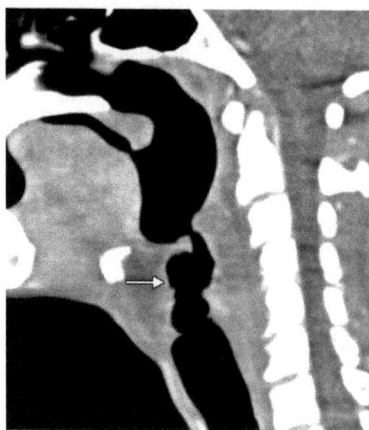

FIG. 20: Corrosive injury. CECT sagittal reformat image shows long-segment mucosal irregularity with ulceration involving the hypopharynx and larynx (arrow).
(CECT: contrast-enhanced computed tomography)

■ CONCLUSION

The abnormalities of the upper airway in the pediatric age group can present with respiratory distress and frequently need emergency management. Imaging has a key role to differentiate between the various etiologies of airway obstruction.

Other Related Chapters that can be Referred to:
- ❑ Chapter 6: Congenital Lung Abnormalities
- ❑ Chapter 15: Central Airway Imaging

■ REFERENCES

1. Daniel SJ. The upper airway: congenital malformations. Paediatr Respir Rev. 2006;7 (Suppl 1):S260-3.
2. Miller CK, Willging JP. The implications of upper-airway obstruction on successful infant feeding. Semin Speech Lang. 2007;28(3):190-203.
3. Men S, Ikiz AO, Topcu I, Cakmakci H, Ecevit C. CT and virtual endoscopy findings in congenital laryngeal web. Int J Pediatr Otorhinolaryngol. 2006;70(6):1125-7.
4. Ho ML, Courtier J, Glastonbury CM. The ABCs (Airway, Blood Vessels, and Compartments) of Pediatric Neck Infections and Masses. Am J Roentgenol. 2016;206(5):963-72.
5. Debnam JM, Guha-Thakurta N. Retropharyngeal and prevertebral spaces: anatomic imaging and diagnosis. Otolaryngol Clin North Am. 2012;45(6):1293-310.
6. Manchanda S, Bhalla AS. Pediatric Neck Lesions. In: Gupta AK, Garg A, Sandhu MS (Eds). AIIMS-MAMC-PGI Imaging Series—Diagnostic Radiology: Paediatric Imaging, 4th edition. New Delhi: Jaypee Brothers Medical Publishers. 2021. pp. 731-51.
7. Seelisch J, De Alarcon PA, Flerlage JE, Hoppe BS, Kaste SC, Kelly KM, et al. Expert consensus statements for Waldeyer's ring involvement in pediatric Hodgkin lymphoma: The staging, evaluation, and response criteria harmonization (SEARCH) for childhood, adolescent, and young adult Hodgkin lymphoma (CAYAHL) group. Pediatr Blood Cancer. 2020;67(9):e28361.
8. Fujioka M, Young L, Girdany B. Radiographic evaluation of adenoidal size in children: adenoidal-nasopharyngeal ratio. Am J Roentgenol. 1979;133(3):401-4.

CHAPTER 15

Central Airway Imaging

Iqbal Bashir, Ashu Seith Bhalla

- ❏ Classification
- ❏ Development and branching anomalies of airways
  - ➢ Congenital anomalies of development of tracheal bud
  - ➢ Disorders of tracheoesophageal septum development and fusion
  - ➢ Disorders of bronchial bud development
  - ➢ Disorders of tracheal and bronchial branching
  - ➢ Abnormality in dimension of large airways
- ❏ Intrinsic (intramural) central airway abnormalities
  - ➢ Iatrogenic strictures and fistulae
  - ➢ Inflammatory airway lesions: stricture
- ❏ Intraluminal obstruction
  - ➢ Foreign body inhalation
  - ➢ Mucus plug obstruction
  - ➢ Masses
- ❏ Extrinsic airway compression
  - ➢ Extrinsic vascular compression
  - ➢ Extrinsic compression: masses

■ INTRODUCTION

Central airway is defined as the trachea, mainstem bronchi, bronchus intermedius, and the lobar bronchi. Peripheral airway refers to the airway beyond this. The central airway is primarily conductive, i.e., it helps in air conduction but not in gas exchange. The peripheral airways are mixed (both conducting and participating in gas exchange). Upper airway is defined as the airway till the level of the thoracic inlet; while lower airway refers to airway beyond that.[1] A host of pathologies may affect the lower central airways, which will be discussed in this chapter. Upper airway disorders will be discussed in a separate chapter.

■ CLASSIFICATION

A classification of major central airway abnormalities is given in **Table 1**.

TABLE 1: Classification of central airway anomalies.	
Development and branching anomalies	• Disorders of development of tracheal and bronchial bud • Disorders of tracheoesophageal septum development and fusion • Disorders of tracheal and bronchial branching
Abnormality in dimension of large airways	• Tracheobronchomalacia • Congenital tracheal stenosis
Intrinsic airway abnormalities	• Iatrogenic or inflammatory stricture • Chronic foreign body-associated stricture • Bronchiectasis
Intraluminal airway obstruction	• Foreign body aspiration • Mucus plug obstruction • Masses
Extrinsic compression	• Vascular • Lymph node/mass causing obstruction

DEVELOPMENT AND BRANCHING ANOMALIES OF AIRWAYS

Congenital Anomalies of Development of Tracheal Bud

- Tracheal atresia, agenesis, stenosis, tracheal web, and bronchopulmonary foregut duplication cyst are rare congenital anomalies of development of tracheal bud, presenting as neonatal respiratory distress.[1]
- Tracheal agenesis is associated with other congenital anomalies (e.g., VATER).
- Tracheal atresia and agenesis are rare congenital anomalies presenting with respiratory distress immediately after birth. Three types (type I–III) of tracheal agenesis are described depending on the severity.
- Congenital tracheal web and stenosis result from failure of complete resorption of epithelium and incomplete recanalization during the development of tracheal bud.
- Tracheal web presents with a membrane encircling the tracheal lumen causing luminal narrowing.
- Congenital tracheal and subglottic stenosis are the most common upper airway anomaly requiring tracheostomy in children.
- Congenital tracheal stenosis can be either generalized (hypoplasia) or segmental stenosis **(Figs. 1A to C)**.

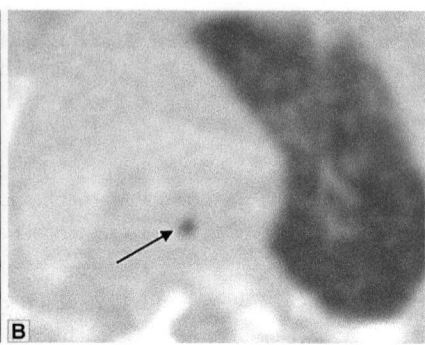
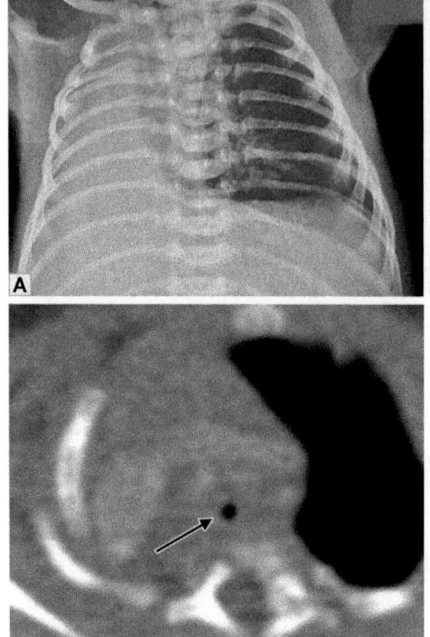

FIGS. 1A TO C: Right-sided pulmonary agenesis with congenital tracheal stenosis. CXR PA (A), axial CECT (B and C). (A) Opaque right hemithorax with ipsilateral mediastinal shift. (B and C) Narrowing of tracheal lumen, with rounded contour (arrows).
(CECT: contrast-enhanced computed tomography; CXR: chest radiograph; PA: posteroanterior)

- Bronchopulmonary foregut duplication cysts can be classified either as bronchogenic or esophageal cyst.
- Bronchogenic cysts are commonly located in right paratracheal or subcarinal location. When large, they may cause airway compression.

Disorders of Tracheoesophageal Septum Development and Fusion

- Primordial respiratory tract arises from a diverticulum of the foregut.
- Tracheoesophageal septum develops between the two and separates the developing upper airway and the pharynx/cervical esophagus.
- Tracheoesophageal fistula is usually associated with esophageal atresia and presents with neonatal respiratory distress, choking, and cyanosis while feeding.
- H-type tracheoesophageal fistula **(Figs. 2A and B)** presents in older children with recurrent respiratory infection.

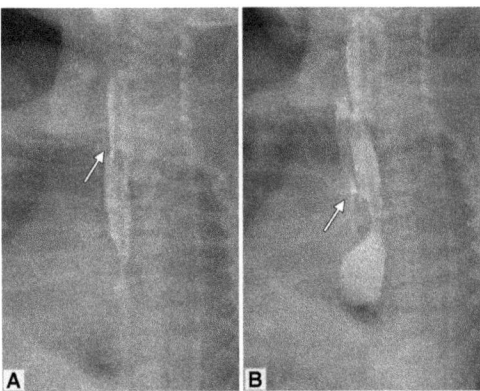

FIGS. 2A AND B: H-type tracheoesophageal fistula. Lateral barium swallow image (A and B). (A) Oblique thin fistulous tract (arrow). (B) Contrast opacification of lower trachea and bronchi (arrow).

Disorders of Bronchial Bud Development

- Pulmonary agenesis results from development of bronchial bud leading to nondevelopment of pulmonary parenchyma **(Figs. 3A to D)**.
- A blind ending bronchial bud and absent pulmonary parenchyma are the usual findings in pulmonary aplasia.
- Pulmonary artery can be absent in both pulmonary agenesis and aplasia.

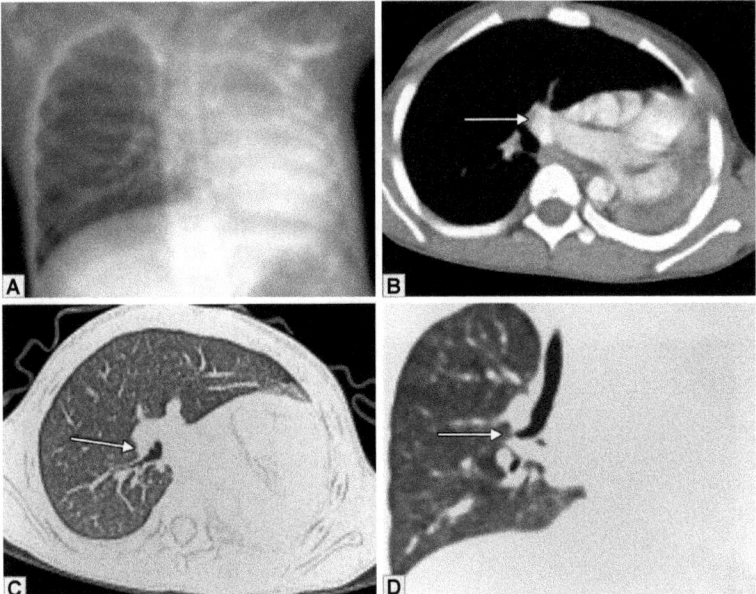

FIGS. 3A TO D: Pulmonary agenesis. CXR PA (A), axial CECT (B and C), and coronal MIP lung window (D). (A) Opaque left hemithorax with ipsilateral mediastinal shift. (B) Right pulmonary artery appears normal (arrow); left pulmonary artery not seen. (C and D) Right lung and bronchial tree normal (arrows).
(CECT: contrast-enhanced computed tomography; CXR: chest radiograph; PA: posteroanterior)

- Pulmonary hypoplasia **(Figs. 4A to C)** can result from absence of segmental bronchus and vessels.
- Congenital bronchoesophageal fistula **(Figs. 5A to D)** is a rare disorder of abnormal communications of the esophagus with the bronchi. It is divided into four types depending on the level of communication.
- Bronchial atresia **(Figs. 6A to D)** is due to segmental obliteration of the lumen of a bronchus leading to proximal mucoid impaction, and is usually asymptomatic.[2]
- Imaging findings are tubular fluid-filled proximal bronchus and distal segmental hyperlucency and reduced vascularity.

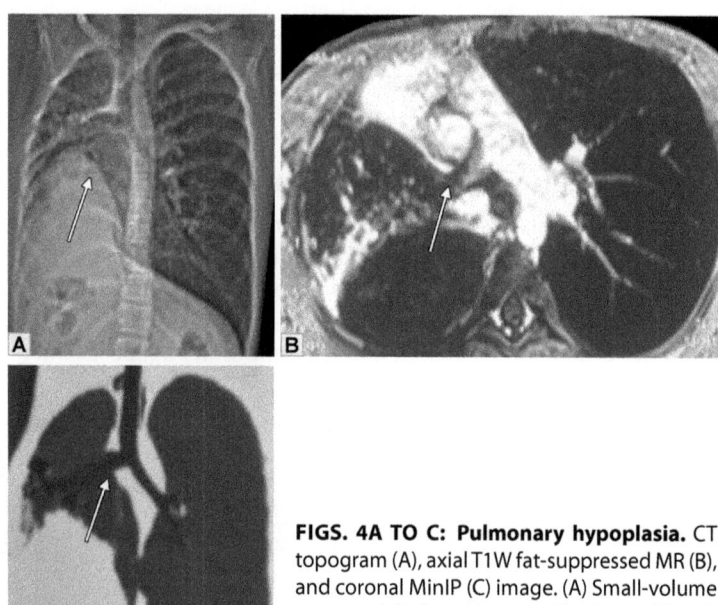

FIGS. 4A TO C: Pulmonary hypoplasia. CT topogram (A), axial T1W fat-suppressed MR (B), and coronal MinIP (C) image. (A) Small-volume opaque right hemithorax with elevated hemidiaphragm (arrow). (B) Small right pulmonary artery (arrow). (C) Bronchiectasis in right lung, and patent right main bronchus (arrow).

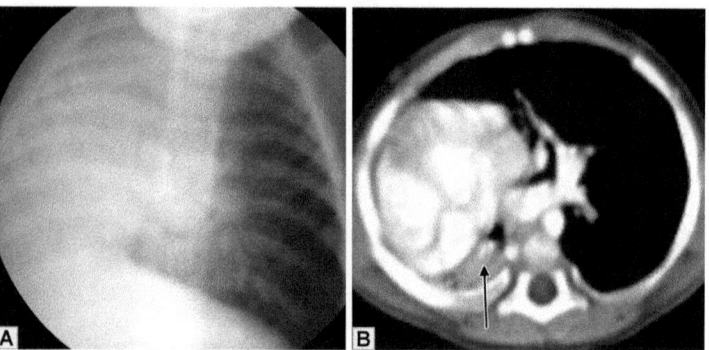

FIGS. 5A TO D: *Continued*

Continued

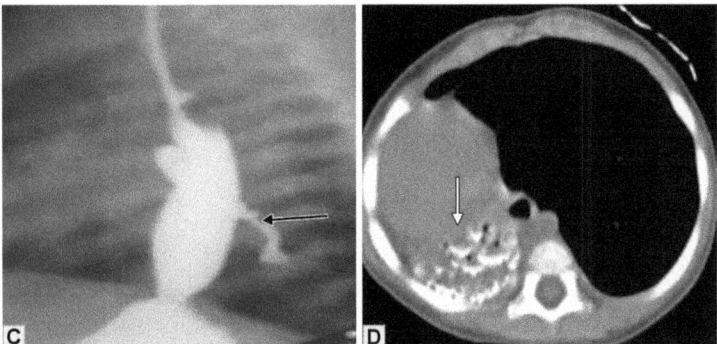

FIGS. 5A TO D: Esophageal lung. CXR PA (A), axial CECT (B), barium image (C), axial CT after barium (D). (A) Opaque right hemithorax with ipsilateral mediastinal shift. (B) Small lung parenchyma at the right posterior costophrenic angle (arrow). (C) Right bronchus originating from the lower esophagus (arrow). (D) Barium in the bronchial tree (arrow).
(CECT: contrast-enhanced computed tomography; CXR: chest radiograph; PA: posteroanterior)

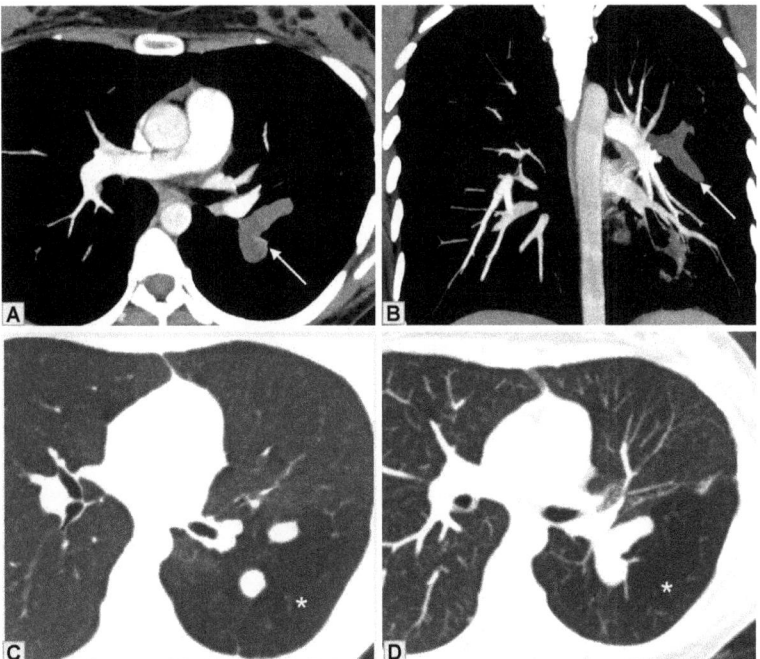

FIGS. 6A TO D: Bronchial atresia. Axial CECT (A), coronal MIP (B), Axial MIP (C), and MinIP (D) images. (A and B) Low-attenuation branching structure close to left hilum (arrows). (C and D) Hyperlucent distal left lower lobe (asterisks).
(CECT: contrast-enhanced computed tomography; MIP: maximum intensity projection; MinIP: minimum intensity projection)

Disorders of Tracheal and Bronchial Branching

- Disorders of tracheal and bronchial branching include a large group of abnormal configuration of the trachea and bronchi. The same has been depicted in **Figure 7**.

1. **Tracheal bronchus**

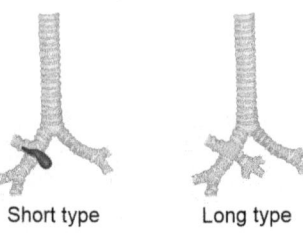

Rudimentary   Displaced   Supernumerary   Anomalous

2. **Accessory cardiac bronchus**

Short type   Long type

3. **Tracheal diverticulum**

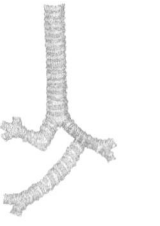

Congenital   Acquired

4. **Bridging bronchus**

Subtype 1   Subtype 2

FIG. 7: *Continued*

Continued

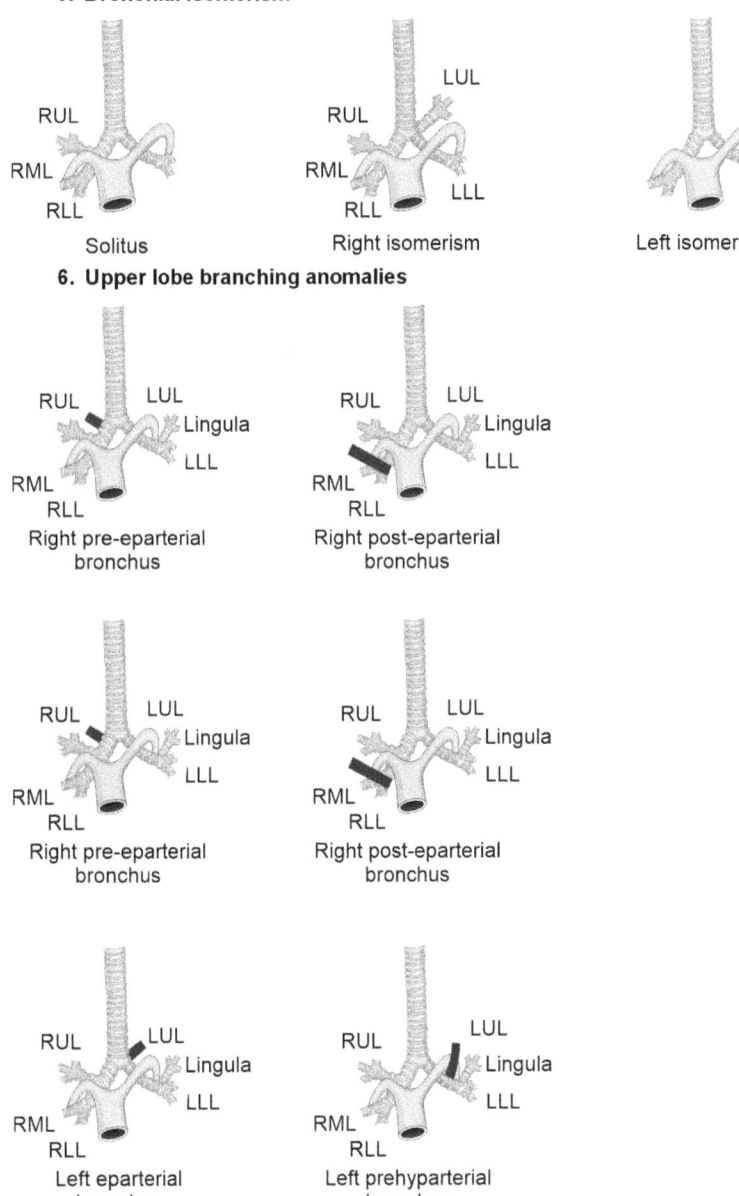

FIG. 7: Anomalies of bronchial branching. Diagrammatic representation.

- Tracheal bronchus (pig bronchus) is an anomalous origin of bronchus above the carina, usually on the right side **(Fig. 8)**.
- Usually incidentally detected, tracheal bronchus can rarely present with recurrent infections of the involved lobe.
- Tracheal trifurcation is an anomalous division of trachea into three segments instead of two segments.

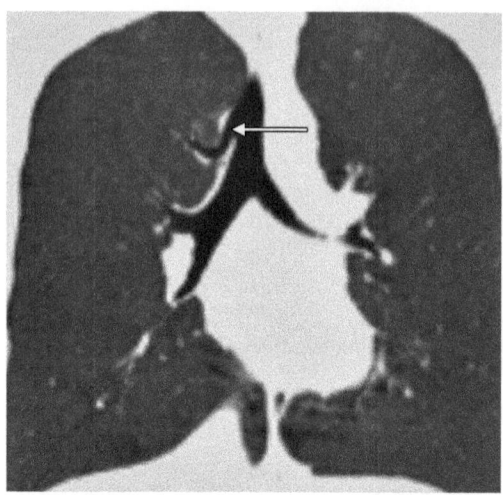

FIG. 8: Tracheal bronchus. Coronal MinIP image. Proximal origin of right upper lobar bronchus from the trachea (arrow).
(MinIP: minimum intensity projection)

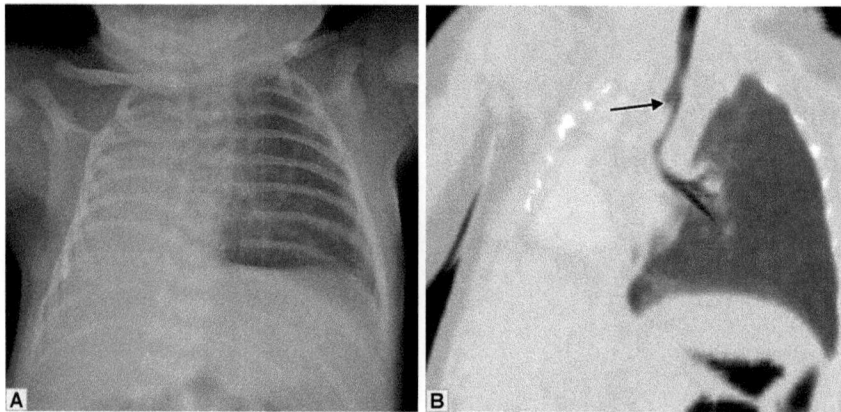

FIGS. 9A AND B: Pulmonary agenesis with tracheal diverticulum. CXR PA (A) and coronal MinIP (B) image. (A) Opaque right hemithorax with ipsilateral mediastinal shift. (B) Absent right main bronchus, and diverticulum arising from upper thoracic trachea (arrow).
(CXR: chest radiograph; MinIP: minimum intensity projection; PA: posteroanterior)

- Tracheal diverticulum is due to abnormal supernumerary branching of trachea. The diverticulum usually is related to the right posterolateral wall of trachea and communicates with tracheal lumen **(Figs. 9A and B)**.
- Bridging bronchus is another uncommon branching anomaly wherein the main bronchus (usually the right main bronchus) originates from the left main bronchus, and has a low carina. On coronal images, the carina appears like an "inverted T" **(Figs. 10A and B)**. It is nearly always associated with pulmonary artery sling and congenital tracheal stenosis.

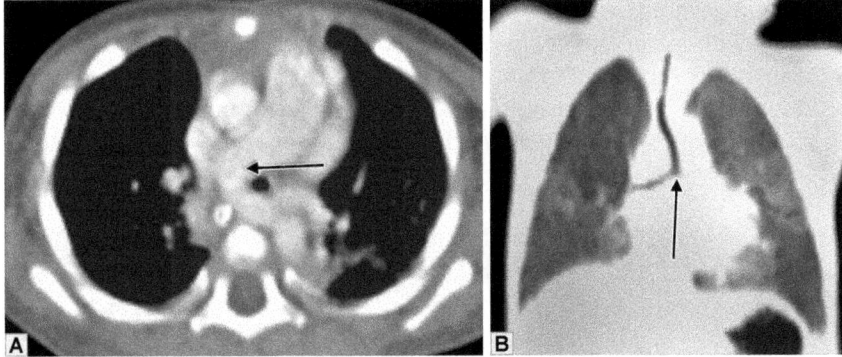

FIGS. 10A AND B: Bridging bronchus and pulmonary artery sling. Axial CECT (A) and coronal MinIP (B). (A) Anomalous origin of left pulmonary artery from the left pulmonary artery (arrow). (B) Low position of carina, with an "inverted T" appearance (arrow).
(CECT: contrast-enhanced computed tomography; MinIP: minimum intensity projection)

Abnormality in Dimension of Large Airways

- Tracheobronchomalacia (TBM) represents an increased collapsibility of the trachea and bronchi that is most pronounced on forced expiration. This entity encompasses unilateral or circumferential airway compression, diffuse or focal weakness of the cartilage with dynamic collapse of the large airways, and exaggerated dynamic motion of the posterior tracheal membrane during forced exhalation. It can occur as an isolated anomaly or in combination, with involvement of different regions of the airway.[3]
- Based on the area involved, TBM can be classified further into tracheomalacia (TM), with isolated involvement of the whole or segments of the trachea, and bronchomalacia, delineating isolated collapse of one or both mainstem bronchi.[1,4] The third entity is small airway malacia, which affects the lobar bronchi and perhaps smaller airways, frequently showing an association with prematurity, bronchopulmonary dysplasia, and other conditions.
- Tracheomalacia results from attenuated stiffness of the tracheal cartilage, with apposition of the anterior and posterior walls, culminating in collapse of the tracheal lumen.
- The lumen of trachea narrows on expiration consequent to the increased intrathoracic/mediastinal pressures relative to the intraluminal airway pressures, leading to compression of the airway with inward bowing of the posterior membranous part.
- A combination of the shape and strength of the cartilage, along with narrow posterior wall and the tone of the pars membranacea, prevents the collapse of healthy trachea, even during accentuated intraluminal pressure with cough and forced exhalation.[4]
- Tracheobronchomalacia is classified as primary (congenital) if there is intrinsic collapse of the trachea, with cartilage malformation being the ubiquitous cause. The abnormal cartilage may be U or bow shaped with

a wide posterior membrane, soft and pliable, or malformed into a narrow plate without an airway support **(Figs. 11A to D)**.
- Secondary (acquired) TBM is a result of extrinsic compression by the esophagus, a major vessel **(Figs. 12A to C)** or a tumor, or an outcome of infection or prolonged mechanical ventilation producing a flaccid trachea.[4]

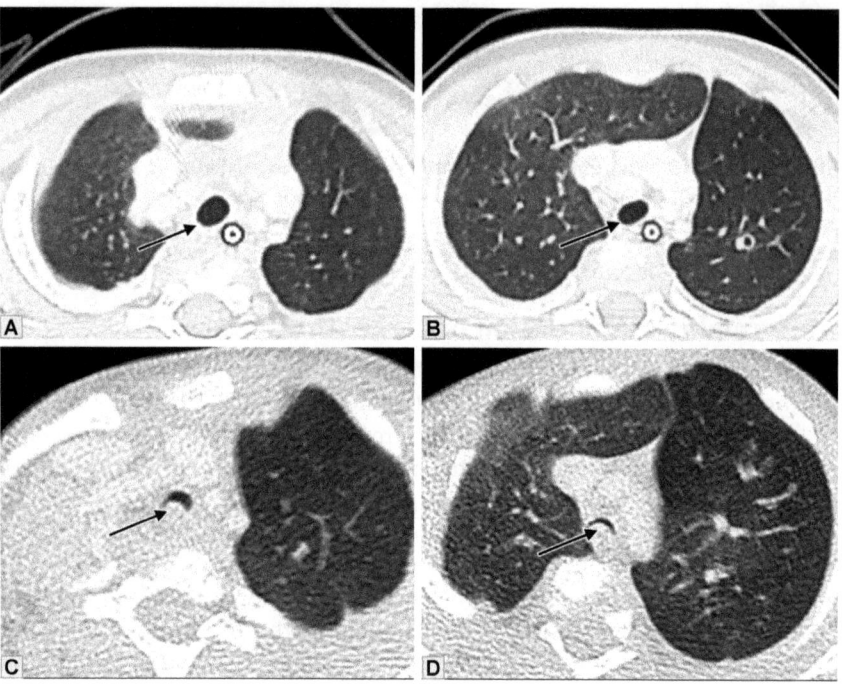

FIGS. 11A TO D: Primary tracheobronchomalacia. Axial CECT inspiratory (A and B) and expiratory (C and D) images. (A and B) Flat posterior wall of the trachea (arrows). (C and D) Inward buckling of the posterior wall (arrows).
(CECT: contrast-enhanced computed tomography)

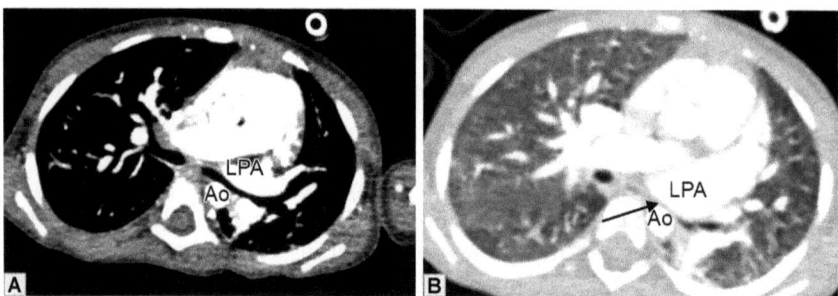

FIGS. 12A TO C: *Continued*

Continued

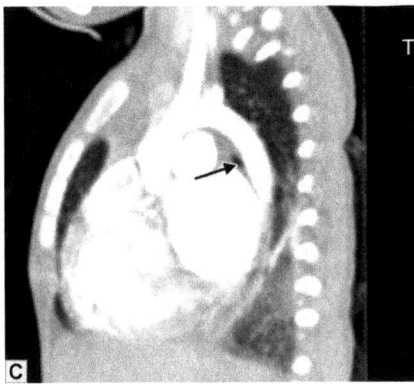

FIGS. 12A TO C: Secondary vascular bronchomalacia in a case of patent ductus arteriosus and pulmonary artery hypertension on echocardiography. Axial CECT images (A and B), sagittal MPR (C). (A) Left main bronchus is compressed between the left pulmonary artery (LPA) and descending thoracic aorta (Ao). (B and C) Near complete occlusion of left main bronchial lumen (arrows).
(CECT: contrast-enhanced computed tomography; MPR: multiplanar reconstructed)

- These are associated with congenital anomalies, including vascular compression from abnormally positioned arteries, vascular rings, or by a dilated esophagus in esophageal atresia. Other causes include tumors, tracheal inflammation, and chronic ventilation leading to compression, injury, weakening, and dilatation of the tracheal walls.[3]
- The estimated incidence of bronchopulmonary dysplasia in patients with between 50 and 72%.[1] Requirement of intubation shortly after birth may mask or delay the diagnosis. Comorbid bronchopulmonary dysplasia requiring intubation at or shortly after birth may mask or delay the diagnosis of TBM.
- Diagnosis of TBM is made through a meticulous history [e.g., barky cough; recurrent respiratory tract infections; BRUEs (brief, resolved, unexplained events) with forced exhalation, laughing, and coughing; exercise intolerance; failure to thrive due to interference with eating/feeding] and physical examination (e.g., barky cough and expiratory rhonchi).
- Imaging methods include dynamic airway computed tomography (CT), which undervalues the degree of airway collapse, and dynamic, 3-phase tracheobronchoscopy, which is the standard for diagnosis of airway structure and dynamic function.[4]
- Medical management comprises nebulizer treatments to enhance airway clearance (normal/hypertonic saline to thin the secretions and ipratropium bromide to decrease the secretions), minimal use of inhaled corticosteroids to prevent aggravation of the airway malacia, gastroesophageal reflux disease therapy to minimize aspiration of inflammatory gastric contents, and chest physiotherapy to assist airway clearance.[4]
- Surgical management consists of tracheotomy to bypass or stent the involved region of the trachea, continuous positive airway pressure (CPAP) to augment the intraluminal airway pressure and ameliorate airway distention, internal airway stents, external airway splints, and anterior aortopexy.[4]

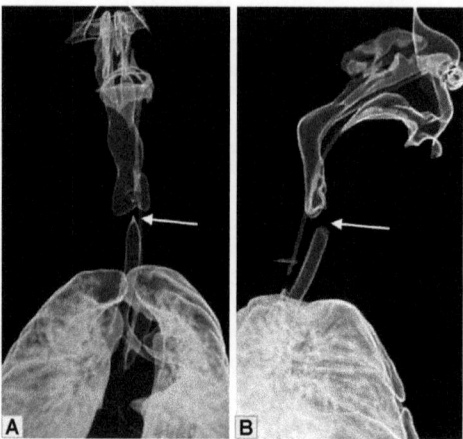

FIGS. 13A AND B: Postintubation tracheal stricture. Volume-rendered images AP (A) and lateral (B) profile. (A and B) Complete occlusion of tracheal lumen in upper thoracic region (arrows).

■ INTRINSIC (INTRAMURAL) CENTRAL AIRWAY ABNORMALITIES

Iatrogenic Strictures and Fistulae

- Prolonged endotracheal intubation may lead to tracheal stenosis and subglottic stenosis.
- Stricture more likely with cuffed endotracheal tube with higher cuff pressure (>30 mm Hg) and prolonged intubation time leading to wall ischemia and fibrosis.
- Clinically presents with inspiratory stridor or monophasic expiratory wheeze on exertion.
- Imaging is helpful in detecting extension of stricture **(Figs. 13A and B)**.
- Treatment modalities include rigid bronchoscopy with balloon dilation, stenting, or surgery.
- Esophagopleural fistula is an uncommon iatrogenic complication of esophageal procedures [nasogastric (NG) tube insertion and balloon dilation] or surgery.

Inflammatory Airway Lesions: Stricture

- Acute inflammatory involvement of the upper airway can be either tracheitis or bronchitis.
- Chronic inflammation can lead to tracheal or bronchial stricture.
- Tuberculosis can involve either trachea or the main bronchi, leading to stricture **(Figs. 14A to D)**.

CHAPTER 15: Central Airway Imaging

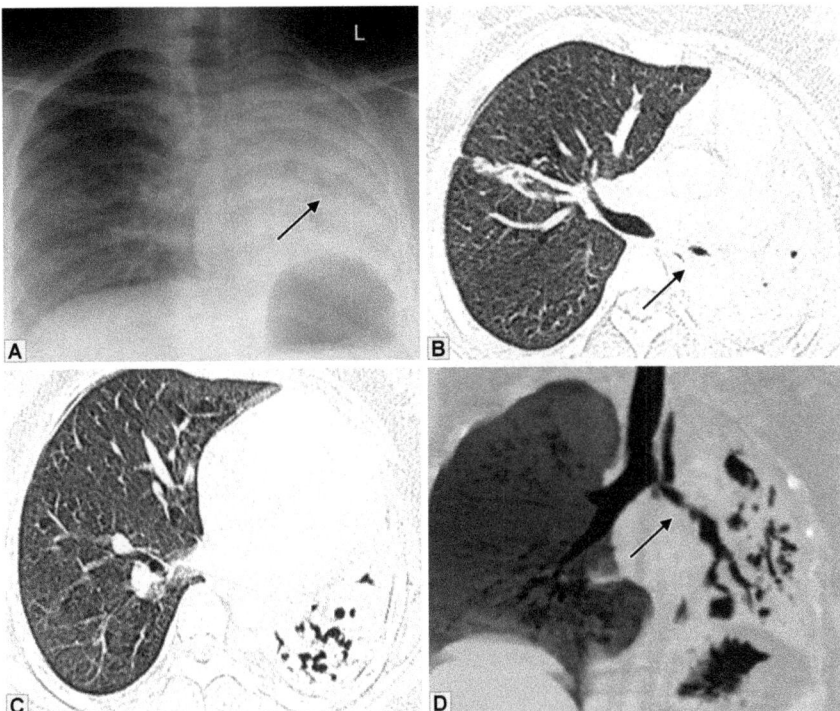

FIGS. 14A TO D: Post-tubercular left main bronchus (LMB) stricture. CXR PA (A), axial CECT (B and C), coronal MinIP lung window image (D). (A) Opaque left hemithorax with ipsilateral mediastinal shift; with bronchiectasis (arrow). (B) Narrow left main bronchus (arrow). (C) Left lower lobe bronchiectasis. (D) Irregular narrowing of LMB (arrow) with distal bronchiectasis.
(CECT: contrast-enhanced computed tomography; CXR: chest radiograph; MinIP: minimum intensity projection; PA: posteroanterior)

▪ INTRALUMINAL OBSTRUCTION

Foreign Body Inhalation

- Common cause of unilateral hyperlucent lung in children.
- Right main bronchus is common area of impaction because of its more straight course.
- Complete obstruction leads to collapse of the lobe subtended by the bronchus.
- Partial obstruction leads to obstructive emphysema.
- Metallic foreign bodies can be visualized on chest radiograph **(Figs. 15A to C)**.
- Organic foreign bodies (e.g., peanut) are the most common to be inhaled and difficult to retrieve as they tend to swell and get fragmented.
- Organic foreign bodies are not detected on chest radiograph; key finding is unilateral hyperlucent lung with air trapping.
- Long-standing foreign body may cause bronchial fibrosis and stricture **(Figs. 16A to C)**.

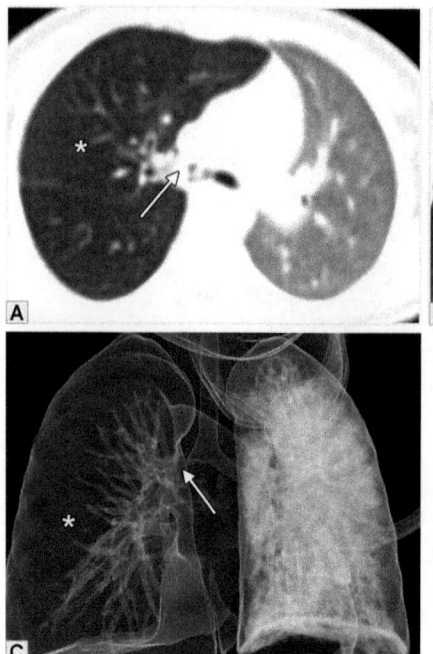
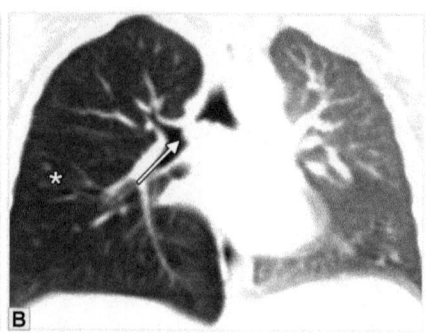

FIGS. 15A TO C: Foreign body in right main bronchus (RMB). Axial CT (A), coronal MPR (B), and volume-rendered (C) images. (A and B) Filling defect in RMB just after carina (arrows); hyperinflated right lung (asterisks). (C) Complete occlusion of RMB (arrow).
(MPR: multiplanar reconstructed)

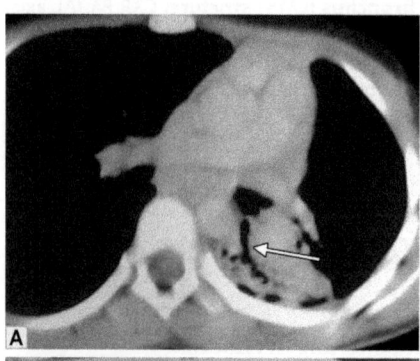
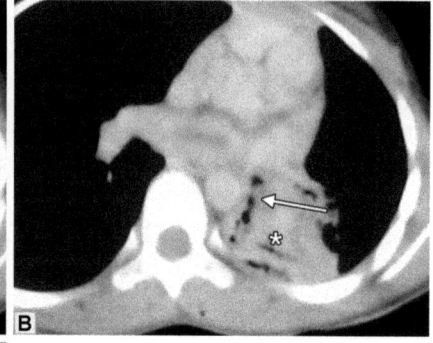
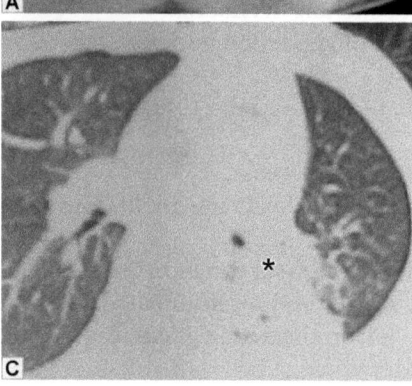

FIGS. 16A TO C: Stricture after chronic retained organic foreign body in left lower lobe bronchus. Axial CECT soft tissue (A and B), and lung (C) window images. Collapsed left lower lobe of lung (asterisks). Irregular lobar bronchus (arrows).
(CECT: contrast-enhanced computed tomography)

Mucus Plug Obstruction

- Mucus plug can cause acute airway obstruction in children, often leading to sudden respiratory distress and cough **(Figs. 17A to E)**.
- This can occur in the setting of viral bronchiolitis, acute exacerbation of asthma, or cystic fibrosis.

Masses

- Intrinsic upper airway obstruction due to masses is uncommon in pediatric age group.
- Subglottic hemangioma is a common cause of neonatal respiratory distress and obstruction at subglottic level.
- Intrabronchial mass **(Figs. 18A to E)** that can cause luminal obstruction in children and adolescents includes adenoma, carcinoid, papilloma, etc.

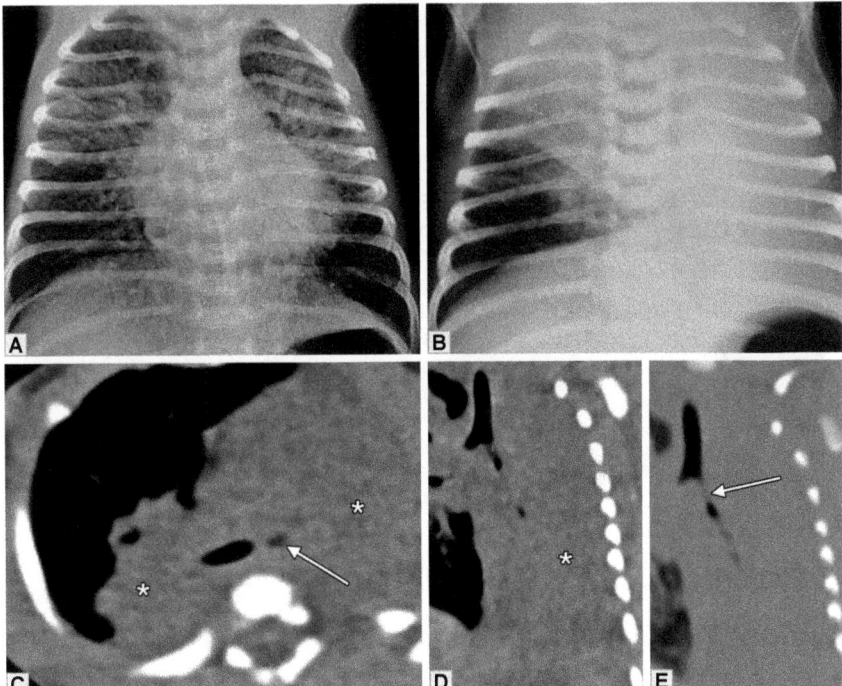

FIGS. 17A TO E: Mucus plug obstruction leading to lung collapse in a child with acute viral bronchiolitis. Serial CXR (A and B), axial NCCT (C), coronal MPR (D), and coronal MinIP (E) images. (A) Diffuse bilateral hyperinflation and peribronchial thickening. (B) Opaque left and right upper hemithorax with left-sided mediastinal shift; suggestive of lung collapse. (C) Intraluminal low-attenuation structure (arrow); HU value—44 (D) with left lung and right upper lobe posterior segment collapse (asterisk). (E) Focal complete occlusion of proximal left main bronchus (arrow).
(CXR: chest radiograph; MinIP: minimum intensity projection; MPR: multiplanar reconstructed; NCCT: noncontrast computed tomography)

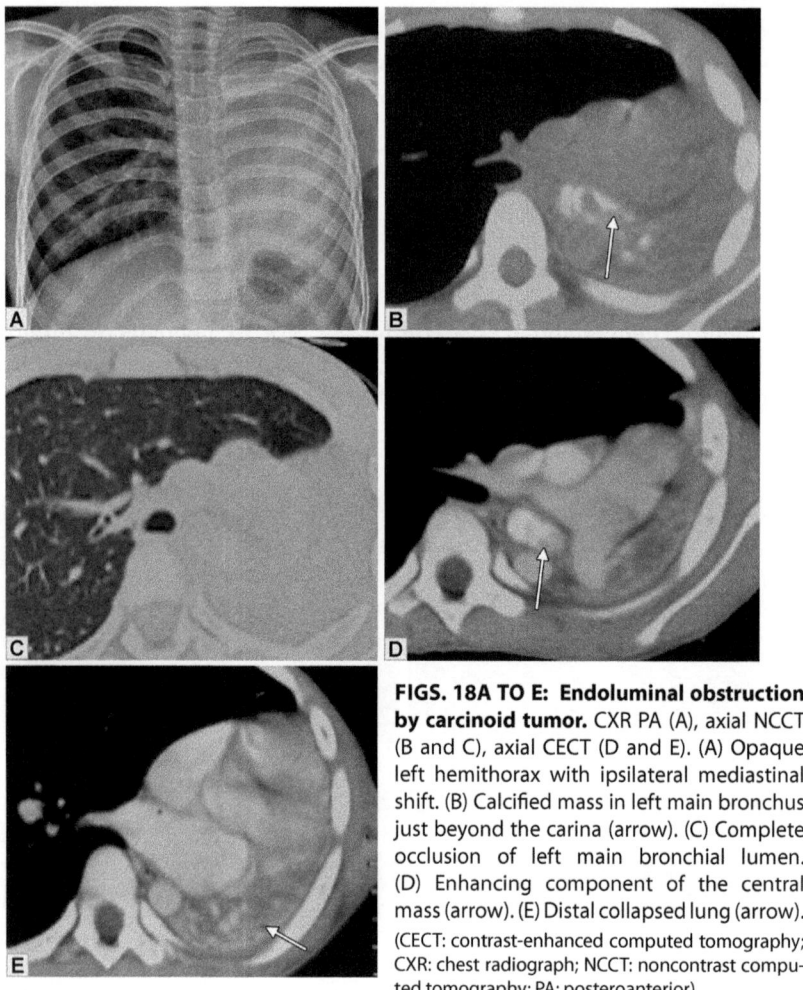

FIGS. 18A TO E: Endoluminal obstruction by carcinoid tumor. CXR PA (A), axial NCCT (B and C), axial CECT (D and E). (A) Opaque left hemithorax with ipsilateral mediastinal shift. (B) Calcified mass in left main bronchus just beyond the carina (arrow). (C) Complete occlusion of left main bronchial lumen. (D) Enhancing component of the central mass (arrow). (E) Distal collapsed lung (arrow).
(CECT: contrast-enhanced computed tomography; CXR: chest radiograph; NCCT: noncontrast computed tomography; PA: posteroanterior)

EXTRINSIC AIRWAY COMPRESSION

Extrinsic Vascular Compression

- Vascular rings causing airway compression include double aortic arch, right aortic arch with aberrant left subclavian artery (SCA), and ligamentum arteriosum.
- Pulmonary artery sling is aberrant origin of the left pulmonary artery (LPA) from the right pulmonary artery (RPA), where the LPA takes a retrotracheal course and causes impression on posterior wall of trachea.
- Innominate artery compression syndrome results from abnormal origin of the innominate artery from the arch of aorta (far left origin), with a long course of the innominate artery in the superior mediastinum anterior to trachea and compression and indentation of anterior tracheal wall.

Enlarged thymus is also implicated to have a role in tracheal compression in this syndrome. The condition is often self-limiting **(Figs. 19A to C)**.
- Other causes of vascular compression on major airways include enlarged main pulmonary artery, RPA, LPA in pulmonary artery hypertension causing main bronchial compression.
- Aberrant right SCA usually does not cause tracheal compression as it has a retroesophageal course **(Figs. 20A and B)**.

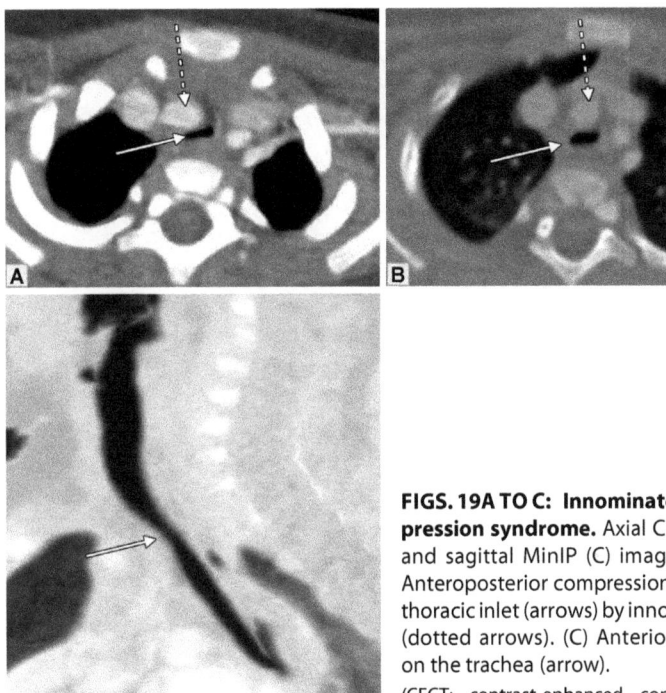

FIGS. 19A TO C: Innominate artery compression syndrome. Axial CECT (A and B) and sagittal MinIP (C) images. (A and B) Anteroposterior compression of trachea at thoracic inlet (arrows) by innominate artery (dotted arrows). (C) Anterior indentation on the trachea (arrow).
(CECT: contrast-enhanced computed tomography; MinIP: minimum intensity projection)

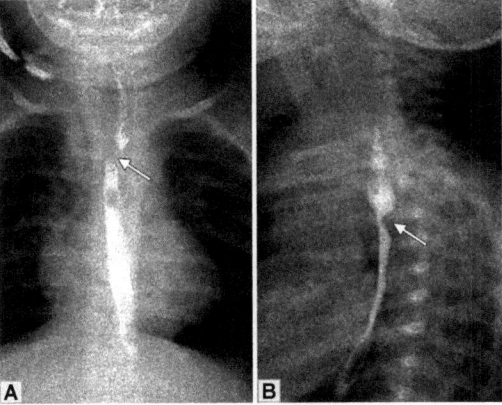

FIGS. 20A AND B: Aberrant right subclavian artery. Fluoroscopic images AP (A) and lateral (B) of barium swallow. (A) Oblique filling defect in upper thoracic esophagus (arrow). (B) Posterior indentation (arrow).

Extrinsic Compression: Masses

- Enlarged mediastinal lymph nodes in tuberculosis or fungal infection can cause extrinsic compression on the trachea or main bronchi.
- Enlarged metastatic mediastinal lymph nodes can also cause extrinsic compression on the trachea or main bronchi **(Figs. 21A to E)**.
- Other causes of extrinsic compression on trachea and main bronchi include mediastinal cystic masses **(Figs. 22A to D)** or unusual mesenchymal tumors.

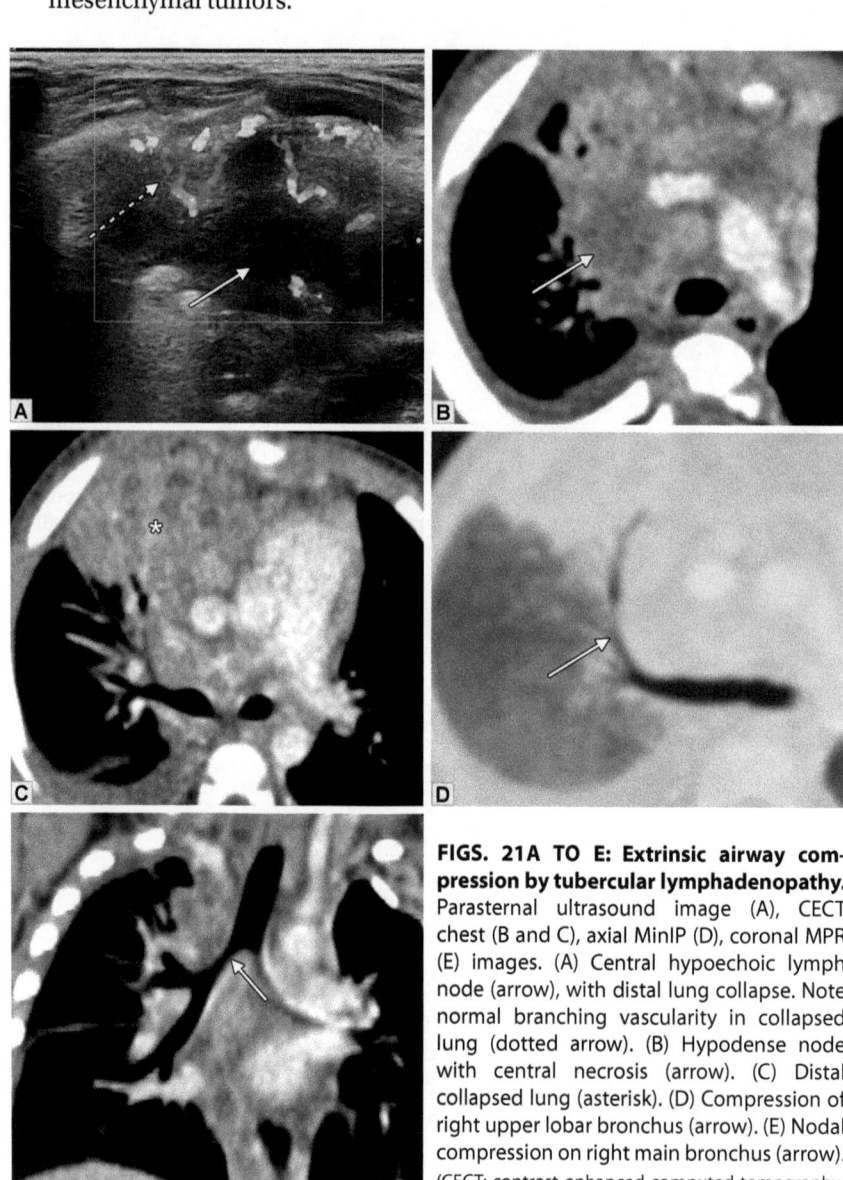

FIGS. 21A TO E: Extrinsic airway compression by tubercular lymphadenopathy. Parasternal ultrasound image (A), CECT chest (B and C), axial MinIP (D), coronal MPR (E) images. (A) Central hypoechoic lymph node (arrow), with distal lung collapse. Note normal branching vascularity in collapsed lung (dotted arrow). (B) Hypodense node with central necrosis (arrow). (C) Distal collapsed lung (asterisk). (D) Compression of right upper lobar bronchus (arrow). (E) Nodal compression on right main bronchus (arrow).
(CECT: contrast-enhanced computed tomography; MinIP: minimum intensity projection; MPR: multiplanar reconstructed)

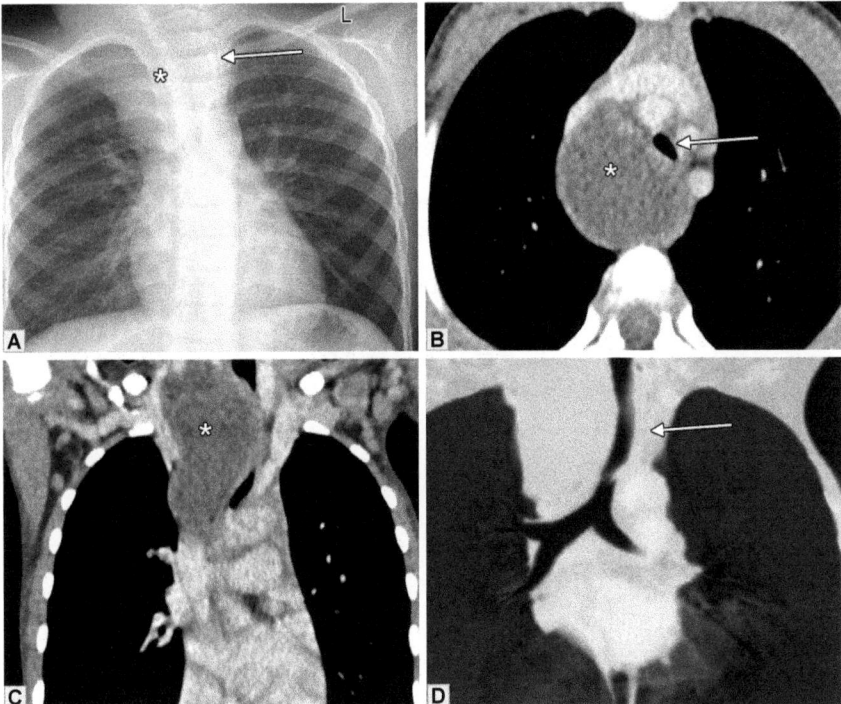

FIGS. 22A TO D: Duplication cyst causing extrinsic tracheal compression. CXR PA (A), axial CECT (B), coronal MPR (C), and coronal MinIP (D) images. (A) Right paratracheal lesion (asterisk) causing contralateral tracheal deviation (arrow). (B) Hypodense cystic lesion causing anterior displacement of trachea (arrow). (C) Craniocaudal extent of the cyst (asterisk). (D) Lateral displacement of trachea (arrow).

(CECT: contrast-enhanced computed tomography; CXR: chest radiograph; MinIP: minimum intensity projection; MPR: multiplanar reconstructed; PA: posteroanterior)

■ CONCLUSION

Pediatric central airway diseases are diverse, and can either be primary, due to intrinsic airway problem, or extrinsic. An adequately performed CT is often the most informative. Depending on the suspected pathology, imaging technique needs to be modified. Dynamic CT is useful in primary TBM; whereas, a CT angiography should be done in suspected vascular causes. Image viewing at the console with proper image restriction is crucial.

Other Related Chapters that can be Referred to:
- Chapter 6: Congenital Lung Abnormalities
- Chapter 23: Thoracic Tumors and Mimics: Part 1
- Chapter 24: Thoracic Tumors and Mimics: Part 2

REFERENCES

1. Prountzos S, Papakonstantinou O, Bizimi V, Velonakis G, Mazioti A, Douros K, et al. Large airway diseases in pediatrics: a pictorial essay. Acta Radiol Open. 2020;9(12):2058460120972694.
2. Alamo L, Vial Y, Gengler C, Meuli R. Imaging findings of bronchial atresia in fetuses, neonates and infants. Pediatr Radiol. 2016;46:383-90.
3. Wallis C, Alexopoulou E, Antón-Pacheco JL, Bhatt JM, Bush A, Chang AB, et al. ERS statement on tracheomalacia and bronchomalacia in children. Eur Respir J. 2019;54(3):1900382.
4. Chassagnon G, Morel B, Carpentier E, Ducou Le Pointe H, Sirinelli D. Tracheobronchial branching abnormalities: lobe-based classification scheme. Radiographics. 2016;36:358-73.

CHAPTER 16

Bronchiectasis

Stuti Chandola, Smita Manchanda

- ❑ Imaging modalities
- ❑ Diagnosis
  - ➤ Diagnosis on chest radiograph
  - ➤ Diagnosis on CT
- ❑ Types of bronchiectasis
- ❑ Etiology and pathogenesis
- ❑ Complications
- ❑ Specific entities
  - ➤ Mucociliary clearance defects
  - ➤ Postinfective bronchiectasis
  - ➤ Post-foreign body stricture and bronchiectasis
- ❑ Management

■ INTRODUCTION

Bronchiectasis refers to irreversible dilatation of the peripheral airways. It is a cause of chronic suppurative lung disease (CSLD) with patients presenting with chronic wet cough. The chronic symptomatology is interspersed with episodes of acute exacerbations. The diagnosis requires the demonstration of bronchial dilatation on imaging, in a patient with a background of chronic wet cough.

■ IMAGING MODALITIES

- Role of imaging is diagnosis, severity assessment, suggesting etiology, identifying extent in surgical candidates and complications, and follow-up.
- Severe forms of bronchiectasis can be diagnosed on chest radiograph (CR) itself; and also, are useful for follow-up, to detect progression and superadded infection. However, CR does not have enough sensitivity to be used for primary diagnosis of bronchiectasis.
- Hence, HRCT [high-resolution computed tomography, reconstructed from multidetector CT (MDCT)] is the modality of choice for the same.
- Magnetic resonance imaging (MRI) has recently been used as an alternative modality for follow-up of these patients.

DIAGNOSIS

Diagnosis on Chest Radiograph

Chest radiographic signs of bronchiectasis are listed in **Box 1**.

BOX 1 | **Chest radiographic signs of bronchiectasis (Figs. 1A to D).**

- In moderate-to-severe cases, a *"tram-track" appearance* of parallel and *ringlike opacities* related to the thickened walls of dilated bronchi
- Later, *obvious cysts* may be seen
- *Tubular densities* related to mucus-filled dilated airways
- Generalized hyperinflation, oligemia in diffuse forms

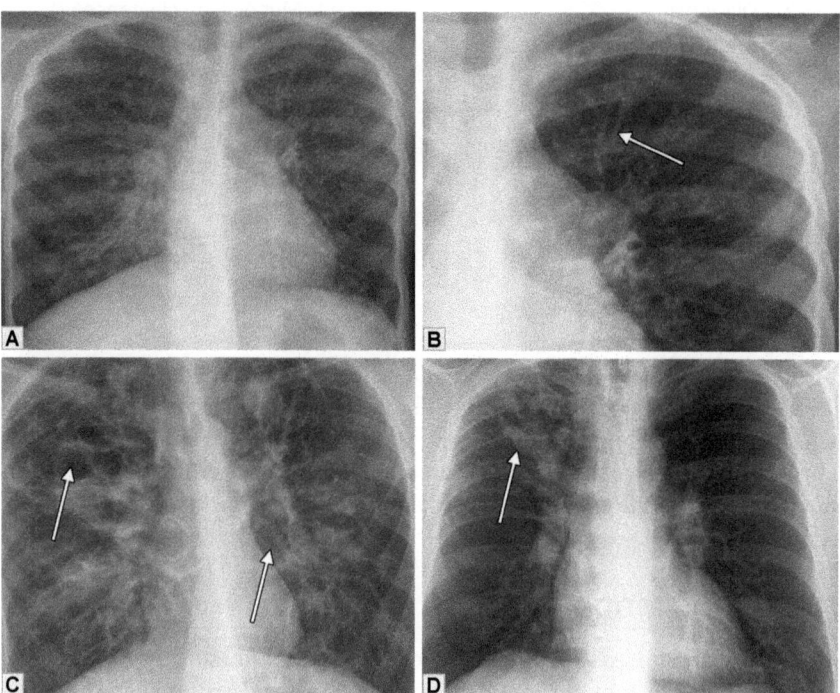

FIGS. 1A TO D: CXR signs of bronchiectasis. (A) Peribronchial thickening; (B) "tram-track" shadows (arrow); (C) cystic bronchiectasis (arrows); and (D) bronchocele (arrow).

Diagnosis on CT

Depending on the severity of bronchiectasis, various features/criteria aid in the diagnosis in CT.

- *Lack of distal tapering of bronchi*: There is no change in caliber at least 2 cm beyond the branching point.
- Visualization of peripheral airways within 1 cm of pleural margin except mediastinal pleura, is another imaging feature **(Figs. 2A and B)**.
- *Signet ring sign*: Visualization of a dilated bronchus in cross-section along with the adjacent artery.[1]
- *Bronchoarterial ratio (BAR)*: In case of marked dilatation, the diagnosis on CT is evident, even without any measurements. In milder cases, BAR is employed. BAR refers to the ratio of inner airway diameter and outer diameter of the accompanying artery **(Figs. 3A and B)**. The artery chosen is the one that is adjoining the artery (within 5 mm). The relation of artery and airway is to be ascertained in a nontangential plane. The cut-offs recommended for diagnosis is BAR >1-1.5 in adults; and BAR >0.8 in children.[1]
- In case of marked dilatation extending to the subpleural region, distinction from cystic lung disease can be challenging. Use of signet ring sign (eccentric location of accompanying artery) and use of multiplanar reformats and minimum intensity projections (MinIPs) can aid in making the distinction.
- Mucoid impaction and mosaic attenuation due to air trapping and air fluid levels within dilated bronchi are some other imaging findings.

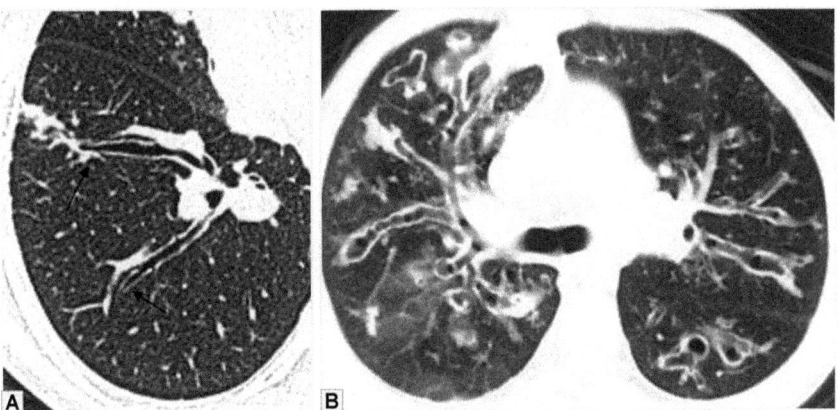

FIGS. 2A AND B: CT signs of bronchiectasis. (A) Lack of distal tapering of bronchi, peribronchial thickening and (B) visualization of distal airways.

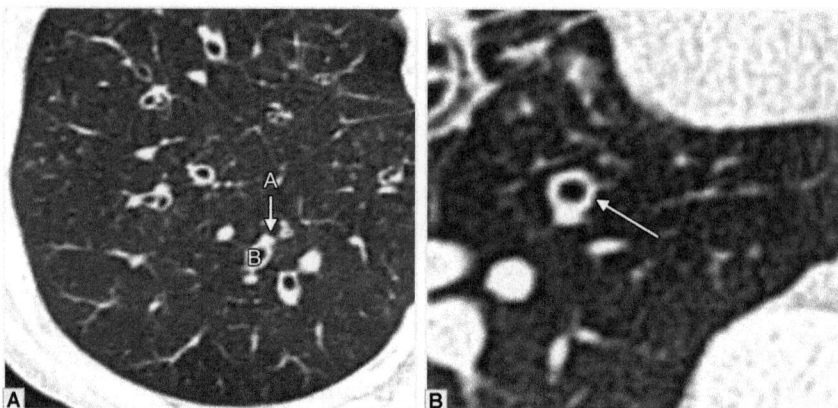

FIGS. 3A AND B: Abnormal bronchoarterial ratio. Dilated bronchi (B) compared to adjacent arterial branch (A); and (B) signet ring sign (arrow).

■ TYPES OF BRONCHIECTASIS

Based on morphology or severity, bronchiectasis has been divided into cylindrical, varicose, and cystic types. While cylindrical bronchiectasis is the least severe type, cystic type **(Figs. 4A to C)** denotes an advanced stage of the process, and often mimics cystic lung disease.

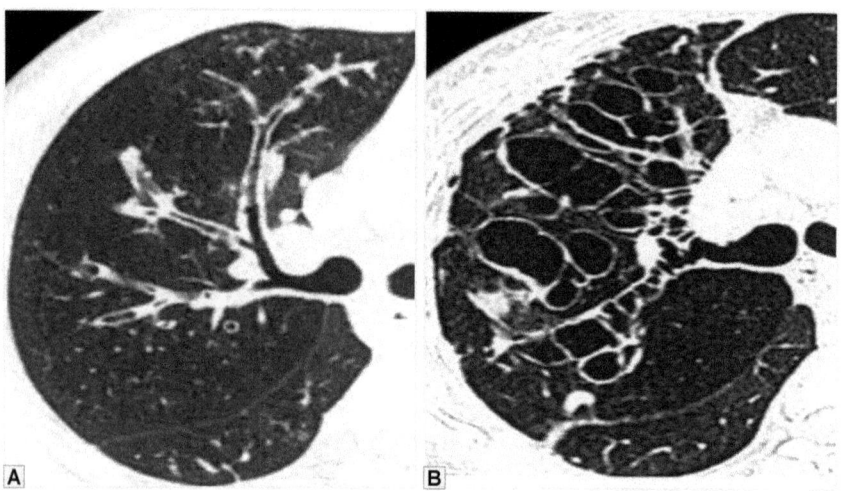

FIGS. 4A TO C: *Continued*

Continued

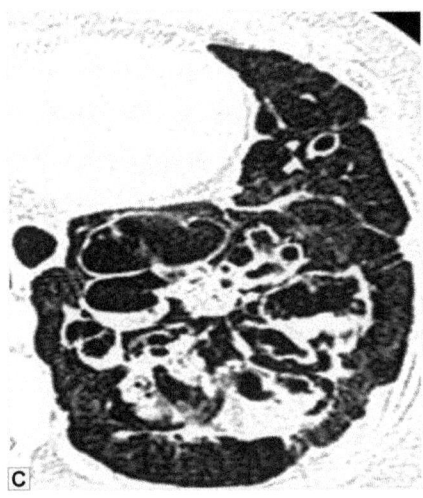

FIGS. 4A TO C: Types of bronchiectasis.
(A) Cylindrical; (B) fusiform; and (C) cystic.

ETIOLOGY AND PATHOGENESIS

- The etiologies of bronchiectasis are heterogeneous and diverse, and vary based on the patient population evaluated. For instance, a dominance of noninfectious causes in higher income groups.
- It can represent the end-stage of several causes. The causes can be focal such as endobronchial obstruction with resultant distal bronchiectasis. Diffuse/extensive bronchiectasis can be the consequence of disorders of mucociliary clearance or immunodeficiency, or even postinfectious.
- Further, there is a vicious cycle of inflammation, infection, and airway dilatation **(Flowchart 1)**.
- The distribution of bronchiectasis and associated findings can help in suggesting the etiology on imaging **(Table 1)**.[2]

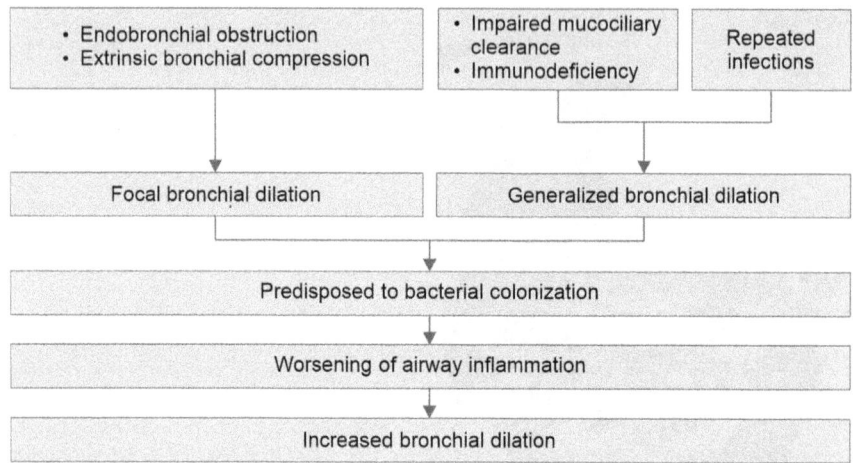

FLOWCHART 1: Vicious cycle of bronchiectasis and inflammation.

TABLE 1: Distribution of bronchiectasis according to etiological causes.		
Focal (lobar/segmental)	**Intraluminal cause**	**Foreign body, mass**
	Mural	*Stricture*: • Postinfective • After foreign body extraction
	Extrinsic compression	• Mass • Lymph nodes
Diffuse	Upper lobar	• ABPA • Cystic fibrosis • TB and sarcoidosis
	Middle lobe and lingula	• Nontubercular mycobacterial infection • Primary ciliary dyskinesia • Asthma

	Lower lobes	• Primary ciliary dyskinesia
		• Aspiration syndromes
		• Primary B-cell immunodeficiency:
		  ○ XLA
		  ○ CVID

(ABPA: allergic bronchopulmonary aspergillosis; CVID: common variable immunodeficiency; TB: tuberculosis; XLA: X-linked agammaglobulinemia)

■ COMPLICATIONS

Complications can be classified as nonvascular and vascular. The most frequent complication is recurrent infection.
- Nonvascular complications include chronic bacterial colonization and infection resulting in vicious cycle, i.e., colonization/infection worsens bronchiectasis and bronchiectasis predisposes to infection.

- Chronic bacterial colonization is an important cause responsible for bronchial wall damage and worsening of bronchiectasis and hence lung function in cystic fibrosis (as also in non-CF bronchiectasis).
    - Colonization refers to the presence of infective organisms within the bronchiectasis in concentrations that can be detected on sampling, however, not causing any symptoms in the patient. Colonization can persist for days to years and its clearance depends on the patient's immune response, other organisms and at times use of antimicrobials.
    - Common bacteria implicated in chronic colonization include *P. aeruginosa, S. aureus, H. influenza,* and *Burkholderia cepacia.*
    - Apart from bacteria secondary infection by mycobacteria/fungi also occurs. Aspergilloma can develop within the dilated bronchi.
    - CF patients are also prone to allergic bronchopulmonary aspergillosis (ABPA)
    - Imaging findings of colonization of the bronchi include presence of centrilobular nodules with tree-in-bud pattern and mucus plugs. It is difficult to distinguish colonization from active infection, however, presence of consolidations, peribronchial thickening, clinical features of exacerbation, and comparison with previous imaging to identify new areas of involvement help to suggest presence of active superadded infection **(Fig. 5)**.
    - There may be bronchiectasis with presence of intraluminal contents, the differentials for which are shown in **Table 2**.
- Vascular complications include pulmonary artery hypertension and bronchial artery enlargement.
- Hemoptysis due to hypertrophy of bronchial arteries, or pulmonary artery hypertension in those with extensive and long-standing disease.

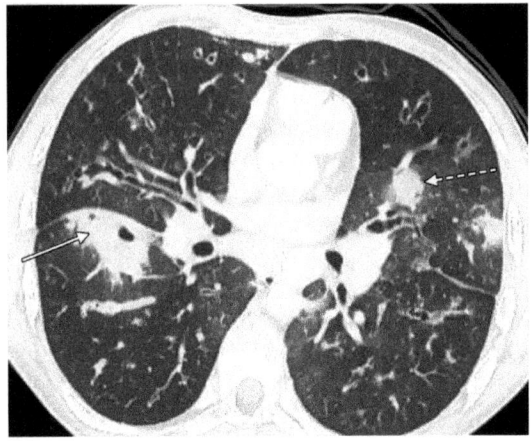

FIG. 5: Colonization and superadded infection in bronchiectasis. Peribronchial consolidation (arrow) and mucus impaction with surrounding ground-glass halo (dotted arrow).

TABLE 2: Differentials for bronchiectasis with intraluminal contents.

Tree-in-bud nodules	Mucus plugs with luminal widening
Nontuberculous mycobacteria (typically affect middle lobe and lingula)	Cystic fibrosis (CF) (low density mucoceles)
Chronic colonization	ABPA (presence of high attenuation mucus)
Aspiration (seen in lower lobes)	CF + ABPA (presence of high attenuation mucus)
Primary ciliary dyskinesia	
Immunodeficiency	

(ABPA: allergic bronchopulmonary aspergillosis)

■ SPECIFIC ENTITIES

Mucociliary Clearance Defects

- Mucociliary clearance (MCC) apparatus comprises the mucus secreted by respiratory epithelium and the cilia. The MCC is a first-line defense mechanism which aids in clearing the airway of inhaled dust particles and bacteria.
- Defects in the MCC mechanism predispose the individual to recurrent infections. These defects could be congenital/acquired.
- Two basic types of defects are those affecting the ciliary mechanism, and those of abnormal mucus secretion **(Table 3)**.

Primary Ciliary Dyskinesia (Figs. 6A and B)

- This is a genetic defect, with autosomal recessive being the most frequent mode of transmission, wherein several gene mutations result in defective ciliary movement.
- Patients present with recurrent sinopulmonary infections, starting in early childhood.
- Other presentations include otitis media and male infertility or subfertility and increased incidence of ectopic pregnancy in females.
- There may be an association with situs inversus in up to half the patients (Kartagener's syndrome) **(Figs. 7A to F)**.
- Less frequent associations include pectus excavatum and congenital heart disease.
- *Diagnosis is based on*:
  - Low nasal NO (nitric oxide) < 250 ppm
  - *Histopathology electron microscopy*: Abnormal ciliary structure and movement
  - Imaging findings include bronchiectasis with a middle and lower lobe predominance. Distribution may be central or diffuse. Bronchial wall thickening, air trapping, and hyperinflation are other imaging findings.

TABLE 3: Causes of abnormal mucociliary clearance.	
Ciliary mechanism	**Abnormal mucus**
Primary ciliary dyskinesia	*Genetic*: Cystic fibrosis
Secondary ciliary dyskinesia	*Acquired*: Asthma

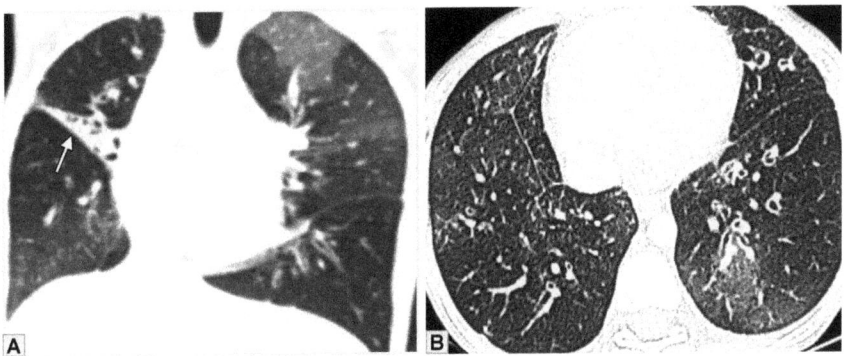

FIGS. 6A AND B: Primary ciliary dyskinesia. (A) Right middle lobe collapse (arrow), generalized hyperinflation and (B) peribronchial thickening and early bronchiectasis of the lower lobes, right middle lobe, and lingula.

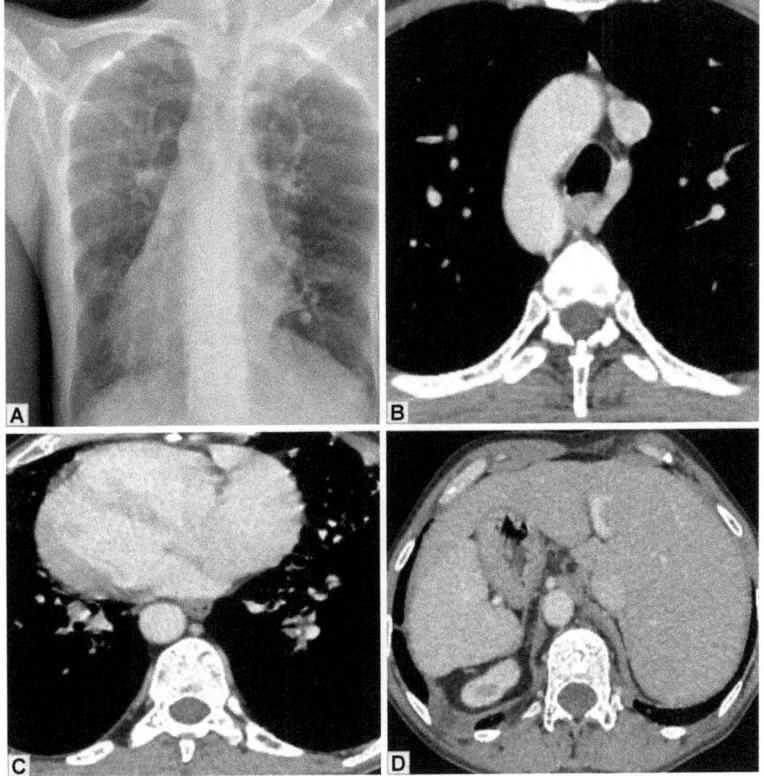

FIGS. 7A TO F: *Continued*

Continued

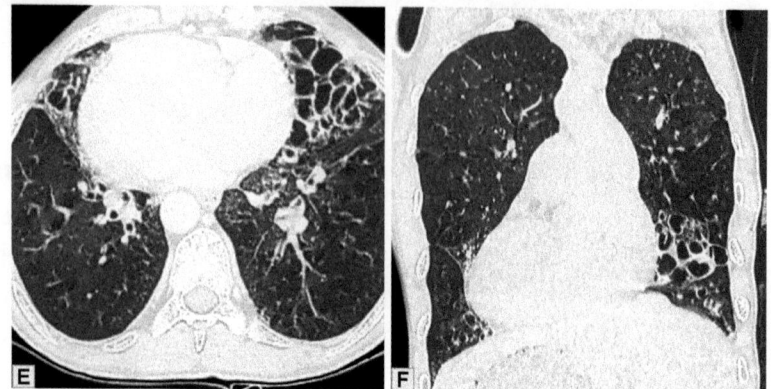

FIGS. 7A TO F: Kartagener's syndrome. (A) Thoracic situs inversus; (B) right-sided aortic arch; (C) dextrocardia; (D) abdominal situs inversus; and (E and F) bronchiectasis in right middle lobe and lingula.

Young's Syndrome/Barry–Perkins–Young Syndrome

It comprises a triad of azoospermia, bronchiectasis, and sinusitis. Its clinical presentation and imaging are similar to CF/primary ciliary dyskinesia (PCD). The pathogenesis is not clear. The cause of azoospermia is thought to be obstructive (epididymis level).

Cystic Fibrosis

- Cystic fibrosis is a multisystem exocrinopathy affecting lungs, pancreas, intestines, and reproductive tract.
- Defect in the *CFTR* protein (CF transmembrane conductance regulator) leads to decreased volume and altered composition of respiratory epithelial secretions resulting in thick, viscous secretions.[3,4]
- CFTR is a gene encoding the chloride (Cl⁻) channel in the epithelial membrane. This abnormal chloride transport results in increased mucus viscosity.
- *Diagnosis*: Sweat electrolyte measurement.
- The mechanism of progression of lung changes in CF is illustrated in **Flowchart 2**.
- *Imaging findings*:
  - Chest X-ray (CXR): Various scoring systems exist for CXRs such as "Wisconsin" and "Brasfield". CXR features are listed in **Box 2**.

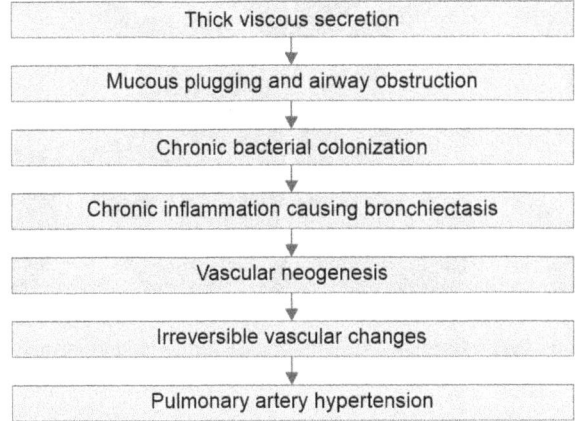

FLOWCHART 2: Pathogenesis of bronchiectasis in cystic fibrosis.

> **BOX 2**   **Chest radiographic features in cystic fibrosis.**
> - Central bronchiectasis with upper lobar predominance
> - Generalized hyperinflation
> - "Tram-track shadows" and "ring shadows (block arrow)" due to peribronchial thickening
> - "Finger in glove" shadows due to mucus impaction
> - Atelectasis

- Similarly various HRCT scoring systems also exist, which are more frequently used, most common amongst them being modified Bhalla and Brody systems.
  - *CT:* Progression of imaging findings **(Figs. 8 and 9)** follows a pattern detailed below:
    - Early findings: Peribronchial thickening with air trapping
    - Intermediate stage findings: Segmental consolidation and atelectasis
    - Advanced stage findings: Bronchiectasis, mucus plugging, lobar consolidation, abscess, and cyst/bullae
    - CF with ABPA **(Figs. 10A to D)**
    - MRI is being increasingly used to monitor patients with CF.

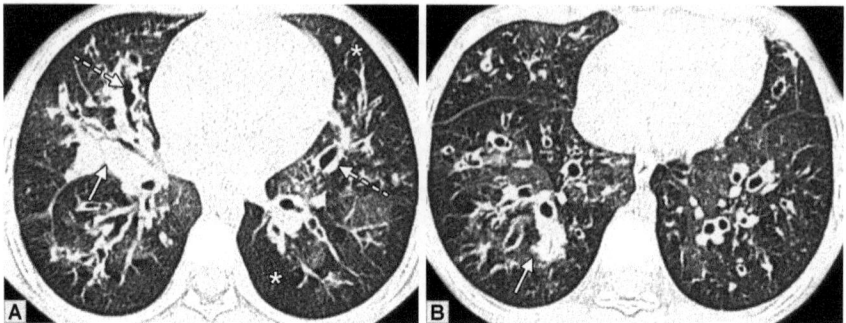

FIGS. 8A AND B: Cystic fibrosis. (A) Peribronchial consolidation (arrow), bronchiectasis (dotted arrows), and air trapping (asterisks) and (B) bronchiectasis with mucus impaction (arrow).

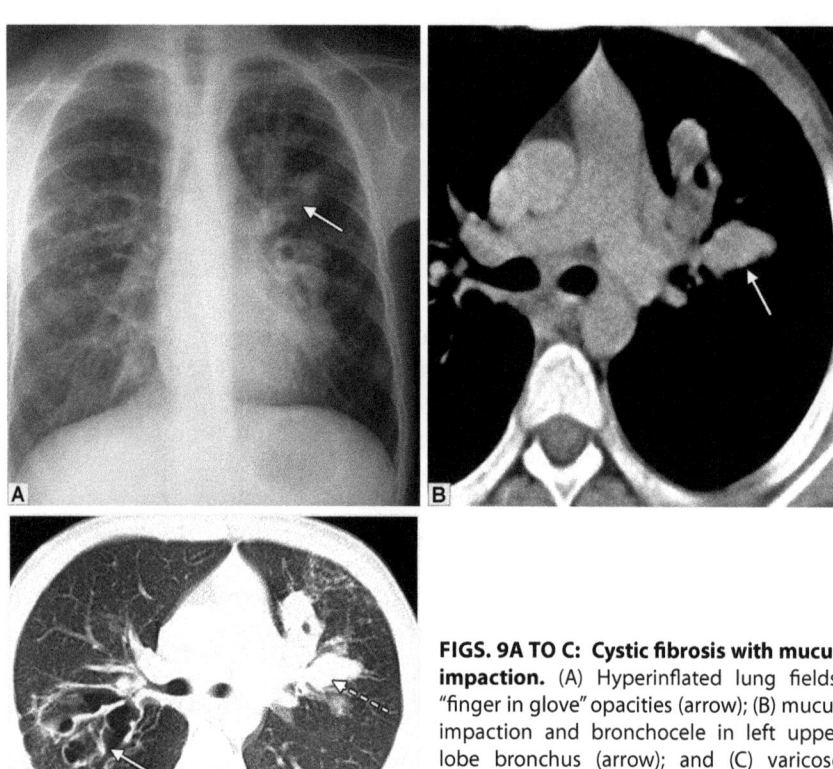

FIGS. 9A TO C: Cystic fibrosis with mucus impaction. (A) Hyperinflated lung fields, "finger in glove" opacities (arrow); (B) mucus impaction and bronchocele in left upper lobe bronchus (arrow); and (C) varicose bronchiectasis in right lower lobe (arrow), bronchocele in left upper lobe (dotted arrow).

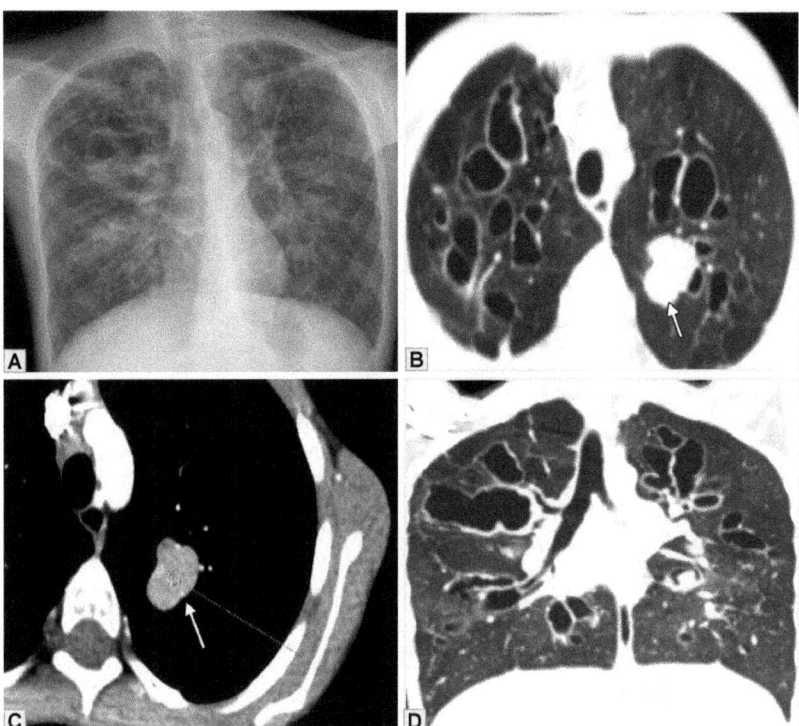

FIGS. 10A TO D: Cystic fibrosis with ABPA. (A) Central cystic and varicose bronchiectasis; (B) left upper lobe mucus impaction; (C) High attenuation in the impacted mucus (arrow); and (D) Central bronchiectasis with upper lobar predominance.

- *MRI (Figs. 11A to C)* can be used for delineating structural abnormality, airway inflammation as well as perfusion abnormality.
    - Peribronchial thickening and airway inflammation can be seen as T2W hyperintensity along the bronchial wall.
    - Air trapping can also be detected on MRI, even though CT is superior in this regards.
    - Inverted mucus impaction signal (IMIS) can be an imaging finding in ABPA superimposed on CF bronchiectasis.
    - Lung perfusion abnormalities can be detected using perfusion MRI.
- *Salient points of Bhalla scoring system*: The abnormalities are scored from 0 (normal) to 3 (most severe).[5] The parameters included are:
    - Severity of bronchiectasis
    - Bronchial wall thickening
    - Extent of bronchiectasis (number of bronchopulmonary segments involved)

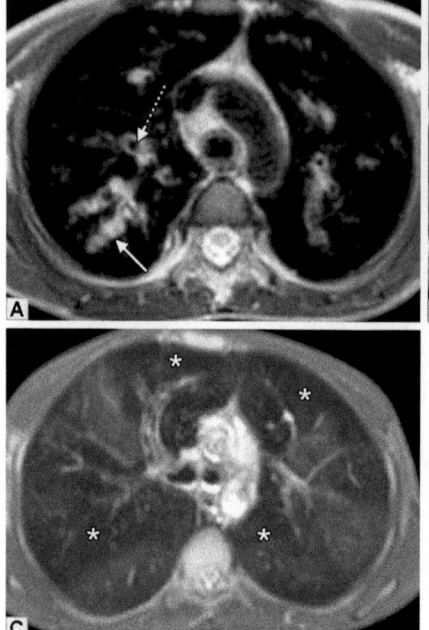
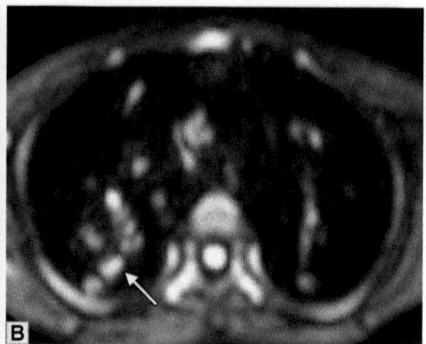

FIGS. 11A TO C: MRI in cystic fibrosis. T2W MVXD (A), DWI (B), and STIR (C)—(A) mucus impaction (arrow) and peribronchial thickening (dotted arrow); (B) mucus impaction seen as 'hotspot' on DWI (arrow); and (C) peribronchial thickening and air trapping (asterisks).

(DWI: diffusion-weighted imaging; STIR: short tau inversion recovery; T2W MVXD: T2-weighted MultiVane-XD)

- Extent of mucus plugging (number of bronchopulmonary segments involved)
- Sacculations/abscesses (number of bronchopulmonary segments involved)
- Emphysema
- Generations of bronchial divisions involved (by bronchiectasis/mucus plugging) grading from 4th to 6th generation
- Number of bullae (< or > 4)
- Collapse/consolidation (subsegmental, segmental, or lobar)
- Acinar nodules (subsegmental, segmental, or lobar)
- Air trapping (subsegmental, segmental, or lobar)

Complete discussion of these systems is beyond the scope of this chapter.

Postinfective Bronchiectasis

- Postinfectious bronchiectasis is seen as an irreversible dilatation of bronchi which contain cartilage.
- Bacteria, tuberculosis, nontubercular mycobacteria, pertussis, and viral infections can lead to bronchiectasis. It may be localized or diffuse forms. Imaging shows either diffuse cylindrical bronchiectasis or localized traction bronchiectasis in the segment of healed fibrotic region (**Figs. 12A to C**).

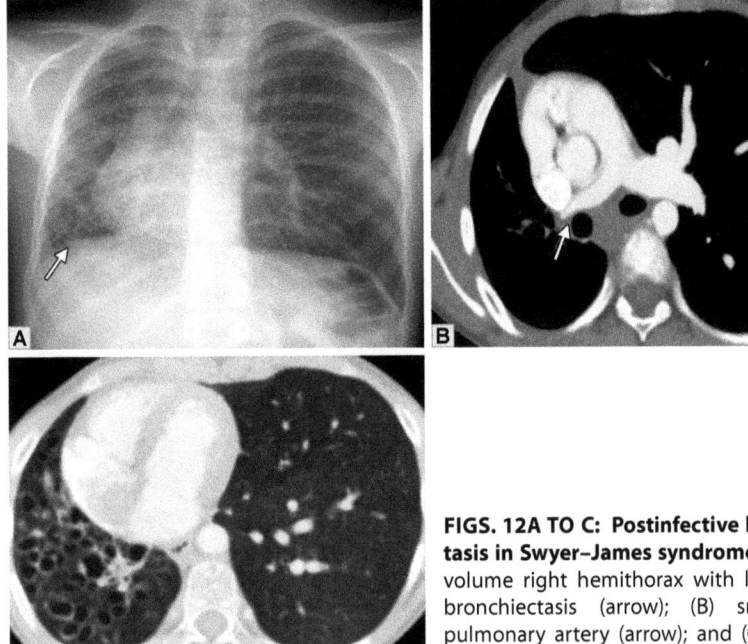

FIGS. 12A TO C: Postinfective bronchiectasis in Swyer–James syndrome. (A) Small volume right hemithorax with lower zone bronchiectasis (arrow); (B) small right pulmonary artery (arrow); and (C) varicose bronchiectasis in right lower lobe.

- Pseudomonas aeruginosa (PA), especially the mucoid phenotype, is particularly implicated in worsening of bronchiectasis of CF and measures to eradicate the organism and prevent exposure are important. The colonization with mucoid PA is associated with more severe bronchiectasis scores, mucus plugging and bronchial wall thickening in patients with CF. Other important organisms are *Burkholderia cepacia* and *Moraxella catarrhalis*.
- Healing of airway infections can be complete or it may heal with fibrosis of the affected region of its wall and lead to strictures or dilatation/bronchiectasis.
- Postinfectious stricture and bronchiectasis has a zonal propensity toward lower lobes. Tubercular strictures can commonly be seen in the right middle lobe bronchus.
- In case of extrinsic compression/endoluminal partial obstruction of a bronchus, it becomes prone to recurrent infections and subsequent development of bronchiectasis.

Post-foreign Body Stricture and Bronchiectasis

- Foreign bodies, especially organic ones, can incite inflammatory response and localized stricture formation in the airway. Recurrent infection in the respective lung segment can lead to bronchiectasis **(Fig. 13)**.

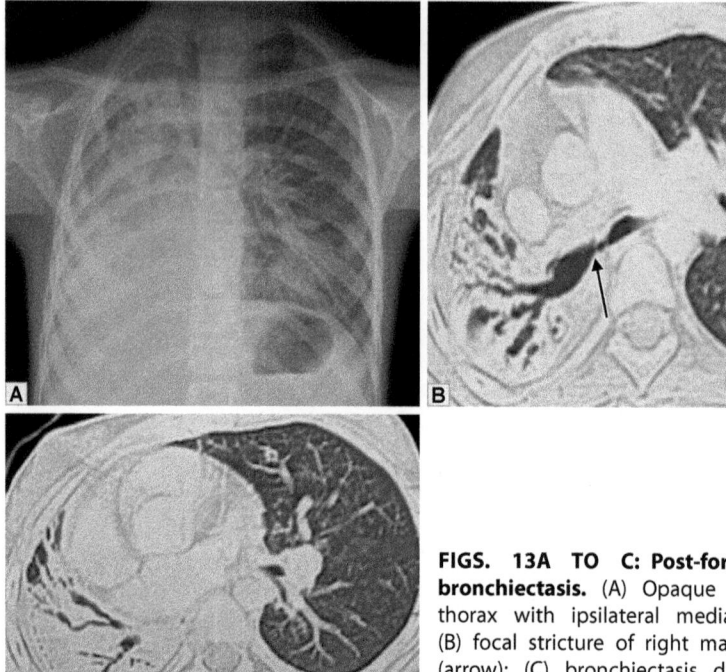

FIGS. 13A TO C: Post-foreign body bronchiectasis. (A) Opaque right hemithorax with ipsilateral mediastinal shift; (B) focal stricture of right main bronchus (arrow); (C) bronchiectasis distal to the stricture.

- While inspiratory-expiratory radiographs are useful for demonstration and detection of air trapping in the acute phase; CT with MinIP reconstructions is essential in chronic stages.
- *Allergic bronchopulmonary aspergillosis (ABPA)*: This has been discussed in detail in Chapter 8.
- *Common variable immunodeficiency (CVID) and X-linked agammaglobulinemia (XLA)* has been discussed in Chapter 10.

MANAGEMENT

Two broad groups of pediatric bronchiectasis are recognized from management point of view—(1) CF and (2) non-CF. The broad principles of management, however, remain similar and include:
- Airway clearance techniques (physiotherapy)
- Use of appropriate antibiotics for prompt treatment of acute exacerbations
- Use of antibiotics as maintenance therapy
- Use of mucolytics and mucokinetics
- Control of responsible factors such as aspiration, repair of tracheoesophageal fistula (TEF), and removal of foreign body
- Replacement therapies as in immunodeficiency, CF.

Novel therapies such as DPP-1 (dipeptidyl peptidase) inhibitors are not validated in children.

CONCLUSION

Bronchiectasis can be the result of multiple causes; the distribution and associated imaging findings can provide a clue to the etiologic diagnosis. Complications can be life-threatening; and imaging techniques need modification according to the presenting symptoms.

Other Related Chapters that can be Referred to:
- Chapter 8: Fungal Chest Infections
- Chapter 10: Chest Infections in Immunocompromised Host

REFERENCES

1. Goyal V, Chang AB. Bronchiectasis in childhood. Clin Chest Med. 2022;43:71-88.
2. Singh A, Bhalla AS, Jana M. Bronchiectasis Revisited: Imaging-based pattern approach to diagnosis. Curr Probl Diagn Radiol. 2019;48(1):53-60.
3. Dournes G, Walkup LL, Benlala I, Willmering MM, Macey J, Bui S, et al. The Clinical Use of Lung MRI in Cystic Fibrosis: What, Now, How? Chest. 2021;159(6):2205-17.
4. Brasfield D, Hicks G, Soong S, Tiller RE. The chest roentgenogram in cystic fibrosis: A new scoring system. Pediatrics. 1979;63:24-9.
5. Bhalla M, Turcios N, Aponte V, Jenkins M, Leitman BS, McCauley DI, et al. Cystic fibrosis: scoring system with thin-section CT. Radiology. 1991;179:783-8.

CHAPTER 17

Small Airway Diseases

Priyanka Naranje, Rajendra K Behera

- ❏ Introduction/Terminology
- ❏ Imaging modalities and signs
- ❏ Classification
  - ➢ Cellular/Inflammatory bronchiolitis
  - ➢ Cellular bronchiolitis: Infectious causes
  - ➢ Cellular bronchiolitis: Noninfectious causes
  - ➢ Constrictive bronchiolitis
- ❏ Asthma versus small airway disease

■ INTRODUCTION/TERMINOLOGY

- The term "small airways" refers to distal airways (bronchioles and their branches) that have diameters between 1 and 2 mm and no cartilage in their wall.
- Bronchioles are further divided into "membranous" and "respiratory" with the former being purely conducting, while respiratory bronchioles have both conducting and gas exchange (including alveoli and alveolar ducts) function.
- Hence, the term small airway disease (SAD) is used synonymously with "bronchiolitis".
- Normally, the small airways make only a minor contribution to airway resistance. However, disorders involving these airways result in increase in the resistance. Eventually patients develop airway obstruction which is not reversible with bronchodilators.

■ IMAGING MODALITIES AND SIGNS

- Chest radiographs (CRs) have limited utility in evaluating SAD as these may be normal in the early/mild involvement.
- High-resolution computed tomography (HRCT) is the modality of choice.
- CT signs suggestive of SAD are well described[1] and have been divided into direct signs and indirect signs **(Table 1; Figs. 1A and B)**.

CHAPTER 17: Small Airway Diseases

TABLE 1: Direct and indirect signs of small airway disease.	
Direct signs	**Indirect signs**
• *Centrilobular nodules* giving tree in bud appearance often described as being V or Y shaped • *Ground glass opacities* which are centrilobular or peribronchiolar in distribution • Bronchiolectasis (in chronic stage)	• Air trapping (best demonstrated on expiratory scans) • Bronchial wall thickening

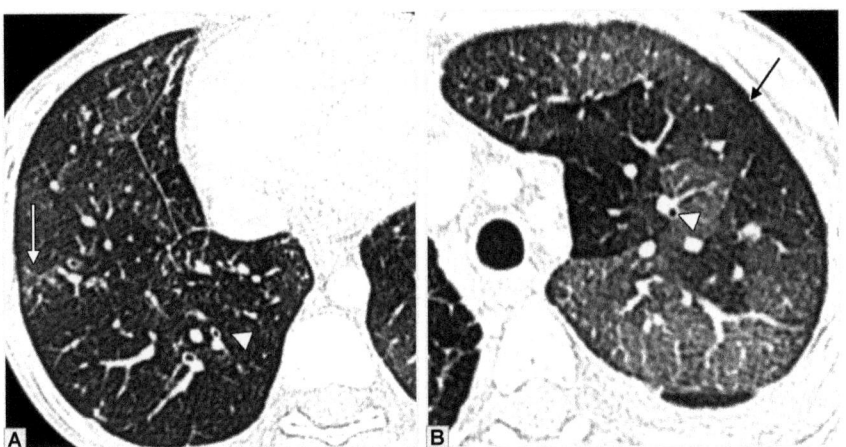

FIGS. 1A AND B: Direct and indirect signs of small airway diseases. (A) Direct signs—centrilobular nodules (arrow) and bronchieolectasis (arrowhead). (B) Indirect signs—air trapping (arrow) and bronchial wall thickening.

■ CLASSIFICATION

The terminology associated with SADs over the years has been confusing and may have different connotations for pathologists, radiologists, and clinicians.
- The most prevalent accepted is based on combined radiopathological approach.
- The classification divides SAD into two major types **(Table 2)**:
  i. Cellular/inflammatory bronchiolitis
  ii. Constrictive/fibrotic bronchiolitis

Acute infectious bronchiolitis encountered in infants and toddlers has been covered under Chapter 7.

Cellular/Inflammatory Bronchiolitis

- The term cellular bronchiolitis is also a pathological term referring to inflammatory response in bronchiolar wall involving infiltration by lymphocytes, neutrophils, or eosinophils.
- Numerous causes include infectious and systemic disorders of immune function (including autoimmune disorders or immune deficiencies).

TABLE 2: Radiopathologic differentiation between two types of bronchiolitis.		
	Inflammatory/cellular bronchiolitis	**Constrictive bronchiolitis**
Pathology	Inflammatory cells (acute chronic or a combination of these) are seen	Bronchiolar lesion resulting in narrowing of bronchiolar lumen due to collagen deposition, fibrosis, and scarring of bronchiolar wall/peribronchiolar area
Etiology/subtypes	• Infectious • Autoimmune/connective tissue disorders • Hypersensitivity pneumonitis • Bronchiectasis-associated bronchiolitis	• Idiopathic • Postinfectious • Inhalation of toxic fumes • Autoimmune/connective tissue disorders • Drug related • Post-transplantation
Imaging	• Centrilobular nodules • Ground glass nodules • Bronchial wall thickening	• Air trapping (characteristic imaging feature) • Bronchiectasis /bronchiolectasis may be seen • Centrilobular nodules are rare

- The term follicular bronchiolitis refers to a form of cellular bronchiolitis associated with disorders of immunity. It is a form of benign lymphoproliferative disorder due to inflammation involving bronchus-associated lymphoid tissue (BALT). The more common specific causes in children are discussed below.

Cellular Bronchiolitis: Infectious Causes

Acute Bronchiolitis
- In children, viruses are the most frequent pathogens causing acute bronchiolitis.
- *Immunocompromised host*: Viral (cytomegalovirus and respiratory syncytial virus), fungal (*Aspergillus* species) and bacteria (*Pseudomonas* species) can all be responsible.
- HRCT: Thickened bronchiolar walls (bronchi become visible on HRCT), well-defined centrilobular nodules, tree in bud nodules and ill-defined centrilobular nodules **(Figs. 2A and B)**.
- Air trapping may be seen but is less frequent.
- In acute bronchiolitis in children CR may be performed to exclude other diagnosis, e.g., consolidation but city is seldom performed. Chest X-ray (CXR) may reveal hyperinflation or may be normal.
- In late stages, bronchial wall thickening with bronchiectasis may be seen.
- Infectious bronchiolitis has more asymmetric or patchy distribution as compared to non-infectious bronchiolitis.
- Associated ground-glass opacity or areas of consolidation may be seen.
- *Differential diagnosis*: Hypersensitivity pneumonitis (HP).

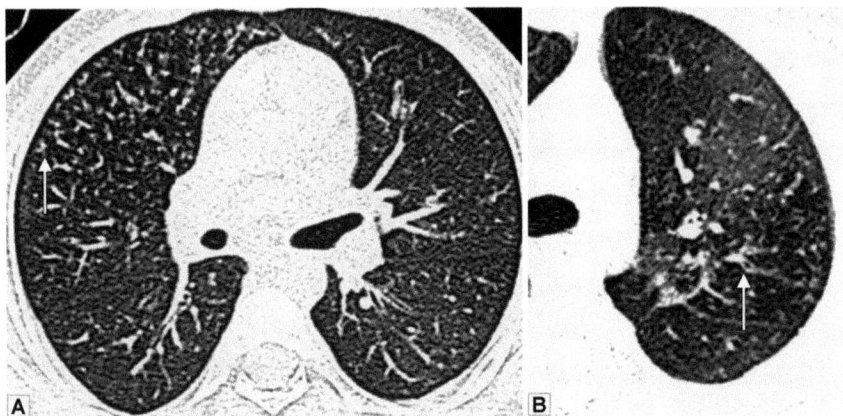

FIGS. 2A AND B: Cellular bronchiolitis. Infectious bronchiolitis in a child presenting with fever and cough. High-resolution computed tomography (HRCT) shows multiple well-defined centrilobular nodules in asymmetric distribution (seen more in right lung), tree in bud nodules (arrows) with bronchial wall thickening (arrow in B).

Chronic Infectious Bronchiolitis
- *Organisms*: Mycobacterium tuberculosis, nontubercular mycobacteria (NTM) (especially *Mycobacterium avium* intracellulare).
- Tuberculosis is associated with centrilobular nodules resulting in tree in bud appearance typically localized to a lobe or segment, although more diffuse involvement may also be seen. Associated consolidation, cavitation, or necrotic lymphadenopathy aids in the diagnosis.
- Superadded infection/chronic colonization of preexisting bronchiectasis is frequent. This form is difficult to differentiate from TB/NTM and is often misdiagnosed as such. The nodules in this setting can persist over long periods.[1]

Cellular Bronchiolitis: Noninfectious Causes
Primary Immunodeficiency Disorders and Small Airway Diseases
- Amongst several clinical presentations of primary immunodeficiencies, respiratory symptoms are typical initial presentation of various primary immunodeficiencies (PIDs) in children.
- Small airway involvement may be in the form of severe infectious bronchiolitis or noninfectious reactive follicular hyperplasia.[2]
- Amongst primary immunodeficiency diseases (PIDDs), selective deficiency of IgA, common variable immunodeficiency (CVID), and severe combined immunodeficiency (SCID) present with small airway involvement.
- Imaging shows numerous centrilobular nodules with bronchial wall thickening distributed in multiple lung segments or diffuse **(Fig. 3A)**.
- Bronchiectasis is commonly associated imaging feature **(Fig. 3B)**.

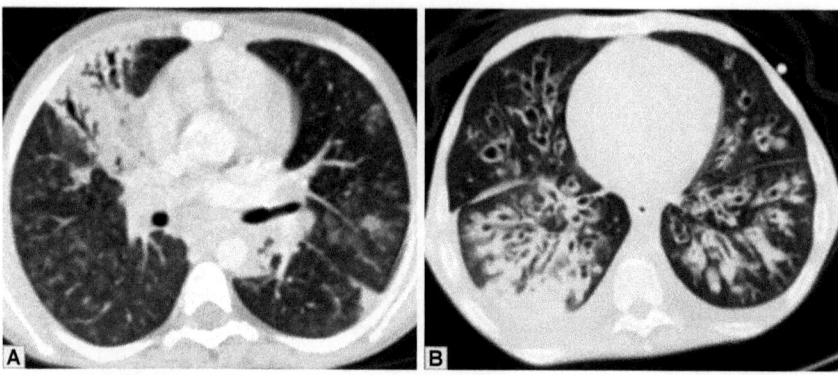

FIGS. 3A AND B: Small airway involvement in primary immunodeficiencies. Two different patients of common variable immunodeficiency (CVID). (A) Numerous centrilobular nodules with consolidation distributed in multiple lung segments. (B) Diffuse lung involvement in later stages of CVID showing bronchiectasis.

Connective Tissue Disorders

- Connective tissue disorders (CTDs) can be a cause of SAD.
- *Pathology*: There is proliferation of lymphoid tissues around the bronchioles which on immunohistochemistry is seen to be polyclonal.
- SAD is characteristically associated with CTDs especially rheumatoid arthritis (RA) and Sjögren's syndrome.
- SAD is seen less frequently in primary Sjögren's syndrome (PSS), SLE, sarcoidosis, and vasculitis.
- *HRCT*: Similar to other causes of cellular bronchiolitis.

Inflammatory Bowel Diseases

- Inflammatory bowel diseases such as ulcerative colitis and Crohn's disease may be associated with SAD.[3]
- While large airway involvement is in the form of bronchiectasis is more frequent, SAD is seen less often.
- Crohn's disease is associated with cellular (granulomatous) bronchiolitis in association with ILD.
- Ulcerative colitis is rarely associated with constrictive bronchiolitis.

Constrictive Bronchiolitis

[*Synonyms*: Obliterative/fibrotic bronchiolitis, bronchiolitis obliterans (BO)].
- Clinical presentation of patients with BO is of dyspnea and air flow obstruction which does not reverse with the use of bronchodilators.
- BO is the consequence of diverse types of insults to the bronchiolar lining, with during the reparative phase result in granulation tissue causing narrowing/obliteration of the airway.
- BO is the term used for the clinical syndrome, while constrictive bronchiolitis is its histopathological correlate.
- Numerous causes include inhalational injury, infections, systemic disorders including CTDs and GVHD, drugs, or idiopathic.[4]

Few specific entities relevant to children are discussed below.

Postinfectious
[*Synonyms*: Postinfectious bronchiolitis obliterans (PIBO)].
- Can occur as a consequence of infections with a variety of organisms
- Adenovirus pertussis tuberculosis measles or mycoplasma
- *HRCT*: Air trapping or mosaic attenuation in patchy distribution. Centrilobular nodules, bronchiectasis, are infrequently seen **(Figs. 4A and B)**.

Swyer–James–MacLeod Syndrome
- This is a sequel of postinfectious constrictive bronchiolitis occurring in children.
- Only difference between PIBO and SJS is the predominant airway obstruction in PIBO, with a bilateral disease
- Classically, described as being unilateral though increasingly recognized that may be bilateral.
- The classic description is of a small unilateral hyperlucent lung with a small pulmonary artery.
- *Pathogenesis*: Infectious bronchiolitis occurring in young children often heals without sequalae or results in fibrosis and narrowing of bronchioles. This impairs subsequent alveolar development.
- *Imaging*: A unilateral or bilateral hyperlucent lung that demonstrates air trapping.
- On HRCT, the air trapping is patchy and lobar/lobular in distribution. Mild bronchiectasis may also be seen. The hyperlucent appearance of the lung is due to a combination of air trapping and diminished vascularity **(Figs. 5A to D)**.
- *Differential diagnosis*: When unilateral needs to be differentiated from pulmonary hypoplasia. Presence of air trapping suggests Swyer-James-MacLeod (SJ) syndrome.

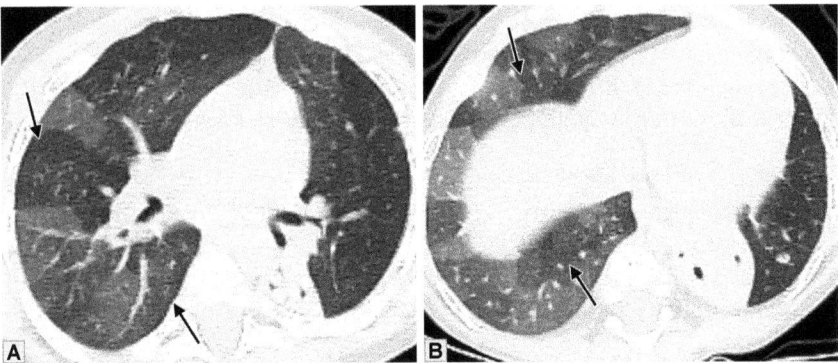

FIGS. 4A AND B: Postinfectious bronchiolitis obliterans (PIBO) in a child presenting with recurrent tachypnea. High-resolution computed tomography (HRCT) shows multifocal areas of air trapping in both lungs (arrows), with collapse of left lower lobe. Centrilobular nodules, bronchiectasis is infrequently seen in PIBO.

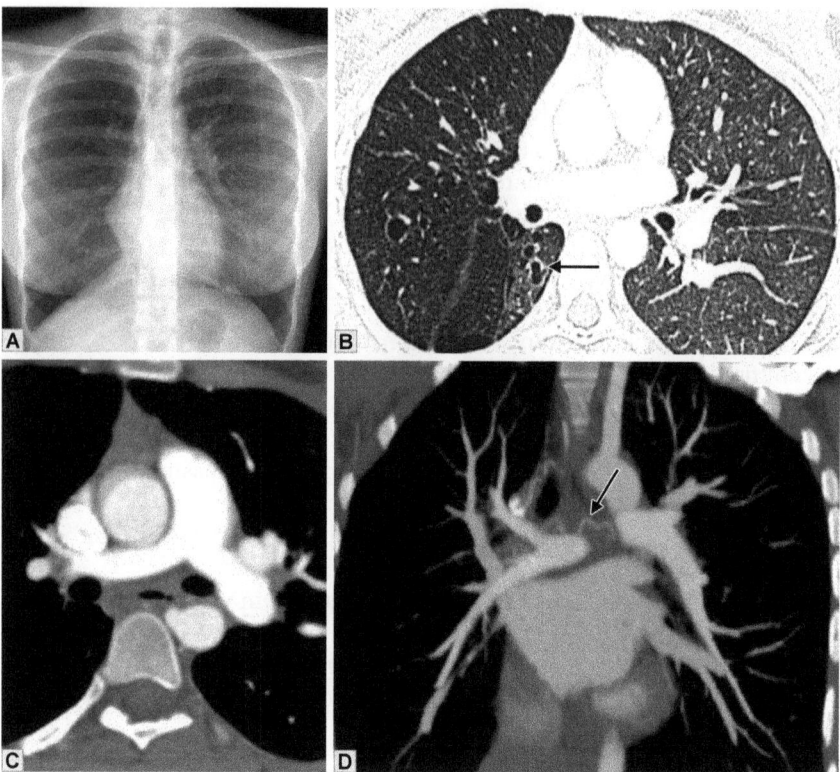

FIGS. 5A TO D: Swyer–James–MacLeod syndrome. (A) Chest X-ray—hyperlucent right lung with flattened diaphragm and diminished pulmonary vascularity; (B) Air trapping in right lung with mild bronchiectasis (arrow); (C) small caliber right PA as compared to left pulmonary artery (LPA); and (D) hypertrophied bronchial arteries (arrow).

Toxic Fume Exposure
- Exposure to noxious fumes may cause acute inflammatory response centered around the bronchiolar walls. Over a 2-6 weeks, subsequent fibrosis can result in obliterative bronchiolitis.
- For example, nitrogen oxide exposure causes silo fillers lung, diacetyl exposure resulting in popcorn flavor manufacturers lung.

Connective Tissue Disorders
- RA and Sjögren's syndrome may be associated with both follicular and obliterative forms of bronchiolitis.
- The two forms may even go exist in the same patient.
- Manifestations of bronchiolitis may even precede articular manifestations.
- *HRCT*: Similar to other causes of obliterative bronchiolitis.

Drug Induced
- *RA treatment*: Follicular as well as constrictive bronchiolitis has been reported with the use of D-penicillamine and infrequently with gold and tiopronin.
- Leads to diagnostic confusion as RA itself can also cause bronchiolitis.
- Busulfan when used prior to allogenic stem cell transplantation to suppress the immune system of the recipient.

Transplantation
- BO can occur as a complication of allogeneic (not of autologous) hematopoietic stem cell transplantation.
- BO is also seen in patients of lung transplantation referred to as BO syndrome.
- The term "BO syndrome" refers to the clinical syndrome occurring in transplant patients, while "BO" is used if there is confirmation on histopathology.
- Clinical presentation is of worsening dyspnea, chronic cough.
- HRCT characteristically demonstrates air trapping and a cut off of air trapping has been used as a criteria for diagnosis.[1]
- Advanced cases may have associated bronchial wall thickening and bronchiectasis.

Hypersensitivity Pneumonitis
Hypersensitivity pneumonitis is a form of inflammation involving both lung parenchyma and small airways with formation of granulomas. It is further discussed in chapter on interstitial lung diseases.

Aspiration-related Bronchiolitis
Chronic/recurrent aspiration results in repeated injury to peripheral and small airways and is a cause of bronchiectasis and possible small airway injury.

Bronchocentric Granulomatosis
This is a form of fungal infection resulting in formation of granulomas more in the peripheral airways but may extend distally to small airways.

■ ASTHMA VERSUS SMALL AIRWAY DISEASE
- Asthma is a differential diagnosis but is not labeled as a SAD, as the air flow obstruction herein is reversible.
- On imaging lung fields may appear hyperinflated but mosaic attenuation is less frequent than bronchiolitis **(Figs. 6A to C)**.
- The hypereosinophilic variant of severe asthma overlaps with obliterative bronchiolitis with similar HRCT features.

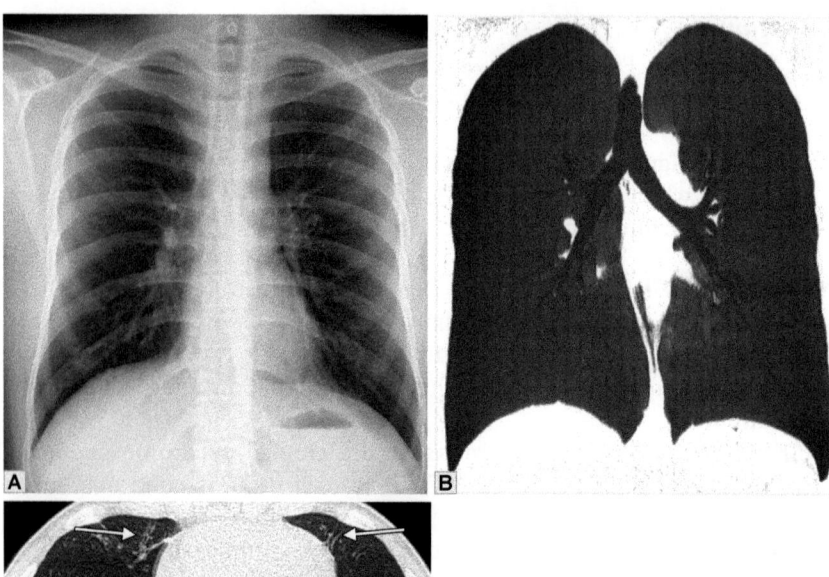

FIGS. 6A TO C: Asthma versus small airway disease (SAD). (A) Chest radiograph and (B) MinIP CT chest show generalized hyperinflation in both lungs rather than mosaic attenuation pattern. (C) Atelectatic bands seen in right middle lobe and lingula (arrows).

■ CONCLUSION

Following the two-pattern approach in SAD helps in forming a differential diagnosis. In an appropriate clinical setting, it is even possible to make a single diagnosis.

■ REFERENCES

1. Pipavath SN, Stern EJ. Imaging of small airway disease (SAD). Radiol Clin North Am. 2009;47(2):307-16.
2. Jesenak M, Banovcin P, Jesenakova B, Babusikova E. Pulmonary manifestations of primary immunodeficiency disorders in children. Front Pediatr. 2014;2:77.
3. Edwards RM, Kicska G, Schmidt R, Pipavath SN. Imaging of small airways and emphysema. Clin Chest Med. 2015;36(2):335-47.
4. Burgel PR, Bergeron A, de Blic J, Bonniaud P, Bourdin A, Chanez P, et al. Small airways diseases, excluding asthma and COPD: an overview. Eur Respir Rev. 2013;22(128): 131-47.

SECTION 6

Vascular and Lymphatic Disorders

CHAPTER 18: Pulmonary Artery Imaging
CHAPTER 19: Pulmonary Veins Imaging
CHAPTER 20: Lymphatic Anomalies: Imaging and Interventions

CHAPTER 18

Pulmonary Artery Imaging

Sneha Goswami, Ashu Seith Bhalla

- ❑ Classification
- ❑ Imaging modalities
  - ➤ Chest radiograph
  - ➤ Echocardiography
  - ➤ CT pulmonary angiography
  - ➤ Magnetic resonance imaging
- ❑ Congenital anomalies
  - ➤ Proximal interruption of the pulmonary artery
  - ➤ Pulmonary artery sling
  - ➤ Idiopathic dilatation of the pulmonary trunk
  - ➤ Pulmonary stenosis
- ❑ Acquired abnormalities
  - ➤ Pulmonary artery hypertension
  - ➤ Pulmonary veno-occlusive disease/pulmonary capillary hemangiomatosis
  - ➤ Pulmonary artery aneurysms
  - ➤ Pulmonary arteriovenous malformation
  - ➤ Hepatopulmonary syndrome
  - ➤ Arteritis
  - ➤ Extrinsic obstruction
  - ➤ Pulmonary thromboembolism

■ INTRODUCTION

Pulmonary arteries (PAs) can be affected by several disorders congenital or acquired, involving the lungs or heart. Multimodality imaging including chest radiograph (CXR), echocardiography, and CT pulmonary angiography (CTPA) forms the cornerstone of diagnosis and follow-up.

■ CLASSIFICATION

Pulmonary artery abnormalities can be classified into congenital and acquired. A broad classification is given in **Table 1**.

SECTION 6: Vascular and Lymphatic Disorders

TABLE 1: Classification of pulmonary artery abnormalities.

Congenital	Acquired
Proximal interruption of PA (PIPA)	Pulmonary artery hypertension (PAH)
PA sling	PA aneurysm
Idiopathic dilation of pulmonary trunk	Pulmonary AVM
Pulmonary stenosis	Hepatopulmonary syndrome
Pulmonary atresia	Arteritis
Pulmonary hypoplasia	Mediastinal fibrosis
	Pulmonary thromboembolism (PTE)

(PA: pulmonary artery)

■ IMAGING MODALITIES

Chest Radiograph

As in other abnormalities, CXR is useful in directing further imaging and follow-up.

Echocardiography

- Vital imaging modality in PA abnormalities.
- PA anomalies are often associated with cardiac anomalies.
- Further, pulmonary artery hypertension (PAH) results in right ventricular strain.
- Complete discussion is beyond the scope of this chapter.

CT Pulmonary Angiography

- Computed tomography pulmonary angiography (CTPA) is the ideal imaging modality in evaluation of most PA abnormalities.
- The protocol used at our institute is given in **Box 1**.

BOX 1   **CTPA protocol.**[1]

- Nonelectrocardiographically gated
- *Injection rate*: 3–4 mL/s with a total contrast material volume of 1.5 mL/kg
- Performed caudocranially using bolus tracking, ROI placed over the right atrium set to a 60-HU threshold
- Images are reconstructed with a 1-mm section thickness and 1-mm reconstruction interval
- Axial maximum intensity projection (MIP) and coronal reformatted MIP used for interpretation
- Dual-energy CT pulmonary angiography may be used in the setting of suspected thromboembolism

(CTPA: computed tomography pulmonary angiography; ROI: region of interest)

Magnetic Resonance Imaging
- Excellent visualization of intracardiac anomalies
- Accurate quantification of volumes and regional right ventricular function
- Provides both anatomical and physiological information

■ CONGENITAL ANOMALIES

For congenital anomalies such as pulmonary atresia, pulmonary hypoplasia; also see Chapter 6.

Proximal Interruption of the Pulmonary Artery
- Proximal interruption of the pulmonary artery (PIPA) is a rare congenital PA with an estimated incidence of approximately 1/200,000.[2,3] It was first described by Doring in 1914. The term "interruption" is preferred over "absence" as only the proximal part of either of the PAs is absent while intrapulmonary vasculature develops normally.[4] It may occur on either side, however, more commonly on the right side.
- *Clinical presentation* is variable with most common symptoms being dyspnea, chest pain, recurrent pulmonary infections, and hemoptysis in severe cases. On examination, reduced breath sounds on the affected side may be found.
- On a plain CXR, there is absence of the right or left PA at the level of hila and underdeveloped ipsilateral lung which manifests as volume loss. Thin reticular opacities may be seen at the periphery which are due to enlarged intercostal and transpleural arteries. Affected lung appears translucent due to oligemia with compensatory hyperinflated contralateral lung which may herniate to the opposite side.
- *CT angiography (CTA) or MR angiography (MRA)* are the preferred imaging modalities as they provide direct and excellent depiction of the vascular anatomy, simultaneous assessment of lung parenchyma and other associated cardiovascular anomalies.
- On *CT angiography*, there is absence or termination within 1 cm of origin of the mediastinal segment of the right or left PA beyond the expected main PA bifurcation while intrapulmonary vasculature on the affected side is normally visualized. There is associated hypertrophy of the systemic bronchial, internal mammary, intercostal, subdiaphragmatic, or coronary artery collaterals with Serrated thickening of the pleura and subpleural parenchymal bands **(Figs. 1A to E)**. Enlargement of the pulmonary trunk and artery on the unaffected side to a variable degree may be seen.

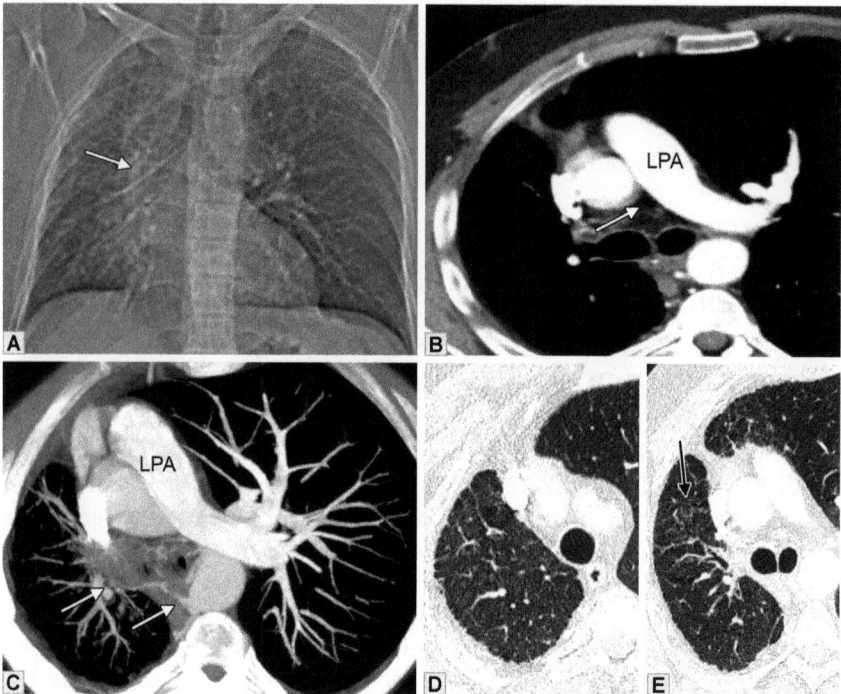

FIGS. 1A TO E: Proximal interruption of pulmonary artery (PIPA). (A) Small-volume right hemithorax with small right hilum. (B) Absent right pulmonary artery at the origin (arrow). (C) Multiple systemic collaterals (arrows). (D and E) Septal thickening secondary to collaterals (arrow).

(LPA: left pulmonary artery)

Pulmonary Artery Sling

- Pulmonary artery sling is a rare vascular anomaly which was first described by Contro et al. in 1958.[6] It is estimated to occur in approximately one in every 17,000 school-aged children, while there is currently no published data regarding its incidence and prevalence in infants.[7] This condition results from a failure of the proximal left sixth arch to properly involute during the development of the adult arterial pattern. As a result, an anastomotic vessel connecting the primitive pulmonary circulations becomes the anomalous left PA, which arises from the right PA. The left PA then travels above the main pulmonary bronchus to reach the left lung hilum by passing between the trachea and esophagus, often causing compression of these structures.[5,6]
- Pulmonary slings are classified into two main categories: (1) type I and (2) type II **(Flowchart 1)**. Type I malformations are less complex and are typically associated with tracheobronchomalacia. However, symptomatic cases can result in significant morbidity and mortality, and are often treated with left PA reimplantation surgery.

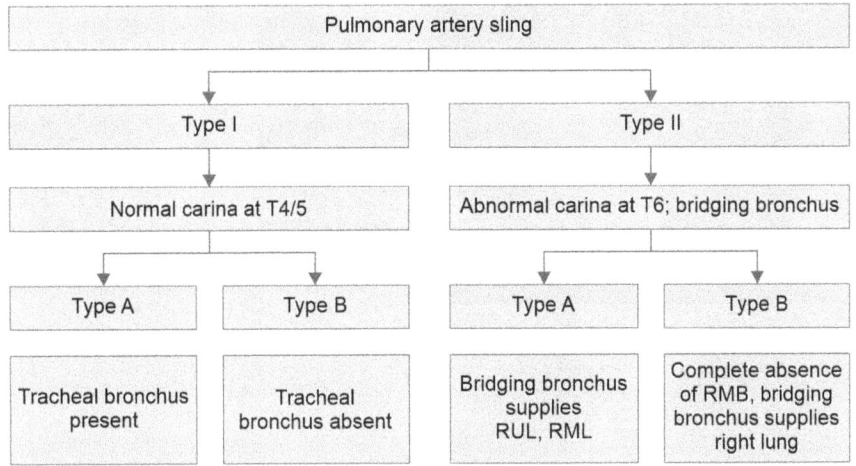

FLOWCHART 1: Classification of PA sling.
(PA: pulmonary artery; RMB: right main bronchus; RML: right middle lobe; RUL: right upper lobe)

- Type II slings refer to a rare congenital abnormality that affects the bronchial tree and PA. This condition is characterized by a hypoplastic lung and an abnormal bridging bronchus and a tracheal bifurcation at 6th thoracic vertebral level.
- Type II slings are frequently associated with other congenital cardiovascular and pulmonary abnormalities. Long-segment tracheal stenosis is also a common complication in type II. Managing this condition requires a multidisciplinary approach involving pediatric pulmonologists, cardiologists, and surgeons to address the various associated abnormalities. In type II, management needs to address not only the aberrant PA but also the airway abnormality.
- *Clinical presentation*: Most patients with PA sling present in early infancy with stridor and signs of respiratory distress. Other clinical manifestations include dysphagia due to compression of the esophagus, failure to thrive, and recurrent chest infections.[10] In some reports, PA sling remained asymptomatic until childhood. Some patients may complain of mild symptoms/signs and present in late childhood or adulthood with nonspecific respiratory symptoms such as chest pain, cough, orthopnea, and exertional symptoms.
- Chest X-ray findings may be nonspecific and can vary depending on the severity of the condition. In some cases, the chest X-ray may appear normal. However, other cases may show abnormal lung vascular markings where the affected lung may appear more opaque due to increased blood flow, abnormal mediastinal contour due to the abnormal location of the left PA, leftward deviation of the trachea due to the abnormal location of the left PA, and cardiomegaly in severe cases. However, these findings are not specific to PAS and may also be seen in other conditions affecting the lungs and heart.

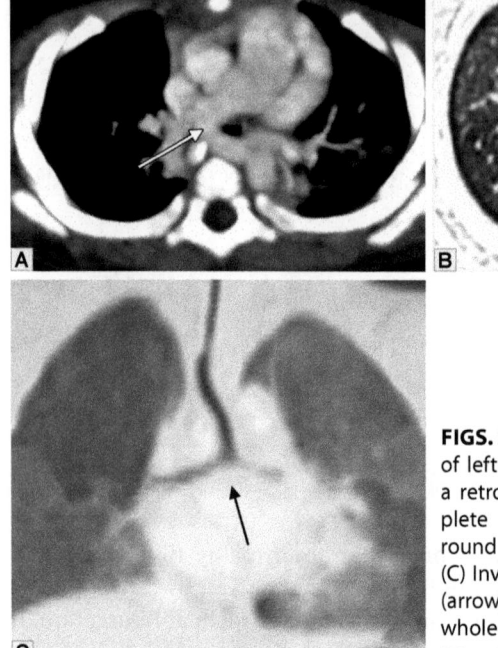
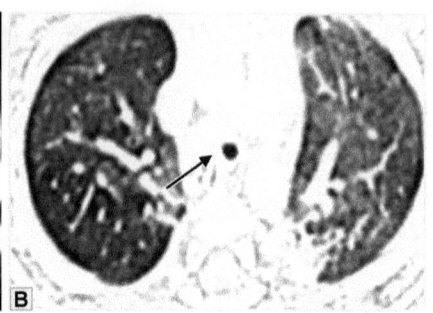

FIGS. 2A TO C: Type-IIB PA sling. (A) Origin of left PA from the right PA (arrow), having a retrotracheal course. (B) Congenital complete tracheal cartilage ring, seen as a round contour of tracheal lumen (arrow). (C) Inverted T-shaped carina at a lower level (arrow), bridging bronchus supplies the whole right lung.
(PA: pulmonary artery)

- On *CT angiography*, an anomalous left PA can be seen originating from the right PA coursing between the esophagus and the vertebral body, forming a vascular ring around the trachea and esophagus. Other findings are a narrowed and elongated trachea, compression of the left main bronchus, and a posterior and leftward deviation of the distal trachea and carina **(Figs. 2A to C)**. Other associated findings may include tracheal stenosis or atresia, bronchial stenosis, and bronchomalacia.

Idiopathic Dilatation of the Pulmonary Trunk

- This refers to a congenitally dilated pulmonary trunk with normal pressures in the absence of other cardiopulmonary disease. It results from an unequal division of the truncus arteriosus or congenital weakness of the arterial wall.
- Patients are usually asymptomatic, although close follow-up is recommended.
- Stable size across serial examinations has been proposed as a diagnostic criterion.
- On CXR, it is seen as a rounded bulge in the left mediastinal border. On CTPA, the pulmonary trunk is dilated.
- Surgical repair is indicated when diameter exceeds 60 mm.

Pulmonary Stenosis

- Pulmonary stenosis (PS) is mostly congenital.
- Mostly associated with congenital heart diseases (CHDs). Discussion of CHD is beyond the scope of this chapter.
- Valvular type is the most common, followed by subvalvular and supravalvular. PS results in restricted opening of leaflets during systole.
- Clinical presentation is variable and depends on the severity which is determined by pressure gradient across the valve. Milder forms may be asymptomatic, whereas severe forms can present with congestive heart failure.
- Imaging findings include thickened and immobile pulmonary valve leaflets, poststenotic dilatation of the pulmonary trunk and the left PA, right ventricular enlargement, and calcification of the valve.

ACQUIRED ABNORMALITIES

Acquired anomalies can be classified based on the PA caliber **(Table 2)**.

Pulmonary Artery Hypertension

- Normal PA pressure ≤25 mm Hg at rest
- Pulmonary hypertension (PAH) is relatively rare in the pediatric population but can be a significant cause of morbidity and mortality in affected individuals
- Adult treatment protocols, targeted to induce pulmonary arterial vasodilation and alleviate right ventricular (RV) pressure, are not necessarily used in pediatric patients because the distinct and diverse causes of pediatric pulmonary hypertension require a tailored approach.
- The 2009 Dana Point Classification at the Fourth World Symposium on Pulmonary Hypertension defined five categories of pulmonary hypertension that were subsequently adapted to comprehensively classify both adult and pediatric patients for the 2015 European Society of Cardiology (ESC) and European Respiratory Society (ERS) guidelines. There is considerable overlap in this classification.[7,8]

TABLE 2: Classification of acquired PA anomalies.

Increased arterial diameter	Reduced arterial diameter	Filling defects
Pulmonary artery hypertension	Takayasu arteritis	Pulmonary thromboembolism
PAVM	Bechet's disease	
PA aneurysm	Mediastinal fibrosis	

(PA: pulmonary artery; PAVM: pulmonary arteriovenous malformation)

Approach

- Echocardiography is the first imaging modality for PAH. The severity assessment of PAH on echocardiography is described in **Flowchart 2**.
- CT angiography might also demonstrate several of these findings, including right atrial and right ventricular enlargement, flattening/bowing of the interventricular septum, and inferior vena cava (IVC) enlargement.
- Main PA and branch PA size are best assessed for enlargement on CT angiography by normalizing measurements to the child's body surface area rather than comparing to the ascending aorta, which could be abnormally small or large in a child with congenital heart disease **(Fig. 3)**.

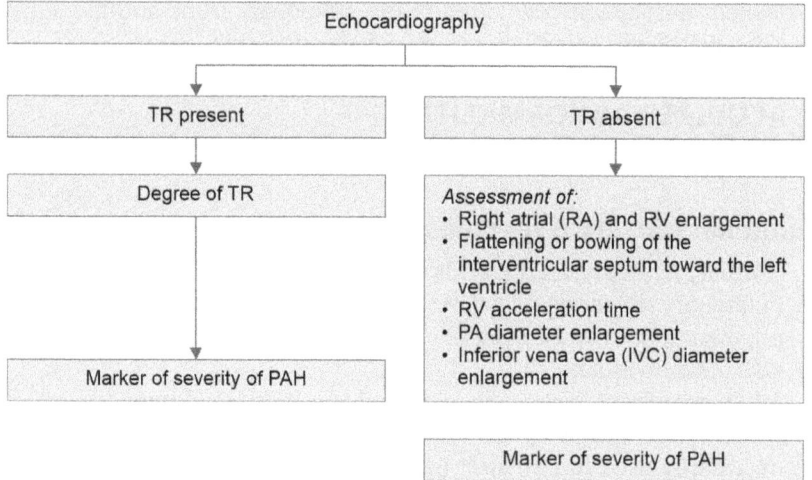

FLOWCHART 2: Approach to diagnosis and severity assessment in pulmonary artery hypertension.
(PAH: pulmonary artery hypertension; TR: tricuspid regurgitation)

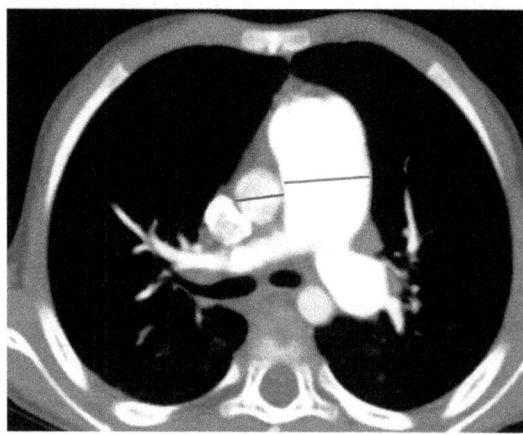

FIG. 3: Pulmonary artery to aorta ratio. Measurement of pulmonary artery (red line), taking ascending aorta (blue line) as internal reference.

- CT angiography is superior to echocardiography for assessing the pulmonary arterial tree and is particularly useful for assessing central and peripheral pulmonary arterial stenoses from heritable arteriopathies such as Williams, Alagille, and Noonan syndromes.

Cause Evaluation
- 57% of pediatric PAH are characterized as idiopathic or hereditary.[10]
- Bone morphogenetic protein receptor type II (BMPR2) mutations are a predominant cause of familial pulmonary hypertension.[11] The BMPR2 gene codes for a transforming growth factor-beta (TGF-β) receptor. When the receptor is defective, apoptosis of endothelial cells and proliferation of smooth muscle cells are increased, causing plexiform lesions in the lungs. In severe pulmonary hypertension, these plexiform lesions might appear at arterial branch points or at the origins of supernumerary arteries. The typical pattern of plexiform lesions on CT is a central enhancing nodule with surrounding ground-glass opacity, although this pattern is not pathognomonic for a BMPR mutation **(Figs. 4A and B)**.
- Other causes are listed in **Box 2**.

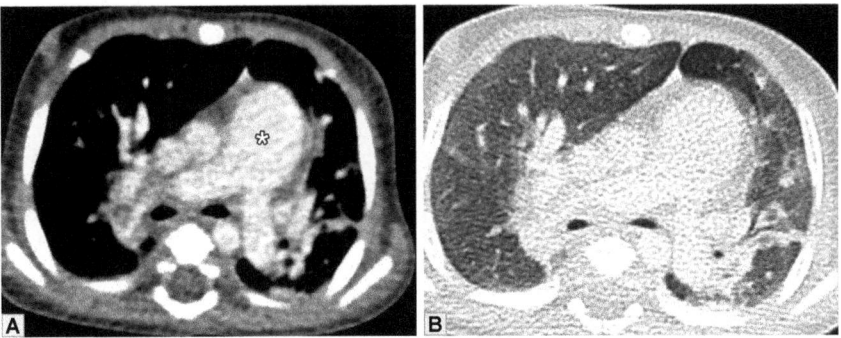

FIGS. 4A AND B: Pulmonary artery hypertension secondary to VSD. (A) Dilated main pulmonary artery (asterisk). (B) Plexiform appearance of the intrapulmonary arteries with surrounding GGO.

BOX 2	Causes of PAH in children.

- Hereditary hemorrhagic telangiectasia (HHT)
- T-box factor 4 (TBX4) mutation
- PVOD/PCH
- Acquired pulmonary hypertension secondary to congenital heart disease
- Portopulmonary hypertension and hepatopulmonary syndrome
- Chronic pulmonary thromboembolism

(PAH: pulmonary artery hypertension; PCH: pulmonary capillary hemangiomatosis; PVOD: pulmonary veno-occlusive disease)

Pulmonary Veno-occlusive Disease/Pulmonary Capillary Hemangiomatosis

- Pulmonary veno-occlusive disease (PVOD) and pulmonary capillary hemangiomatosis (PCH) are two uncommon causes of postcapillary PA hypertension.[9]
- In PVOD, there is occlusion of the venules, which in turn leads to dilation of the capillaries, lymphatics, and results in interlobular septal thickening.
- In PCH, there are discrete areas of capillary proliferation without lymphatic of venular changes.
- Both lead to unexplained PAH, which does not respond to vasodilators. On administration of vasodilators, pulmonary edema can precipitate.
- On high-resolution computed tomography (HRCT), PVOD presents with smooth interlobular septal thickening, with ground-glass opacities.
- PCH shows evidence of ground-glass nodules, without any septal thickening **(Figs. 5A to C)**.

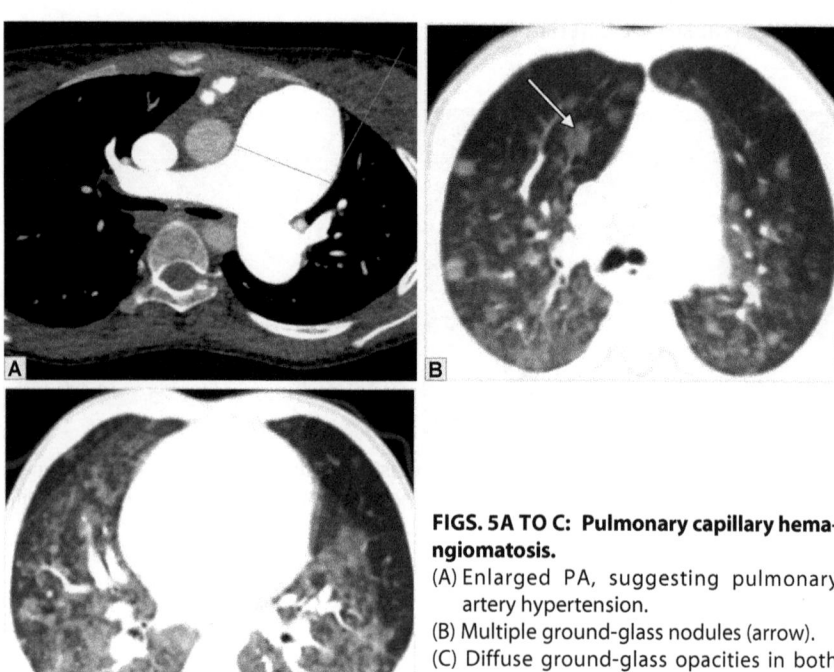

FIGS. 5A TO C: Pulmonary capillary hemangiomatosis.
(A) Enlarged PA, suggesting pulmonary artery hypertension.
(B) Multiple ground-glass nodules (arrow).
(C) Diffuse ground-glass opacities in both lower lobes.
(PA: pulmonary artery)

Pulmonary Artery Aneurysms

- The PA aneurysms can be congenital (associated with congenital heart diseases) or acquired. Causes of acquired aneurysms include trauma, infection, vascular abnormality (Marfan's, Ehler Danlos, Behcet's, Takayasu, and cystic medial necrosis) and PAH.
- Mostly these are clinically asymptomatic and incidentally detected. Sometimes, they might present with hemoptysis.
- On CXR, they might present as hilar enlargement/focal mass that remains stable or increases with size in serial scans.
- Computed tomography pulmonary angiography is the ideal imaging modality. PA aneurysms are seen as saccular or fusiform areas of dilation, and show homogeneous contrast filling, simultaneous with PA **(Figs. 6A to C)**.
- Early diagnosis is crucial, as a ruptured aneurysm has a mortality close to 100%.

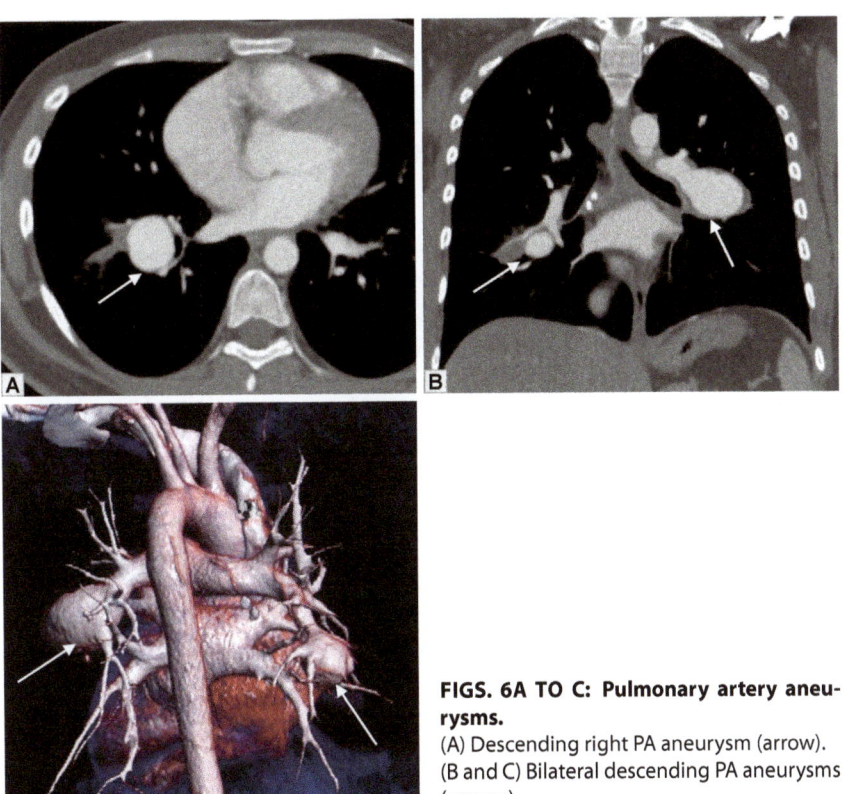

FIGS. 6A TO C: Pulmonary artery aneurysms.
(A) Descending right PA aneurysm (arrow).
(B and C) Bilateral descending PA aneurysms (arrows).
(PA: pulmonary artery)

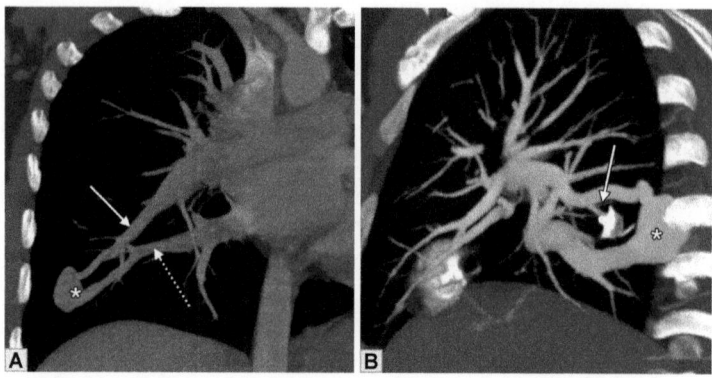

FIGS. 7A AND B: Pulmonary AVM (PAVM). (A) Simple PAVM: one arterial feeder (arrow) and one venous drainage (dotted arrow); Nidus (n). (B) Complex PAVM: Multiple arterial feeders, of which one occluded by Amplatzer device (arrow).
(PAVM: pulmonary arteriovenous malformation)

Pulmonary Arteriovenous Malformation

- Abnormal direct communication between PA and vein.
- Can be either congenital (most common) or acquired.
- May be associated with hereditary hemorrhagic telangiectasia (35%).
- Clinical features include left to right shunt (hemoptysis and paradoxical embolus).
- Can be morphologically classified into simple, complex, and diffuse **(Figs. 7A and B)**:
  - *Simple*: Consists of one arterial feeder and one draining vein.
  - *Complex*: Consists of multiple arterial feeders.
  - *Diffuse*: One lung segment or lobe affected.

Hepatopulmonary Syndrome

- Chronic liver dysfunction associated with pulmonary manifestations due to alterations in the production or clearance of circulating cytokines and other mediators.[10]
- Hypoxemia due to pulmonary vasodilatation with significant arteriovenous shunting and ventilation-perfusion mismatch.
- Clinically presents with dyspnea and platypnea.
- CT imaging findings include pulmonary vasodilation in the peripheral subpleural lung regions **(Figs. 8A to C)**.

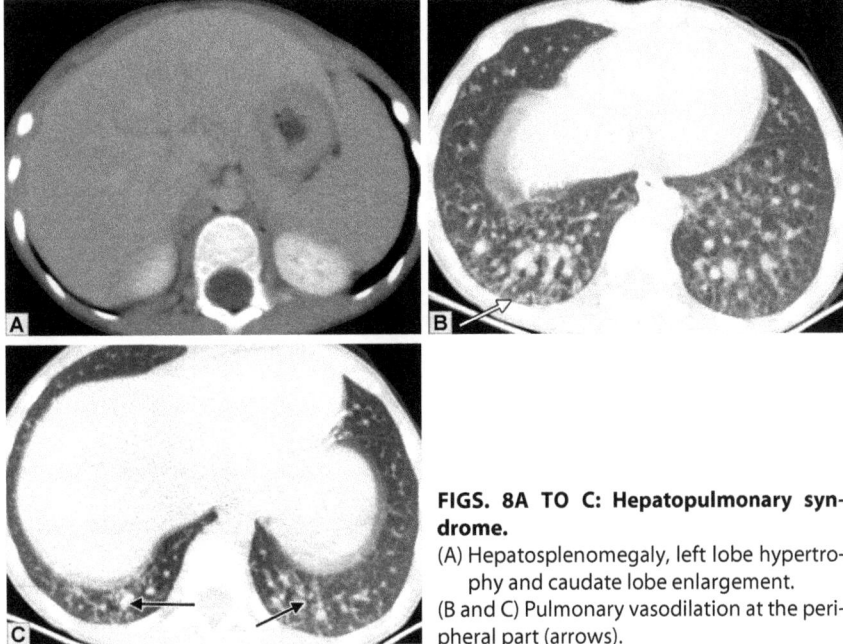

FIGS. 8A TO C: Hepatopulmonary syndrome.
(A) Hepatosplenomegaly, left lobe hypertrophy and caudate lobe enlargement.
(B and C) Pulmonary vasodilation at the peripheral part (arrows).

Arteritis

Takayasu's Arteritis

- This is an idiopathic arteritis affecting the large-vessel (elastic) arteries; wherein, the aorta and its major branches are commonly affected.
- Pulmonary artery involvement is seen in 50–80% patients, and might be in the form of stenosis or occlusion **(Figs. 9A and B)**. Segmental or subsegmental branches are more frequently affected than lobar or main arteries.
- CT angiography can show both luminal and mural changes in the form of arterial wall thickening. In the early phase, wall thickening and enhancement can be expected. Later, mural calcification of occlusion may be seen.

Bechet's Disease

- This is an idiopathic chronic inflammatory disease presenting with recurrent oral and genital ulcers, uveitis, and vascular manifestations in pulmonary and nonpulmonary systems.
- PA aneurysms are commoner, seen in 65% cases, followed by occlusion (35%).
- The PA aneurysms in Bechet's disease can be either single or multiple, preferentially affect central PAs and pertain a poor prognosis **(Figs. 10A and B)**.
- On CT, mural thrombus is frequently observed.

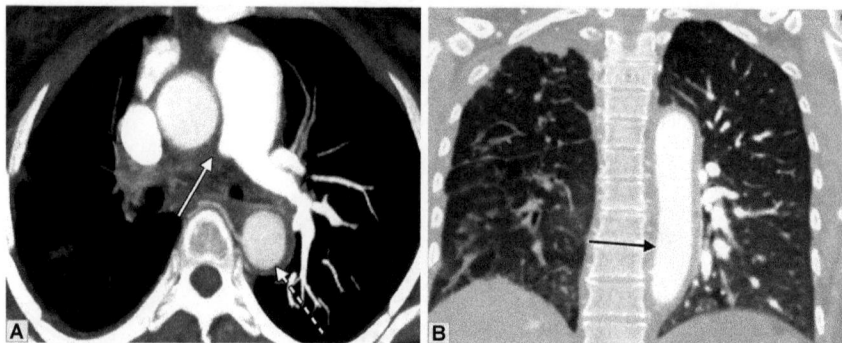

FIGS. 9A AND B: Takayasu's arteritis. (A) Occlusion of right pulmonary artery (arrow), descending thoracic aorta wall thickening (dotted arrow). (B) Wall thickening of the descending thoracic aorta (arrow).

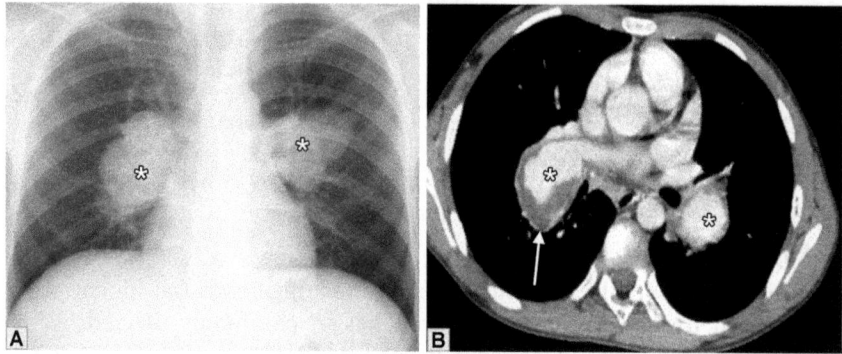

FIGS. 10A AND B: Bechet's disease. (A) Bilateral lobulated hilar masses (asterisks). (B) Aneurysms of RPA and LPA (asterisks), eccentric thrombus in RPA aneurysm (arrow).
(LPA: left pulmonary artery; RPA: right pulmonary artery)

Extrinsic Obstruction

Extrinsic obstruction can be caused by nodes, masses, or mediastinal fibrosis **(Figs. 11A to C)**.

Pulmonary Thromboembolism

- Uncommon in children
- Risk factors include hypercoagulable states, indwelling central venous catheters, infections, inflammatory and autoimmune disorders, and antiphospholipid antibody syndrome **(Figs. 12A to C)**.
- Imaging findings of acute and chronic pulmonary thromboembolism (PTE) are listed in **Table 3**.
- Chronic PTE can result in pulmonary hypertension (CTEPH).

CHAPTER 18: Pulmonary Artery Imaging

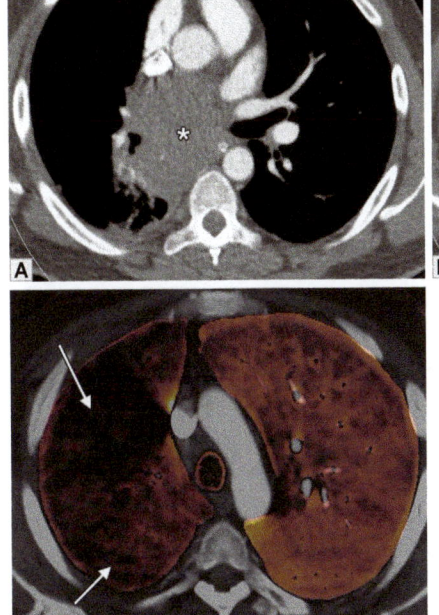
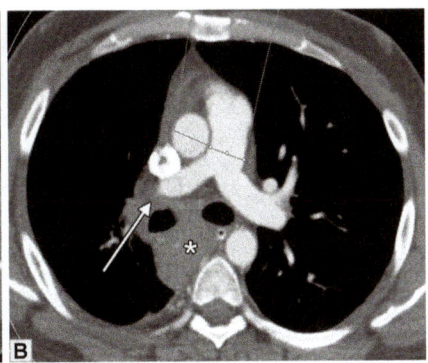
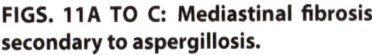

FIGS. 11A TO C: Mediastinal fibrosis secondary to aspergillosis.
(A) Multicompartmental mediastinal soft tissue (asterisk).
(B) Right PA narrowing (arrow).
(C) Reduced perfusion in right lung on iodine map images (arrows).

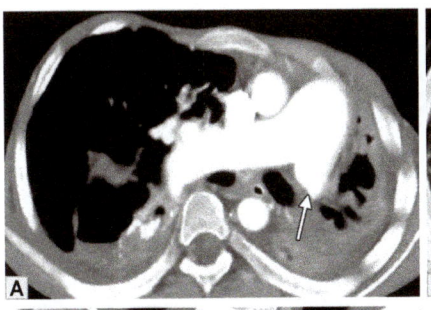
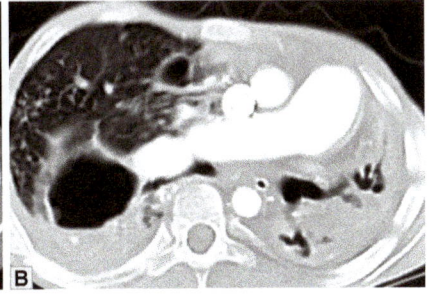
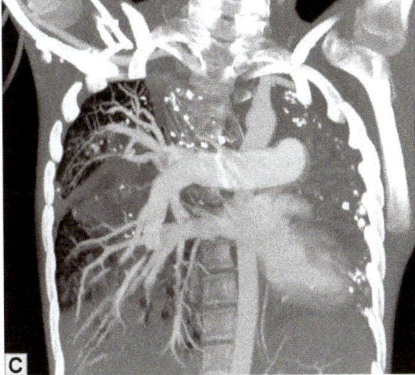

FIGS. 12A TO C: Acute pulmonary arterial thrombus in tuberculosis. (A) Abrupt occlusion of left pulmonary artery (arrow). (B) Left upper lobe bronchiectasis and right upper lobe cavity. (C) Parenchymal calcification in left lung, volume loss and non-visualized intrapulmonary branches of left pulmonary artery.

TABLE 3: Imaging findings in acute and chronic PTE.	
Acute PTE	**Chronic PTE**
• Filling defect within artery • Perfusion defect on dual-energy iodine map images • Right ventricular strain (displaced interventricular septum to the left)	• Pruning of peripheral vessels • Eccentric filling defect within artery • Linear central filling defect within artery • Focal eccentric thickening of arterial wall • Perfusion defect on dual-energy iodine map images
(PTE: pulmonary thromboembolism)	

CONCLUSION

Standardized CT scan acquisition is key to a comprehensive report, as suboptimal CTPAs are common and often result in missed information.

REFERENCES

1. Bhalla AS, Das A, Naranje P, Irodi A, Raj V, Goyal A. Imaging protocols for CT chest: A recommendation. Indian J Radiol Imaging. 2019;29(3):236-46.
2. Williams EA, Cox C, Chung JH, Grage RA, Rojas CA. Proximal interruption of the pulmonary artery. J Thorac Imaging. 2019;34(1):56-64.
3. Aypak C, Yıkılkan H, Uysal Z, Görpelioğlu S. Unilateral absence of the pulmonary artery incidentally found in adulthood. Case Rep Med. 2012;2012:942074.
4. Kieffer SA, Amplatz K, Anderson RC, Lillehei CW. Proximal interruption of a pulmonary artery. Am J Roentgenol Radium Ther Nucl Med. 1965;95(3):592-7.
5. Newman B, Cho Y Ah. Left pulmonary artery sling—anatomy and imaging. Semin Ultrasound CT MR. 2010;31(2):158-70.
6. Wells TR, Gwinn JL, Landing BH, Stanley P. Reconsideration of the anatomy of sling left pulmonary artery: the association of one form with bridging bronchus and imperforate anus. Anatomic and diagnostic aspects. J Pediatr Surg. 1988;23(10):892-8.
7. Galiè N, Humbert M, Vachiery JL, Gibbs S, Lang I, Torbicki A, et al. ESC/ERS guidelines for the diagnosis and treatment of pulmonary hypertension: the joint task force for the diagnosis and treatment of pulmonary hypertension of the European Society of Cardiology (ESC) and the European Respiratory Society (ERS). Eur Heart J. 2015;37: 67-119.
8. Hansmann G, Apitz C. Treatment of children with pulmonary hypertension. Expert consensus statement on the diagnosis and treatment of paediatric pulmonary hypertension. The European Paediatric Pulmonary Vascular Disease Network, endorsed by ISHLT and DGPK. Heart. 2016;102:ii67-ii85.
9. Woerner C, Cutz E, Yoo SJ, Grasemann H, Humpl T. Pulmonary veno-occlusive disease in childhood. Chest. 2014;146:167-74.
10. Machicao VI, Fallon MB. Hepatopulmonary syndrome. Semin Respir Crit Care Med. 2012;33:11-6.
11. Newman B, Feinstein JA, Cohen RA, Feingold B, Kreutzer J, Patel H, et al. Congenital extrahepatic portosystemic shunt associated with heterotaxy and polysplenia. Pediatr Radiol. 2010;40:1222-30.

CHAPTER 19

Pulmonary Veins Imaging

Manisha Jana, Ashu Seith Bhalla

- ❑ Normal anatomy
- ❑ Disorders of pulmonary veins
- ❑ Classification based on morphological changes
- ❑ Classification based on etiology
- ❑ Congenital pulmonary vein anomalies
  - ➢ Anomalous venous connections
  - ➢ Total anomalous pulmonary venous connections
  - ➢ Partial anomalous pulmonary venous connection
  - ➢ Pulmonary vein atresia
- ➢ Pulmonary vein stenosis
- ➢ Pulmonary varix
- ➢ Meandering pulmonary vein
- ➢ Pulmonary arteriovenous malformations
- ❑ Acquired pulmonary vein anomalies
  - ➢ Pulmonary vein obstructive syndrome
  - ➢ Pulmonary artery hypertension

■ INTRODUCTION

- Pulmonary veins (PVs) can be involved in a myriad of abnormalities, both congenital and acquired. These abnormalities are often overlooked on routine computed tomography (CT) reporting, and hence, these disorders remain under-diagnosed.
- Further, in case of absence of obstruction, collateral pathways are limited; and result in left-to-right shunting.
- Computed tomography angiography (CTA) is the modality of choice for evaluating PVs.

■ NORMAL ANATOMY

The typical arrangement encountered in the majority of people (>60%) comprises four PVs which drain into the left atrium. These are right upper pulmonary veins (PUPV), right lower pulmonary veins (RUPV), left upper pulmonary veins (LUPV), and left lower pulmonary veins (LLPV) **(Figs. 1A to C)**.

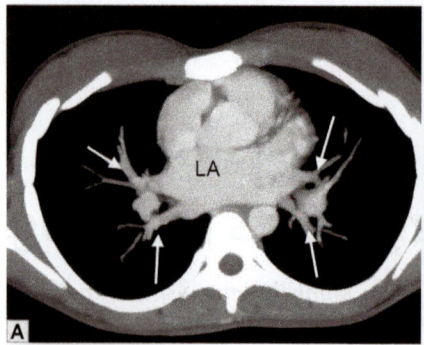
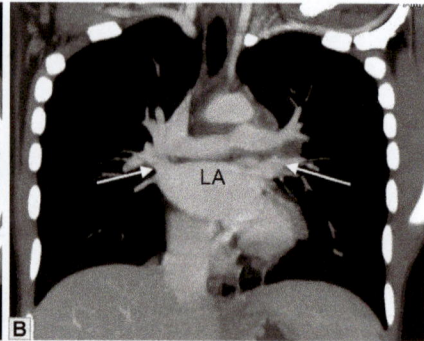
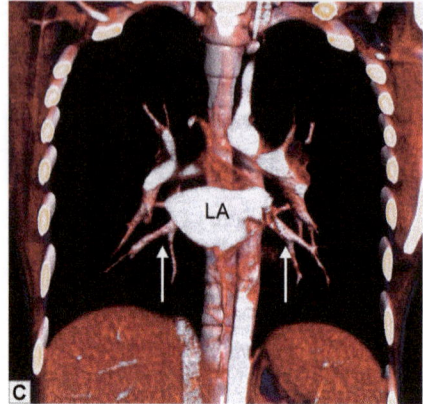

FIGS. 1A TO C: Normal pulmonary vein anatomy. (A) Axial and (B) coronal maximum intensity projection (MIP), (C) coronal thin VR images.
Normal inferior pulmonary veins (arrows in A and C).
Normal superior pulmonary veins (arrows in B).
(LA: left atrium)

DISORDERS OF PULMONARY VEINS

Disorders of PVs can result in either absence or narrowing, dilatation, or anomalous connections. Etiology wise, these can be either congenital or acquired.[1-4] The more frequently encountered entities are being discussed below.

CLASSIFICATION BASED ON MORPHOLOGICAL CHANGES

These can be classified into three broad groups—(1) narrowing/absence, (2) dilation, and (3) anomalous connections **(Table 1)**.

TABLE 1: Morphology-based classification of pulmonary vein (PV) anomalies.		
Narrowing/absence	Dilation	Anomalous connection/course
PV atresia	PV varix	PAPVC
PV stenosis	Arteriovenous malformation (AVM)	TAPVC
Pulmonary vein obstructive syndrome		Meandering pulmonary vein
(PAPVC: partial anomalous pulmonary venous connection; TAPVC: total anomalous pulmonary venous connection)		

TABLE 2: Etiology-based classification of pulmonary vein anomalies.	
Congenital	Acquired
Total anomalous pulmonary venous connection (TAPVC)	Meandering pulmonary vein
Partial anomalous pulmonary venous connection (PAPVC)	Pulmonary hypertension due to pulmonary vein causes
Cor triatriatum	
Pulmonary vein atresia	
Pulmonary vein stenosis	
Pulmonary varix	
Meandering pulmonary vein	

CLASSIFICATION BASED ON ETIOLOGY

These are listed in **Table 2**.

CONGENITAL PULMONARY VEIN ANOMALIES

Anomalous Venous Connections

- Anomalous venous connections vary from complex cardiac malformation [total anomalous pulmonary venous connection (TAPVC)] to a meandering PV.
- Complete discussion of the cardiac anomaly is beyond the scope of the chapter, which focuses on those connections which can be even diagnosed on nongated CTA/contrast-enhanced CT (CECT) in patients presenting with respiratory symptoms.

Total Anomalous Pulmonary Venous Connections

- TAPVC is a cardiac anomaly wherein the PVs do not have a normal drainage into LA, and instead drain elsewhere into the systemic vasculature.
- This results in a left-to-right shunt, to compensate which there is presence of an intracardiac right-to-left shunt.
- The major subtypes are briefly mentioned in **Table 3**. Further discussion of this condition is beyond the scope of this chapter.

TABLE 3: Subtypes of total anomalous pulmonary venous connections.		
Type	Name	Drainage
1	Supracardiac	Systemic vessel above heart
2	Cardiac	Right heart (through coronary sinus)
3	Infracardiac	Systemic vessel below heart/portal vein
4	Mixed	Combination

Partial Anomalous Pulmonary Venous Connection

- Similar to TAPVC, partial anomalous pulmonary venous connection (PAPVC) refers to anomalous PV drainage resulting in a left-to-right shunt.
- PAPVC can result in pulmonary artery hypertension (PAH). Several of these patients are however asymptomatic, and the condition remains underdiagnosed on imaging too. Symptoms also depend on associated cardiac anomalies.
- The drainage pattern depends on the affected PV **(Flowchart 1; Figs. 2 and 3)**.
- Some of the specific entities are discussed in detail.

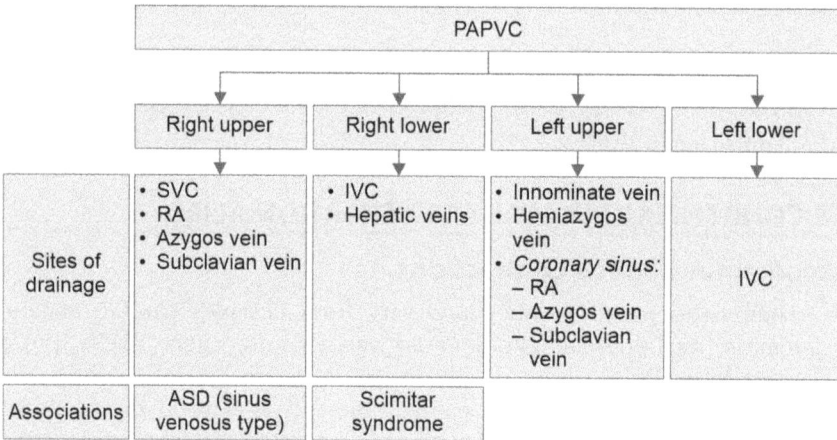

FLOWCHART 1: Types of PAPVC.
(ASD: atrial septal defect; IVC: inferior vena cava; PAPVC: partial anomalous pulmonary venous connection; RA: right atrium; SVC: superior vena cava)

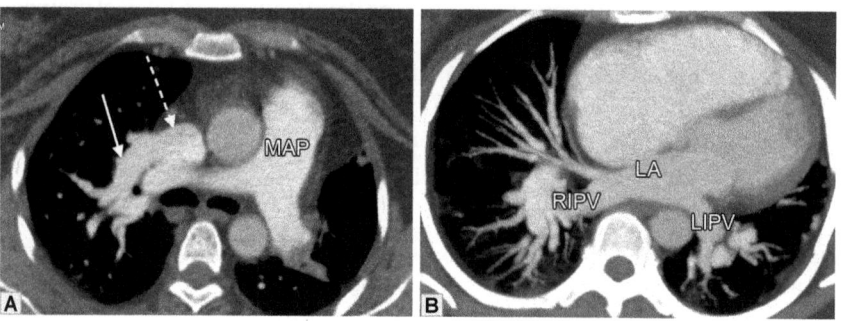

FIGS. 2A TO C: *Continued*

Continued

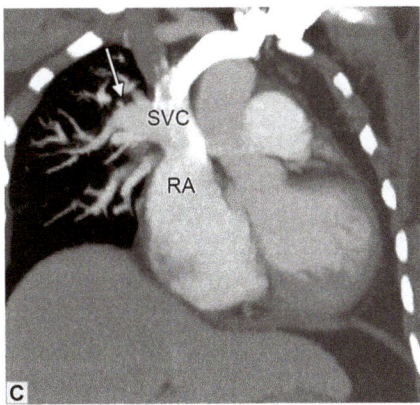

FIGS. 2A TO C: Right upper lobe PAPVC: (A) axial mediastinal window, (B) axial maximum intensity projection (MIP), and (C) coronal MPR images—RUPV (arrow) draining to SVC (dotted arrow in A) and normal RIPV and LIPV draining to LA.

(LA: left atrium; LIPV: left inferior pulmonary vein; MPR: multiplanar reformation; PAPVC: partial anomalous pulmonary venous connection; RIPV: right inferior pulmonary vein; RUPV: right inferior pulmonary vein; SVC: superior vena cava)

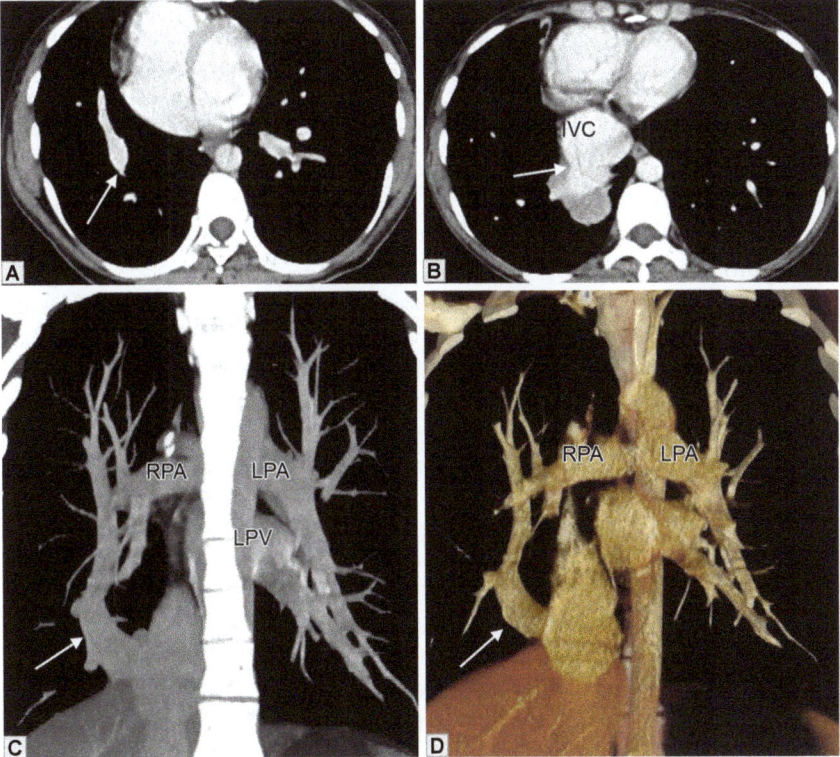

FIGS. 3A TO D: Right infrahepatic PAPVC. (A and B) axial soft tissue window, (C) coronal MIP, and (D) VR images. Anomalous vein draining right lung, draining into IVC (arrows). Note normal RPA, LPA, and LPV.

(LPA: left pulmonary artery; LPV: left pulmonary vein; RPA: right pulmonary artery)

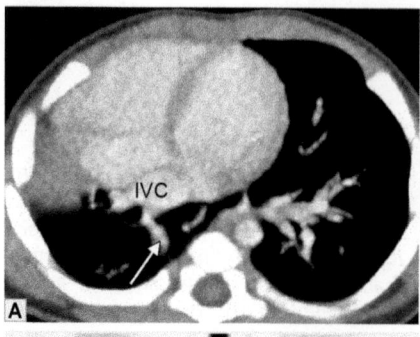
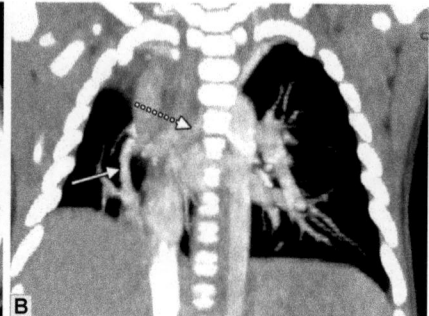
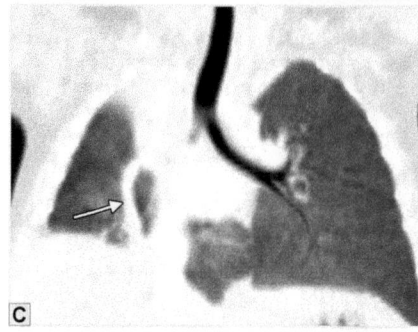

FIGS. 4A TO C: Scimitar syndrome. (A) axial soft tissue window, (B) coronal MIP, (C) coronal MinIP images. A curvilinear lower lobe pulmonary vein "scimitar vein" (arrow) draining into IVC; small right pulmonary artery (dotted arrow in B); and small right lung and right main bronchus (C).

(MinIP: minimum intensity projection; MIP: maximum intensity projection)

Scimitar Syndrome

- *Synonym*: Hypogenetic lung syndrome and congenital venolobar syndrome.
- This syndrome refers to the combination of right lower PAPVC with pulmonary hypoplasia.
- The anomalous vein draining the right lung (or sometimes right middle and lower lobe) resembles a Turkish sword (scimitar) as it comes down to drain into inferior vena cava (IVC)/hepatic veins **(Figs. 4A to C)**.
- Associated pulmonary, diaphragm, and cardiac anomalies are also reported.
- *Differential diagnosis*: Meandering vein.

Left Upper PAPVC

- In this subtype, there is an anomalous ventral vein which courses in the prevascular space and drains into the innominate vein **(Figs. 5A to D)**.
- Differential diagnosis is a left-sided SVC, which drains into the coronary sinus and often the innominate vein is absent or hypoplastic **(Figs. 6A to C)**.

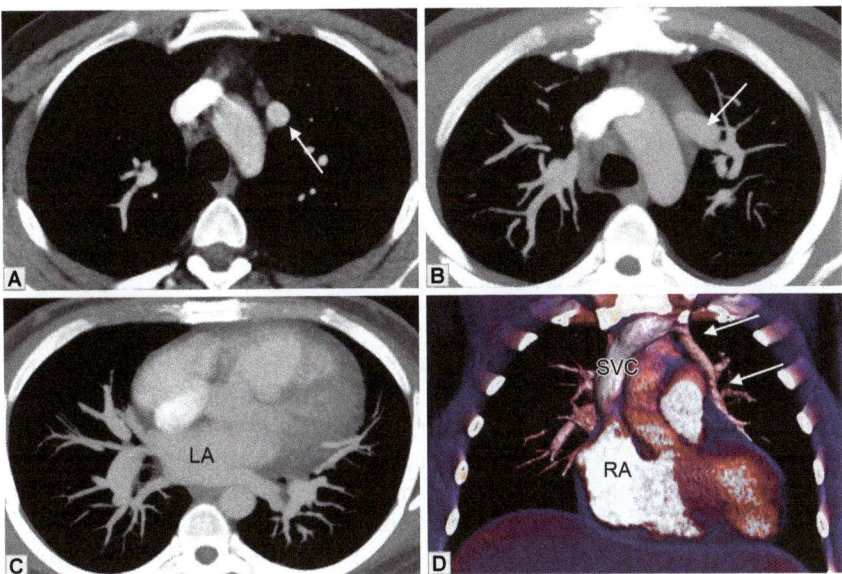

FIGS. 5A TO D: Left upper lobe PAPVC: (A) axial soft tissue window, (B and C) axial MIP, and (D) coronal thin VR images. A contrast filled structure in the prevascular space (arrow in A). Drainage of LUPV into the venous structure/vertical vein (arrows in B and D). LIPV drains normally into the LA.

(LA: left atrium; LIPV: left inferior pulmonary vein; LUPV: left upper pulmonary vein; MIP: maximum intensity projection; PAPVC: partial anomalous pulmonary venous connection)

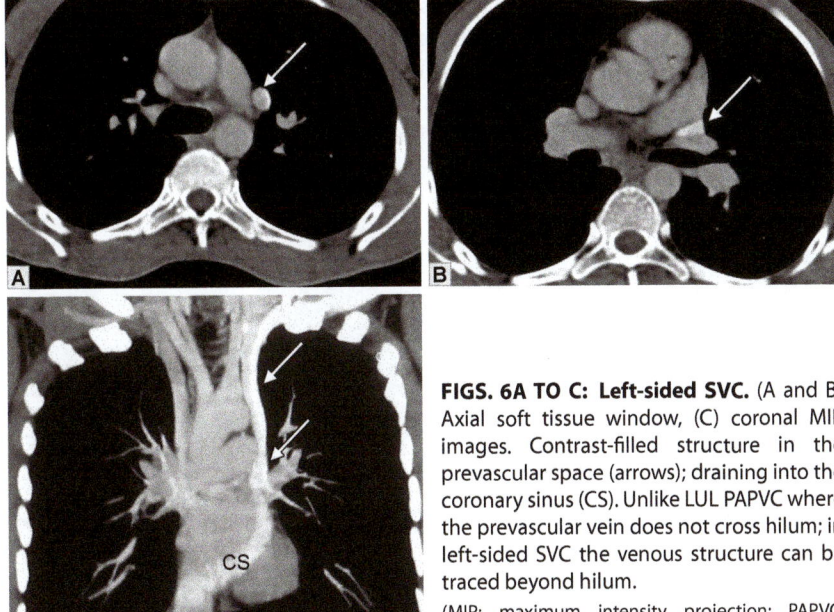

FIGS. 6A TO C: Left-sided SVC. (A and B) Axial soft tissue window, (C) coronal MIP images. Contrast-filled structure in the prevascular space (arrows); draining into the coronary sinus (CS). Unlike LUL PAPVC where the prevascular vein does not cross hilum; in left-sided SVC the venous structure can be traced beyond hilum.

(MIP: maximum intensity projection; PAPVC: partial anomalous pulmonary venous connection; SVC: superior vena cava)

TABLE 4: Causes of abnormal vessels in prevascular space.	
Anomaly	**Drainage**
Left upper PAPVC with vertical veins	Vertical vein drains to innominate vein
Persistent vertical vein	Similar course but normal PV
Persistent left SVC	Drains to coronary sinus
Venovenous collaterals	In case of SVC obstruction often drain into azygos/hemiazygos vein

Persistent Vertical Vein

- A persistent vertical vein may be seen even in absence of PAPVC (normal PV drainage).
- This occurs in several cardiac anomalies such as left heart hypoplasia.
- In these situations, this vein serves as an additional channel for decompression of pulmonary venous siphon.
- It connects the pulmonary and systemic venous returns.

Differentials of anomalous vessel in prevascular/preaortic space are listed in **Table 4**.

Pulmonary Vein Atresia

- PV atresia is mostly congenital and occurs as a consequence of non-fusion of the common PV with the left atrium during development **(Figs. 7A to D)**. There is however no persistent systemic venous connection (unlike anomalous venous connections).
- PV atresia can be of these subtypes **(Table 5)**.
- CTA in all cases of atresia will demonstrate changes of venous edema, with the distribution depending on the involved vessels.
- The findings include septal thickening with ground-glass opacities (GGO) with or without pleural effusion **(Figs. 8A to C)**.

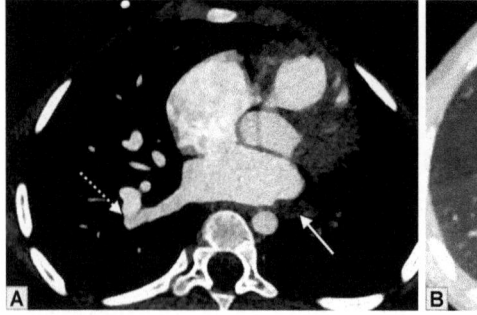
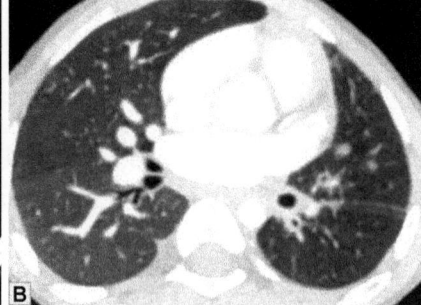

FIGS. 7A TO D: *Continued*

Continued

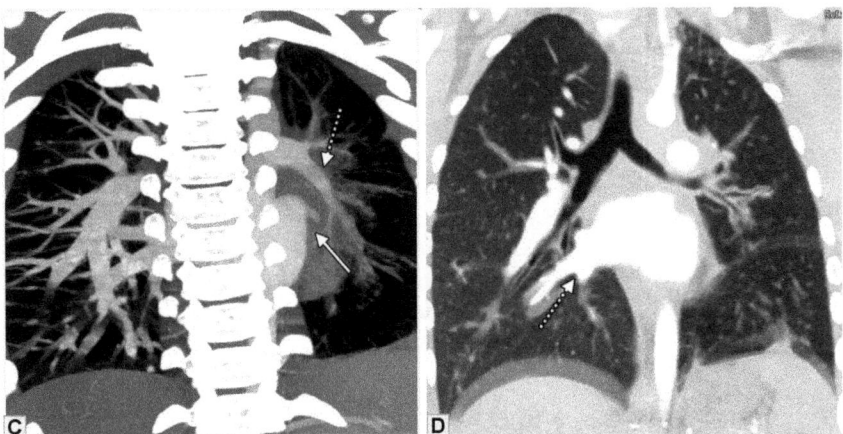

FIGS. 7A TO D: Complete pulmonary vein atresia in pulmonary hypoplasia: (A) axial MIP, (B) axial lung window, (C) coronal MIP, and (D) coronal lung window images. Small volume left lung, with less vascularity; Absence of all pulmonary veins on left side, smooth convex outline of left atrium (arrow); and normal RIPV (dotted arrow).
(MIP: maximum intensity projection; RIPV: right inferior pulmonary vein)

TABLE 5: Subtypes of PV atresia.			
	Common	**Unilateral**	**Individual**
Extent	All PVs involved	All PVs of one lung	Individual PV, rare
Time of presentation	Soon after birth (<48 h)	Childhood	Late childhood/ adulthood
Clinical presentation	Cyanosis, metabolic acidosis, and poor systemic perfusion	Hemoptysis, recurrent pulmonary infections, and PAH	• Often asymptomatic • Similar to unilateral
CTA	• Pulmonary edema • CPV confluence separate from LA	• Long segment unilateral PV atresia • No LA outpouching (no ostia) • Pulmonary hypoplasia • Small PA • Hilar mass • Soft tissue*	Variable changes depending on PV involved
Management	• Difficult • High mortality • Depending on gap between CPV confluence and LA • ECMO for stabilizing	• Mostly conservative • Persistent symptoms—pneumonectomy	Conservative

*Represents dilated lymphatics or venous channels.
(CTA: CT angiography; CPV: common pulmonary vein; ECMO: extracorporeal membrane oxygenation; LA: left atrium; PV: pulmonary veins; PA: pulmonary artery)

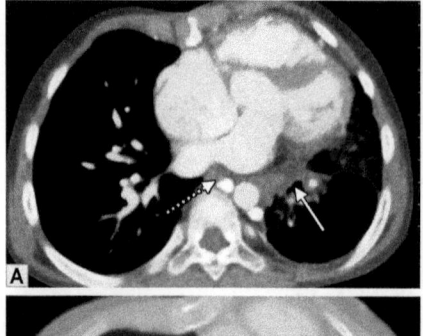
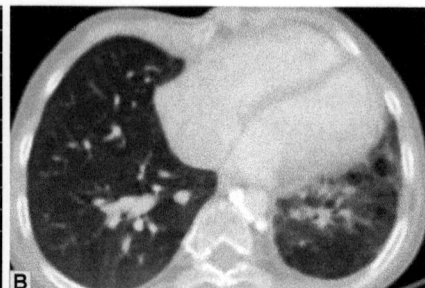
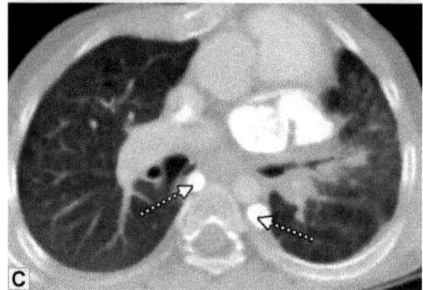

FIGS. 8A TO C: Left lower pulmonary vein (LLPV) atresia. (A) Axial soft tissue window and (B and C) axial lung window images. Nonvisualized left lower lobe pulmonary veins, smooth convex outline of left atrium (arrow). Septal thickening of left lower lobe (B) and prominent azygous venous system (dotted arrows in A and C) as a collateral venous drainage pathway. Note the left hilar hypodense soft tissue.

Pulmonary Vein Stenosis

- Pulmonary vein stenosis is different from atresia in that the development and connection with LA is normal, but narrowing is present/develops overtime.
- It may be primary or secondary to cardiac surgery (postrepair PV stenosis).
- The "primary" form is no longer referred to as "congenital" as it is seen to be progressive.
- Severity and timing of presentation are variable depending on the cause and number of veins involved, with several patients being asymptomatic or having minor symptoms.
- Similar to venous atresia, patients can have tachypnea, recurrent infections or hemoptysis, and PAH.
- On CTA, the extent of stenosis varies from short segment to long segment to diffuse narrowing. There are no standard normal PV diameters below while a vessel is labeled as stenosed.
- Management is endovascular (angioplasty or stenting) and surgical depending on extent of stenosis. Restenosis and progression are frequent, with poor long-term outcomes.

Pulmonary Varix

- Pulmonary varix refers to abnormal dilatation of a PV.
- Causes include congenital or acquired.

- The most common cause of an acquired varix is elevated left atrial pressure resulting in pulmonary venous hypertension (e.g., mitral stenosis/regurgitation). These are reversible if the primary etiology is corrected. Acquired varix can also be post-traumatic.
- These are often asymptomatic. Rarely, these present with rupture, recurrent infections, or result in emboli.
- Several conditions which give an appearance of a dilated pulmonary vessel need to be differentiated from each other on CTA.
- Unlike varices, pulmonary arteriovenous malformations (PAVMs) have an abnormally dilated feeding artery also. PAVMs are more symptomatic and need to be evaluated.
- Pulmonary varices on the other hand are not associated with any AV shunting, and show persistent enhancement on a later phase.

Differentials of dilated pulmonary vessels on CTA include:
- Pulmonary varix
- Pulmonary AVM
- PAPVC
- Anomalous single pulmonary artery
- Pulmonary vein thrombosis
- Bronchial varix

Meandering Pulmonary Vein

- Meandering PV refers to a vein which has an abnormal curved course but drains normally into the atrium **(Figs. 9A to C)**.
- It is more frequent on right side.
- Associated systemic supply to the affected lung is also reported.
- *Differential diagnosis*: Scimitar syndrome.

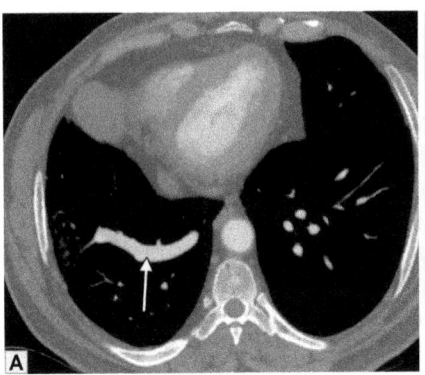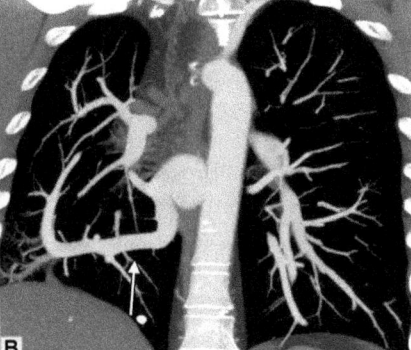

FIGS. 9A TO C: *Continued*

Continued

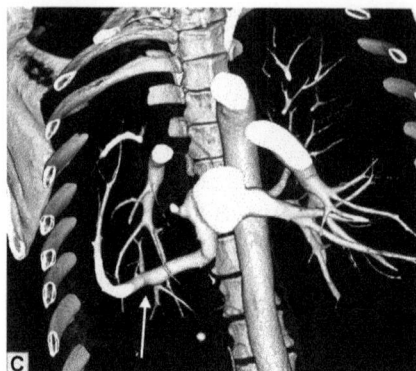

FIGS. 9A TO C: Meandering pulmonary vein:
(A) axial MIP,
(B) coronal MIP, and (C) coronal thin VR images. An elongated tortuous right lower pulmonary vein (arrows), draining normally into the LA.
(LA: left atrium; MIP: maximum intensity projection; VR: virtual reality)

Pulmonary Arteriovenous Malformations

Pulmonary arteriovenous malformations result in dilatation of the draining veins. These are discussed under the pulmonary arterial disorders section.

■ ACQUIRED PULMONARY VEIN ANOMALIES

Pulmonary Vein Obstructive Syndrome

- Pulmonary vein obstructive syndrome (PVOS) refers to narrowing or obstruction of PVs occurring as a result of external compression or mural inflammation.
- CTA reveals compression or narrowing or intraluminal filling defects with nonopacification of the affected PV.
- The affected pulmonary lobe shows changes of venous edema in the form of smooth interlobular septal thickening **(Figs. 10A to D)**.

The causes encountered in children include:[5,6]

- *Infections*: Contiguous spread of infection from lung can result in thrombosis and narrowing. This situation can be challenging to differentiate from venous stenosis/atresia. Only the presence of consolidation, often necrotizing encasing the PV aids in the distinction.
- Mediastinal fibrosis, occurring as a result of conglomerate tubercular nodes or immunoglobulin G4 (IgG4)-related disease can also result in compression as well as infiltration and resultant thrombosis of affected PV.
- Malignant masses including nodal, e.g., lymphoma causing extrinsic compression.
- PVOD

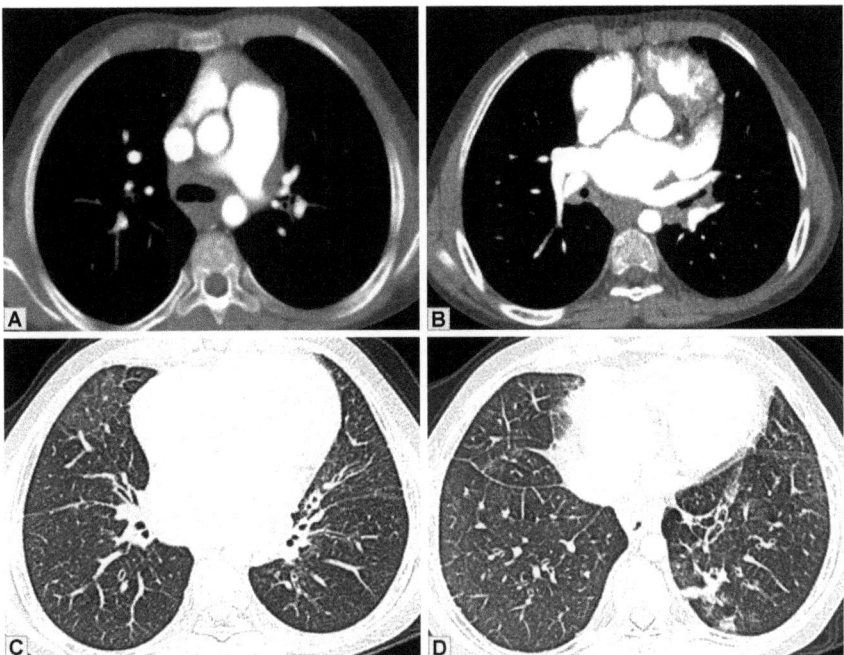

FIGS. 10A TO D: Pulmonary veno-occlusive disease (PVOD). (A) Dilated main pulmonary artery, (B) Normal pulmonary veins. (C and D) Smooth septal thickening and dependent consolidation in left lung lower lobe.

Pulmonary Artery Hypertension

One cause of PAH can be pulmonary venous disorders. A good quality CTA performed for PAH should look for these specifically, because if missed, it is a potential cause of erroneous labelling of PAH as idiopathic. PV disorders which can result in PAH include OV narrowing/stenosis, PAPVC, PAVM, small vessel disorders, and PVOD.

CONCLUSION

Pulmonary vein anomalies in children can be seen as isolated abnormality; or associated with other cardiopulmonary conditions. Meticulous reporting of all the venous drainage can avoid misinterpretation.

Other Related Chapters that can be Referred to:
- Chapter 6: Congenital Lung Abnormalities
- Chapter 18: Pulmonary Artery Imaging
- Chapter 27: Hemoptysis: Imaging and Interventions

REFERENCES

1. Romberg EK, Stanescu AL, Bhutta ST, Otto RK, Ferguson MR. Computed tomography of pulmonary veins: review of congenital and acquired pathologies. Pediatr Radiol. 2022;52:2510-28.
2. Abdel Razek AAK, Al-Marsafawy H, Elmansy M, El-Latif MA, Sobh D. Computed tomography angiography and magnetic resonance angiography of congenital anomalies of pulmonary veins. J Comput Assist Tomogr. 2019;43(3):399-405.
3. Pandey NN, Sharma A, Jagia P. Imaging of anomalous pulmonary venous connections by multidetector CT angiography using third-generation dual source CT scanner. Br J Radiol. 2018;91(1092):20180298.
4. Türkvatan A, Güzeltaş A, Tola HT, Ergül Y. multidetector computed tomographic angiography imaging of congenital pulmonary venous anomalies: A pictorial review. Can Assoc Radiol J. 2017;68(1):66-76.
5. Saad EB, Marrouche NF, Saad CP, Ha E, Bash D, White RD, Rhodes J, et al. Pulmonary vein stenosis after catheter ablation of atrial fibrillation: emergence of a new clinical syndrome. Ann Intern Med. 2003;138: 634-8.
6. Liaw CC, Chang H, Yang TS, Wen MS. Pulmonary venous obstruction in cancer patients. J Oncol. 2015;2015:210916.

CHAPTER 20

Lymphatic Anomalies: Imaging and Interventions

Ishan Gupta, Priyanka Naranje

- ❏ Normal anatomy
  - ➢ Right lymphatic duct
  - ➢ Thoracic duct
- ❏ Imaging
  - ➢ Magnetic resonance lymphangiography
  - ➢ Intranodal conventional lymphangiography
  - ➢ Lymphatic vessel disorders
- ❏ Management in lymphatic malformations in chest
  - ➢ Complex lymphatic malformations: Role of interventional radiology
  - ➢ Simple lymphatic malformations: Role of sclerotherapy
  - ➢ Medical management
  - ➢ Surgery

■ INTRODUCTION

- The lymphatic system is a part of the circulatory system, which fulfills multiple functions by carrying excess fluids and proteins from interstitium back to circulatory system through veins. It also removes debris from tissues, and performs the important function of transporting fat from the intestines. The basic outline of lymphatic system is illustrated in **Figure 1**.
- It comprises peripheral fine lymphatic ducts which are interspersed in the capillaries which form larger ducts which drain into the central veins. The intervening organs such as lymph nodes, spleen, and thymus that mount a response to the pathogens detected.
- This chapter discusses imaging of the lymphatic vessels as relevant to thoracic disorders and not the lymphoid organs (nodes, spleen, thymus, and bone marrow).

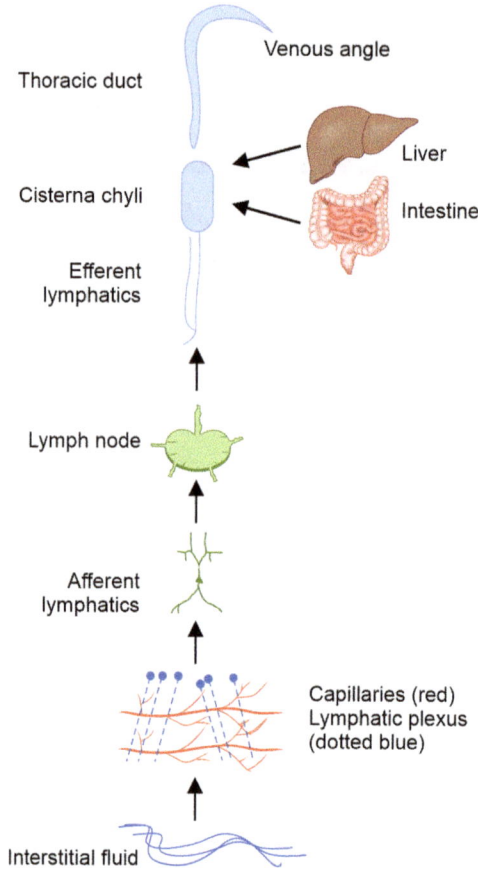

FIG. 1: The normal anatomy of the lymphatic system.

■ NORMAL ANATOMY

Lymphatic vessels comprise three levels:
1. Lymphatic capillaries form a fine network which is located in the interstitium.
2. Collecting vessels which carry lymph from the capillaries through lymph nodes (afferent and efferent).
3. *Lymphatic ducts*: The two large lymphatic ducts, thoracic duct and right lymphatic duct which open into the venous system. A diagrammatic representation of lymphatic ducts and their drainage is shown in **Figure 2**.

Lymphatics can also be considered as peripheral or central. Central conducting lymphatics (CCLs) comprise thoracic duct, cisterna chyli, and retroperitoneal lymphatics, and imaging of these is most relevant to thoracic disorders and is discussed further.

CHAPTER 20: Lymphatic Anomalies: Imaging and Interventions

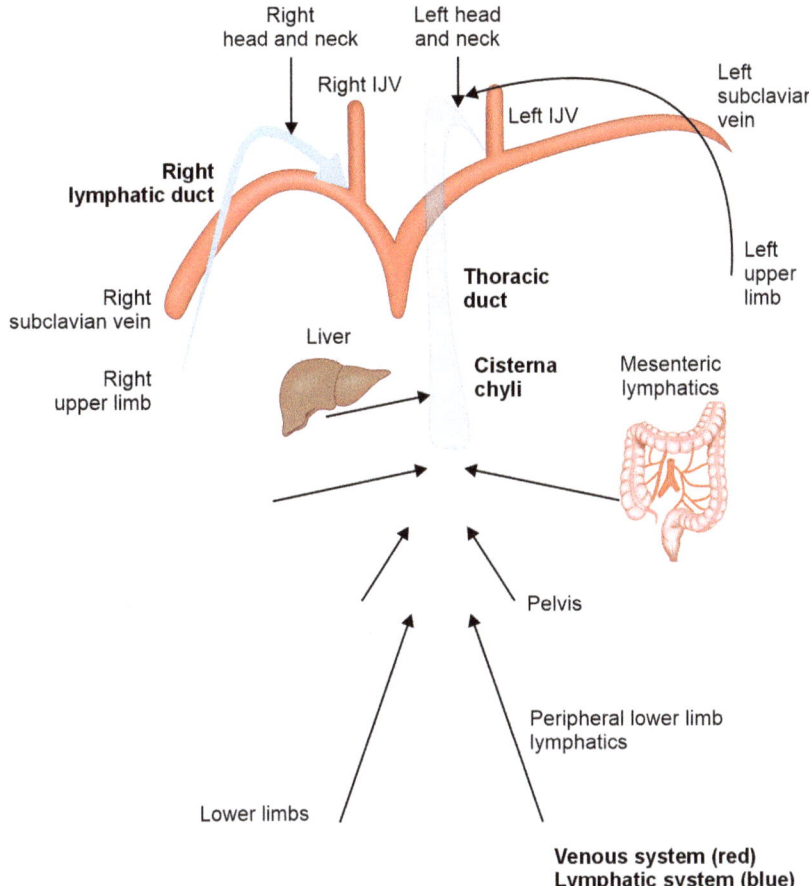

FIG. 2: Lymphatic ducts and their drainage into venous system.
(IJV: internal jugular vein)

Right Lymphatic Duct

It is a short channel which opens at the junction of right internal jugular vein and subclavian vein. It drains right head and neck, right upper limb, and right side of chest including lung and part of heart.

Thoracic Duct

- It is a long channel which opens at the junction of left internal jugular vein and subclavian vein (venous angle). It drains rest of the body which includes lower limbs, liver, intestine, left upper limb, left side of chest, and left head and neck.
- The anatomy of the cisterna chyli and thoracic duct is variable in different individuals based on different embryological development. Cisterna chyli can appear as a single straight tube-like structure, short sausage shaped,

V- or Y-shaped structure, or sometimes cannot be identified and replaced by a focal lymphatic plexus. Similarly, thoracic duct can also show a variable anatomy and diameter, can appear tortuous or beaded, can be interrupted or discontinuous at places and sometimes appear as more than a single lymphatic trunk in the thorax.

IMAGING

- Imaging of central lymphatic ducts is challenging, especially in children. Traditional direct lymphangiography involved injection of ethiodized oil-based contrast into the peripheral lymphatics of the feet through the web spaces. Similarly, lymphoscintigraphy techniques used injection of radiotracer agents into the web spaces of hand and feet and imaging the peripheral lymphatics.
- However, these techniques are technically challenging and time-consuming and are inadequate for the visualization of central lymphatics which include retroperitoneal lymphatics, cisterna chyli, and thoracic duct and associated abnormalities, and do not provide optimal diagnostic quality anatomic details and resolution.
- Recently, noncontrast and dynamic contrast-enhanced magnetic resonance (MR) techniques have been developed for imaging the central lymphatics and we focus on these techniques further.

Magnetic Resonance Lymphangiography

Position, Anesthesia, and Hardware

Magnetic resonance imaging can be done on 1.5 or 3T imaging systems (3T systems have the advantage of better signal and thus provide better anatomic details) and depending upon the age of the child can be performed under local or general anesthesia. MR imaging is done in supine position and anatomic coverage is from lesser trochanter to the level of mid neck to cover from the level of inguinal nodes up to the level of drainage of thoracic duct into venous angle.[1]

Technique

The two components of MR lymphangiography are noncontrast MR lymphangiography (T2W imaging) and dynamic postcontrast MR lymphangiography (postcontrast dynamic T1W imaging). The sequences used in MR lymphangiography are shown in **Table 1**.[1]

Noncontrast MR lymphangiography: The commonly used sequences are:
- T2W [echo time (TE) 80–100 ms] (with or without fat suppression) for an overall evaluation of anatomy and for gross abnormalities such as pleural effusions, ascites, and large lymphatic anomalies.
- Heavily T2W 3D sequences [e.g., MR cholangiopancreatography (MRCP)] (TE 700–800 ms) for visualization of smaller lymphatic channels.

CHAPTER 20: Lymphatic Anomalies: Imaging and Interventions

TABLE 1: MR lymphangiography protocol sequences.

Sequences	Acquisition plane	TR	TE	Matrix	Slice thickness (mm)	Pixel band width	Flip angle (degrees)	NSA	Time (approximately)
T2W	Axial	1,000	80	268 × 189	4	672	90	1	4 minutes
Heavily T2W 3D sequence (MRCP)	Coronal	1,315	650	404 × 324	2 (1-mm voxel recon)	399	90	1	5 minutes
HASTE SPAIR	Coronal	961	80	300 × 223	5	641	90	2	1 minute 30 seconds
STIR	Coronal	1,391/140 (TI)	60	264 × 236	5	673	180	2	2 minutes
STIR	Axial	1,491/140 (TI)	60	208 × 200	4	641	180	3	6 minutes
mDIXON T1W pre- and postgad	Coronal	5.9	1.8/4	236 × 199	5 (2.5-mm voxel recon)	543	15	1	11 seconds

(3D: three-dimensional; FSE: fast spin-echo; HASTE: half-fourier single-shot turbo spin echo; MRCP: MR cholangiopancreatography; NSA: number of signal averages; TE: echo time; TR: repetition time; SPAIR: spectral attenuated inversion recovery; STIR: short tau inversion recovery; T2W: T2 weighted; TR: repetition time)

- Single-shot fast spin echo (FSE) T2W sequences [e.g., half-Fourier turbo spin echo (HASTE)] (intermediate TE 160 ms) with fat suppression and/or short-tau inversion recovery (STIR) to evaluate thoracic duct and cisterna chyli and smaller lymphatics which are difficult to evaluate with heavily T2W sequences.

Dynamic contrast material-enhanced MR lymphangiography (DCE MR Lymphangiography): T1W 3D gradient echo (GRE) sequences with fat suppression [e.g., volumetric interpolated breath-hold examination (VIBE), modified Dixon (mDIXON) T1W turbo field echo (TFE)] are acquired in coronal plane. After that cannulation of inguinal nodes is done, followed by intranodal contrast injection.

Technique of intranodal contrast injection:
- After prior assessment of bilateral inguinal regions for suitable sized nodes, inguinal regions are sterile prepared and draped. The inguinal node is accessed under ultrasonography (USG) guidance with a thin 22–25-G needle and the tip of the needle is positioned within the central part of node. A 21-inch long tubing with a 3-way stopcock can be connected to the needle to provide stability. Saline injection under USG guidance can be used to confirm needle tip position as with injection, the node increases in diameter and no perinodal leak should be demonstrated **(Figs. 3A and B)**. Following needle placement, dilute gadolinium (1:1–1:2 dilution) can be injected with a dose of 0.1 mmol/kg body weight. Bilateral nodes are injected, and the total volume of contrast divided.
- After injection of contrast into the inguinal lymph node, T1W 3D sequences are again acquired in the coronal plane every 30 seconds until the contrast reaches the thoracic duct drainage site into the venous angle of neck. Axial images can be acquired if necessary. Maximum intensity projection (MIP) reformation can be done to better evaluate the small lymphatic ducts **(Figs. 4 and 5)**.

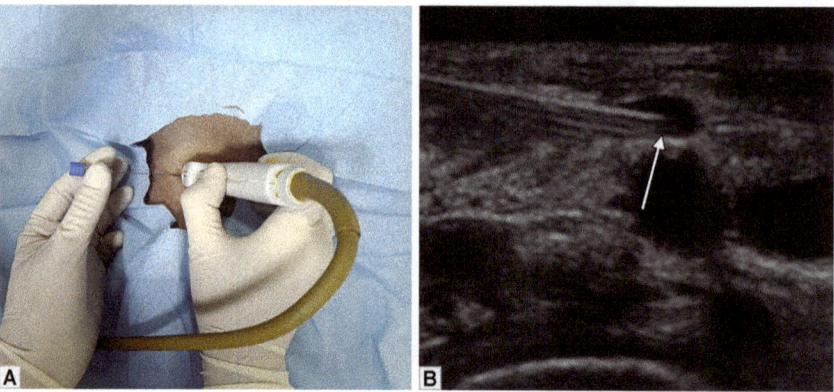

FIGS. 3A AND B: Groin lymph node cannulation for magnetic resonance (MR) lymphangiography. (A) sterile-draped groin region with 23-G needle used to access lymph node under USG guidance and (B) longitudinal ultrasound (US) images of the groin shows needle tip in situ within the lymph node (arrow).

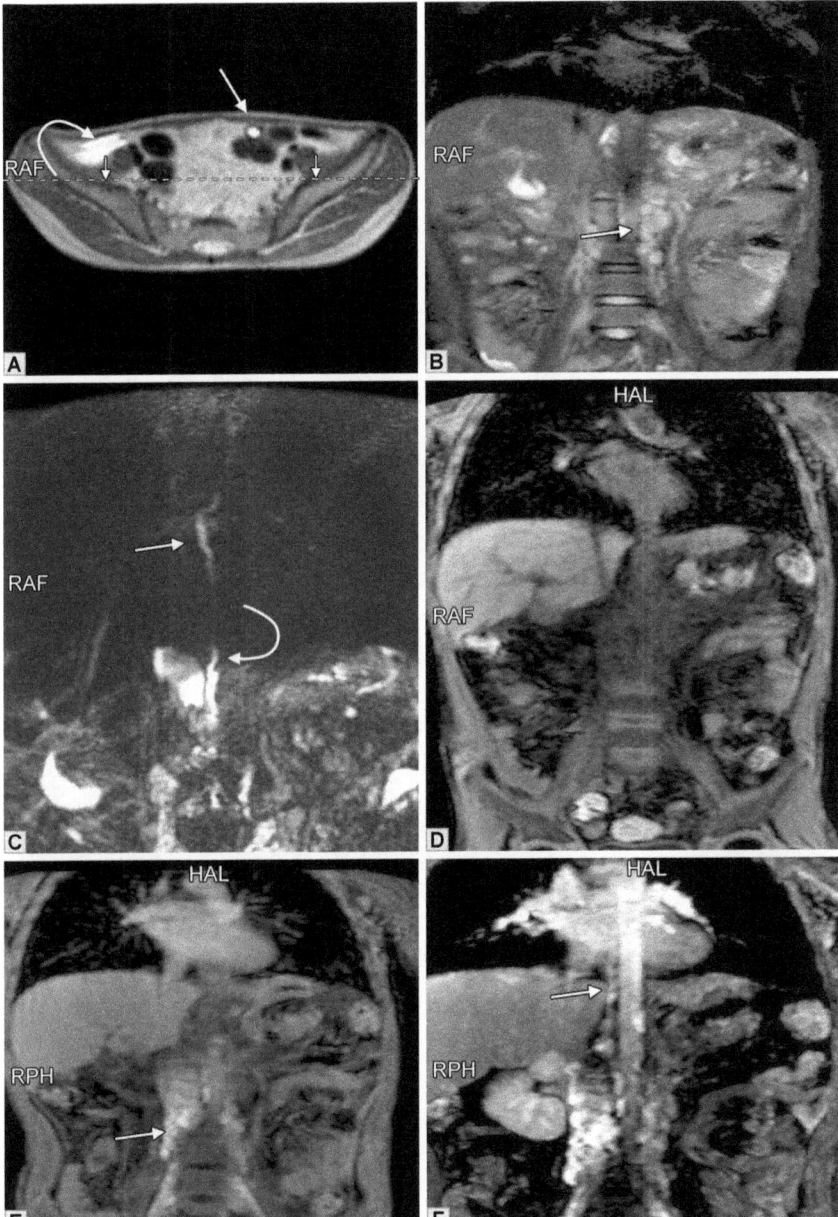

FIGS. 4A TO F: DCE-MRI in a 10-year-old male child with chylous ascites. (A) T2W axial image showing ascites (curved arrow) and a drainage tube (arrow) in situ. (B) Coronal STIR image showing few retroperitoneal nodes (arrow). (C) 3D MRCP cor image showing normal caliber thoracic duct (arrow) and cisterna chyli (curved arrow). Coronal precontrast (D) and dynamic postcontrast MR images (E and F) showing contrast opacification of retroperitoneal lymphatic channels (arrow in E) and proximal thoracic duct (arrow in F). No active contrast leak was identified on DCE-MRI.

(DCE-MRI: dynamic contrast-enhanced magnetic resonance imaging; MRCP: magnetic resonance cholangiopancreatography; STIR: short-tau inversion recovery)

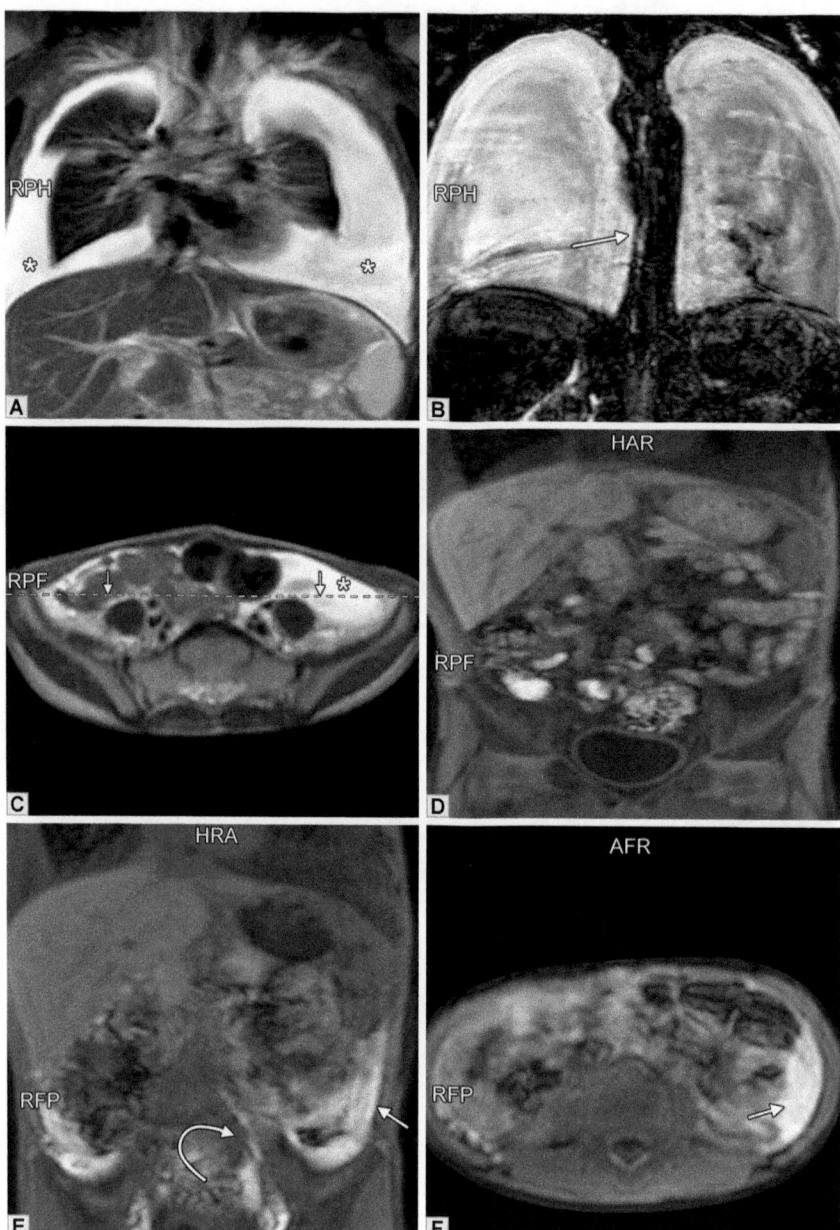

FIGS. 5A TO F: DCE-MRI in an 8-year-old male child with chylous effusion and ascites.
(A) Coronal STIR image showing bilateral pleural effusion (asterisks). (B) 3D MRCP cor image showing normal caliber thoracic duct (arrow). (C) T2W axial image at the level of lower abdomen showing ascites (asterisk). Coronal precontrast (D) and dynamic postcontrast MR images, coronal (E) and axial (F) showing contrast opacification of retroperitoneal lymphatic channels (curved arrow in E) and postcontrast enhancement of ascites (arrow in E and F) suggestive of lymphatic leak.

(DCE-MRI: dynamic contrast-enhanced magnetic resonance imaging; MRCP: magnetic resonance cholangiopancreatography; STIR: short-tau inversion recovery)

Intranodal Conventional Lymphangiography
- In this technique, oil-based contrast material (lipiodol) is injected into the inguinal nodes and imaging is performed under fluoroscopic guidance. It also serves as an important step prior to lymphatic embolization procedures. Imaging can be performed under local or general anesthesia.
- Technique of accessing the inguinal nodes is similar as with contrast-enhanced MR lymphangiography. The inguinal nodes are accessed with 22-25-G thin needle under USG guidance followed by saline injection to confirm the position of the needle tip within the node. After needle tip placement, lipiodol is slowly administered through handheld injections using a 1-3 mL syringe. Single or video fluoroscopic or digital subtraction angiography (DSA) clips are recorded at different intervals till the central lymphatic channels of interest are visualized and anatomic abnormality adequately demonstrated. The maximum lipiodol dose injected should not exceed 0.25 mL/kg.

Lymphatic Vessel Disorders
Following clinical manifestations/disorders have overlapping features and are discussed below:
- Pulmonary lymphatic perfusion syndrome (PLPS)
- Plastic bronchitis
- Chylothorax
- Neonatal lymphatic flow disorders
- Lymphatic malformations

Pulmonary Lymphatic Perfusion Syndrome
- An important concept that has emerged in understanding these disorders based on DCE MR lymphangiography is that of PLPS.
- The normal flow of lymphatics in the chest is from the lungs and mediastinum toward the thoracic duct.
- In PLPS, the flow is reversed and goes retrograde toward the lung/mediastinum **(Figs. 6A and B)**.
- This occurs due to congenital distal stenosis of thoracic duct with development of abnormal collateral channels.
- Though the stenosis is congenital, the clinical presentation is variable from neonatal presentation to patients remaining asymptomatic.
- Symptoms develop when the collaterals around the bronchi or pleura or pericardium rupture resulting in plastic bronchitis, chylothorax, or chylopericardium, respectively.
- Rupture occurs as a result of an insult such as a severe lower respiratory tract infection or trauma. This can also occur with increased central venous pressures, e.g., due to thrombosis or post-Fontan procedure.
- DCE-MRI shows the retrograde flow typical of PLPS, along with thoracic duct narrowing or stenosis.

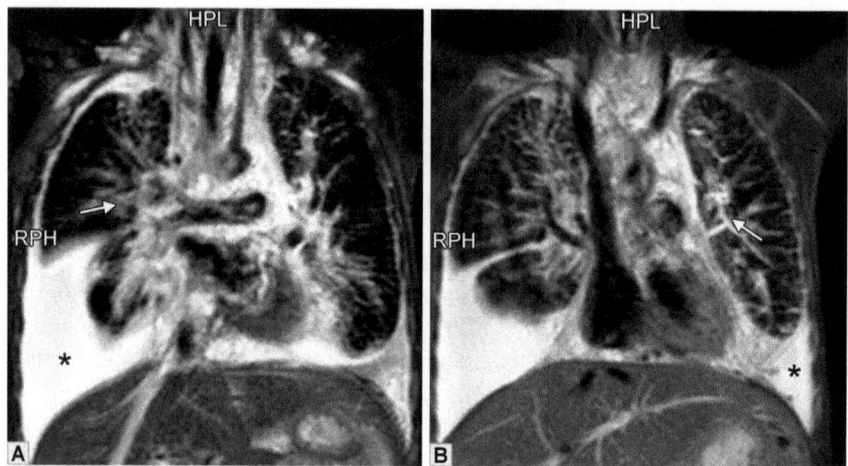

FIGS. 6A AND B: STIR cor images in a patient with bilateral chylothorax (asterisks) demonstrating abnormal hyperintense linear structures radiating from the hila toward lung parenchyma suggesting abnormal lymphatic perfusion.
(STIR: short-tau inversion recovery)

Plastic Bronchitis
- Plastic bronchitis refers to a condition where there is exudation of protein rich material into the airways resulting in the formation of "casts".
- These branching casts obstruct the airways and are also expectorated by the patient.
- The cause of exudation of this material is PLPS resulting in retrograde flow of lymph.
- The most common conditions predisposing to this are cardiac surgeries that result in elevated central venous pressure such as Fontan procedure. These procedures which establish direct cavopulmonary connections result in elevated venous pressures.
- Other predisposing conditions include cystic fibrosis, sickle cell anemia, or asthma.
- DCE-MRI aids in the diagnosis by demonstrating PLPS.
- Lymphoscintigraphy reveals increased uptake of tracer in the lungs.
- Management includes medical therapy (mucolytics, steroids, and phosphodiesterase 5 inhibitors) or interventional radiology.
- However, in those conditions which are post cardiac surgery, predisposing abnormal flow mechanism needs to be corrected, which may entail even cardiac transplantation.

Idiopathic Chylothorax
Dynamic contrast material-enhanced MR lymphangiography can be helpful in demonstrating anatomy in idiopathic chylothorax when there is no other demonstrable cause. It also demonstrates abnormal lymphatic flow from the thoracic duct toward the pulmonary parenchyma along with dilatation of thoracic duct, which is commonly seen.

Neonatal Lymphatic Flow Disorders
- Neonatal flow disorders include chylothorax, chylous ascites, and hydrops fetalis (associated with congenital lymphatic dysplasia).
- Dynamic MR lymphangiography can be used to differentiate between these conditions.
- In isolated neonatal chylothorax, there is absence of upper thoracic duct on MR lymphangiography and lymphatic flow is directed toward the lungs which manifest as nutmeg appearance of lungs on MRI. This abnormal lymphatic flow can be embolized with ethiodol resulting in complete resolution of chylothorax.
- Congenital lymphatic dysplasia/hydrops manifest on MR imaging as absence or nonvisualization of central lymphatic ducts and abnormal dermal lymphatic flow which can manifest as soft tissue edema, pleural or pericardial effusions, and ascites in various combinations. Embolization is contraindicated and microsurgical techniques attempting thoracic duct to venous connection can be tried for treatment.
- Isolated neonatal chylous ascites can manifest as enhancing high signal masses or with frank contrast extravasation into ascitic fluid on DCE MRI.

Lymphatic Malformations
- Lymphatic anomalies are nonneoplastic developmental lesions characterized by abnormally formed lymphatic channels, which may present as diffuse abnormalities or localized lesions.[2]

  They can be classified as:
  - *Simple*: These include macrocystic (cystic spaces > 1 cm), microcystic (cystic spaces < 1 cm) or mixed malformations. These usually manifest as fluid intensity chest wall or mediastinal masses, and are not discussed further.
  - *Complex*: These include poorly defined developmental anomalies involving the central lymphatics and include generalized lymphatic anomaly (GLA), kaposiform lymphangiomatosis, CCL anomaly (channel type lymphatic malformation), and lymphatic malformation in Gorham–Stout disease. Clinically, these conditions usually manifest with deteriorating lung function and respiratory difficulty. On MR imaging, these malformations present as pleural effusions, features of PLPS, and thoracic duct abnormalities. These can also manifest as interstitial lung disease on imaging. The salient points of these entities are elaborated further.
    - *Generalized lymphatic abnormality*: It is a congenital condition characterized by abnormal proliferation of lymphatic channels resulting in abnormal thin walled and dilated lymphatics. It usually present in the first two decades of life with multiple site involvement with the most common being lung and bone and others being spleen, liver, retroperitoneum, and kidney.[3]

On imaging, it can present with PLPS features mentioned above with effusions, ascites, pulmonary interstitial thickening, and nodules. On MR lymphangiography, pulmonary lymphangiectasia, thoracic duct abnormalities, and sites of leakage can be found.

Associated bone abnormalities include lucent lesions, which can progress to fractures and bone fragmentation **(Figs. 7 and 8)**.

- *Kaposiform lymphangiomatosis*: It is differentiated from other CLAs by frequent occurrence of consumptive coagulopathy characterized by hypofibrinogenemia and thrombocytopenia (Kasabach–Merritt syndrome) resulting in more severe and rapidly progressive abnormalities, and high morbidity and mortality.

Imaging findings overlap with GLA, although retroperitoneal and mediastinal involvement by soft tissue masses is more extensive and hemorrhagic pleural and pericardial effusions and ascites are more common than GLA. Presence of spindle cells on biopsy is a characteristic histological feature **(Figs. 9A and B)**.

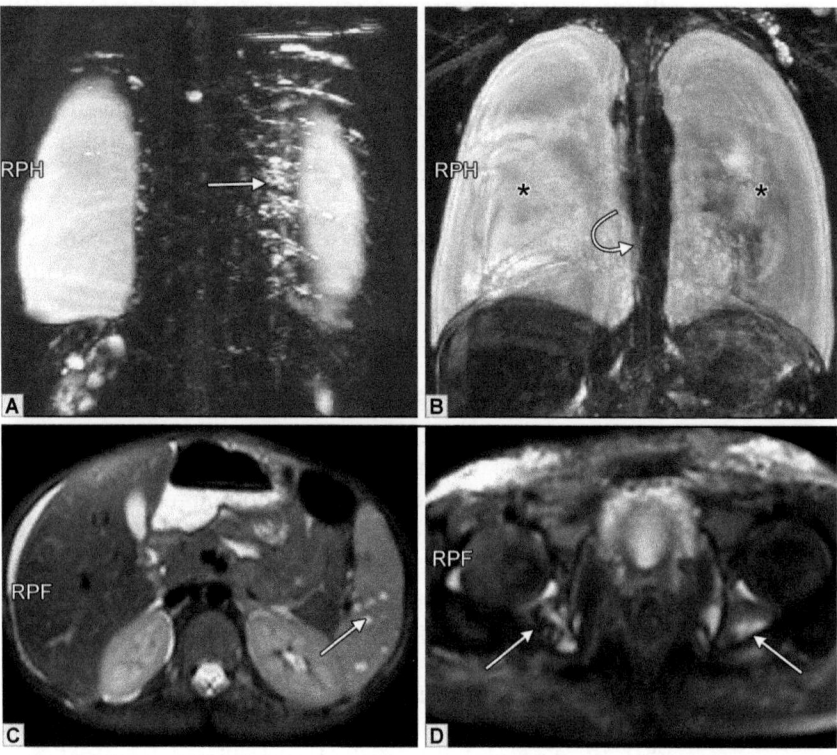

FIGS. 7A TO D: DCE-MRI in a 7-year-old male child with generalized lymphatic anomaly. (A) and (B) 3D MRCP cor images showing bilateral pleural effusion (asterisks) and dilated left chest wall lymphatic channels (arrow in A). Thoracic duct (curved arrow in B) is partly visualized and shows normal caliber. (C) T2 FS axial image shows chylous ascites and small splenic T2 hyperintense lesions (arrow). (D) T2FS axial images through the pelvis demonstrate small hyperintense lesions in ischium bilaterally (arrows).

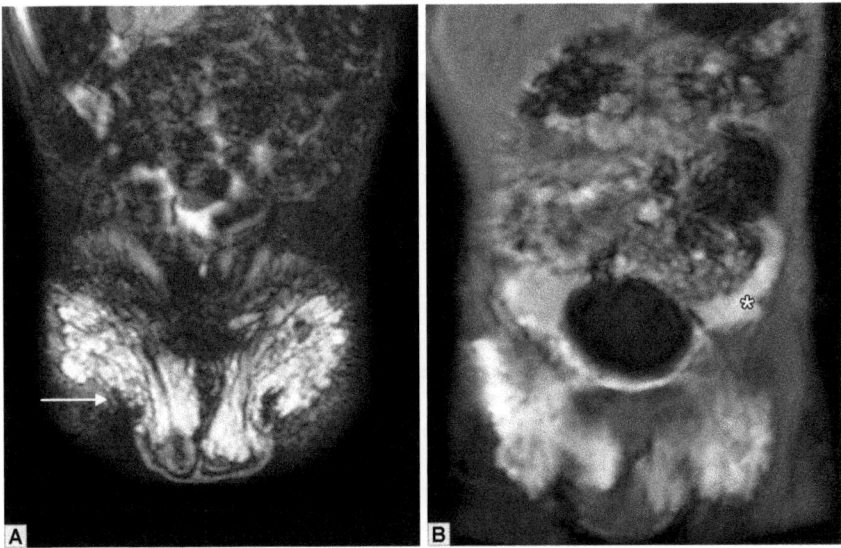

FIGS. 8A AND B: DCE-MRI in a 7-year-old male child with generalized lymphatic anomaly. (A) coronal T2 FS images show dilated lymphatic channels in bilateral inguinoscrotal regions (arrow) and (B) postcontrast DCE MRI (mDIXON) image showing enhancement of the inguinoscrotal lymphatic channels and contrast opacification of ascites (asterisk) suggestive of lymphatic leak.

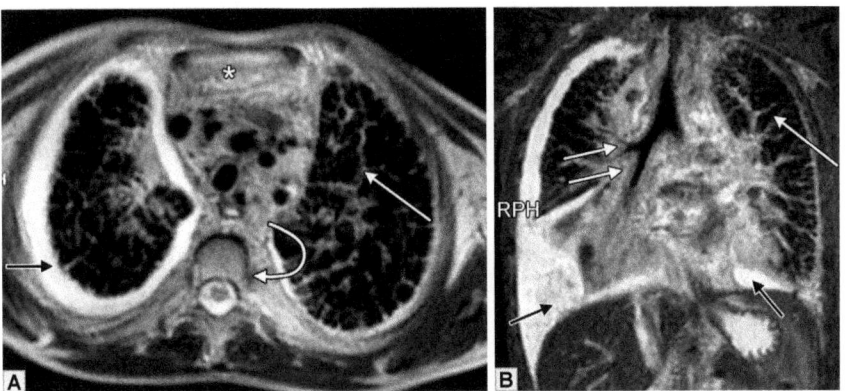

FIGS. 9A AND B: Axial T2 (A) and coronal STIR (B) MR images in a 12-year-old male with Kaposiform lymphangiomatosis. MR imaging findings include extensive hyperintense mediastinal soft tissue (asterisk) encasing the mediastinal vascular structures, bronchial wall thickening (white arrows), prevertebral soft tissue (curved arrow), diffuse septal thickening in bilateral lungs (long white arrows) and bilateral pleural effusions (black arrows).

- *Central conducting lymphatic anomaly*: It encompasses the disorders of central lymphatics, i.e., thoracic duct and cisterna chyli resulting from atretic or poorly formed/dysplastic channels. It can manifest as a part of other CLAs or can present as an isolated abnormality of its own. It can present with effusions, ascites,

protein losing enteropathy, or recurrent infections, and MR lymphangiography reveals central lymphatic channel disruption.
- *Gorham–Stout disease associated LA*: A characteristic feature of this entity is progressive osteolysis caused by abnormal proliferation of bone lymphatics. Axial skeleton is more commonly affected and can lead to pathological fractures, limb dysfunction or even spinal disability if vertebrae are involved. Pleural effusions and splenic lesions can also be associated. Radiography or CT can show lucent/lace-like lesions, fractures, vanishing bones, or a sucked candy appearance whereas MR lymphangiography is usually normal.

MANAGEMENT IN LYMPHATIC MALFORMATIONS IN CHEST

The management of lymphatic malformations requires a multidisciplinary approach as they often require multimodality treatment in the form of medical or systemic therapy, minimally invasive interventional management as well as surgical treatment. The primary goal of treatment is to reduce infection risk, improve function as well as aesthetic preservation.

Complex Lymphatic Malformations: Role of Interventional Radiology

Thoracic or lymphatic duct embolization can be performed in lymphatic flow disorders such as chylothorax and chylous ascites, plastic bronchitis, and complex lymphatic anomalies where there is demonstration of a chylous leak. Embolization is preceded by oil-based (Lipiodol) lymphangiography which is often used to demonstrate abnormal lymphatic flow and chyle leaks in these disorders which are subsequently embolized **(Fig. 10)**.[4]

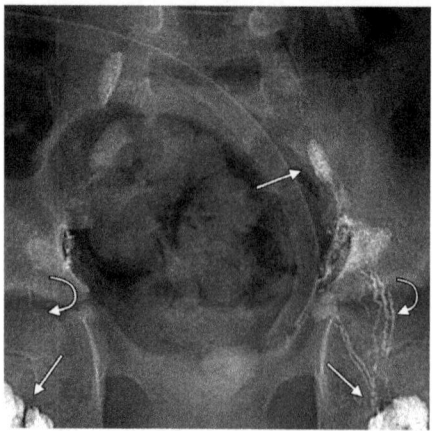

FIG. 10: Spot fluoroscopic image in a child with chyle leak demonstrating opacification of bilateral inguinal and iliac nodes (arrows) and lymphatic channels (curved arrows) visualized up to the retroperitoneum.

However, due to rarity and complex nature of these disorders as well as technical challenges encountered due to the small size and difficult visualization of lymphatic ducts in children, the treatment approaches are not standardized.

Hardware
The equipment needed for thoracic duct embolization includes:
- 22–25-G needle for percutaneous lymph node access
- Short-extension tubing
- Syringes
- 22-G Chiba needle
- 0.018 guidewire
- Microcatheters (2.4–2.7 F)
- 0.018 microcoils
- N-butyl-2-cyanoacrylate (NBCA) glue
- Lipiodol

Technique of Embolization
- Technique can be performed under sedation or general anesthesia. Bilateral inguinal regions are prepared and sterile draped. Likewise, left upper neck and chest are prepared so as to allow for sonographic evaluation and access of thoracic duct at venous angle, if required. Chest and abdomen are also prepared, if there is a possibility of direct access of thoracic duct, cisterna chyli, or retroperitoneal lymphatics for direct embolization.
- Under US guidance, direct access of inguinal lymph nodes is obtained bilaterally using 22–25G needle, which is then connected to extension tubing prepared and primed with lipiodol. After confirming the position of the needle tip within the node, contrast is slowly injected under fluoroscopy which demonstrates filling of efferent vessels. Contrast is injected slowly (approximately 1 mL every 5–10 minutes) with a max dosage of 0.25 mL/kg. Intermittent fluoroscopy is done to look for contrast progression. Saline can also be used to flush the contrast if needed.
- Then fluoroscopic images are carefully assessed for slow or poor flow, duct ectasia, collaterals, evaluation of cisterna chyli and thoracic duct, and its drainage into the venous angle and do demonstrate site of any abnormal leakage.
- If any abnormal site of contrast leakage is demonstrated, direct percutaneous lymphatic duct or thoracic duct access is done using a thin 22-G Chiba needle. If duct access is unsuccessful, repeat punctures can be done (thoracic duct disruption sometimes is enough to resolve leaks) or another site selected. Then a 0.018 guidewire is advanced over which a microcatheter is advanced and iodinated contrast injected through the microcatheter to confirm and demonstrate leak site. The leak site is then embolized using 0.018 microcoils and completed using N-butyl cyanoacrylate in a 1.1 or 1.2 mixture with lipiodol.

Complications

Complications are uncommon with oil-based lymphangiography and include hypersensitivity to contrast agents, oil embolization to lungs. Systemic oil embolization is rare in absence of right-to-left shunts. Percutaneous lymphatic or thoracic duct access can occasionally cause bile leaks and hematoma. Nontarget glue embolization is another potential complication.

Simple Lymphatic Malformations: Role of Sclerotherapy

Sclerotherapy has become popular as the initial management technique due to its relative ease, low cost, efficacy, and safety. It involves instillation of sclerosing agents which promote scarring and fibrosis by causing damage to the endothelium of the lymphatic malformations. It can be used to treat simple lymphatic malformations involving the chest wall and cervicothoracic regions.[5]

Commonly Used Agents

Bleomycin, doxycycline, polidocanol, and sodium tetradecyl (STS) foam are used. Bleomycin is commonly reconstituted in normal saline and mixed with air in a ratio of 1:2-1:4 so as to form foam medium to increase the endothelial surface contact. Commonly used dose of bleomycin is 0.5-1 mL/kg with maximum single session dose of 15 mg. It is an ideal sclerosing agents for lesions close to the airway as it causes minimal postprocedural inflammation and swelling. Polidocanol is also administered as a foam and the maximum dose is 2 mg/kg. Doxycycline can be reconstituted with normal saline or iodinated contrast and administered up to a maximum single session dose of 150 mg in neonates, 300 mg in infants and 1,200 mg in other patients.[6]

Technique

- Depending upon the patient's characters and location, procedure can be done under sedation or general anesthesia.
- Under USG guidance, access is maintained typically with 22-24-G needles. Larger needles or catheters can be used for large lesions. The cyst fluid is aspirated first for confirmation of lymphatic malformation and cyst fluid sent for cytology. Then under fluoroscopic guidance, cystography is performed using iodinated contrast to exclude any venous connections. Then sclerosant is instilled with a typical volume of 50-75% of aspirated fluid volume **(Figs. 11A to D)**. Depending upon the size and the distribution of lymphatic malformation, multiple sessions which are typically scheduled 6-8 weeks apart may be required. Microcystic, multiseptated and large malformations are usually more difficult to treat and require more treatment sessions. To reduce postprocedure inflammation and swelling, systemic steroids can be administered.

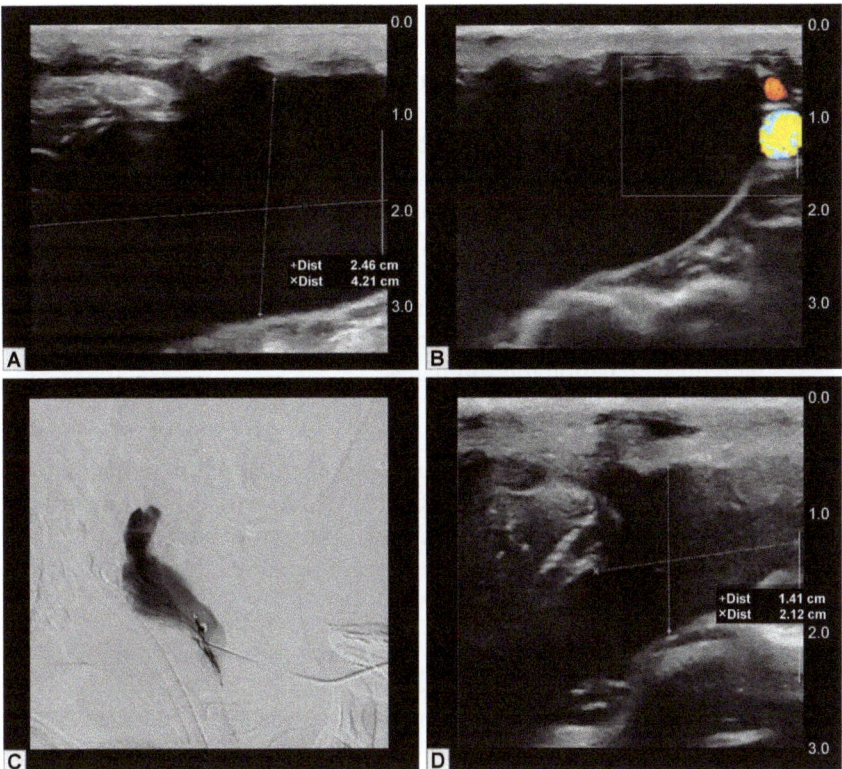

FIGS. 11A TO D: USG in a 3-year-old female child with simple lymphatic malformation treated with bleomycin sclerotherapy. (A and B) a simple anechoic lesion in cervical region with no internal contents or vascularity; (C) DSA image after contrast injection with needle in situ and no communication with venous channels; and (D) follow-up USG image showing significant reduction in the size of lymphatic malformation.

Complications

Sclerotherapy can cause scarring, fibrosis, nerve damage, skin ulceration, and superinfection. Hypersensitivity reactions can occur to the sclerosing agents used. In addition, bleomycin-induced pneumonitis progressing to fibrosis can occur with increased cumulative dose of the drug.

Medical Management

- *Sirolimus*: It is a mechanistic target of rapamycin (mTOR) inhibitor, which is a serine/threonine kinase which is involved in cellular growth, protein synthesis and is overactive in most lymphatic malformations and some complex lymphatic anomalies. It is effective and commonly used as the first-line drug in the medical management of lymphatic malformations. Initial dose is 0.8 mg/m^2 twice daily and requires frequent monitoring for dose titration. Side effects include increased risk of infection due to

immunosuppressive effects, bone marrow and blood toxicity causing anemia, low platelet and white blood cell (WBC) cell counts, and gastrointestinal (GI) and dermatological manifestations.
- *Other targeted therapies*:
  - *Tyrosine kinase inhibitors [RAS/mitogen-activated protein kinase (MAPK) pathway]*: This pathway is frequently activated in CLAs and drugs such as sunitinib and trametinib have been shown to be effective in management of CLAs.
  - Vascular endothelial growth factor (VEGF) inhibitors such as pegylated interferon-alpha cause downregulation of VEGF resulting in inhibition of angiogenesis and thus cause clinical improvement in patients with lymphatic anomalies.

Surgery

Surgical debulking can be done in large lymphatic malformations. In sites where lymphatic disruption is identified in CCLA, surgical lymphovenous anastomosis can be created to improve the lymphatic flow. Further, pleurodesis can be done for symptomatic improvement in cases of recurrent or nonresolving pleural effusions.

■ REFERENCES

1. Chavhan GB, Amaral JG, Temple M, Itkin M. MR lymphangiography in children: Technique and potential applications. Radio Graphics. 2017;37:177590.
2. International Society for the Study of Vascular Anomalies. (2018). ISSVA classification 2018. [online] Available from https://www.issva.org/UserFiles/file/ISSVA-Classification-2018.pdf [Last accessed August, 2023]
3. Snyder EJ, Sarma A, Borst AJ, Tekes A. Lymphatic Anomalies in Children: Update on Imaging Diagnosis, Genetics, and Treatment. AJR Am J Roentgenol. 2022;218:1089-101.
4. Majdalany BS, Saad WA, Chick JFB, Khaja MS, Cooper KJ, Srinivasa RN. Pediatric lymphangiography, thoracic duct embolization and thoracic duct disruption: a single-institution experience in 11 children with chylothorax. Pediatr Radiol. 2018;48(2):235-40.
5. Chaudry G. Complex lymphatic anomalies and therapeutic options. Tech Vasc Interv Radiol. 2019;22(4):100632.
6. Cronan J, Gill AE, Shah JH, Hawkins CM. The role of interventional radiologists in the treatment of congenital lymphatic Malformations. Semin Intervent Radiol. 2020;37(3):285-94.

SECTION 7

Mediastinum Imaging

CHAPTER 21: Approach to Mediastinal Lesions: Part 1
CHAPTER 22: Approach to Mediastinal Lesions: Part 2

CHAPTER 21

Approach to Mediastinal Lesions: Part 1

Shruti Badkhane, Manisha Jana

- ❏ Compartments of mediastinum
- ❏ Role of imaging
  - ➢ Chest radiograph
  - ➢ Role of computed tomography
  - ➢ Role of ultrasonography
- ➢ Role of MRI
- ➢ Role of positron emission tomography-CT (PET-CT)
- ❏ Mediastinal masses
  - ➢ Anterior mediastinal masses (Prevascular compartment)

■ INTRODUCTION

Mediastinum refers to the space between the two lungs, lined by mediastinal pleura on both sides and containing fat. It extends from the thoracic inlet to the diaphragm. Besides containing the heart, it is a passage for tubes passing from neck to chest or to abdomen—trachea, aorta, inferior vena cava (IVC), esophagus, thoracic duct, and sympathetic chain. It also houses lymph nodes and lymphatics.

The approach to a mediastinal mass is based on several factors, which include:
- Location on imaging
- The likelihood of a particular mass depends on the age and sex of the patient; and the clinical presentation may guide the etiology (e.g., myasthenia gravis), while several lesions are incidentally detected.
- *Computed tomography (CT) morphology*: Solid, cystic, fat containing, calcification, and enhancement also help.

■ COMPARTMENTS OF MEDIASTINUM

- Typically, a compartment-based approach has been used while discussing/dividing lesions of the mediastinum; although there are no fascial planes that divide it into compartments; or actually limit the disease spread. Location broadly aids characterization and is hence widely used by both surgeons and radiologists.[1]

- Different methods have been used for this division, the most frequently used among them being Felson's method **(Fig. 1)**, anatomists' traditional method, and the recently advocated cross-sectional imaging-based system developed by International Thymic Malignancy Interest Group (ITMIG). A comparative detail is given in **Table 1**.
- Borders and structures within the various compartments are described in **Table 2**.
- The superior and inferior boundaries of all compartments are the thoracic inlet and diaphragm, respectively.
- For the purpose of this chapter, the terms anterior, middle, and posterior are retained due to familiarity of most readers, but the divisions have been aligned according to the ITMIG recommendations.

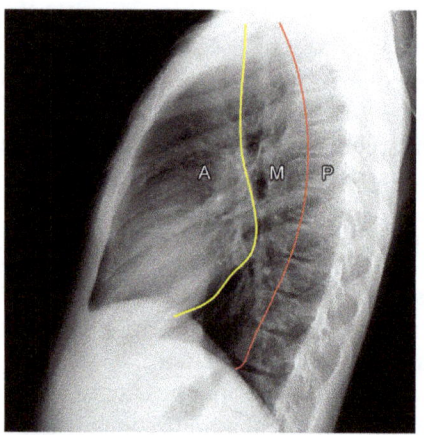

FIG. 1: Division of mediastinum (Felson's method). Space between sternum and yellow line is anterior mediastinum (A); middle mediastinum (M); and posterior to red line—posterior mediastinum (P).

TABLE 1: Compartments of mediastinum.		
	Felson's system	**ITMIG**
Primary imaging modality	CXR	CT
Number of compartments	3	3
Anterior compartment terminology	Anterior mediastinum	Prevascular
Middle compartment terminology	Middle mediastinum	Visceral
Posterior compartment terminology	Posterior mediastinum	Paravertebral

CHAPTER 21: Approach to Mediastinal Lesions: Part 1

TABLE 2: Boundaries and contents of mediastinum (Felson's system).			
Boundaries	Anterior	Middle	Posterior
Anterior	Sternum	Pericardium	Line drawn 1 cm posterior to the anterior vertebral margin
Posterior	Pericardium (anterior aspect)	Line drawn 1 cm posterior to the anterior vertebral margin	
Lateral	Mediastinal pleura (parietal) wrapped around the heart		Lateral margin of transverse processes
Important structure included	• Thymus • Fat • Nodes • Left brachiocephalic vein	• Trachea and carina • Nodes • Esophagus	Vertebrae and paravertebral soft tissues

ROLE OF IMAGING

Chest radiograph (CXR) is often the first imaging performed; but CT is the most important modality for characterization and extent assessment.

Chest Radiograph

Signs of mediastinal mass on CXR: Mediastinal pathologies result in mediastinal widening or a mass lesion. Mediastinal mass on CXR shows following signs **(Box 1)**. Compartmentalization of mediastinal masses can be done on the following radiographic signs **(Table 3)**.

BOX 1 CXR signs of mediastinal masses.
- Sharply marginated
- Broad base to mediastinum
- Central mass, often bilateral
- Tapering superior and inferior borders
- Medial margin not defined
- Obtuse angle with mediastinum
- Wide paravertebral shadow
- Involvement of spine, ribs

TABLE 3: Radiographic signs for compartmentalization of mediastinal masses.

Anterior mediastinal mass *(Fig. 2)*	Middle mediastinal mass *(Fig. 3)*	Posterior mediastinal mass *(Fig. 4)*
Silhouette sign: Loss of definition of ascending aorta, heart border	Widening of right paratracheal stripe	Widening of paraspinal stripes
Cervicothoracic sign: Seen in anterior mediastinal mass having a cervical extension and vice versa	Convex contour of aortopulmonary window	*Silhouette sign*: Loss of definition of aortic knuckle
Hilum overlay sign: Present	Widening of the carinal angle in case of subcarinal lesions	Scalloping of posterior ends or ribs/vertebral body destruction
Hilum convergence sign: Absent	*Lateral projection*: "Doughnut sign" in hilar adenopathy	Widened posterior intercostal spaces
Loss of retrosternal lucency on lateral CXR		Retrocardiac mass
		Spine sign: Increased density overlying lower thoracic vertebrae on lateral projection

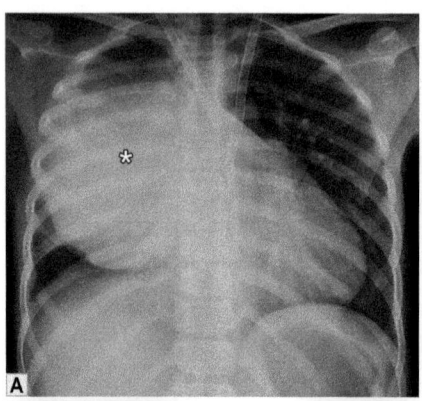
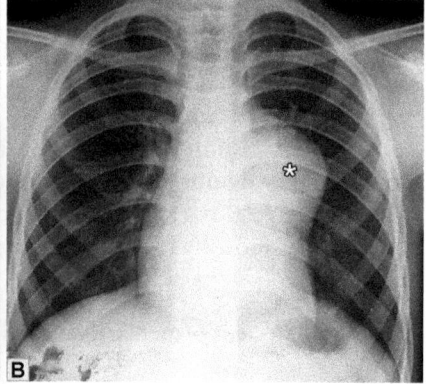
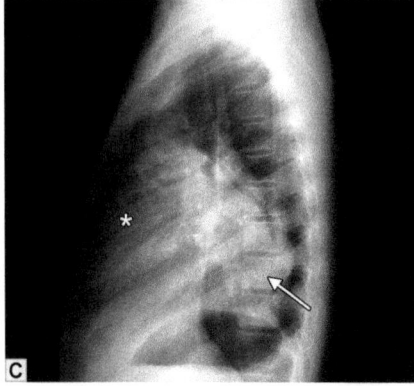

FIGS. 2A TO C: Radiographic features of anterior mediastinal mass (asterisk) in three different patients.
(A) Loss of silhouette of right cardiac border and superior vena cava;
(B) Hilum overlay sign; and
(C) Loss of retrosternal lucency. Posterior mediastinal component seen as "spine sign" (arrow).

CHAPTER 21: Approach to Mediastinal Lesions: Part 1

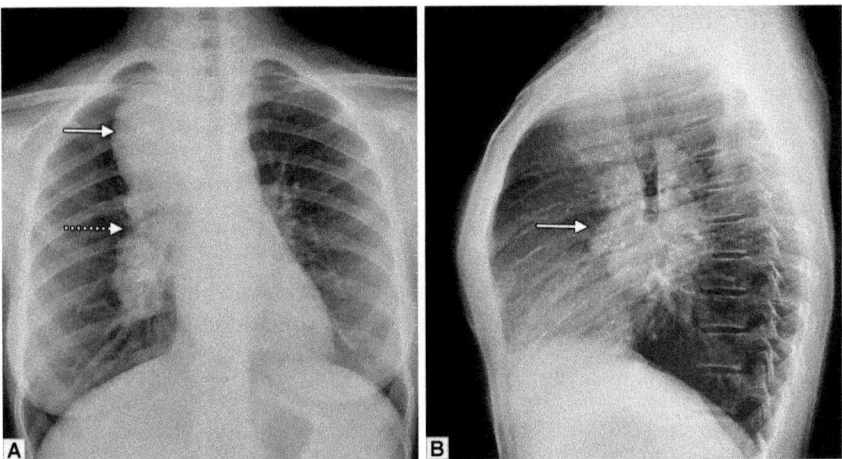

FIGS. 3A AND B: Radiographic features of middle mediastinal mass. (A) Widened right paratracheal stripe (arrow), hilar enlargement (dotted arrow); (B) doughnut sign (arrow).

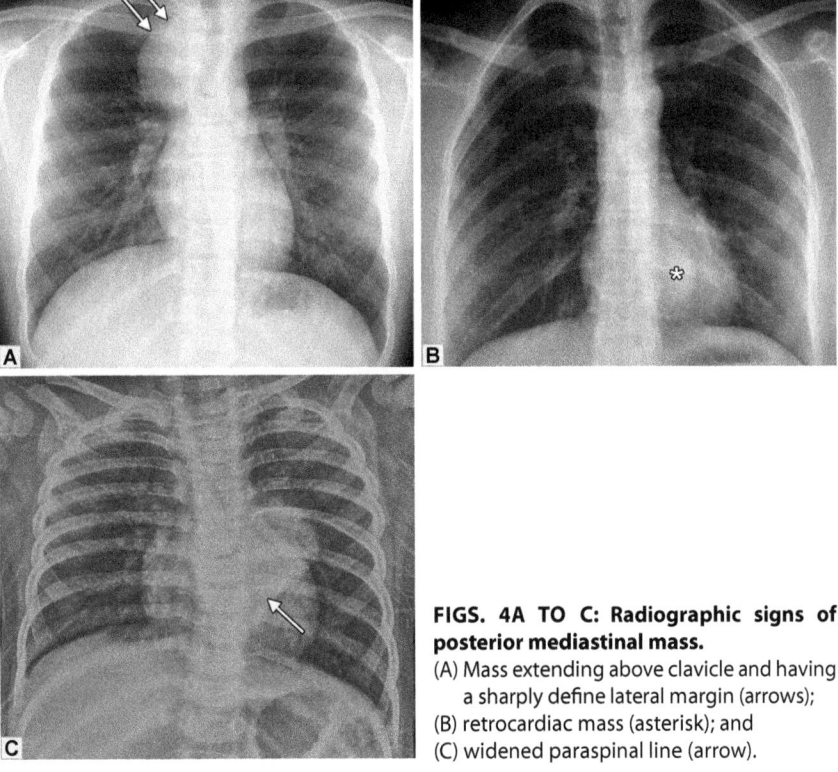

FIGS. 4A TO C: Radiographic signs of posterior mediastinal mass.
(A) Mass extending above clavicle and having a sharply define lateral margin (arrows);
(B) retrocardiac mass (asterisk); and
(C) widened paraspinal line (arrow).

Role of Computed Tomography
- Contrast-enhanced CT (CECT) is the workhorse of imaging in mediastinal masses.
- Useful for characterization and extent evaluation of masses.

Role of Ultrasonography
- Applicable to superficial lesions. It is particularly relevant in children due to the presence of a better acoustic window.
- Most often conclusive in differentiating anterior mediastinal mass from an enlarged thymus in infants, also cystic vs solid differentiation.

Role of MRI
- Cystic versus solid differentiation, especially in lesions not accessible to ultrasonography (USG)
- *Assessing solid component of complex cystic lesions or thymic hyperplasia versus thymoma*: Chemical shift imaging (CSI), diffusion-weighted imaging (DWI), and magnetic resonance (MR) perfusion useful.
- Spinal extension of posterior mediastinal lesions
- Cine MRI for equivocal cardiac or vascular invasion
- In renal failure, noncontrast MRI gives more information than non-contrast CT where iodinated CT contrast cannot be administered
- Patients allergic to iodinated contrast

Role of Positron Emission Tomography-CT (PET-CT)
- Positron emission tomography-CT (PET-CT) is not required for characterization of mediastinal masses, except in the uncommon thymic carcinoids where DOTA-NOC PET is useful.
- 18F-fluorodeoxyglucose (18F-FDG) PET-CT is used for staging of several malignancies.
- FDG uptake can be seen in infective and inflammatory lesions, and even in hyperplastic thymus, hence its limited utility in characterization.

MEDIASTINAL MASSES

The largest proportion of mediastinal masses occurs in the anterior mediastinum (prevascular compartment) (50% or more), with an equal proportion of the remaining being present in the middle or posterior mediastinum. Multicompartmental masses are also common.

Anterior Mediastinal Masses (Prevascular Compartment)
- Anterior mediastinal lesions can arise from thymus, or retrosternal extension of thyroid, or lymph nodal in origin. Also, several neck masses may extend to the anterior mediastinum cervicothoracic masses. And also cardiophrenic angle masses on CXR are anterior mediastinal in location.

- Whereas masses like GCTs project on one side of the mediastinum, lymphoma appears as a mass projection on both the sides **(Fig. 2)**.
- *Mediastinal widening or mass projecting on both sides of mediastinum (Fig. 2)*: Nodal enlargement due to any causes (e.g., lymphoma). The outline is lobulated in nodal enlargement.

Cross-sectional Imaging-based Approach to Anterior Mediastinal Masses (Prevascular Compartment)

- The ITMIG in 2014 presented an algorithmic approach to anterior mediastinal masses.[2] While most of the features are applicable to CT, MRI should preferably be performed for all cystic lesions for adequate characterization.
- Normal structures and the pathologies are listed in **Table 4**. Approach to cystic and solid masses is discussed in **Flowcharts 1 and 2** and **Figures 5 and 6**.[2,3]

TABLE 4: Normal structures and pathologies of the anterior mediastinum.

Normal structure	Pathologies
Thymus	Thymic hyperplasia, thymic cyst, germ cell tumor, lymphoma, and thymoma
Fat and lymph nodes	Lymphoma
Thyroid	Goiter
Heart, pericardium	
Ascending aorta	
Azygos arch, superior vena cava	
Internal mammary vessels	

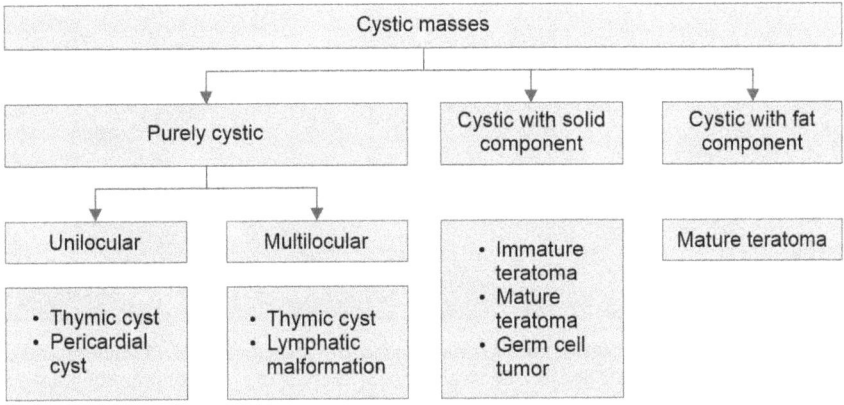

FLOWCHART 1: Imaging approach to cystic anterior mediastinal masses.

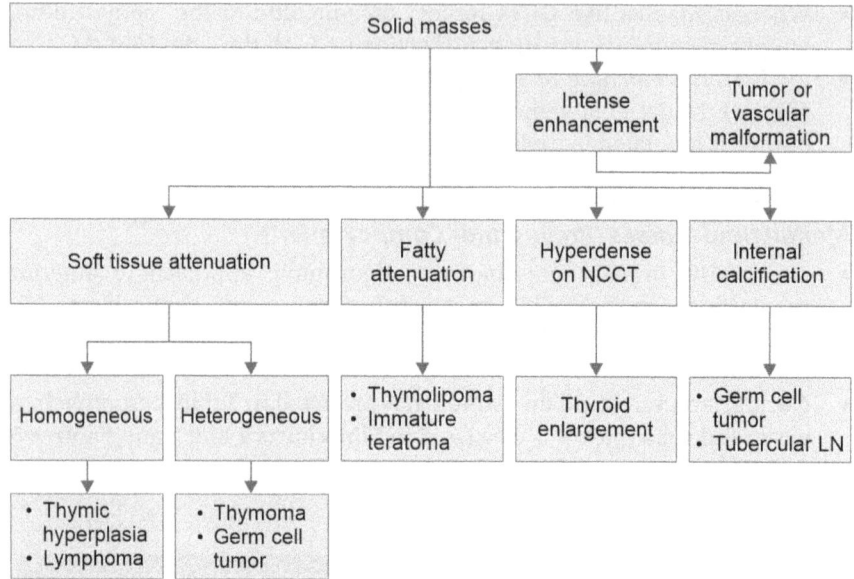

FLOWCHART 2: Imaging approach to solid anterior mediastinal masses.
(LN: lymph node; NCCT: noncontrast computed tomography)

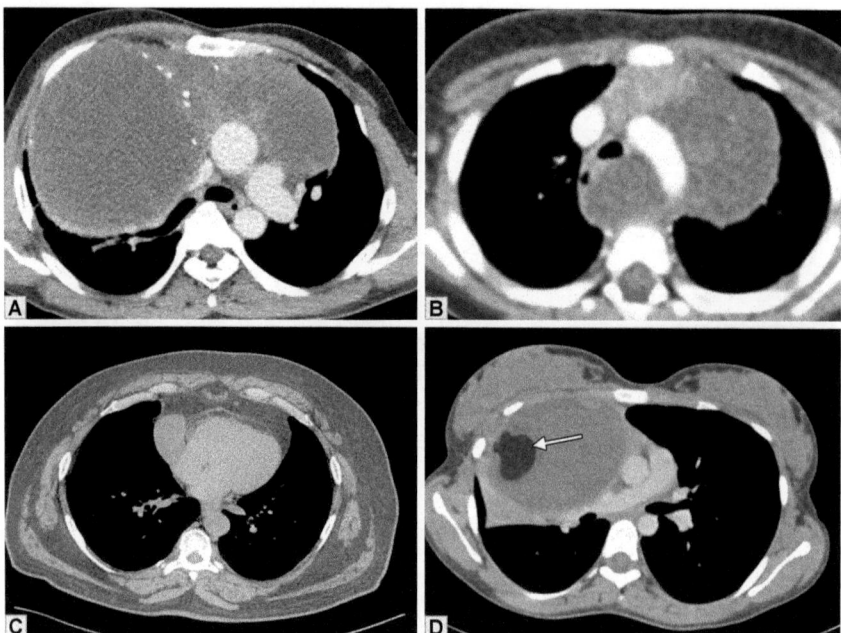

FIGS. 5A TO D: Cystic anterior mediastinal masses (prevascular space). (A) Multiseptated cystic with thin rim calcification in *teratoma*; (B) Multilocular, transcompartmental in *lymphatic malformation*; (C) unilocular cyst at cardiophrenic angle: *Pericardial cyst*; and (D) cyst with fat attenuation (arrow): *Dermoid cyst*.

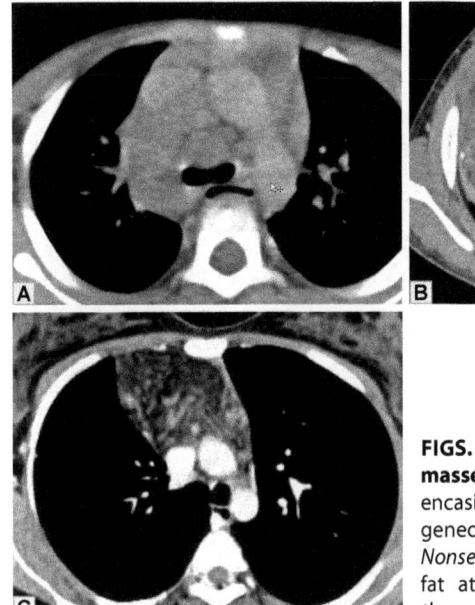
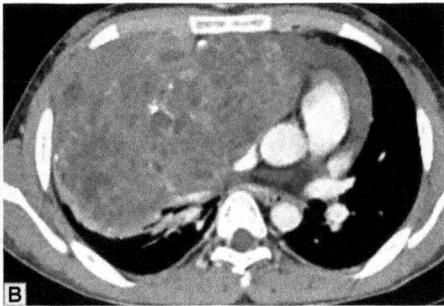

FIGS. 6A TO C: Solid anterior mediastinal masses. (A) Conglomerate homogenous mass encasing vessels in *lymphoma*; (B) heterogeneous solid mass with specks of calcifiation: *Nonseminomatous germ cell tumor;* and (C) fat attenuation with interspersed septae in *thymolipoma*.

Normal Thymus

The size of normal thymus is variable and depends on age of the child. The signs associated with normal thymus on radiograph and ultrasound are listed in **Table 5**. Attenuation of thymus varies with age, and also in various disease processes. In infants (<1 year), the thymus is usually denser than chest wall muscles and the heart. Several disease processes (e.g., hemosiderosis) might also result in a hyperdense thymus **(Fig. 7)**. The density declines with increasing age in normal children.[4]

TABLE 5: Imaging signs of normal thymus.	
Sign	Description
Wave sign	Indentation on thymus by anterior ends of ribs
Sail sign	Lateral concave contour of thymic lobes, and an acute angle with the cardiac border
Starry sky sign	Speckled appearance of thymus on ultrasound

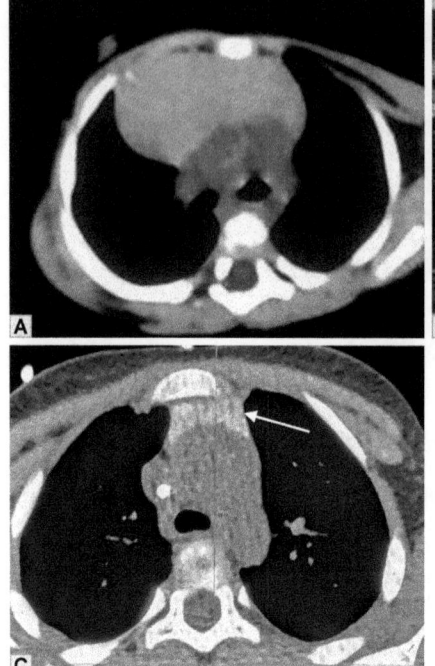
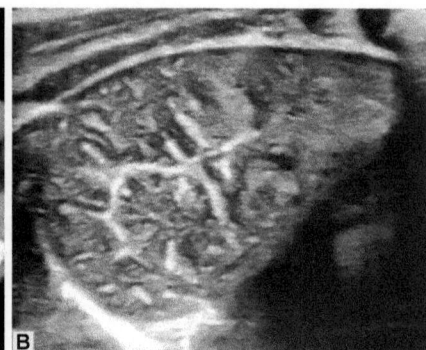

FIGS. 7A TO C: Hyperdense thymus.
(A) Normal thymus in an 8-month-old infant, which appears hyperdense;
(B) Normal speckled appearance on ultrasound;
(C) Hyperdense thymus (arrow) in an older child with hemosiderosis.

Thymic Hyperplasia

- Thymic hyperplasia can be either true or lymphoid hyperplasia. True hyperplasia can be seen in patients recovering from stress-induced thymic involution. This is known as rebound thymic hyperplasia. Hyperthyroidism, sarcoidosis, and pure red cell aplasia are other conditions that can be associated with thymic hyperplasia.[5] On imaging, the thymus is enlarged but internal architecture is preserved. On ultrasound, the "starry sky" pattern of a normal thymus is retained **(Fig. 8)**. On chemical shift MR imaging, there is signal drop on opposed phase T1 gradient-echo image.
- Lymphoid hyperplasia is associated with immune-mediated diseases such as systemic lupus erythematosus, vasculitis, Grave's disease, myasthenia gravis, rheumatoid arthritis, and thyrotoxicosis. The size of thymus may not be enlarged.
- Differentiating thymic hyperplasia from thymic neoplasms can be done with reasonable certainty on imaging **(Table 6)**.

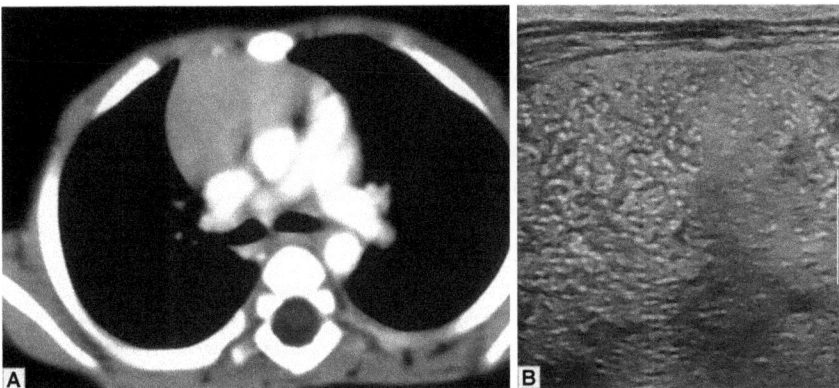

FIGS. 8A AND B: Thymic hyperplasia in a 7-year-old boy. (A) Asymmetric right lobe enlargement of thymus, homogeneous in attenuation and (B) starry sky pattern on ultrasound.

TABLE 6: Differentiating thymic hyperplasia from mass.		
	Thymic hyperplasia	**Thymic mass**
Outline	"Sail sign" "Wave sign"	Lobulated, asymmetrical
USG	Normal starry sky pattern	Heterogeneous
Vascularity	Normal	Distorted/encased vessels
Necrosis/calcification	Absent	May be seen
MRI	Signal drop on dual echo T1W gradient-echo images	No signal drop

Thymic Cyst

Thymic cysts are uncommon benign lesions in children. They can either be congenital or acquired. Congenital cysts can be seen wither in the mediastinum or in the neck. Acquired cysts can be seen after treatment in Hodgkin's lymphoma, cystic change in thymic tumors, or in autoimmune disorders. On imaging, they are usually unilocular, hypodense on CT, with occasional thin rim calcification.

■ CONCLUSION

Imaging of mediastinal tumors often requires multiple imaging modalities. Description of the other compartments is given in the subsequent chapter.

Other Related Chapters that can be Referred to:
- Chapter 20: Lymphatic Anomalies: Imaging and Interventions
- Chapter 22: Approach to Mediastinal Lesions: Part 2
- Chapter 23: Thoracic Tumors and Mimics: Part 1
- Chapter 24: Thoracic Tumors and Mimics: Part 2

REFERENCES

1. Carter WB, Okumura M, Detterbeck FC, Marom EM. Approaching the patient with an anterior mediastinal mass: A guide for radiologists. J Thorac Oncol. 2014;9:S110-8.
2. Carter WB, Benveniste MF, Madan R, Godoy MC, de Groot PM, Truong MT, et al. ITMIG Classification of Mediastinal Compartments and Multidisciplinary Approach to Mediastinal Masses. Radiographics. 2017;37:413-36.
3. Whitten CR, Khan S, Munneke GJ, Grubnic S. A diagnostic approach to mediastinal abnormalities. Radiographics. 2007;27:657-71.
4. Sklair-Levy M, Agid R, Sella T, Strauss-Liviatan N, Bar-Ziv J. Age-related changes in CT attenuation of the thymus in children. Pediatr Radiol. 2000;30:566-9.
5. Manchanda S, Bhalla AS, Jana M, Gupta AK. Imaging of the pediatric thymus: Clinicoradiologic approach. World J Clin Pediatr. 2017;6(1):10-23.

CHAPTER 22

Approach to Mediastinal Lesions: Part 2

Ashu Seith Bhalla, Manisha Jana

- ❏ Middle mediastinal masses (Visceral compartment)
- ❏ Posterior mediastinal masses (Paravertebral compartment)
- ❏ Multicompartmental masses
- ❏ Masses where biopsy is not indicated
- ❏ Specific entities
  - ➢ Congenital lesions
  - ➢ Nodal enlargement
- ❏ Fibrosing mediastinitis

■ INTRODUCTION

Anterior mediastinal lesions are discussed in Chapter 21. This chapter will cover middle and posterior mediastinal lesions.

■ MIDDLE MEDIASTINAL MASSES (VISCERAL COMPARTMENT)

Middle mediastinal masses can be considered based on the organ of origin. Common masses are listed in **Box 1**.

BOX 1 Middle mediastinal masses.

- Duplication cyst
- Bronchogenic cyst
- Rosai–Dorfman disease
- Castleman disease
- Lymphadenopathy:
  ○ Sarcoidosis
  ○ Infective
  ○ Lymphoma
- Fibrosing mediastinitis
- Cardiac masses:
  ○ Rhabdomyoma
  ○ Angiosarcoma
  ○ Chamber enlargement
  ○ Thrombus

The International Thymic Malignancy Interest Group (ITMIG) recommendations divide the visceral compartment masses into two categories—(1) those which can be diagnosed on imaging alone (e.g., esophageal duplication cyst); and (2) those where combined clinical and imaging information are required to make a diagnosis (e.g., paraganglioma, Castleman's disease, and esophageal lesions).[1,2] An approach has been summarized in **Table 1**.

TABLE 1: Middle mediastinal masses based on morphology and attenuation.		
Attenuation	**Neoplastic**	**Nonneoplastic**
Cystic		• Duplication cyst **(Figs. 1A to C)** • Bronchogenic cyst • Neurenteric cyst
Solid		
Solid intensely enhancing	Rosai–Dorfman disease	Castleman diseases
Solid homogeneous enhancing	• Lymphoma • Metastasis **(Figs. 2A to D)**	• Sarcoidosis • Infective LN
Solid heterogeneous		• Inflammatory/infective • Fibrosing mediastinitis
Cardiac masses	• Rhabdomyoma • Angiosarcoma	Chamber enlargement thrombus

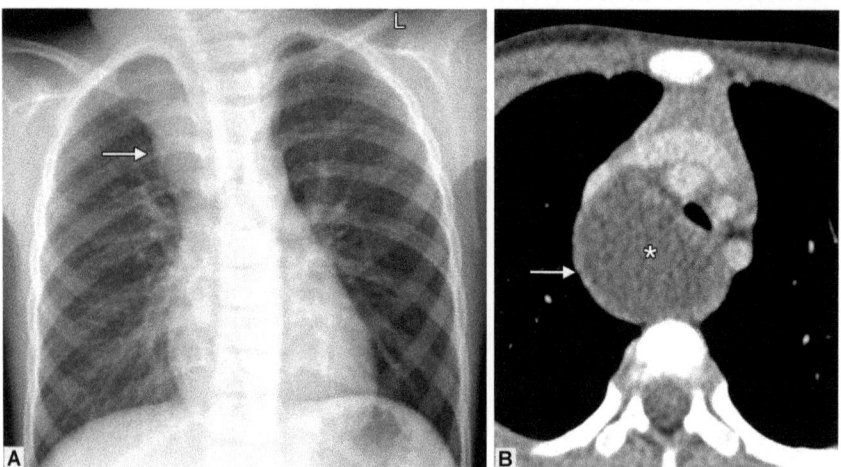

FIGS. 1A TO C: *Continued*

Continued

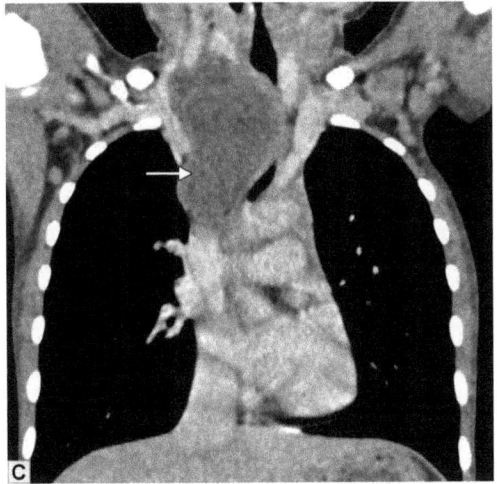

FIGS. 1A TO C: Cystic middle mediastinal (visceral compartment) mass. Duplication cyst in a 4-year-old boy with respiratory distress— (A) Widened right paratracheal stripe (arrow); (B) retroesophageal fluid attenuation lesion (asterisk) with thick wall (arrow); and (C) craniocaudally elongated nature of the lesion (arrow).

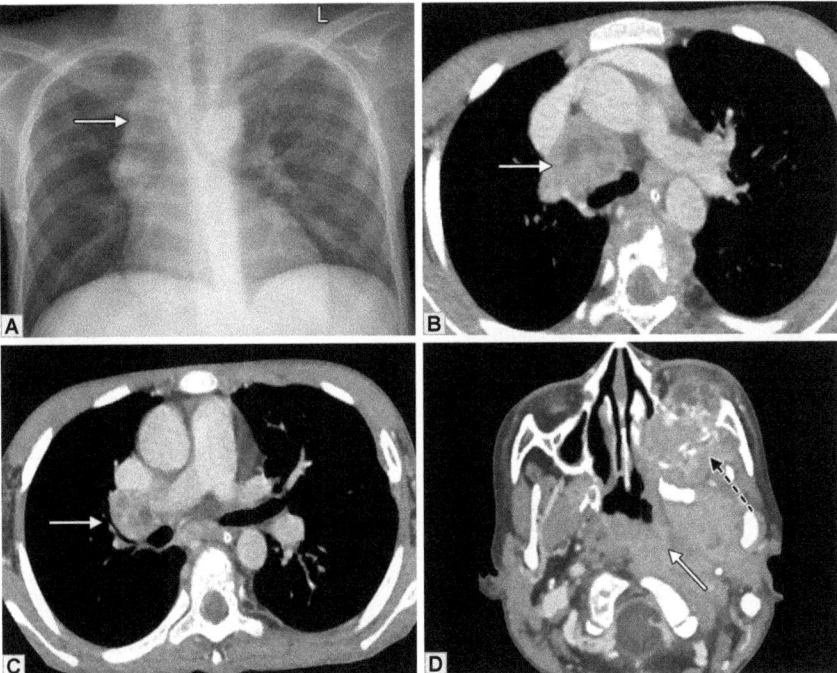

FIGS. 2A TO D: Solid middle mediastinal (visceral) mass. Metastatic lymphadenopathy from nasopharyngeal carcinoma in a 12-year-old boy—(A) Mediastinal widening extending till right hilum (arrow); (B) necrotic precarinal node (arrow); (C) necrotic right hilar lymph node (arrow); and (D) nasopharyngeal mass (arrow) with extension to left maxilla (dotted arrow).

POSTERIOR MEDIASTINAL MASSES (PARAVERTEBRAL COMPARTMENT)

- Chest radiographic signs are listed in Chapter 21.
- If the ITMIG compartment model is adopted then posterior mediastinum essentially includes only the vertebrae and paravertebral soft tissues.
- The most common masses are neurogenic tumors which may either arise from the peripheral nerves (nerve sheath tumors) or from the sympathetic ganglia. Paraganglioma is a rare tumor arising from chromaffin cells around the sympathetic ganglia.
- Neurogenic tumors comprise neurofibroma or schwannoma, neuroblastoma, ganglioneuroblastoma, or ganglioneuroma.
- Posterior mediastinal masses have limited differential diagnoses. An approach based on attenuation/morphology is listed in **Table 2**.

TABLE 2: Posterior mediastinal masses based on morphology and attenuation.		
Attenuation	**Neoplastic**	**Non-neoplastic**
Cystic	Cystic schwannoma	• Intrathoracic meningocele • Neurenteric cyst **(Figs. 3A to D)** • Spondylitis with collection abscess • Postoperative seroma • Pancreatic pseudocyst • Bochdalek's hernia
Solid		
Solid masses with moderate enhancement	• Ganglion cell tumors **(Figs. 4A to C)** • Peripheral nerve sheath tumors	
Intensely enhancing solid masses: • Unilateral • Bilateral	Paraganglioma	Extramedullary hematopoiesis

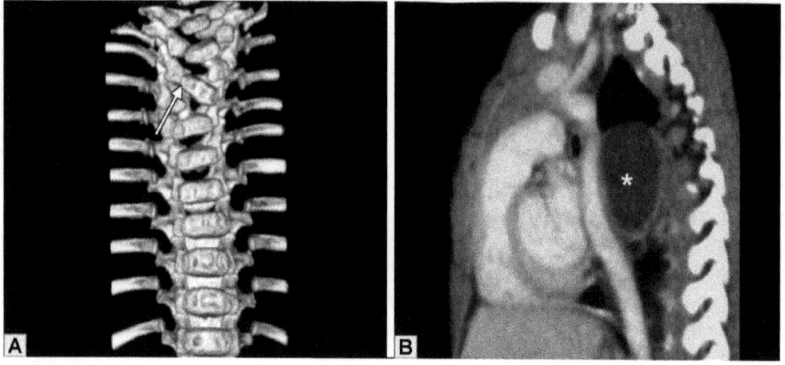

FIGS. 3A TO D: *Continued*

Continued

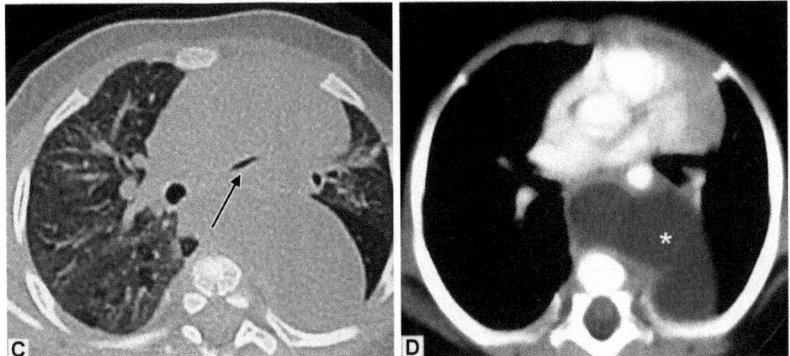

FIGS. 3A TO D: Cystic posterior mediastinal (paravertebral) mass. Neurenteric cyst in an infant—(A) Vertebral segmentation anomalies (arrow); (B) cystic lesion with thick wall (asterisk); (C) mass effect on left main bronchus (arrow); and (D) cyst located posterior to thoracic aorta, in the paravertebral space (asterisk).

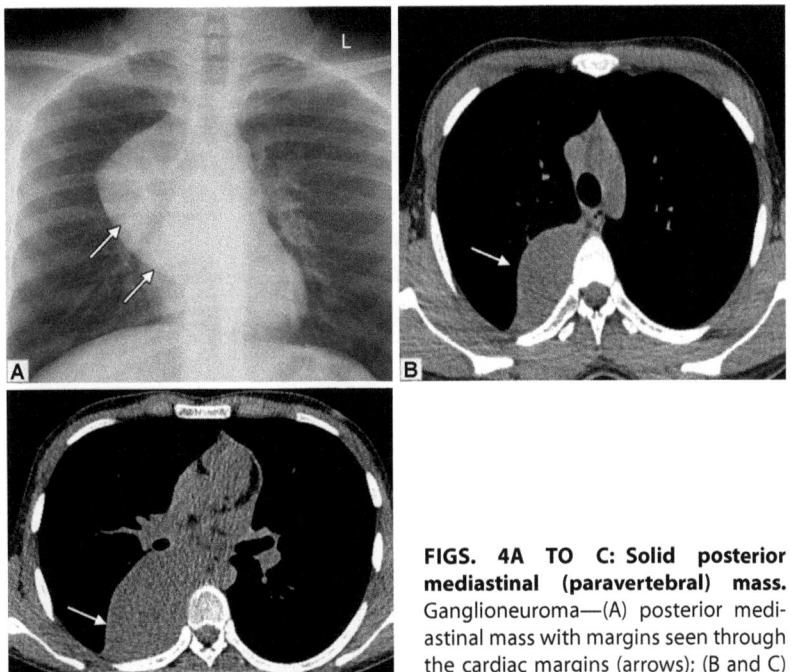

FIGS. 4A TO C: Solid posterior mediastinal (paravertebral) mass. Ganglioneuroma—(A) posterior mediastinal mass with margins seen through the cardiac margins (arrows); (B and C) solid paravertebral mass (arrow).

■ MULTICOMPARTMENTAL MASSES

Chest radiographic findings of multicompartmental masses include a combination of the findings of different mediastinal compartments **(Figs. 5A and B)**. The classification of multicompartmental masses based on their morphology is listed in **Table 3**.

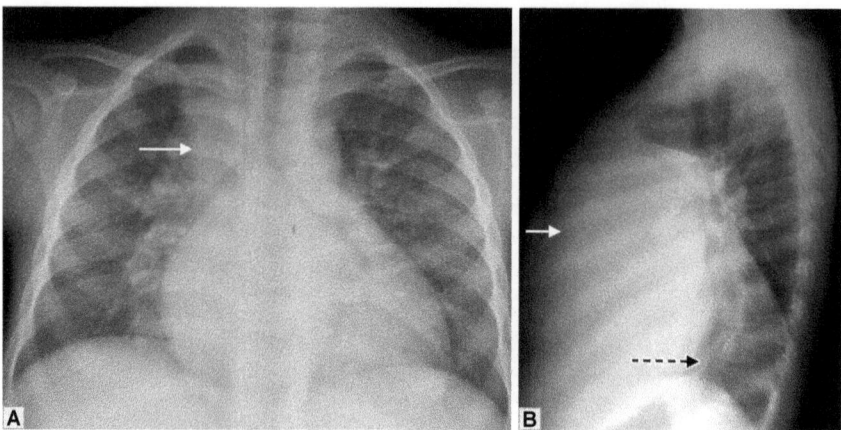

FIGS. 5A AND B: Multicompartmental mass on chest X-ray (A) posteroanterior (CXR PA) and (B) lateral view. (A) Mediastinal mass (arrow) and (B) loss of retrosternal lucency (arrow); spine sign (dotted arrow).

TABLE 3: Multicompartmental masses.		
Attenuation	**Neoplastic**	**Non-neoplastic**
Cystic		• Lymphatic malformation • Abscess
Solid		
Solid masses with moderate enhancement	• Infections (nodal/extranodal) **(Figs. 6A to C)** • Fibrosing mediastinitis • Immunoglobulin G4 (IgG4)-related diseases	• Infections (nodal/extranodal) • Fibrosing mediastinitis • IgG4-related diseases

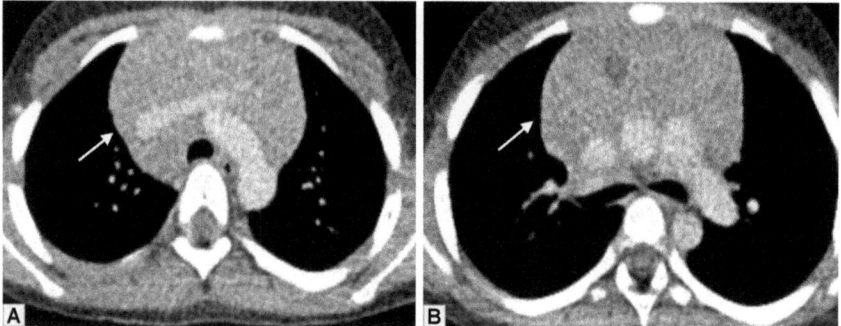

FIGS. 6A TO C: *Continued*

Continued

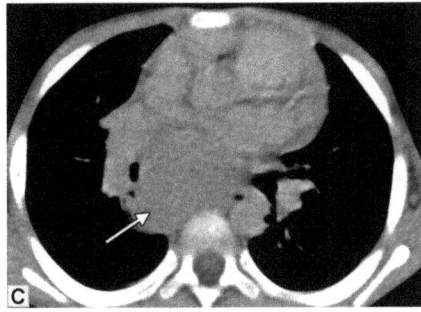

FIGS. 6A TO C: Multicompartmental masses on CT. Non-Hodgkin's lymphoma in a 5-year-old girl—(A and B) conglomerate prevascular nodal mass (arrow) and (C) subcarinal nodal mass (visceral compartmental) (arrow).

■ MASSES WHERE BIOPSY IS NOT INDICATED

- Some mediastinal masses have a characteristic imaging finding; hence biopsy is not indicated. Biopsy may even be detrimental due to risk of hemorrhage or introduction of infection.
- Mediastinal extension of goiter does not need to be sampled; however, sampling is required if a thyroid malignancy is suspected. A malignancy is suspected if a mass shows indistinct margins, or is associated with enlarged nodes (cervical/thoracic).
- Benign mature teratoma (dermoid cyst) with typical imaging features in young patients.
- Purely cystic, thymic cyst with no solid component. However, a mixed cystic-solid lesion or a cystic lesion with thick walls could represent a cystic teratoma.
- *Vascular mass (e.g., vascular malformation)*: Biopsy should be avoided (**Figs. 7A and B**).

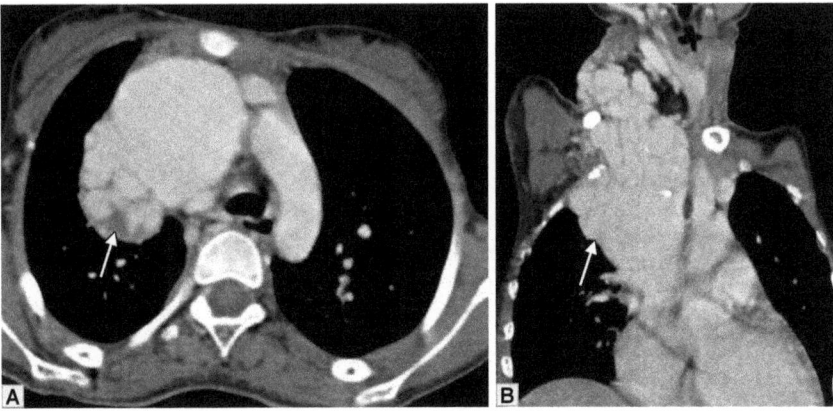

FIGS. 7A AND B: Mass where biopsy to be avoided. Intensely enhancing vascular malformation having cervicothoracic extension (arrow).

SPECIFIC ENTITIES

Tumors have been covered in Chapter 23.

Congenital Lesions

Developmental Cysts
- Developmental foregut cysts can be bronchogenic or enteric.
- Bronchogenic cysts are lined by respiratory epithelium. They are commonly located in the subcarinal or right paratracheal area in close proximity to the trachea or bronchus.
- Enteric duplication cysts are lined by gastrointestinal mucosa. Common locations include paraspinal position in the middle to posterior mediastinum near the esophagus **(Fig. 1)**. On ultrasound, a thick wall with layered appearance (gut signature) is considered characteristic of this entity **(Table 4)**.
- They might contain ectopic gastric mucosa, and cause hematemesis or melaena. Tc99m pertechnetate scan can detect ectopic gastric mucosa.
- Imaging findings of neurenteric cysts include a posterior mediastinal/multicompartmental thick-walled cystic lesion associated with vertebral anomalies **(Fig. 3)**. The intraspinal component of neurenteric cyst may be small and not well detected on imaging.

TABLE 4: Developmental cysts.

	Bronchogenic	Duplication	Neurenteric
Location	Right paratracheal, mediastinal, and rarely intrapulmonary	Subcarinal, close to esophagus	Posterior mediastinal, subcarinal
Wall	Thin	Thick, gut signature	Thick
Associated abnormality		Abdominal duplication cyst, ectopic gastric mucosa	Vertebral segmentation defects
Tc99m pertechnetate scan	No uptake	May show uptake due to presence of ectopic gastric mucosa	May show uptake due to presence of ectopic gastric mucosa

Nodal Enlargement
- Several infections can cause enlargement of mediastinal lymph nodes. Significant enlargement of mediastinal lymph nodes is considered when short axis diameter is >10 mm.
- *Infectious causes include*:
    - *Common organisms*:
        - Tuberculosis
        - Fungi such as histoplasmosis and coccidioidomycosis
        - Human immunodeficiency virus-acquired immunodeficiency syndrome (HIV-AIDS)

- Uncommon organisms:
  - Bacteria: *Streptococcus*, *Fusobacterium* species, *Corynebacterium* species, *Streptococcus milleri*, *Pseudomonas aeruginosa*, and *Burkholderia cepacia*
  - Viruses: Epstein–Barr virus (EBV), varicella-zoster virus, influenza viruses, dengue virus, and hantaviruses
  - Aspergillus, nontuberculous mycobacteria, and *Pneumocystis jirovecii* (rare, nodal involvement in immunocompromised individuals, especially AIDS)
- *Imaging features of common infectious causes*:
  - *Tuberculosis*:
    - Increased size of nodes (generally >2 cm diameter) with central hypodensity due to caseous necrosis.
    - The rim of inflammatory granulation tissue of the lymph node enhances on postcontrast images.
    - Perinodal fat stranding and conglomeration of the nodes are other characteristics.
    - Calcification within the nodes is also a common feature.
  - *Bacterial infections*: There is mild lymph node enlargement (generally <2 cm diameter), usually homogenous with maintained fatty hilum.
  - *Histoplasmosis*:
    - Enlarged low density lymph nodes with calcification associated with lung parenchymal nodules.
    - Mediastinal mass composed by enlarged caseous/liquified nodes with surrounding thin fibrous capsule forming mediastinal granuloma which occurs due to direct infection of lymph nodes by *Histoplasma capsulatum*. This can lead to fibrosing mediastinitis.
- *Noninfectious causes of mediastinal lymphadenopathy include*:
  - *Benign*: Sarcoidosis, rheumatoid arthritis, systemic lupus erythematosus (SLE), idiopathic pulmonary fibrosis, silicosis, drug-induced (phenytoin and methotrexate), chronic left heart failure, and Castleman's disease
  - *Malignant*: Lymphoma and metastases **(Figs. 8A to D)**
- Differentiating infectious from noninfectious causes of enlargement of mediastinal lymph nodes is challenging **(Tables 5 and 6)**. Clinical features and associated other lung parenchymal, pleural, or extrathoracic abnormalities should be taken into consideration.

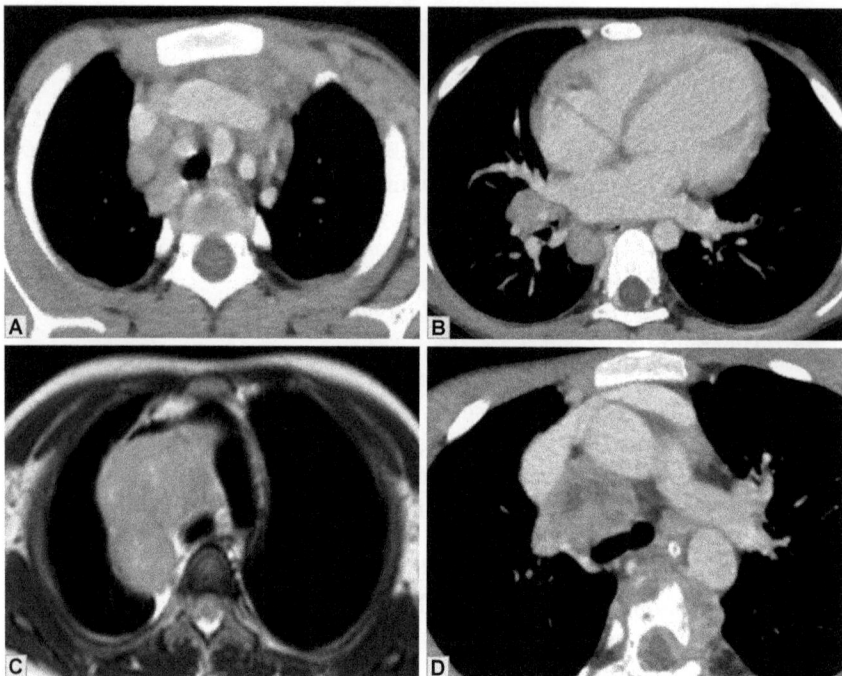

FIGS. 8A TO D: Nodal masses, three different patients. (A and B) Homogeneous discrete nodes in Hodgkin lymphoma; (C) T2W hyperintense conglomerate nodal mass in Hodgkin lymphoma; and (D) necrotic nodes in metastatic nasopharyngeal carcinoma.

TABLE 5: Features differentiating infectious from noninfectious causes of mediastinal lymphadenopathy.	
Features favoring infectious etiology	**Features favoring noninfectious etiology**
Presence of necrosis	May or may not show necrosis
Perinodal fat stranding	Less common
Conglomeration	Less common
• Calcification is a common feature • Coarse pattern	Uncommon in untreated metastases or lymphoma (when present, may be fine and rarely seen in metastases from thyroid carcinomas)
Associated lung changes include consolidation, cavity, and centrilobular nodules	Associated lung changes include primary mass and metastatic random nodules
Clinical features of fever, leukocytosis	Clinical features of primary malignancy, weight loss

TABLE 6: Differentiating features between tuberculosis, sarcoidosis, and lymphoma.

Attribute	Tuberculosis	Sarcoidosis	Lymphoma
Distribution pattern	Right hilar, right paratracheal, and subcarinal regions are involved more frequently	• Symmetrical bilateral hilar lymph nodes are involved most frequently • Bronchopulmonary node involvement is characteristic • Right paratracheal and subcarinal nodes are also seen	• Prevascular, para-aortic and paratracheal regions are typically involved • Subcarinal, pretracheal, aortopulmonary window, paraesophageal, internal mammary, retrocrural, epiphrenic nodes are also seen • Bilateral hilar region involvement is rare
Enhancement	• Peripheral or multilocular enhancement patterns (most common) • Homogenous enhancement (uncommon)	Homogeneous	• Homogeneous enhancement mostly • Homogenous enhancement mixed with peripherally enhancing nodes may be seen in some cases
Size	Usually, <4 cm	<4 cm	Usually, >4 cm
Conglomeration	Conglomeration present	Discrete, noncoalescent	• Discrete • Contiguous nodes involved
Calcification	Common, coarse, focal, and central	Icing sugar/egg-shell patterns are characteristic	Note seen in untreated cases
Perinodal fat	Obscured	Clean	Clean
Lung involvement	Centrilobular nodules, cavities	Perilymphatic nodules	• Uncommon • Large nodules/consolidation appears contiguous to the enlarged nodes

■ FIBROSING MEDIASTINITIS

- Fibrosing mediastinitis refers to a benign inflammatory process resulting in fibrosis and obstruction of mediastinal structure. It is a chronic inflammation of mediastinal connective tissue characterized by excessive proliferation of soft tissue composed of fibroblasts. It can be focal or diffuse; and a result of a host of infection (e.g., tuberculosis, histoplasmosis, cryptococcosis, and blastomycosis) or inflammatory diseases [e.g., immunoglobulin G4 (IgG4)-related diseases].

- On imaging, it appears a diffuse sheet-like mediastinal soft tissue and obstruction/compression of mediastinal vessels and/or aerodigestive tract.[3]
- Magnetic resonance imaging (MRI) has additional benefits over computed tomography (CT) in characterizing the mediastinal soft tissue. Mediastinal fibrosis usually appears as T1W and T2W hypointense, and shows homogeneous contrast enhancement.
- Two patterns of involvement of the mediastinum are described:
  1. *Focal*: There is a localized hilar or mediastinal (mostly subcarinal or right paratracheal region) soft tissue which frequently shows calcification **(Figs. 9A to D)**. This form is mostly associated with infectious causes.
  2. *Diffuse*: Homogenous soft tissue throughout the mediastinum. Calcification is less common in this form. This form is mostly associated with noninfectious causes or is idiopathic.
- *On CT*, the appearance is of a homogenous, infiltrative soft tissue density lesion in the mediastinum with or without calcification. Occlusion or narrowing of the critical mediastinal structures is seen which leads to various imaging findings tabulated in **Table 7**.
- *On MRI*, the soft tissue shows hypointense signal on T2-weighted image **(Figs. 9A to D)**, when the tissue is densely fibrotic, whereas areas of active inflammation show hyperintense signal. On T1-weighted images, the soft tissue shows intermediate signal intensity. Enhancement on postcontrast images is variable and depends on the amount of active inflammation which shows mild enhancement, while dense fibrotic regions show no enhancement.

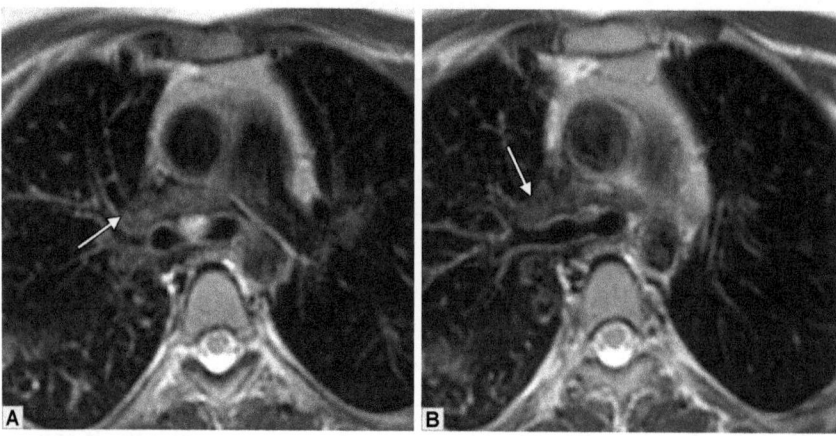

FIGS. 9A TO D: *Continued*

Continued

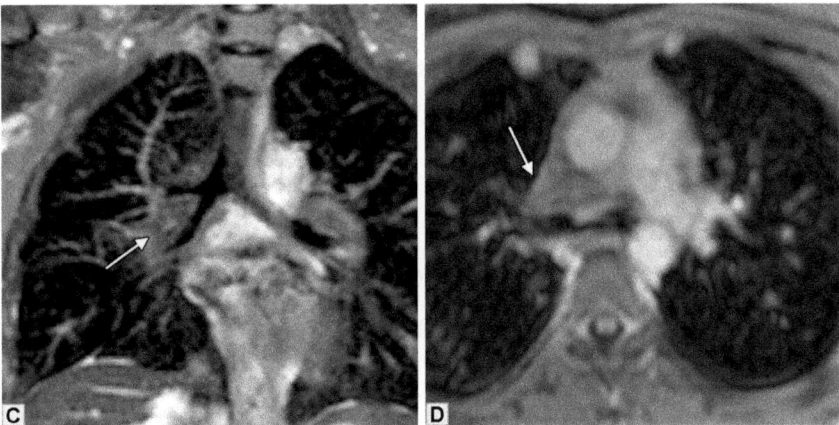

FIGS. 9A TO D: Fibrosing mediastinitis secondary to IgG4-related disease in a 13-year-old girl. (A and B) T2W hypointense soft tissue anterior to carina (arrow); (C) right hilar soft tissue contiguous to the mediastinal lesion (arrow); and (D) homogeneous postcontrast enhancement (arrow).

TABLE 7: CT findings of the secondary effects of fibrosing mediastinitis.

Encased structure	CT findings
Pulmonary artery (PA)	• Narrowing • Proximal dilatation • Distal oligemia or infarction
Superior vena cava (SVC)	• Extrinsic compression or thrombosis leading to SVC syndrome • Engorged venous collaterals
Trachea	Smooth stenosis
Major bronchi	• Smooth stenosis • Postobstructive pneumonitis or collapse
Pulmonary veins and lymphatics	Smooth interlobular septal thickening in lungs
Cardiac chamber	Compression or infiltration of the walls by the soft tissue
Aorta	• Narrowing of origin of major vessels • Wall thickening of aorta contiguous with mediastinal soft tissue
Esophagus	• Wall thickening • Barium swallow shows smooth long segment narrowing

■ CONCLUSION

Imaging based approach helps to reach reasonable differentials avoiding unnecessary biopsy.

Other Related Chapters that can be Referred to:
- Chapter 6: Congenital Lung Abnormalities
- Chapter 21: Approach to Mediastinal Lesions: Part 1
- Chapter 23: Thoracic Tumors and Mimics: Part 1
- Chapter 24: Thoracic Tumors and Mimics: Part 2

REFERENCES

1. Carter WB, Benveniste MF, Madan R, Godoy MC, de Groot PM, Truong MT, et al. ITMIG Classification of mediastinal compartments and multidisciplinary approach to mediastinal masses. Radiographics. 2017;37:413-36.
2. Whitten CR, Khan S, Munneke GJ, Grubnic S. A diagnostic approach to mediastinal abnormalities. Radiographics. 2007;27:657-71.
3. Garrana SH, Buckley JR, Rosado-de-Christenson ML, Martínez-Jiménez S, Muñoz P, Borsa JJ. Multimodality Imaging of focal and diffuse fibrosing mediastinitis. Radiographics. 201939:651-67.

SECTION 8

Tumors and Mimics

CHAPTER 23: Thoracic Tumors and Mimics: Part 1
CHAPTER 24: Thoracic Tumors and Mimics: Part 2

CHAPTER 23

Thoracic Tumors and Mimics: Part 1

Deeksha Bhalla, Akshay Baheti

- ❑ Spectrum of pediatric chest tumors
- ❑ Unique pediatric tumors
- ❑ Thoracic tumors with syndromic association
- ❑ Tumors presenting in neonates
- ❑ Imaging of region-specific tumors in children
  - ➤ Mediastinal tumors

■ INTRODUCTION

- The spectrum of chest tumors encountered in older children may be similar to adults, however, neonates, and younger children are afflicted by several unique entities. Amongst the primary thoracic neoplasms, mediastinal tumors are far more common than primary lung tumors.
- Also, there is a frequent delay in diagnosis in children, with several patients being treated for pneumonia for long.

■ SPECTRUM OF PEDIATRIC CHEST TUMORS

The spectrum of pediatric chest tumors is enlisted in **Table 1**.

■ UNIQUE PEDIATRIC TUMORS

- Certain neoplasms arise during differentiation of developing tissues and are encountered only in the pediatric age group. Several of them are "congenital tumors" and are detected either in utero or soon after birth.
- The terms "embryonal/dysembryonic/dysontogenetic tumors" are used for tumors arising from developing organs or tissues, e.g., neuroblastoma (NB), pleuropulmonary blastoma (PPB), and rhabdomyosarcoma.[1,2] Some of the nonthoracic tumors in this group for instance include Wilms tumor, hepatoblastoma, and pancreatoblastoma.

TABLE 1: Spectrum of pediatric thoracic tumors.		
Compartment	Benign	Malignant
Mediastinum	• GCT • Hemangioma • Schwannoma • Neurofibroma	• Lymphoma, leukemia • GNB, neuroblastoma • MPNST • Malignant GCTs
Lung	• Pulmonary hamartoma (<adults) • Sclerosing pneumocytoma (rare)	• Pleuropulmonary blastoma (PPB) • IMT • CPMT • Adenocarcinoma • LAM • Kaposi sarcoma (AIDS defining malignancy)
Airway	• Hemangioma • RRP (squamous papilloma)	• Carcinoid • MEC
Pleura	SFT	PPB
Chest wall	• Hemangioma • Lipoblastoma • Lipoma • Osteochondroma • Mesenchymal hamartoma	• Ewing's sarcoma family of tumors • Osteosarcoma • Infantile fibrosarcoma

(CPMT: congenital peribronchial myofibroblastic tumor; GCT: germ cell tumor; GNB: ganglio-neuroblastoma; IMT: inflammatory myofibroblastic tumor; MEC: mucoepidermoid carcinoma; MPNST: malignant peripheral nerve sheath tumor; RRP: recurrent respiratory papillomatosis; SFT: solitary fibrous tumor)

■ THORACIC TUMORS WITH SYNDROMIC ASSOCIATION

- Several of the pediatric tumors are associated with syndromes referred to as "cancer predisposition syndromes". While these constitute only a minority of pediatric tumors, the majority being sporadic; it is important to be aware of these to facilitate early recognition and planning screening in susceptible individuals.[3]
- Though inherited, all of these tumors may not present in childhood and often occur in adults.
- The thoracic tumors associated with the common syndromes are summarized in **Table 2**. The complete listing or discussion of the extrathoracic manifestations of these syndromes is beyond the scope of this chapter.

TABLE 2: Thoracic tumors with syndromic association.

Syndrome	Synonym	Inheritance mutation	Thoracic tumors	Nonthoracic manifestations
DICER1 syndrome	Pleuropulmonary blastoma—familial tumor dysplasia syndrome	Variable DICER1 gene	PPB	• Multilocular cystic nephroma (CN) • Wilms tumor • Ovarian Sertoli–Leydig tumor • Pituitary blastoma
Tuberous sclerosis	Bourneville disease	Autosomal dominant TSC1 or TSC2 genes	• LAM • Multifocal micronodular Pneumocyte hyperplasia (MMPH) • Cardiac rhabdomyomas	• Neurological • Renal • Cutaneous • Dental
Neurofibromatosis (NF) type 1	von Recklinghausen disease	Autosomal dominant NF-1 gene (on chromosome 17)	• Nerve sheath tumors • Rhabdomyosarcoma • PNET • MPNST	• Cutaneous neurofibromas • Optic nerve gliomas • Café-au-lait spots
Multiple endocrine neoplasia (MEN) type 2	MEN2-A or B	RET protooncogene	• Paragangliomas • Carcinoid tumors (infrequent association)	• Medullary thyroid carcinoma • Pheochromocytoma • Parathyroid hyperplasia or adenomas

(LAM: lymphangioleiomyomatosis; MPNST: malignant peripheral nerve sheath tumor; PNET: primitive neuroendocrine tumor; PPB: pleuropulmonary blastoma; RET: rearranged during transfection; TSC: tuberous sclerosis)

TUMORS PRESENTING IN NEONATES

- Tumors in the neonatal period are often distinct from those encountered in older children. Several of these are detected antenatally and cause significant fetal morbidity. Moreover, the majority of these tumors are benign. The knowledge of their characteristic locations and appearance is essential to avoid misdiagnosis.
- Thoracic tumors encountered in neonates include:
  - *Anterior mediastinum*: Teratoma (immature) and hemangioma
  - *Middle mediastinum*: All tumors rare in this age group

- *Cardiac*: Rhabdomyomas
- *Posterior mediastinum*: NB
- *Pulmonary*: PPB and congenital peribronchial myofibroblastic tumor (CPMT)
- *Chest wall*: Hemangioma, lipoma, lipoblastoma/lipoblastomatosis, and congenital mesenchymal hamartoma

■ IMAGING OF REGION-SPECIFIC TUMORS IN CHILDREN

Region specific division for the purpose of discussion is done as follows:
- Mediastinal tumors (Part I)
- Pulmonary, airway and chest wall tumors (Chapter 24)
- Brief discussion of disorders will also be present other chapters such as Chapters 21 and 22.

Mediastinal Tumors

Mediastinum is the most common thoracic compartment involved by primary neoplasms, with anterior mediastinum being the most frequent site.

Germ Cell Tumors
Teratomas

Teratomas are tumors that have elements derived from all three germinal layers (ectoderm, mesoderm, and endoderm).

Mature teratoma (MA):
- Greek word "terato"; means a monster. MTs are the most frequent mediastinal germ cell tumor (GCT) (up to 75%). These occur within or close to the thymus. About 3% MTs may occur in posterior mediastinum.
- *Synonyms*: "Dermoid cyst"—this term is used when ectoderm elements predominate, wherein there is a cyst containing mucous and hair.

Pathology: These tumors contain *mature* elements arising from the three germinal layers (at least 2 out of 3). These elements include:
- *Ectoderm*: Skin, hair, dermal appendages, and squamous epithelium-lined cysts
- *Endoderm*: Pancreatic tissue
- *Mesoderm*: Bone, cartilage, and muscle
- *Rokitansky protuberances*: This is the solid component of tumor, comprising of varying histology seen in up to 80% of tumors.
- In presence of other GCT elements, the tumor is labeled as mixed GCT and is treated as nonseminomatous GCT (NSGCT).

- An important concept is that while testicular MAs have potential to metastasize, same lesions in the mediastinum behave as benign tumors.

Clinical features:
- MTs are encountered in children or young adults, who are often asymptomatic with lesions being incidentally detected in chest radiograph (CXR).
- Huge tumors result in compression of adjoining structures with symptoms of cough or dyspnea, or even chest pain.
- Tumors can rupture into bronchus, lung, pleural, or pericardial space, with resultant symptoms. A typical symptom is expectoration of hair (trichoptysis) or oily substances.

Imaging findings:
- *CXR:* MTs appear as well-defined anterior mediastinal masses, projecting to one side usually **(Fig. 1)**. Calcification is reported in up to 40% cases and is due to either tumor calcification or teeth/mature bone in tumor. Rarely a fat-fluid level is seen on CXR itself.
- *Ultrasonography (USG)*: Demonstrate the cystic content and fat **(Figs. 2A and B)**; although computed tomography (CT) is superior for extent assessment.

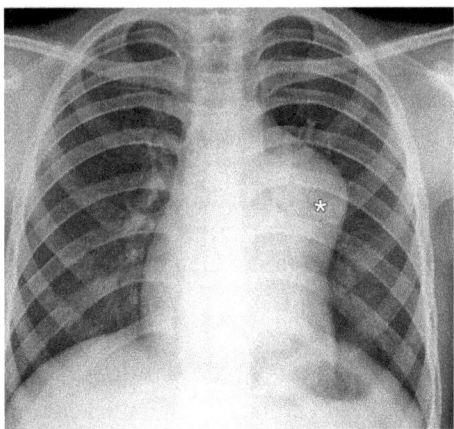

FIG. 1: Anterior mediastinal (prevascular) mature teratoma in a 10-year-old boy. Mass (asterisk) with a broad base towards the mediastinum and silhouetting of left heart border. The mass projects on one side of the mediastinal contour (compared to seminoma which extends on both the sides).

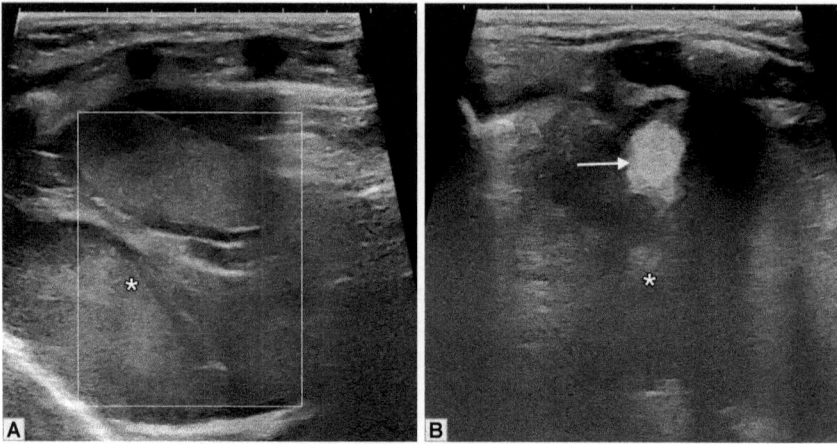

FIGS. 2A AND B: Anterior mediastinal (prevascular) cystic mature teratoma in a **newborn.** (A) USG chest: cystic lesion (asterisk) and (B) echogenic focus of fat (arrow) in nondependent location.

Computed tomography:
- CT appearance shows all three components of fluid, fat, and calcification.
- The tumor is often mainly cystic, with interspersed soft tissue component.
- The content of the cysts may be of fluid attenuation or more frequently of high density.
- Fat component is variable, with a fat nodule or large areas of fat **(Figs. 3A and B)**. Fat-fluid levels may be seen.
- Calcification is present in the capsule or within the tumor; and is linear/punctate. Teeth or even bone such as structures may be seen.
- The tumor is located in prevascular space, in close relation to the pericardium.
- On contrast administration, there is enhancement of the cyst wall and septae.

Complications:
- Following rupture, the cyst shows air-fluid levels, with adjoining consolidation, pleural/pericardial effusion, thickening and enhancement, depending on the site of rupture **(Figs. 4 and 5)**.
- Due to the prevascular location, a common site of rupture is the right middle lobe bronchus with lobar consolidation.
- Malignant transformation in mediastinal MTs is extremely rare; unlike the MTs elsewhere in the body.
- However, the presence of a suspicious solid component from the wall, especially showing infiltration into adjacent fat, should raise suspicion.

CHAPTER 23: Thoracic Tumors and Mimics: Part 1

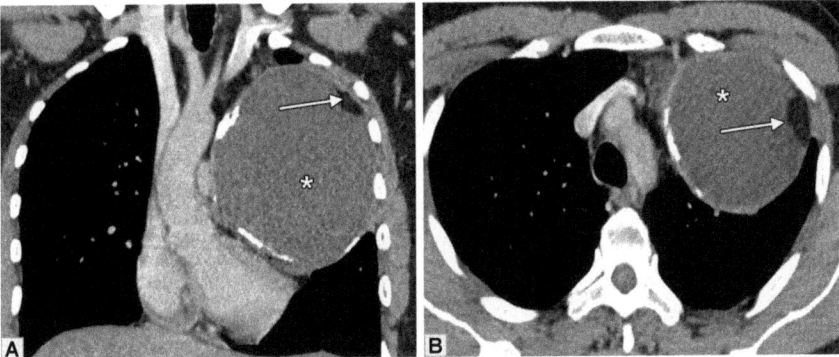

FIGS. 3A AND B: Mature cystic teratoma/dermoid cyst of anterior mediastinum (prevascular space). Well-defined cystic attenuation mass in anterior mediastinum (asterisks) and rim calcification and fat component (arrows).

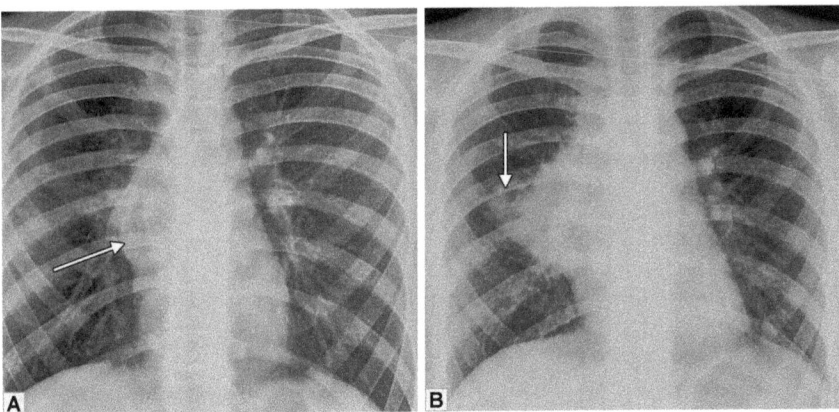

FIGS. 4A AND B: Ruptured dermoid cyst on CXR. (A and B) Intrabronchial rupture of anterior mediastinal dermoid in a 15-year-old male—(A) anterior mediastinal mass (arrow) on baseline image and (B) apparent increase in size with irregular margins; adjacent consolidation (arrow).

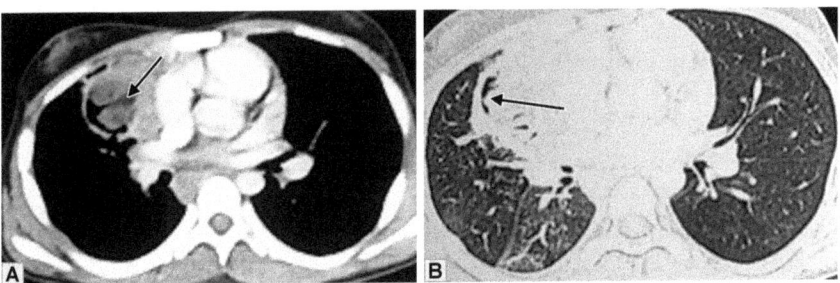

FIGS. 5A TO F: *Continued*

Continued

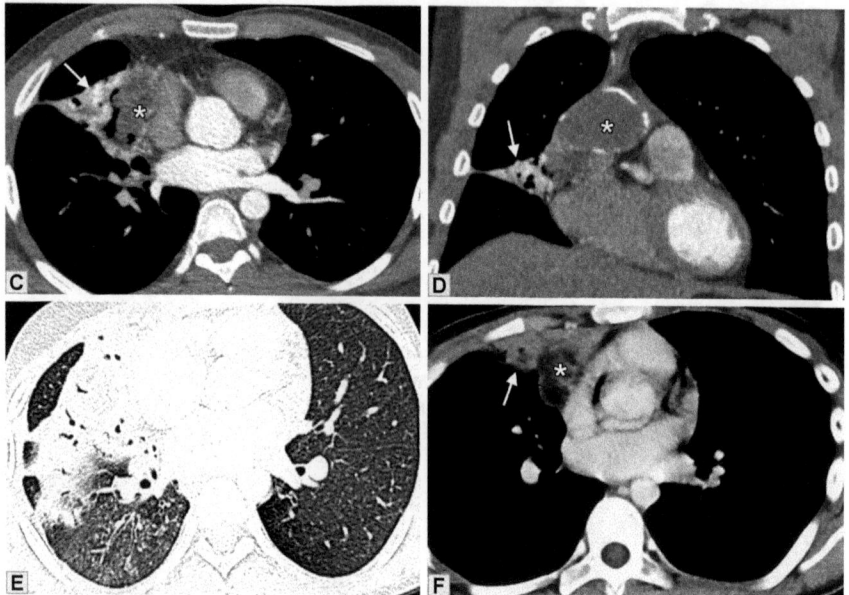

FIGS. 5A TO F: Ruptured Dermoid cyst on CT. Intrabronchial rupture of anterior mediastinal (prevascular) dermoid—(A) prevascular space mass (arrow) with fat density and (B) air crescent sign (arrow). Intrabronchial rupture leading to middle lobe collapse—(C) cystic mass with rim calcification (asterisk) with right middle lobe collapse; (D) right middle lobe collapse (arrow); (E) extensive consolidation of right middle lobe and centrilobular nodules in lower lobe; and (F) pleural spread (arrow) in ruptured anterior mediastinal teratoma (asterisk).

Magnetic resonance imaging (MRI) **(Box 1)**:
- On MRI, the tumors appear heterogeneous, with solid areas, and cystic areas of variable signal intensity.
- While the solid areas are isointense to muscle, cystic areas usually show variable T1 signal intensity and can be hypo- or hyperintense depending on the amount of sebaceous material. On T2-weighted image (T2WI), these are hyperintense.
- Contrast-enhanced MRI (CEMRI) shows peripheral and septal enhancement.
- Adjoining inflammation may be seen even in unruptured tumors.

BOX 1 | **Magnetic resonance imaging features of mature teratoma (Figs. 6A to C).**

- Sebaceous fat in cyst (hyperintense cyst on T1-weighted image)
- Fat–fluid level
- *Chemical shift imaging*: Dark line between fat and fluid
- Rokitansky protuberances appear as "palm tree like" areas projecting inside from the cyst lining
- *Focal thickening/extramural extension*: Suspect malignancy

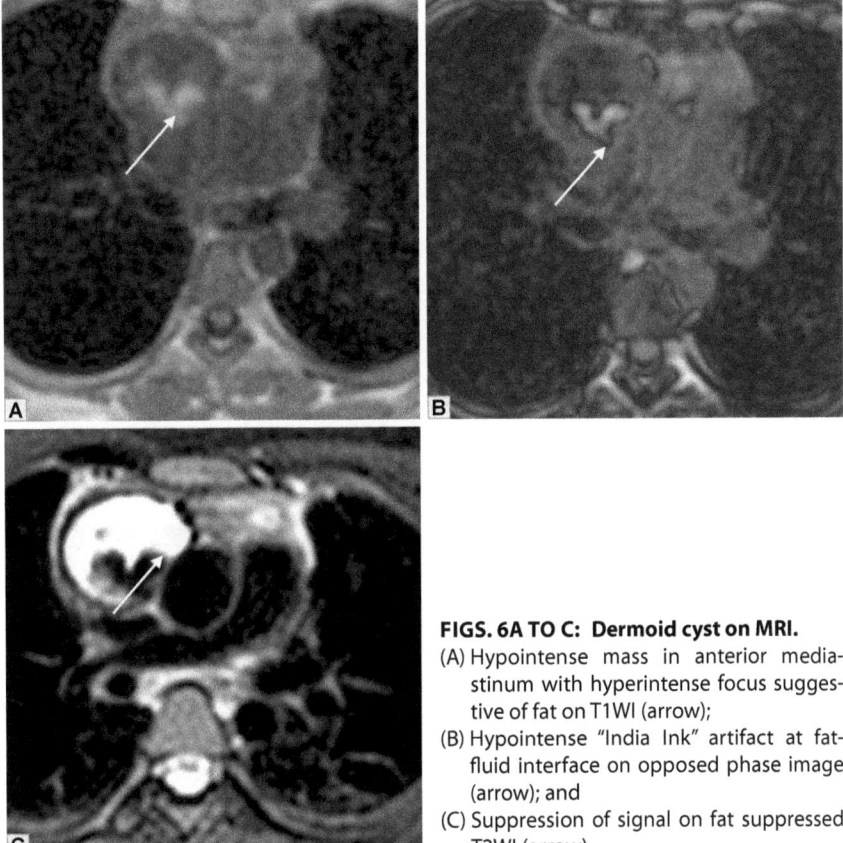

FIGS. 6A TO C: Dermoid cyst on MRI.
(A) Hypointense mass in anterior mediastinum with hyperintense focus suggestive of fat on T1WI (arrow);
(B) Hypointense "India Ink" artifact at fat-fluid interface on opposed phase image (arrow); and
(C) Suppression of signal on fat suppressed T2WI (arrow).

Management:
- Surgical resection is the treatment of choice for MTs.
- In ruptured MTs, surgery often requires resection of involved adjoining lung.

Immature teratomas:
- Immature teratomas are rare tumors, containing elements from the three germinal layers, admixed with immature foci. The immature elements can be small, or involve almost the entire tumor.
- The immature elements in these tumors are predominantly neuroectodermal. These form the "solid" component of tumor.
- Immature teratomas are encountered in infants and young children, wherein even the immature elements show a benign behavior **(Figs. 7A and B)**. However, immature elements if present in adults are aggressive in behavior similar to NSGCTs, with a poorer prognosis.
- The diagnostic criteria for these tumors are not clear, as these are rare. On imaging, these present with predominantly multilocular cystic masses with smaller foci of fat and septal/mural calcifications **(Figs. 8A to C)**.
- Differentiating mature from immature teratoma is challenging. The key points are highlighted in **Box 2**.

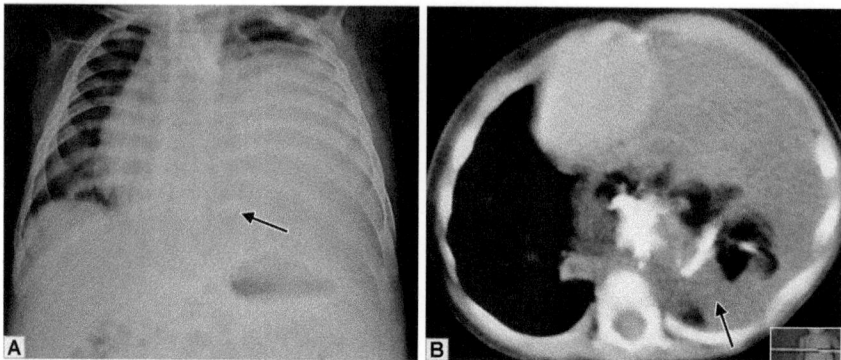

FIGS. 7A AND B: Immature teratoma of the posterior mediastinum (prevascular space) in an infant. (A) Large mass in left hemithorax with area of calcification (arrow) and (B) mass having calcification and fat as well as large soft tissue component (arrow).

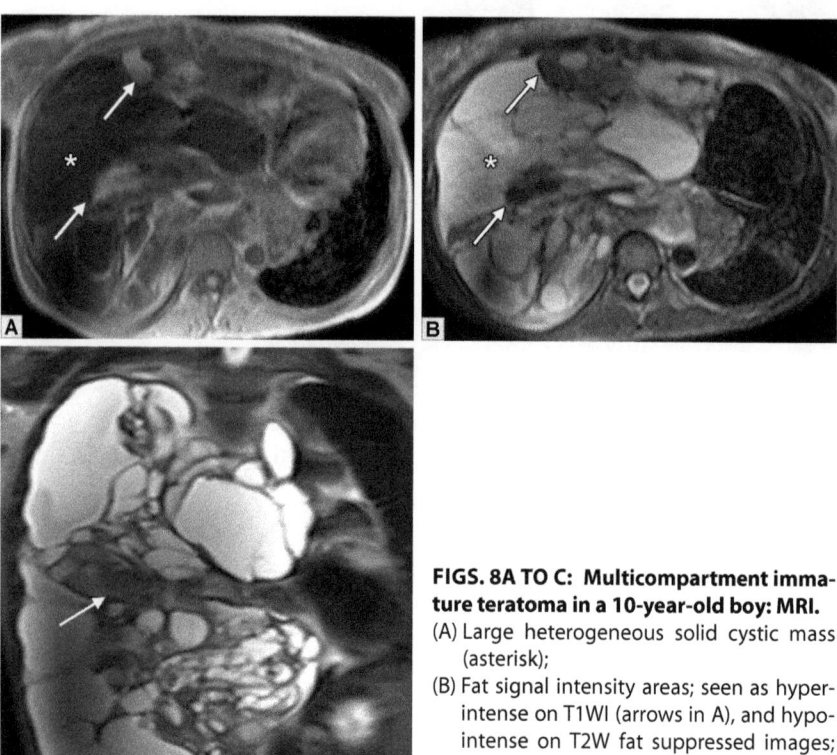

FIGS. 8A TO C: Multicompartment immature teratoma in a 10-year-old boy: MRI.
(A) Large heterogeneous solid cystic mass (asterisk);
(B) Fat signal intensity areas; seen as hyperintense on T1WI (arrows in A), and hypointense on T2W fat suppressed images; and
(C) Thick internal septations and soft tissue components (arrow in C).

> **BOX 2 Immature versus mature teratomas.**
> - Both are encapsulated, large tumors
> - Solid component is larger in immature teratoma. MTs have Rokitansky protuberances showing as solid component
> - Immature teratomas have scattered foci of fat/calcification, MTs show larger areas with more evolved differentiation (teeth, bone, etc.)
> - Alpha-fetoprotein (AFP) is raised in almost half of immature teratomas, not in MTs

Seminoma:
- Seminomas comprise up to 40% of all mediastinal GCTs, and are the most common malignant form of these tumors. Tumor cells of this neoplasm are very similar to the primordial germ cells.
- These are slow-growing tumors that are often large at the time of diagnosis.
- Seminomas typically affect males, usually in adolescent or older age groups. The equivalent tumor in girls is termed as dysgerminoma.

Laboratory investigations:
- Beta human chorionic gonadotropin (hCG) is known to be elevated in NSGCTs, but can be increased (>1,000 IU/L) in about a third of seminomas.
- AFP is not elevated.

Imaging:
- Characteristic of seminomas is their uniform, homogenous appearance reflecting their pathology.
- Seminomas are large anterior mediastinal masses, often extending to both sides of the mediastinum.

Nonseminomatous Germ Cell Tumors

Among the mediastinal NSGCTs, yolk sac tumor is the most frequent entity comprising about 60% of the cases. This is unlike the gonads and retroperitoneum, where embryonal carcinoma is more common.

Clinical presentation:
- Age profile is same as seminomas (second to fourth decade) are more frequent in males.
- An important clinical association is between mediastinal NSGCTs and hematological manifestations. The reported hematological disorders include leukemia (myelogenous/megakaryocytic), myelodysplasia, mastocytosis, and histiocytosis.
- Unlike seminomas, most patients are symptomatic which include systemic and local manifestations, including SVC syndrome.
- Gynecomastia is seen in choriocarcinoma (due to hCG).

The pathological features of major subtypes is shown in **Table 3**.

SECTION 8: Tumors and Mimics

TABLE 3: Pathological features of NSGCT subtypes.

Entity	Tumor cells	Hemorrhage/ necrosis	Laboratory investigation
Embryonal carcinoma	Anaplastic embryonal cells Ill-defined margins	Punctate	Increased AFP
Yolk sac tumor	Primitive cells with bizarre, hyperchromatic nucleus	++	Increased AFP
Choriocarcinoma	• Trophoblastic cells (cyto or syncytio) • Often mixed cell types	++	Increased beta-hCG

(AFP: alpha-fetoprotein; hCG: human chorionic gonadotropin; NSGCT: nonseminomatous germ cell tumor)

Imaging:
- NSGCTs are large, anterior mediastinal masses, similar to seminoma.
- However, areas of hemorrhage and necrosis are far more frequent in NSGCTs (especially yolk sac tumor and choriocarcinoma).
- Also, these tumors may have infiltrative margins with involvement of surrounding structures **(Figs. 9A to F)**.
- Pleural and lymph nodal enlargements are also seen.
- MRI demonstrates no specific features except the hemorrhage, necrosis, and resultant heterogeneous enhancement better seen. It may be performed to evaluate their relationship with adjacent large vessels and the heart, for presurgical planning.
- Solid components can exhibit restricted diffusion (similar to seminomas).

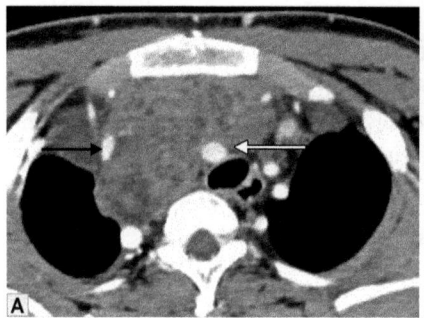
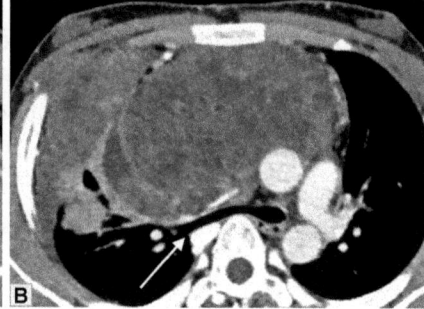

FIGS. 9A TO F: *Continued*

Continued

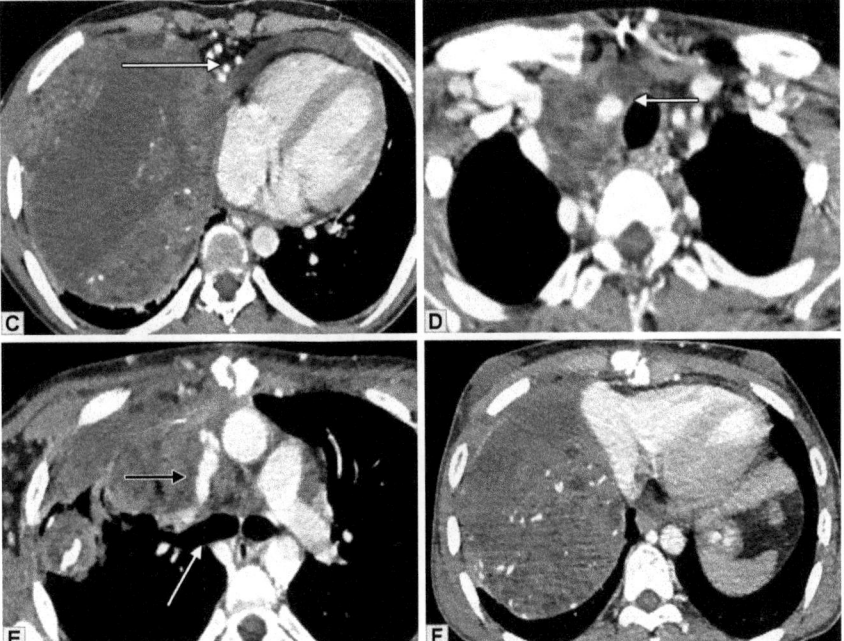

FIGS. 9A TO F: Nonseminomatous germ cell tumor in a 16-year-old boy. (A to C) Baseline imaging—(A) heterogeneous anterior mediastinal mass encasing brachiocephalic artery (BCA), superior vena cava (SVC); (B) airway compression (arrow); and (C) pericardial thickening (arrow). (D to F) Postchemotherapy—(D and E) Shrunken mass with persistent encasement of BCA, SVC (arrow). (F) Airway compression and pericardial thickening have resolved.

Neuroblastoma

- Neuroblastoma that arises primarily in the thorax from the sympathetic ganglia is referred to as thoracic neuroblastoma (TNBL). Adrenal NB may also extend into the chest through the retrocrural space, but these tumors are not labeled as TNBL.
- While TNBL account for less than one-fifth of all NBs, these are the most frequent solid mediastinal masses in children under 2 years.
- TBNLs have an earlier age of presentation and a better prognosis than abdominal NB. TNBLs disseminate less frequently, and in children <2 years may show spontaneous resolution.
- Some key features of TNBL are summarized in **Box 3 (Figs. 10A to C)**.

BOX 3 | **Features of thoracic neuroblastoma.**

- Earlier age of presentation
- Higher incidence of opsoclonus-myoclonus
- Less dissemination
- Better prognosis
- Commonest location is paraspinal (posterior mediastinum)
- Less frequent site is anterior mediastinum
- Calcification is less commonly seen as compared to abdominal neuroblastomas

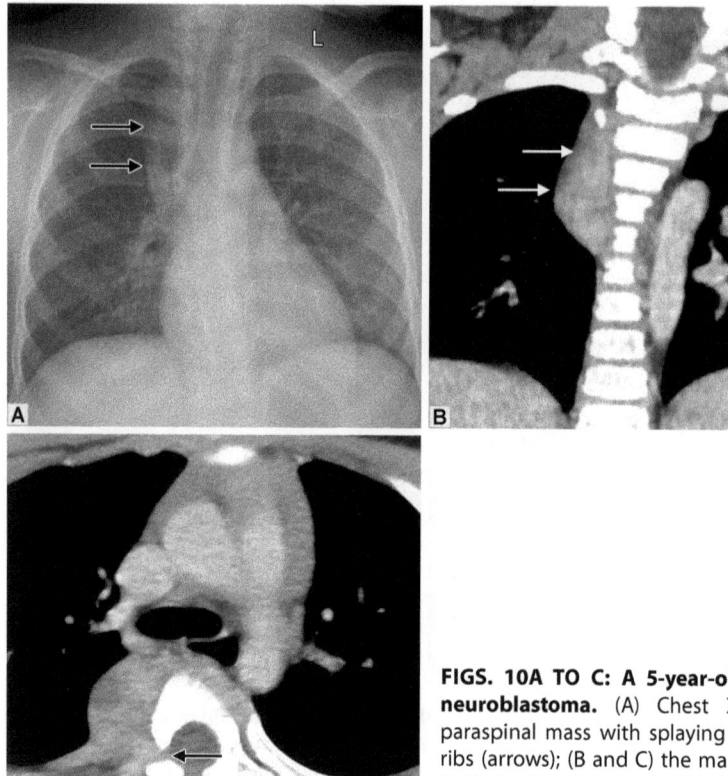

FIGS. 10A TO C: A 5-year-old girl with neuroblastoma. (A) Chest X-ray: Right paraspinal mass with splaying of posterior ribs (arrows); (B and C) the mass has longitudinal > transverse extension (white arrows) as well as intraspinal extension (black arrow).

- The complete discussion of diagnosis, staging, and management of NB is beyond the scope of this book. Some key points relevant to thoracic involvement have been highlighted here and in Chapter 22.
- The imaging features of NB are further discussed in Chapter 22.
- The staging system employed for staging of NB is the International Neuroblastoma Risk Group Staging System (INRGSS).
- INRGSS has defined some imaging-based features, the presence of which places the tumor in L2 stage (Vs L1). These are referred to as image-defined risk factors (IDRFs).
- For thoracic disease, the *IDRFs* include encasement by the tumor of the following structures—aorta, its major branches; compression of trachea and main bronchi and/or costovertebral junction involvement (at levels T9-T12). Intraspinal extension for more than one-third of its cross-sectional diameter or cord compression also constitute IDRFs.[4]
- For disease at level of thoracic inlet (cervicothoracic disease), the IDRFs include compression of trachea or encasement of any one the following structures—subclavian vessels, carotid artery, vertebral artery, or brachial plexus roots.

Nerve Sheath Tumors

- Benign entities include schwannoma and neurofibroma, while malignant lesions are represented by malignant peripheral nerve sheath tumor (MPNST).
- Uncommon in the pediatric population except in the setting of Neurofibromatosis 1 (NF1).
- Typical imaging manifestation of neurofibroma is a homogenous posterior mediastinal mass oriented perpendicular to the spinal axis rather than parallel (unlike NB, which is oriented along the longitudinal axis) which may have intraspinal extension along spinal nerves. In the setting of NF1, multiple neurofibromas arising from intercostal as well as peripheral nerves are present.[4]
- Plexiform neurofibroma, a lesion characteristic of NF1 (**Figs. 11A to C**). There is contiguous infiltration of skin, subcutaneous tissue, muscle, and bone, causing diffuse mediastinal widening. On MR, the lesions are hyperintense on T2 with characteristic central hypointense dot due to collagen deposition. Homogeneous low attenuation is seen on CT. Cervicothoracic extension is also not uncommon.

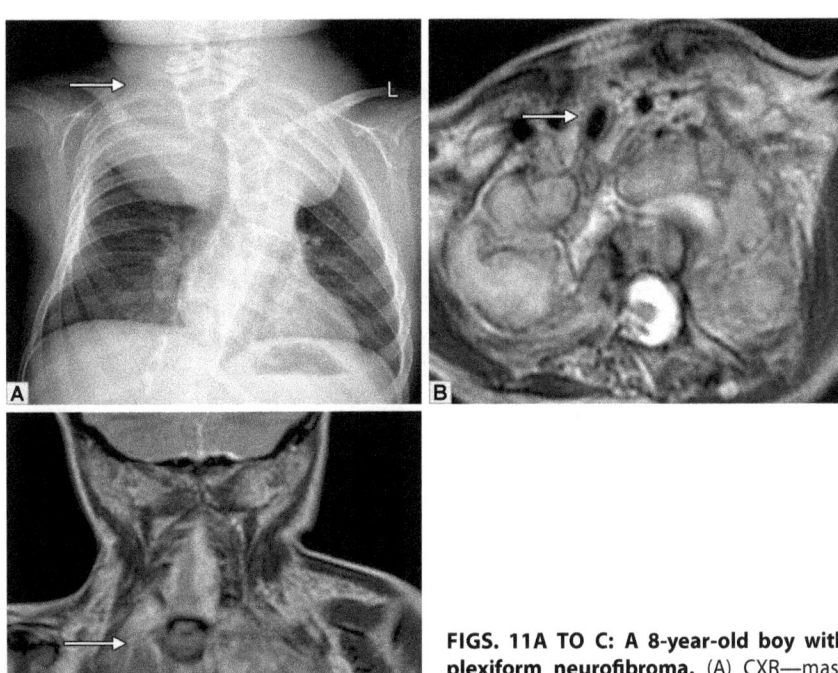

FIGS. 11A TO C: A 8-year-old boy with plexiform neurofibroma. (A) CXR—mass with symmetric extension on both side of mediastinum with cervicothoracic extension (arrow) and scoliosis. (B and C) T2W MRI—lobulated, homogenous mass at thoracic inlet with airway displacement and cervical extension (arrow).
(CXR: chest X-ray; MRI: magnetic resonance imaging)

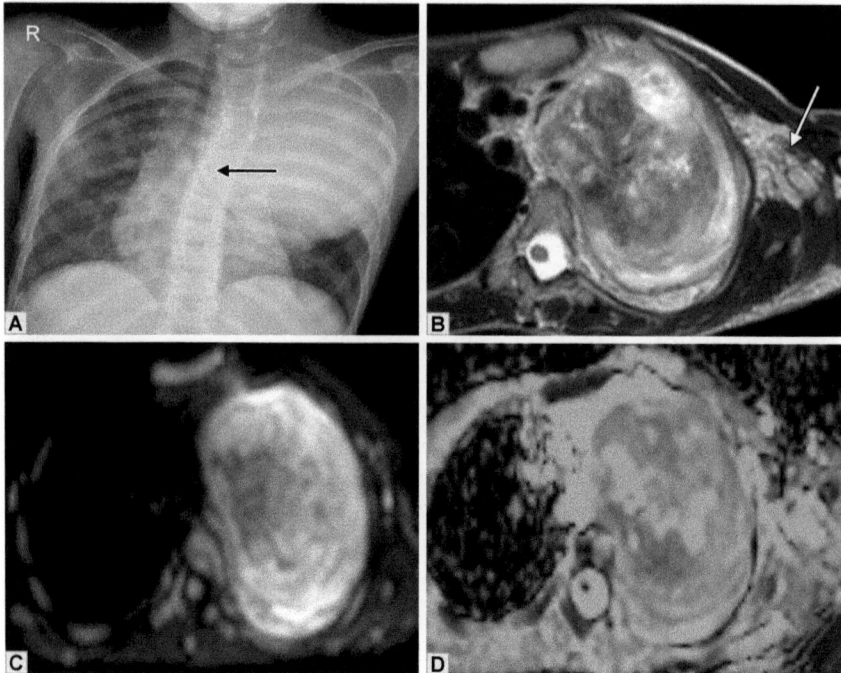

FIGS. 12A TO D: A 9-year-old boy with malignant peripheral nerve sheath tumor.
(A) CXR—eccentric mediastinal mass with scoliosis, rib splaying, and narrowing of left main bronchus (arrow); (B) T2W MRI—heterogeneous tumor; (C and D) DWI and ADC—peripheral diffusion restriction. Plexiform NF seen in axilla (white arrow in B).

(ADC: apparent diffusion coefficient; CXR: chest X-ray; DWI: diffusion-weighted images; NF: neurofibromatosis; MRI: magnetic resonance imaging)

- The incidence of MPNST in NF1 is 2–5%, compared to general population incidence of 0.001%. Deep plexiform neurofibromas themselves predispose to the development of MPNST.[5]
- On imaging, large size, intratumoral heterogeneity and irregular margins are suggestive **(Figs. 12A to D)**. Peripheral enhancement, perilesional edema, and intratumoral cysts are other factors suggesting malignant transformation.

Lymphoma/Leukemia

- Lymphoma is not only the most common malignant mass in thorax, but also the most common mediastinal mass encountered in children.
- Non-Hodgkin lymphoma (NHL) forms of lymphoma are more frequent than Hodgkin lymphoma (HL). In addition, even leukemia may sometimes present with anterior mediastinal masses, particularly patients with T-cell type acute lymphoblastic leukemia (T-ALL).[6-8]
- The most common location is the anterior mediastinum, followed by both anterior and superior mediastinal extension. Anterior and middle mediastinal extension is also a potential pattern of involvement.

- In HL, mediastinal masses are of nodal origin while in NHL, they are due to thymic infiltration.
- The subtype of lymphoma affects the imaging manifestations. High-grade tumors often show central necrosis **(Figs. 13 and 14)**. The pointers to specific pathological diagnosis are mentioned in **Table 4**.
- In addition, superior vena cava (SVC) syndrome and superior mediastinal syndrome (SMS), which refers to SVC as well as airway compression are medical emergencies that must be reported, if found at imaging. Rather, airway compression must be evaluated on radiographs prior to CT imaging since supine positioning can worsen the compromise.
- The Ann Arbor staging system is used for HL. For NHL, the St. Jude's system is preferred in children over the Lugano system due to predominant extranodal involvement.

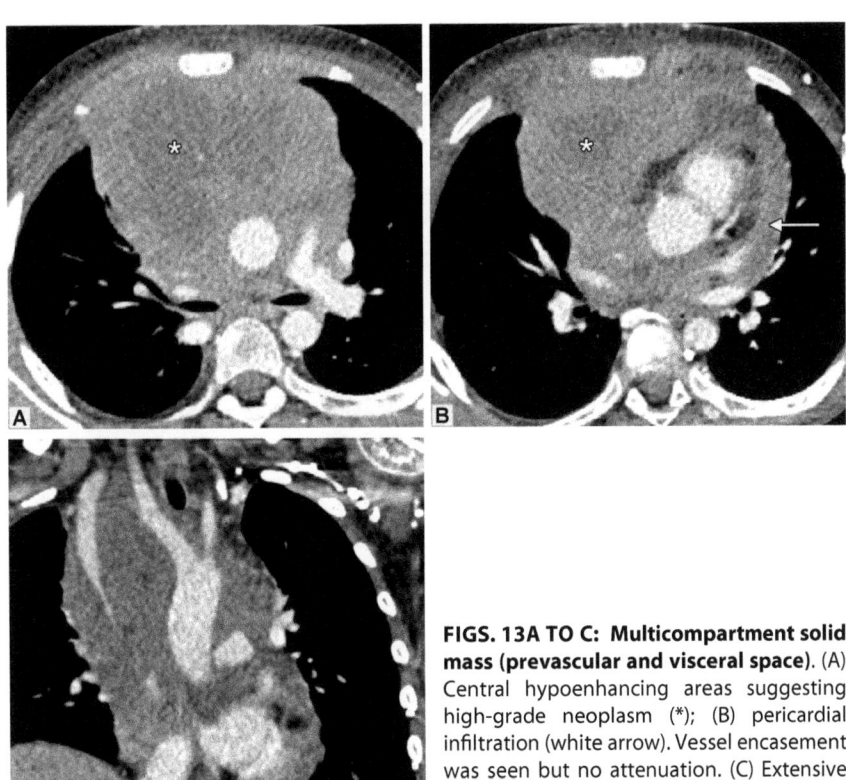

FIGS. 13A TO C: Multicompartment solid mass (prevascular and visceral space). (A) Central hypoenhancing areas suggesting high-grade neoplasm (*); (B) pericardial infiltration (white arrow). Vessel encasement was seen but no attenuation. (C) Extensive vascular encasement with maintained caliber, characteristic of *hematolymphoid neoplasms*.

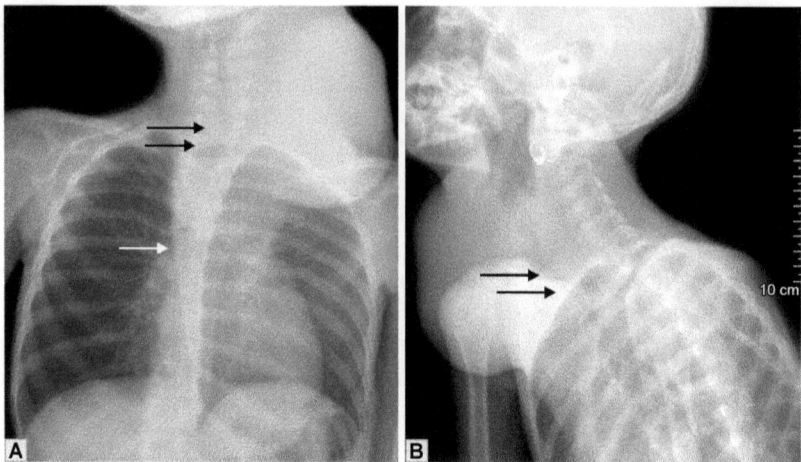

FIGS. 14A AND B: A 13-year-old girl with diffuse large B-cell lymphoma. (A) Large neck mass causing narrowing of the airway (black arrows) (B) Azygoesophageal stripe displacement suggesting mediastinal component (black arrows).

TABLE 4: Imaging features of lymphoma subtypes.	
Imaging features	**Lymphoma subtype**
Bulky disease (more than one-third of transthoracic diameter; >10 cm diameter)	T-ALL and T-lymphoblastic lymphoma > HL
Pleural effusion	T-ALL, T-lymphoblastic lymphoma, and Burkitt lymphoma (mediastinal/abdominal)
Cervical lymphadenopathy: • Isolated • With mediastinal mass	 • HL • NHL>HL
Discrete nodal masses	HL
Localized mediastinal involvement	Primary mediastinal large B-cell lymphoma
Multisystem involvement	Diffuse large B-cell lymphoma **(Fig. 15)** and Burkitt lymphoma
Lung masses	NHL
Posttreatment: • Residual fibrotic tissue • No residual tissue	 • HL • NHL
(HL: Hodgkin lymphoma; NHL: non-Hodgkin lymphoma; T-ALL: T-cell acute lymphoblastic leukemia)	

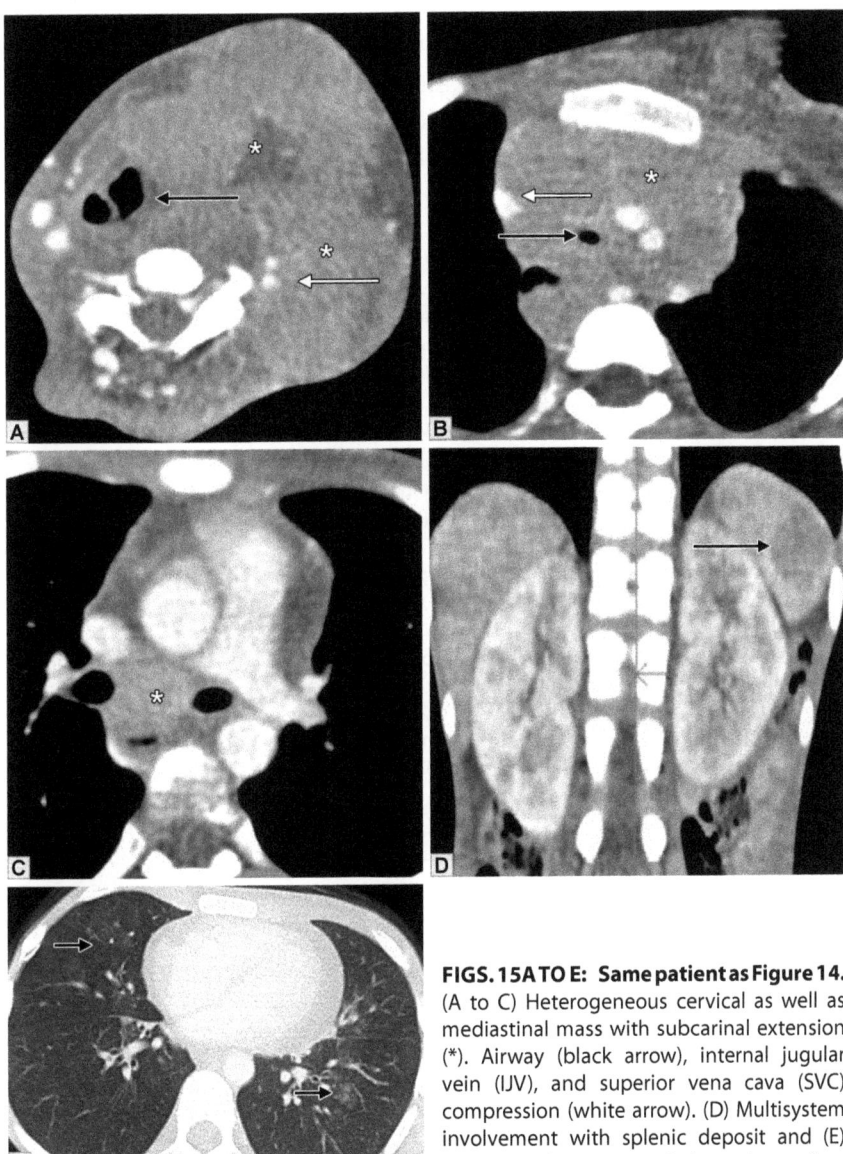

FIGS. 15A TO E: Same patient as Figure 14. (A to C) Heterogeneous cervical as well as mediastinal mass with subcarinal extension (*). Airway (black arrow), internal jugular vein (IJV), and superior vena cava (SVC) compression (white arrow). (D) Multisystem involvement with splenic deposit and (E) aspiration changes seen in lungs (arrows).

CONCLUSION

When a mass is detected on chest radiograph, cross-sectional imaging is required to delineate the extent and nature of the mass. Mediastinal mass imaging requires a compartment-wise approach. A complete knowledge of the pediatric mediastinal tumors is imperative to reach a final imaging diagnosis.

Other Related Chapters that can be Referred to:
- Chapter 21: Approach to Mediastinal Lesions: Part 1
- Chapter 22: Approach to Mediastinal Lesions: Part 2
- Chapter 24: Thoracic Tumors and Mimics: Part 2

REFERENCES

1. Zapala MA, Ho-Fung VM, Lee EY. Thoracic neoplasms in children: Contemporary Perspectives and Imaging Assessment. Radiol Clin North Am. 2017;55(4):657-76.
2. Sood S, Hryhorczuk AL, Rissmiller J, Lee EY. Spectrum of syndromic disorders associated with pediatric tumors: Evolving role of practical imaging assessment. Radiol Clin North Am. 2017;55(4):869-93.
3. Swift CC, Eklund MJ, Kraveka JM, Alazraki AL. Updates in diagnosis, management, and treatment of neuroblastoma. Radiographics. 2018;38:566-80.
4. Suh JS, Abenoza P, Galloway HR, Everson LI, Griffiths HJ. Peripheral (extracranial) nerve tumors: correlation of MR imaging and histologic findings. Radiology. 1992;183(2):341-6.
5. Wasa J, Nishida Y, Tsukushi S, Shido Y, Sugiura H, Nakashima H, et al. MRI features in the differentiation of malignant peripheral nerve sheath tumors and neurofibromas. AJR Am J Roentgenol. 2010;194(6):1568-74.
6. Chen L, Wang M, Fan H, Hu F, Liu T. Comparison of pediatric and adult lymphomas involving the mediastinum characterized by distinctive clinicopathological and radiological features. Sci Rep. 2017;7(1):2577.
7. McCarten KM, Nadel HR, Shulkin BL, Cho SY. Imaging for diagnosis, staging and response assessment of Hodgkin lymphoma and non-Hodgkin lymphoma. Pediatr Radiol. 2019;49(11):1545-64.
8. Marie E, Navallas M, Katz DS, Farajirad E, Punnett A, Davda S, et al. Non-Hodgkin lymphoma imaging spectrum in children, adolescents, and young adults. Radiographics. 2022;42(4):1214-38.

CHAPTER 24

Thoracic Tumors and Mimics: Part 2

Ashu Seith Bhalla, Vasundhara Patil

- ❑ Primary pulmonary tumors
  - ➤ Benign neoplasms
  - ➤ Malignant neoplasms
- ❑ Airway tumors
  - ➤ Benign
  - ➤ Malignant
- ❑ Chest wall tumors
  - ➤ Benign
  - ➤ Malignant

■ INTRODUCTION

Mediastinal masses are covered in Chapters 21 to 23. The current chapter focuses on imaging features of some key pulmonary, pleural, and chest wall masses.

■ PRIMARY PULMONARY TUMORS

Benign Neoplasms

Benign primary pulmonary tumors encountered in children include pulmonary hamartoma, hamartoma/chondroma **(Figs. 1 and 2)**, hemangioma **(Fig. 3)** and diffuse pulmonary lymphangiomatosis (DPL). All these are uncommon tumors.[1]

Pulmonary Hamartomas

Pulmonary hamartomas are benign tumors comprising of varying combinations of tissue elements such as cartilage, fat, calcium, or mature connective tissue. These are mostly incidental lesions. On imaging, these are well-defined, intrapulmonary masses. Margins appear smooth or lobulated, internal coarse "popcorn calcification" on radiograph is characteristic. Besides showing calcification (in up to 50% cases), computed tomography (CT) also frequently demonstrates fat (in up to 60% cases), and is diagnostic **(Figs. 1A and B)**.

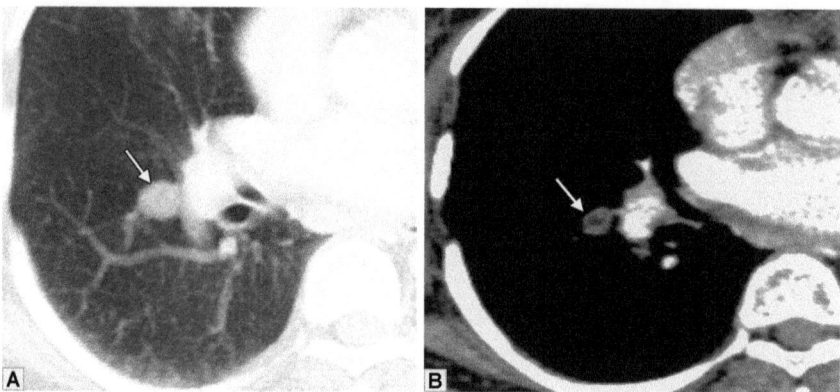

FIGS. 1A AND B: Pulmonary Hamartoma. (A) CT lung window shows a solitary well-defined nodule with mildly lobulated margins (arrow). (B) Mediastinal window demonstrates the low-fat density within the nodule (arrow) suggestive of benign nature.

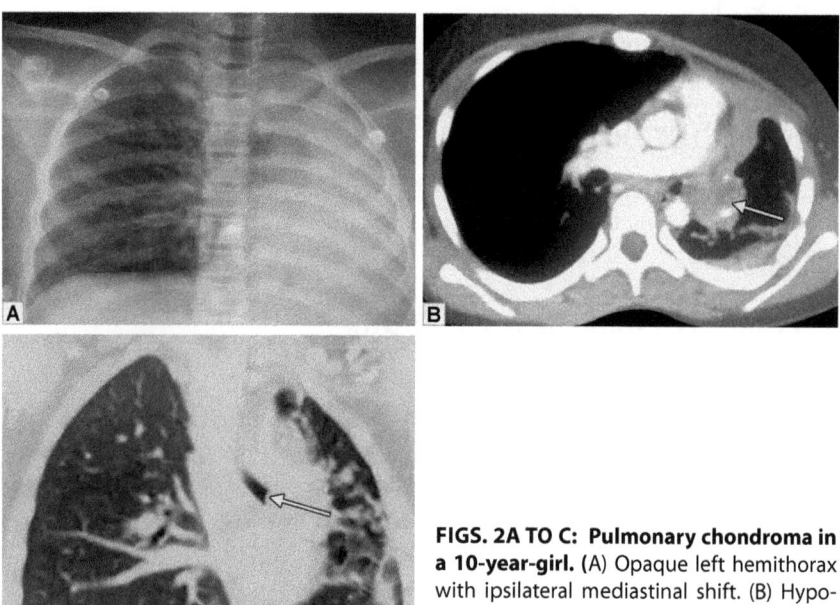

FIGS. 2A TO C: Pulmonary chondroma in a 10-year-girl. (A) Opaque left hemithorax with ipsilateral mediastinal shift. (B) Hypodense left hilar mass with foci of calcification (arrow). (C) Abrupt cut-off in left main bronchus (arrow).

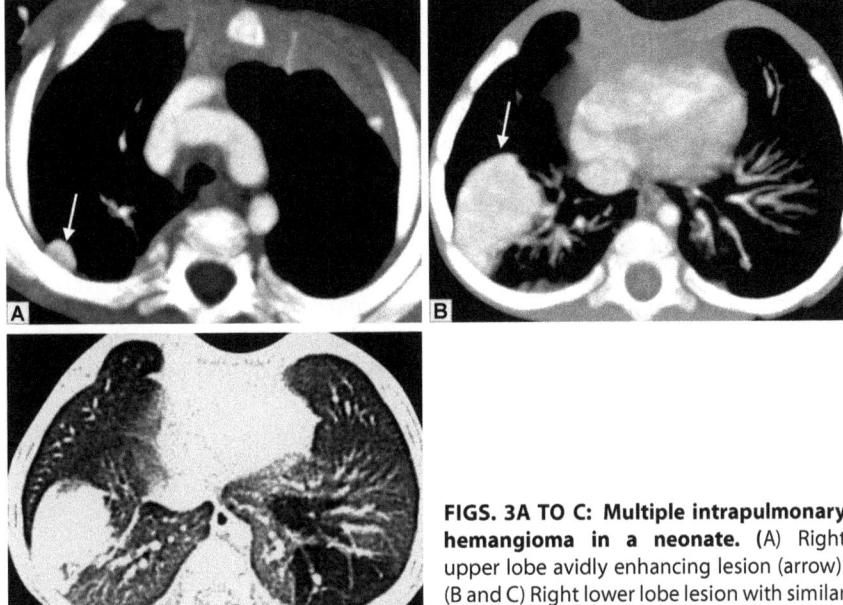

FIGS. 3A TO C: Multiple intrapulmonary hemangioma in a neonate. (A) Right upper lobe avidly enhancing lesion (arrow). (B and C) Right lower lobe lesion with similar enhancement (arrow).

Diffuse Pulmonary Lymphangiomatosis

- DPL is a rare disease characterized by infiltration of the lung, pleura, and mediastinum with thin-walled lymphangiomas.
- It is classified in WHO classification of lung tumors 2021 under mesenchymal tumors of the lung.
- It is predominantly identified in children and young adults, and affects both gender equally.
- Clinical symptoms occur because of the mass effect from infiltrative disease, restrictive and/or obstructive physiology, chylous effusions, and respiratory failure.
- CT shows peribronchovascular and interlobular septal thickening, diffuse cystic lesions causing infiltration of the mediastinal soft tissue and pleural effusions.[2]
- DPL is distinct from lymphangioleiomyomatosis (LAM) because there is no infiltration into the alveoli of the lung parenchyma and disease affects the lymphatic system and predominantly the peribronchovascular interstitium.

Lymphangioleiomyomatosis/Tuberous Sclerosis
- LAM may be sporadic or tuberous sclerosis (TS) associated, and is present in about a third of TS patients. TS is an autosomal dominant disease associated with *TSC1* and *TSC2* gene mutations.[3]
- TS-LAM presents with diffuse cystic disease in affected females with pulmonary involvement in patients beyond 15 years of age.
- In TS associated LAM, other associated lesions of LAM are seen—cranial (subependymal nodules and cortical tubers), cardiac rhabdomyomas, and renal angiomyolipomas.
- *Multifocal micronodular pneumocyte hyperplasia (MMPH):* This is a rarer association of TS, and is seen as multiple, tiny randomly distributed nodules. It is more frequent adult females with TS, rather males in children.
- *Cardiac rhabdomyomas*: These are benign tumors occurring in infants (<1 year). Several of these involute/regress overtime.

Malignant Neoplasms
- Unlike other thoracic sites (e.g., chest wall), primary lung neoplasms are uncommon in children, and the majority are malignant.
- However, the spectrum of these malignant lesions is different from adults, with common carcinomas such as squamous cell carcinoma (SCC) and adenocarcinomas being distinctly rare in children.

Pleuropulmonary Blastoma
Pleuropulmonary blastoma (PPB) is a rare primary lung tumor encountered only in children, being extremely rare in adults.

Background/Genetics
- PPB is a dysembryonic type of tumor and is associated with *DICER1* gene mutation. *DICER1* gene is located on chromosome 14q and the mutation affects 5p mature micro-RNA.
- Up to one-fourth of children with PPB have this mutation, screening (with chest CT) of *DICER1* gene mutation positive children for PPB is recommended.
- Although only 10% of those with the mutation may develop PPB, and a large number never develop the tumor.
- Those with *DICER-1* gene mutation may also show a multilocular cystic nephroma (CN), concurrently with a PPB. Conversely, the presence of this combination is a highly strong association with the mutation.
- Majority of PPB originate in the lung, although a minority may arise from the parietal pleura.
- PPB is divided into three types. It is believed that the three types may represent an evolution from type 1 to type III, with increased proliferation of the primitive malignant cells, which are mainly mesenchymal.
- Some of the type I PPBs may remain stable or even regress.

Clinical Presentation
- The median age of presentation is 3 years.
- PPB may be an incidentally detected lesion or patients may present with respiratory symptoms or chest pain.

Imaging
- PPBs are located in the periphery of the lung, and are more frequent on the right side.
- On CT, the tumors have a solid/cystic/mixed appearance.
- The size is variable, with the bigger tumors even occupying an entire hemithorax.
- Cystic lesions can also expand the lobe that they occupy. In addition, hemorrhage may be seen within with resultant air-fluid (A-F) levels.
- Type I PPB are purely cystic lesions.
- Type II PPB may show characteristic enhancing nodules along the cyst walls **(Figs. 4A and B)**.
- Type III PPB appears as completely solid masses **(Figs. 5A to C)** and differentiation from rhabdomyosarcomas is difficult on imaging.
- Type II and II can disseminate with metastases to the brain, bone, or liver.
- Differentiating features between various types of PPB are summarized in **Table 1**.
- Differentiation of type I and II PPB from congenital pulmonary airway malformations (CPAM) can be challenging. The following features aid in the differentiation:
    - CPAMs are present antenatally and hence a lesion detected on prenatal imaging is a CPAM rather than PPB.
    - Lesion involving multiple lobes favors PPB.
    - Differentiation of type II PPB from other solid tumors such as rhabdomyosarcoma is difficult on imaging.
- Contrast-enhanced CT (CECT) is the modality of choice. MRI if performed shows heterogeneous enhancement of solid component. Also solid portions are F-fluorodeoxyglucose (FDG) avid on positron emission tomography-CT (PET-CT).

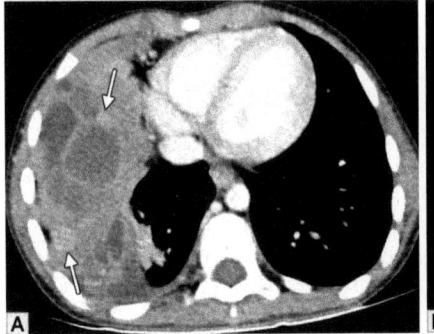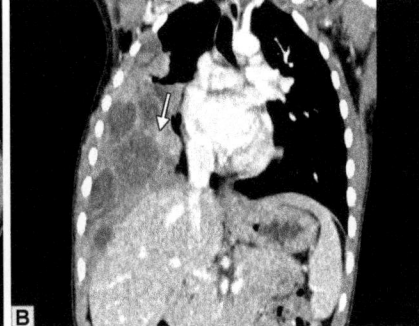

FIGS. 4A AND B: Pleuropulmonary blastoma type II. Axial and coronal CECT image shows multicystic mass in right hemithorax with solid heterogenous components (arrows).

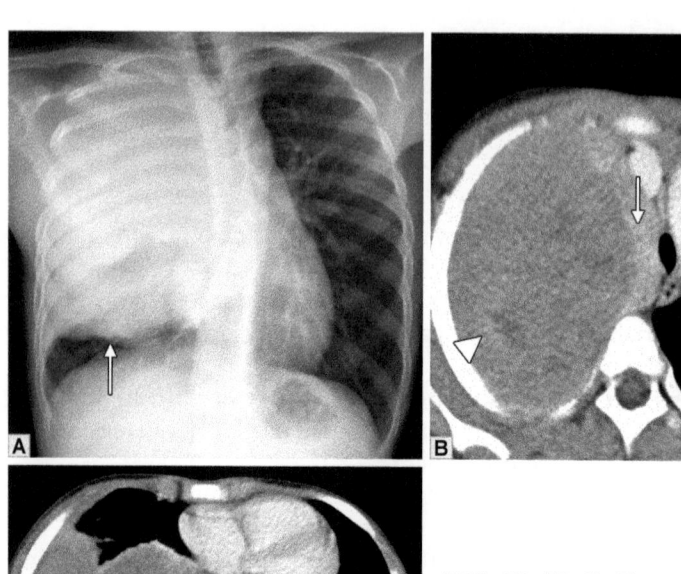
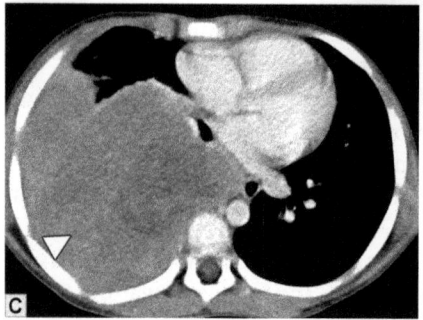

FIGS. 5A TO C: Pleuropulmonary blastoma type III. (A) CXR. Opacity in right hemithorax with lobulated inferior margin (arrow) and shift of mediastinum and trachea to left. (B and C) CT shows solid heterogeneously enhancing mass (arrowhead) in right hemithorax (predominantly pleural based) with compression of lung parenchyma (arrow).

TABLE 1: Differentiating features of types of PPB.			
Type	I	II	III
Age of presentation	• Median—10 months • Mostly < 3 years	After first year	• After first year • Median—4 years
Pathology	A lining of benign respiratory epithelium covers underlying primitive malignant cells	Mixed solid and cystic tumor with variable thickened or nodule-like areas	Heterogenous tumor with one or more of: • Primitive blastema-like small cells • Spindle and ovoid cells • Malignant chondroid elements • Clusters of large anaplastic cells
Morphology	Purely cystic	Mixed solid and cystic components	Purely solid
Additional imaging features	Few internal septations ±	Enhancing nodules along cyst wall	Heterogeneous enhancement
Size	Variable	Variable	Often large
Pneumothorax	Maybe +	Maybe +	Absent

Continued

Continued

Type	I	II	III
Pleural effusion	Maybe +	Maybe +	Maybe +
Metastases	Absent	Maybe +	Maybe +
Additional imaging required	Screen for renal tumors	Screen for renal tumors plus metastatic work-up	Screen for renal tumors plus metastatic work-up
Prognosis	• Better survival • May regress spontaneously	Intermediate prognosis	Poorer prognosis
Management	Surgical resection	Surgical resection with adjuvant chemotherapy	Surgical resection with adjuvant chemotherapy

Inflammatory Myofibroblastic Tumor

- Inflammatory myofibroblastic tumor (IMT) is one of the most common primary lung neoplasm in children. It is categorized as a mesenchymal tumor under the WHO classification. Previously considered a benign lesion, it is now recognized as a low-grade malignancy as occasionally these tumors can metastasize.
- *Synonyms*: Previously called inflammatory pseudotumor, plasma cell granuloma, and fibroxanthoma.
- On histopathologic examination (HPE) several types of cells are visualized including spindle-shaped fibroblasts, myofibroblasts, histiocytes, and plasma cells.
- Tumors can be peripheral or central (in <15% cases).

Clinical Presentation
- Inflammatory myofibroblastic tumor occurs in children or young adults.
- Those with endobronchial tumors present earlier with respiratory symptoms including hemoptysis.

Imaging
- Peripheral tumors appear as a solitary pulmonary nodule (SPN) or a mass, which have a benign appearance. Their margins are usually well-defined. Multiple lesions are occasional (5%).
- Central masses (as in all endobronchial lesions) often have associated atelectasis **(Figs. 6A to D)**.
- Calcifications can be present, and are more frequent in children. The reported patterns of calcification being amorphous or fleck-like.
- Also in children, lesions often assume large sizes.
- Pleural effusion can be seen.
- On MRI, the tumors are hypointense on both T1 and T2W imaging **(Figs. 7A to D)**.
- There is a combination of "inflammatory" and "fibrotic" components. The inflammatory portion shows contrast enhancement, and similarly can be FDG avid on PET-CT.

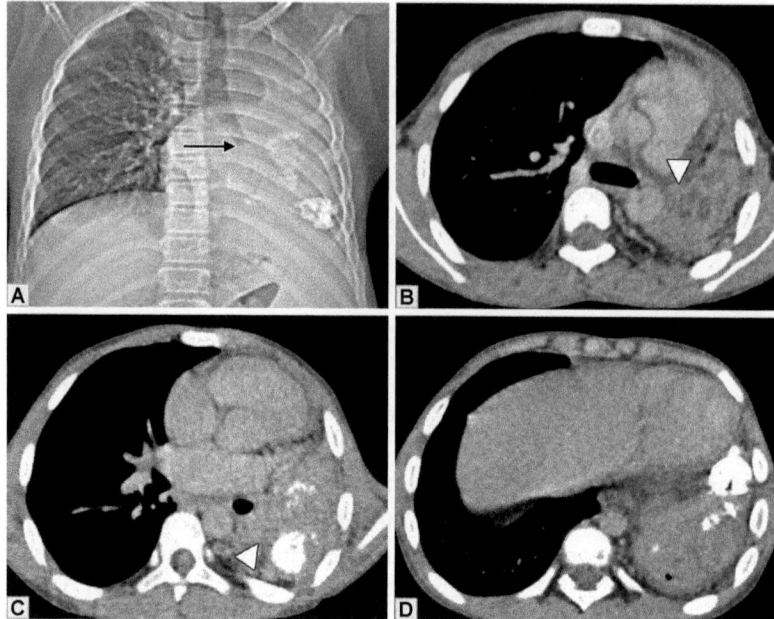

FIGS. 6A TO D: Inflammatory myofibroblastic tumor. A 12-year-old male. (A) Chest radiograph and (B to D) axial CECT: Enhancing mass with chunky calcifications in left lower lobe, bronchial encasement with collapse of left upper lobe and fluid-filled bronchi within.

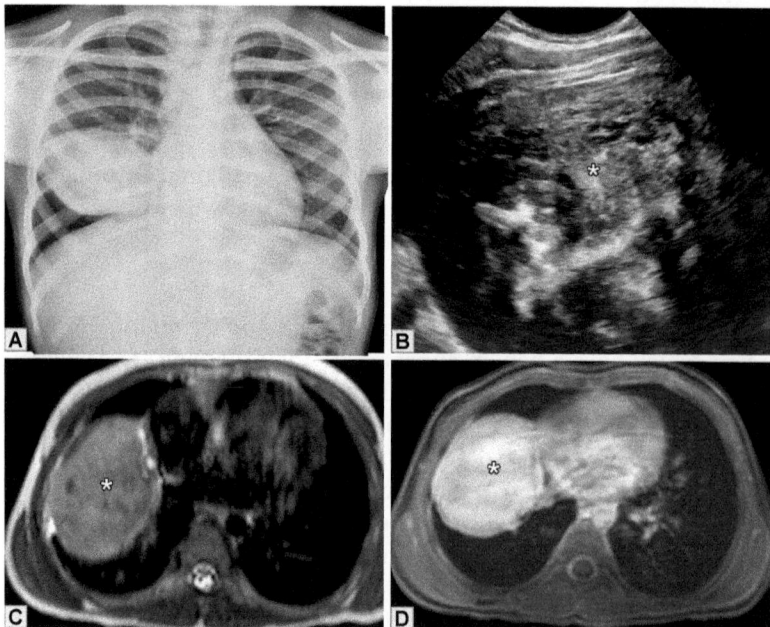

FIGS. 7A TO D: Inflammatory myofibroblastic tumor in a 5-year-old boy. (A) Well-defined right lower zone pulmonary mass (arrow); (B) solid mass on ultrasound (asterisk); (C) T2W isointense right lower lobe mass (asterisk); and (D) intense homogenous postcontrast enhancement.

Congenital Peribronchial Myofibroblastic Tumor

- *Synonyms*: Previously called congenital pulmonary myofibroblastic tumor, congenital mesenchymal malformation.
- Congenital peribronchial myofibroblastic tumors (CPMTs) are rare mesenchymal tumors arising from the mesenchyme around the central bronchi and further differentiating into spindle cells (fibroblasts/myofibroblasts) with areas of cartilage formation.
- The description of these tumors is confined to case reports, with most presenting in perinatal period, and rarely in infancy.
- In the prenatal period, CPMT has been described as causing hydrops fetalis, in the neonatal period presenting with respiratory distress; or rarely in infancy with other chest symptoms.
- Imaging features are of a solid, heterogeneous mass, with necrotic or cystic areas.
- Its main differential diagnosis is a PPB.
- Surgical resection is the primary management.

Adenocarcinoma

- Adenocarcinoma is rare in children. It may occur in a setting of underlying CPAM, or even more rarely as a primary tumor.
- The type of adenocarcinoma developing in CPAM is the *mucinous form*, exclusively, as walls of type I CPAM also have proliferating mucinous cells resembling adenocarcinoma of the same type.
- Another variant is the *"fetal adenocarcinoma"* which is so called due to its similarity with the epithelial lining found in the fetal lung.
  - These tumors can be peripheral or central, with central ones presenting with postobstructive changes.
  - There are no specific imaging features and these can present as areas of nodules, consolidation, or central masses.

AIRWAY TUMORS

Benign

Hemangioma

- Hemangiomas are one of the most benign pediatric neoplasms. These comprise vascular endothelial cells which show abnormal proliferation.
- Based on age at presentation and clinical behavior, they are divided into various subtypes; the two major pediatric forms being, congenital and infantile forms.
- The infantile hemangiomas (IH) express glucose transporter 1 (GLUT-1), and are more common than the congenital form.
- Subglottis is the most frequent site of airway involvement, with trachea and major bronchi being far less common.
- Subglottic hemangiomas (SH) are typically IH. Since subglottic airway is involved, patients present with stridor.

- IH displays a typical clinical course with the following phases:
  - *Age of onset*: Neonatal period
  - *Proliferating phase*: 3–6 months
  - *Involuting phase*: 1–5 years, may continue to regress up to 10 years, and typically show complete resolution.
  - On laryngoscopy/bronchoscopy, the lesion is submucosal with overlying mucosa showing bluish appearance.

Imaging
- Plain radiographs are the initial imaging modality employed in children with stridor.
- Soft tissue neck (STN) anteroposterior (AP) and lateral views reveal narrowing of the subglottic, which is asymmetric, with or without direct visualization of the "mass" lesion.
- The common differential diagnosis of infantile stridor is croup or subglottic stenosis; wherein the narrowing is symmetric and no additional soft tissue is seen.
- *Ultrasonography (USG)* should be performed if SH is suspected and it shows a solid, echogenic lesion. Though typically homogeneous, larger lesions may be heterogeneous. IH shows vascularity in the proliferating phase and Doppler waveforms are of arterial as well as venous patterns **(Figs. 8A and B)**.
- USG is diagnostic, differentiating SH from papillomas and lymphatic malformations.
- *Multidetector CT (MDCT)*: MDCT is required for mapping extent of the lesion. CECT reveals an intensely enhancing lesion **(Figs. 9A to D)** that usually has well-defined margins.
- MRI reveals a T2 hyperintense intensely enhancing mass lesion which has multiple flow voids. While MRI cannot be performed in an acute setting, it can be performed once the patient is on tracheostomy.
- It is a useful radiation-free modality in patients who are placed on medical therapy. For smaller lesions, USG should be employed for this purpose.

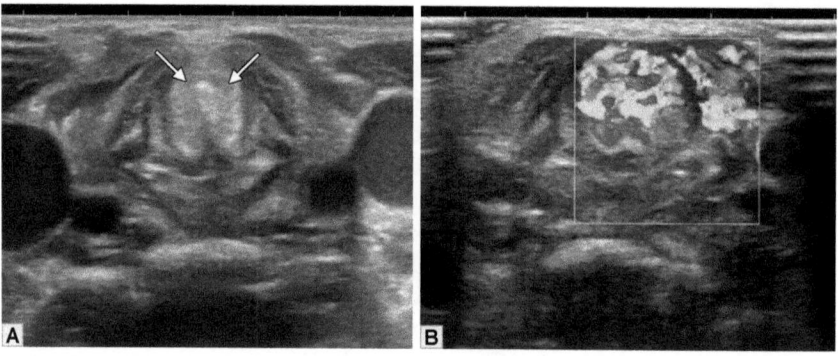

FIGS. 8A AND B: Subglottic hemangioma. USG shows *hyperechoic* mass (arrows) in subglottic airway in a neonate. Color Doppler shows intense vascularity with the mass s/o hemangioma.

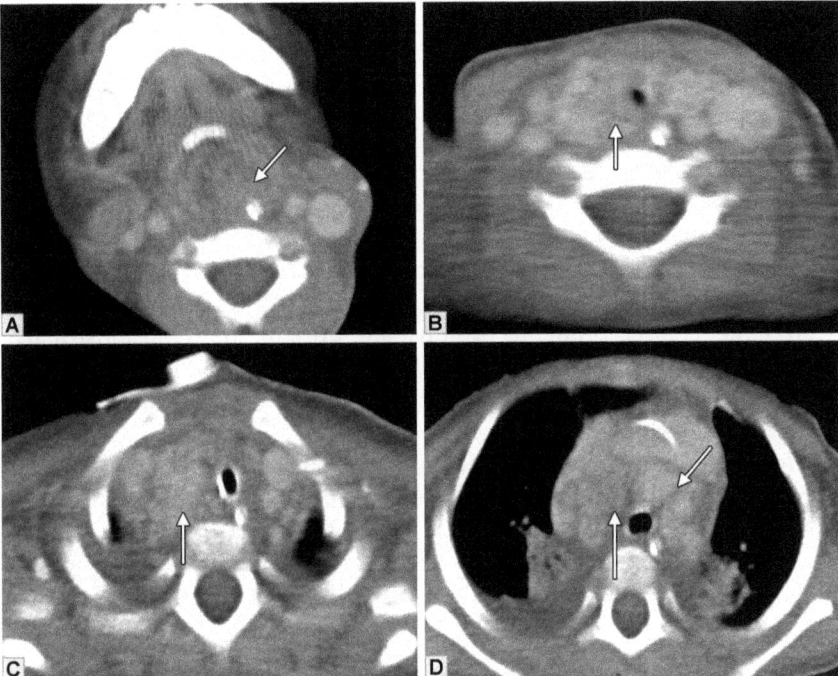

FIGS. 9A TO D: Hemangioma with mediastinal extension. (A) Intensely enhancing lobulated soft tissue in the subglottic region obliterating its lumen. (B) The soft tissue is extending in right paratracheal space and in the middle mediastinum surrounding the airway (arrows) (C and D).

Management
- Medical therapy includes systemic beta-blockers (propranolol), steroids, or intralesional steroids.
- Surgery is performed in case of significant airway obstruction or residual lesions postmedical therapy.

Recurrent Respiratory Papillomatosis
- Recurrent respiratory papillomatosis (RRP) is a human papillomavirus (HPV)-related disease. The virus is transmitted from the mother to the baby during vaginal delivery.
- It results in the formation of multiple, recurrent papillomas (or "warts") in the respiratory epithelium of the central airway.
- The "papilloma" comprises a frond-like projection of the respiratory epithelium which is lined by stratified squamous epithelium.
- RRP is the most common neoplasm affecting the large airways in children.
- Not only are the lesions recurrent, but are also prone to malignant transformation into SCC in 1–4% cases.[4]

Clinical Presentation
- The most common age of presentation is 2–4 years.
- Patients present with hoarseness of voice or stridor as larynx is most frequently involved.

Imaging
- *Sites of involvement*: Larynx (most common), trachea, and main bronchi. The peripheral airways and lung parenchyma are involved less frequently.
- *Central lesions* appear as nodular growths in the larynx or trachea. Trachea may show multiple, nodular excrescences arising from the epithelium.
- If large central bronchial lesions are present, then postobstructive changes will also be seen.
- The *peripheral lesions* present as nodules in peribronchial location which cavitate **(Figs. 10 and 11)**.
- In presence of SCC of larynx, following malignant transformation of a papilloma, the parenchymal cavitary lesions can be challenging to differentiate from metastases.
- FDG uptake is variable, and is seen not only once SCC develops but also in some of the benign lesions.

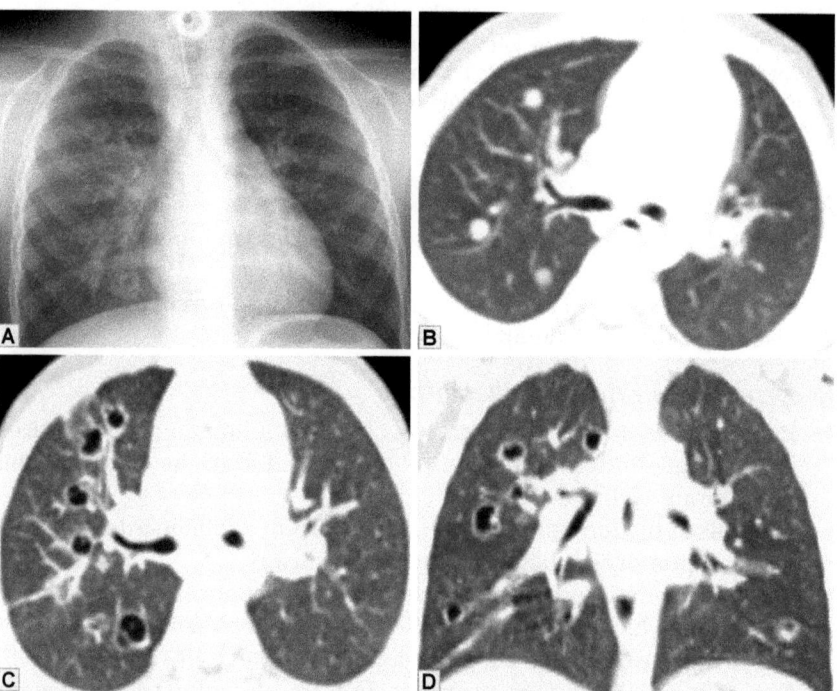

FIGS. 10A TO D: Recurrent respiratory papillomatosis (RRP) in a 3-year-old girl. (A) Multiple solid nodules in both lungs; and (B to D) Coexistent solid and cavitary lung nodules bilaterally.

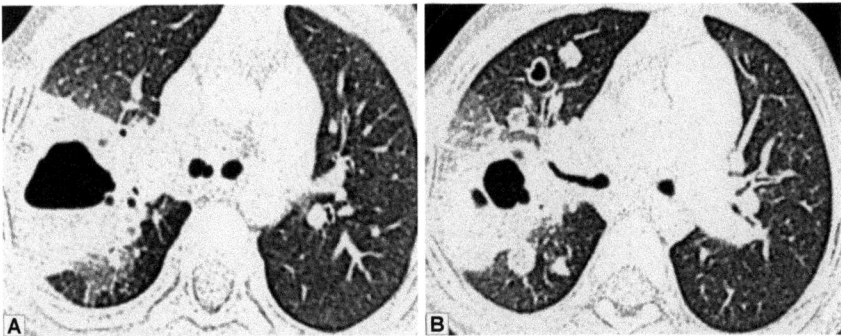

FIGS. 11A AND B: Recurrent respiratory papillomatosis with superadded infection in a cavity. (A) right upper lobe cavity with a thick wall. (B) Multiple nodules in right lung, one showing cavitation.

Management
- The management of RRP depends on the degree of airway obstruction, and severity of resultant respiratory symptoms. An emergency tracheostomy is often required in those with large laryngeal lesions followed by debulking.
- Microsurgical techniques are often employed, e.g., laser ablation or microdebridement for reduction of tumor bulk.
- Cidofovir can be injected locally following the surgery.
- Once SCC develops then radical resection is required.

Malignant
Carcinoid and mucoepidermoid carcinomas (MEC) are the malignant airway tumors which can be seen in children, amongst which MEC is rare. Squamous cell carcinoma as mentioned can be seen in RRP.

■ CHEST WALL TUMORS

Benign
Benign chest wall masses are frequent in children (especially infants), with majority being of soft tissue origin. Longstanding benign soft tissue lesions cause pressure effects on the developing chest wall.

Hemangioma
- Clinical phases and imaging features are similar to those of hemangiomas in other sites (as discussed above in airway lesion). In addition, IH can bleed during proliferating phase either spontaneously or following trivial trauma.
- USG and MRI form the mainstay of diagnosis.
- IHs are differentiated from arteriovenous malformations (AVMs) by the presence of large, solid, enhancing soft tissue component as the major imaging feature.

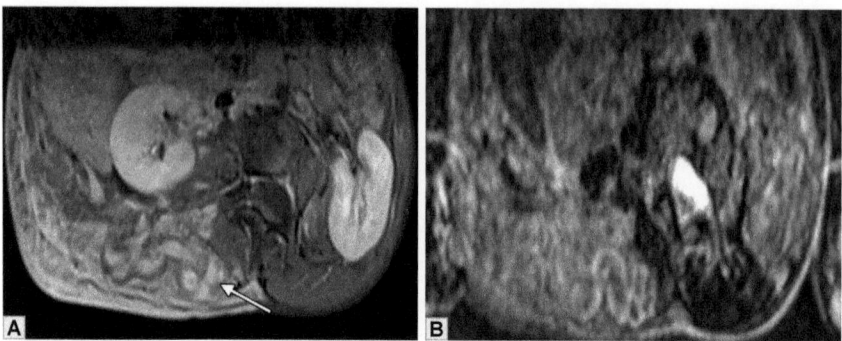

FIGS. 12A AND B: Plexiform neurofibroma of chest wall. (A) Serpiginious T2W hyperintense lesion along right chest wall (arrow). (B) Peripheral enhancement after contrast administration.

- Management is mostly medical (as discussed above). Endovascular embolization can be done if lesions are rapidly enlarging and causing cardiac compromise, or in case of bleeding.

Neurofibroma
- Can be seen in neurofibromatosis 1 **(Figs. 12A and B)**.
- Well-defined solid masses in the chest wall.

Mesenchymal Hamartoma of the Chest Wall
- Mesenchymal hamartoma of the chest wall (MHCW) is previously called infantile cartilaginous hamartoma and infantile osteochondroma.
- These are rare benign congenital chest wall masses that present in the perinatal period, and arise from the ribs.
- On HPE, there is proliferation of primitive mesenchymal tissues with cartilaginous components. There may be areas of secondary aneurysmal bone cyst (ABC) formation.

Clinical Presentation

Neonates present with chest wall deformity, swelling, or respiratory symptoms. The respiratory symptoms may be consequent to underlying lung compression, however, an unrelated pulmonary cause should be excluded.

Imaging
- On imaging, these appear as well-circumscribed masses involving multiple ribs.
- The ribs show changes in the form of scalloping or smooth erosion.
- The tumor has a solid component with calcification or matrix mineralization (chondroid pattern) **(Figs. 13A and B)**.
- The tumor can also show large cystic areas with fluid-fluid levels.
- The age of onset and the characteristic imaging appearance enable a specific diagnosis.

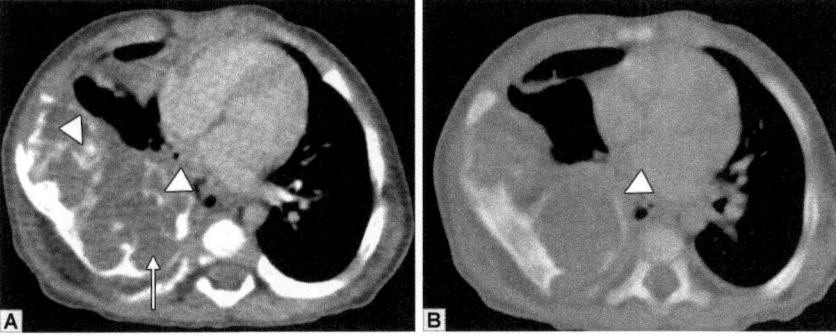

FIGS. 13A AND B: Mesenchymal hamartoma of the chest wall (MHCW). Though common in neonates, this child was 5 years old presenting with chest wall deformity since birth. (A) Solid heterogeneous mass seen in right chest wall with intrathoracic extension (arrow). (B) Curvilinear areas of calcification/matrix mineralization of chondroid pattern (arrowhead) was noted in the mass along with chest wall deformity.

Management
- Management is dependent on the patient's symptoms. If there are no significant respiratory effects, the lesion can be left alone and can show gradual regression.
- Surgical resection is indicated in those with respiratory consequences.

Lipoblastoma and Lipoblastomatosis
- Lipoblastoma is rare benign soft tissue tumor, typically occurring in infants or children < 3 years of age.
- The encapsulated form is referred to as lipoblastoma, while the diffuse infiltrative form is called lipoblastomatosis. Lipoblastomatosis can infiltrate into deeper tissues.
- Its tissue of origin is the embryonic fat (white fat).
- On HPE, the tumor shows immature adipocytes with intervening septae, lipoblasts, and myxoid stroma.
- On pathology, the lesion can be indistinguishable from liposarcoma; and the age of presentation helps, with liposarcoma being rare in children <10 years. Also atypical nuclei/mitoses are not seen in lipoblastoma.
- Lipoblastomas can subsequently mature into lipomas with age.

Clinical Presentation
Sites of the tumor include extremities, trunk, and neck. It presents in infancy or early childhood (< 3 years age) as a superficial mass that is rapidly growing.

Imaging
- Imaging reveals a well-defined fat containing lesions. It can, however, contain soft tissue components (corresponding to myxoid stroma) **(Figs. 14A and B)**.

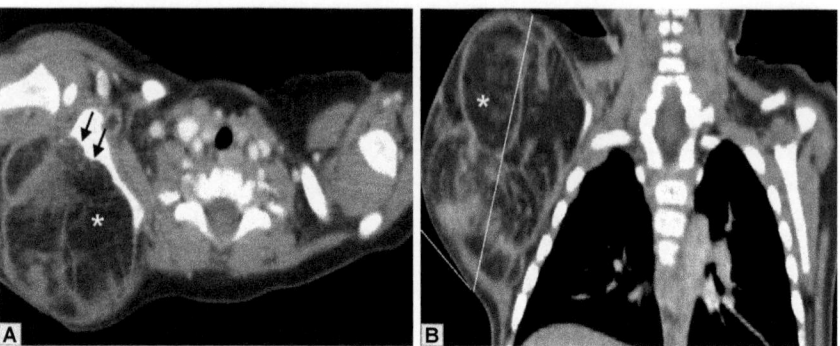

FIGS. 14A AND B: Lipoblastoma of chest wall. CT shows large well defined/encapsulated (asterisks), predominantly fat containing mass in right posterolateral chest wall causing scalloping of the scapula (black arrows in A).

- Lipoblastoma appears as well-defined mass located in subcutaneous mass.
- Lipoblastomatosis, however, extends into intermuscular planes or even intramuscular.
- Imaging appearance is similar to liposarcoma, only age of presentation aids in the differentiation.

Malignant

Malignant chest wall masses in children are mostly mesenchymal tumors arising from the soft tissues (rhabdomyosarcomas/infantile fibrosarcoma) or from the ribs (Ewing's sarcoma family of tumors and osteosarcoma). Ewing's sarcoma family of tumors is the most common amongst these occurring in older children.

Infantile Fibrosarcoma

- Infantile fibrosarcoma/congenital fibrosarcoma are rare, malignant soft tissue tumor arising in the chest wall. These typically present in neonates and are usually detected at birth (30% cases) or in first year of life. It is the most common soft tissue tumor among children under 1 year of age.[5] Also, these present as rapidly enlarging soft tissue masses, which even ulcerates and fungates.
- Most common site is extremities, and other sites include head and neck region and trunk regions. Chest wall is an uncommon site of involvement. There is a high incidence of TEL gene rearrangement and TEL/TRKC fusion gene, which can be utilized in diagnosis.
- Imaging shows well defined, solid heterogenous mass in the chest wall in subcutaneous/intermuscular planes.

- It is predominantly a locally invasive tumor and metastasis is rare. Local recurrence rates are high after surgery.
- Management consists of surgical excision along with neoadjuvant/adjuvant chemotherapy.

▮ CONCLUSION

When a thoracic mass is detected on chest radiograph, cross-sectional imaging is often required to accurately localize and characterize the lesion and narrow the differential diagnosis. Knowledge of differential possibilities for a thoracic tumor in children is imperative since certain tumors are unique to pediatric age group and present with characteristic imaging appearances.

Primary pulmonary parenchymal tumors such as PPB, CPMT, IMT, and chest wall tumors such as lipoblastomas and MHCW are some of the unique ones. Syndromic associations of some of the thoracic tumors warrant further genetic workup for various mutations.

Other Related Chapters that can be Referred to:
- Chapter 23: Thoracic Tumors and Mimics: Part 1
- Chapter 25: Chest Wall Imaging
- Chapter 26: Pleural Disorders: Imaging

▮ REFERENCES

1. Zapala MA, Ho-Fung VM, Lee EY. Thoracic neoplasms in children: Contemporary perspectives and imaging assessment. Radiol Clin North Am. 2017;55(4):657-76.
2. DU MH, Ye RJ, Sun KK, Li JF, Shen DH, Wang J, et al. Diffuse pulmonary lymphangiomatosis: A case report with literature review. Chin Med J (Engl). 2011;124(5):797-800.
3. Sood S, Hryhorczuk AL, Rissmiller J, Lee EY. Spectrum of syndromic disorders associated with pediatric tumors: Evolving role of practical imaging assessment. Radiol Clin North Am. 2017;55(4):869-93.
4. Jeong WJ, Park SW, Shin M. Presence of HPV type ysplasialasia and carcinoma arising from recurrent respiratory papillomatosis. Head Neck. 2009;31:1095-101.
5. Gupta SS, Singh O, Sharma SS, Mathur RK. Congenital fibrosarcoma of the chest wall: Report of a Case. J Cutan Aesthet Surg. 2010;3(3):177-80.

SECTION 9

Chest Wall and Pleural Disorders

CHAPTER 25: Chest Wall Imaging
CHAPTER 26: Pleural Disorders: Imaging

CHAPTER 25

Chest Wall Imaging

Poonam Sherwani, Ashu Seith Bhalla

- ❑ Imaging modalities
- ❑ Classification
- ❑ Specific entities
  - ➢ Congenital or developmental abnormalities
  - ➢ Infections
  - ➢ Trauma
  - ➢ Metabolic disorders
  - ➢ Neoplasms
  - ➢ Diffuse periosteal reaction of thoracic cage bones in children

■ INTRODUCTION

- Chest wall is composed of the thoracic cage (formed by the sternum, costal cartilages, ribs, and thoracic vertebrae), intercostal muscles, vessels, lymphatics and fascia, and skin. Chest wall pathologies can arise from any of the components.
- Few chest wall diseases are common in adults and children; however, several entities are exclusively seen in the pediatric population.[1-3]
- In the case of bony lesions, radiographs are extremely useful, followed by computed tomography (CT) with volume rendering technique (VRT).

■ IMAGING MODALITIES

- Radiographs are the initial investigation performed.
- Often followed by ultrasound (especially valuable) as it has real-time ability to examine the patient.
- CT or magnetic resonance imaging (MRI) are required for confirmation and further characterization of a chest wall lesion.
- 18F-fluorodeoxyglucose positron emission tomography CT (18F FDG PET-CT) is employed in case of metabolic activity assessment of chest wall tumors (e.g., Ewing's sarcoma family of tumors (ESFT)).

■ CLASSIFICATION

The broad classification of chest wall lesions is tabulated in **Table 1**. *Based on etiology, chest wall lesions can be classified as follows:*

TABLE 1: Classification of chest wall lesions.	
Congenital or developmental	• Pectus excavatum • Pectus carinatum • Skeletal dysplasias
Infection	• Bacterial infection • Tuberculosis • Fungal infection
Inflammatory	• Chronic nonbacterial osteomyelitis (CNO) • Infantile cortical hyperostosis (Caffey's disease)
Trauma	• Accidental trauma • Nonaccidental injury (child abuse)
Metabolic	• Rickets • Scurvy
Hematological	Hemolytic anemias
Storage disorders	Mucopolysaccharidosis and mucolipidosis
Benign osseous tumors	• Osteochondroma • Fibrous dysplasia • Mesenchymal hamartoma
Malignant soft-tissue tumors	• Rhabdomyosarcoma • Osteosarcoma • Ewing sarcoma family of tumors
Metastatic diseases (most common)	• Neuroblastoma • Rhabdomyosarcoma • Lymphoma or leukemia

■ SPECIFIC ENTITIES

Congenital or Developmental Abnormalities

The more common conditions are described below.

Pectus Excavatum

- It refers to depression of the sternum relative to the rest of the anterior chest **(Figs. 1A to C)**.
- In most cases, deformity is purely cosmetic. Severe cases can result in pain, dyspnea, restrictive lung disease, and right atrium compression.
- Anterior indentation and deformity of right ventricle.
- Heart may be rotationally displaced into the left hemithorax.
- Mitral valve prolapsed might result from the deformity of mitral valve annulus.
- Chronic hypoxia secondary to poor respiratory function might result in pulmonary hypertension.

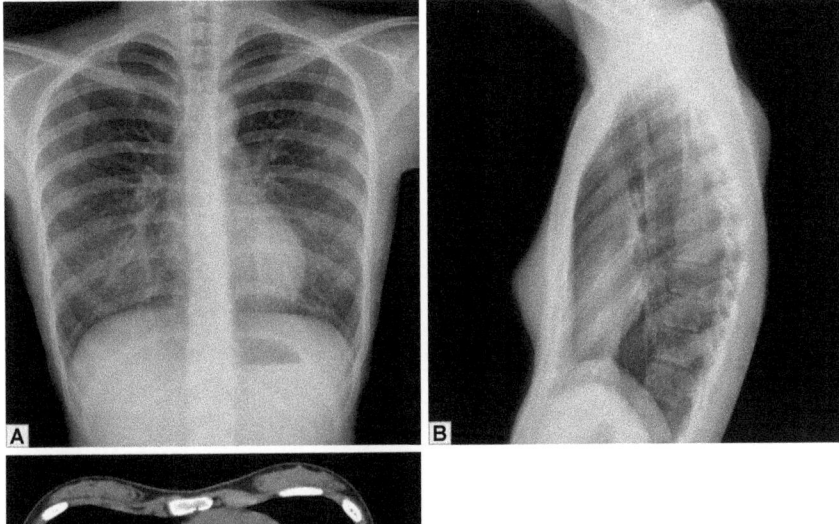

FIGS. 1A TO C: Pectus excavatum. (A) Chest PA, (B) lateral radiograph, and (C) axial CT. (A) Mild leftward shift of heart with the mild blurring of the right heart border. Anterior ribs are sloping. (B) Depression of the sternum with decreased AP diameter. (C) Haller index was 2.95.

Imaging
- Reduced thoracic anteroposterior diameter can result in compression of trachea leading to tracheomalacia.
- Apparent pseudo infiltrates to the right of the cardiac silhouette related to greater visibility of the hilar vessels and displacement of cardiac silhouette to the left.
- The sternal depression can be directly visualized on the lateral radiograph.
- Quantify the severity by the *Haller index* (maximal transverse diameter of chest/AP diameter from vertebral body to the sternum)—<2.56 is considered normal; >3.25 often requires surgical correction.

Pectus Carinatum
- It refers to anterior protrusion of the sternum **(Figs. 2A and B)**.
- It has a male predominance.
- Associations—Marfan disease, Noonan syndrome, Prune belly, Morquio syndrome, osteogenesis imperfecta, mitral valve prolapse, homocystinuria, and rickets.
- It can manifest clinically as shortness of breath and exercise intolerance.

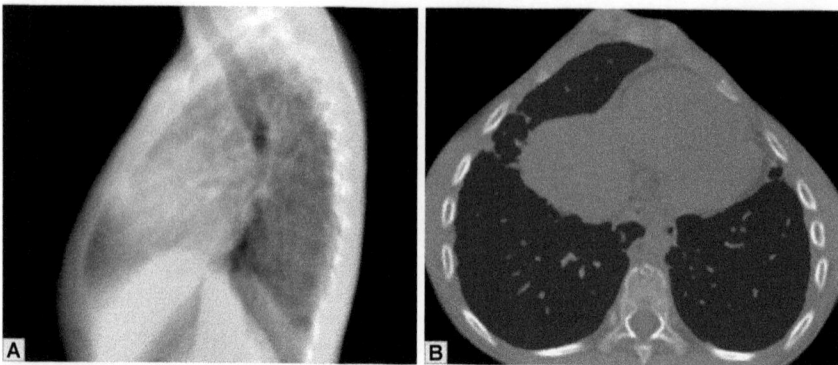

FIGS. 2A AND B: Pectus carinatum. (A) Chest lateral radiograph and (B) axial CT. (A) Outward protrusion of the lower thoracic wall and (B) asymmetric prominence of the right lower sternocostal joints.

Imaging: Increased anteroposterior diameter of the chest and anterior protrusion of the sternum—Haller index <1.98.

Skeletal Dysplasias

Thoracic abnormalities associated with common thoracic dysplasias are listed in **Table 2**.

TABLE 2: Thoracic manifestations of skeletal dysplasias.	
Thoracic imaging findings	**Associated skeletal dysplasia**
Decreased bone density, thin ribs	Osteogenesis imperfecta
Decreased bone density, poor ossification of vertebral body	Achondrogenesis (**Figs. 3A to C**)
Increased bone density, marrow cavity obliterated	• Osteopetrosis (**Figs. 4A and B**) • Pyknodysostosis
Hypoplastic/absent clavicles	Cleidocranial dysostosis
Short ribs, narrow thorax	• Jeune's syndrome • Short rib polydactyly syndromes • Ellis–van Creveld syndrome • Thanatophoric dysplasia (**Figs. 5A to C**)
Handlebar clavicles, hypoplastic scapula	Campomelic dysplasia
Short humeri	• Achondroplasia • Other rhizomelic dysplasias
Paddle-shaped ribs	Mucopolysaccharidosis

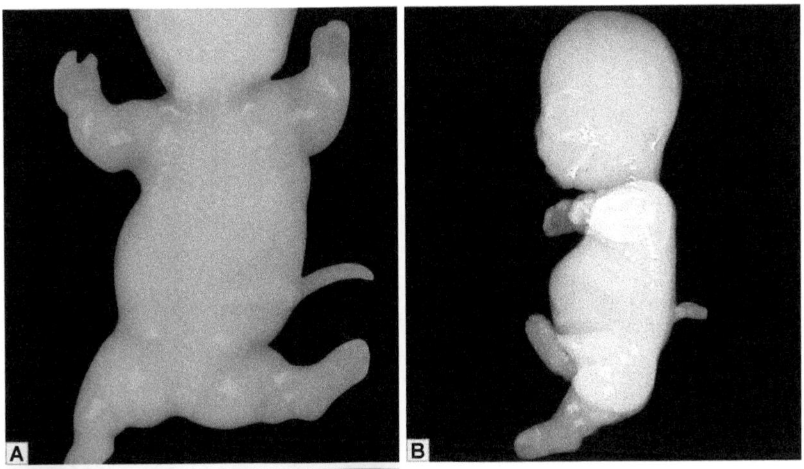

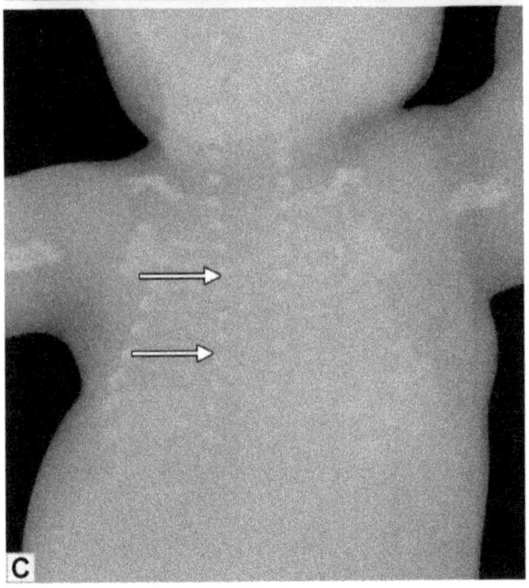

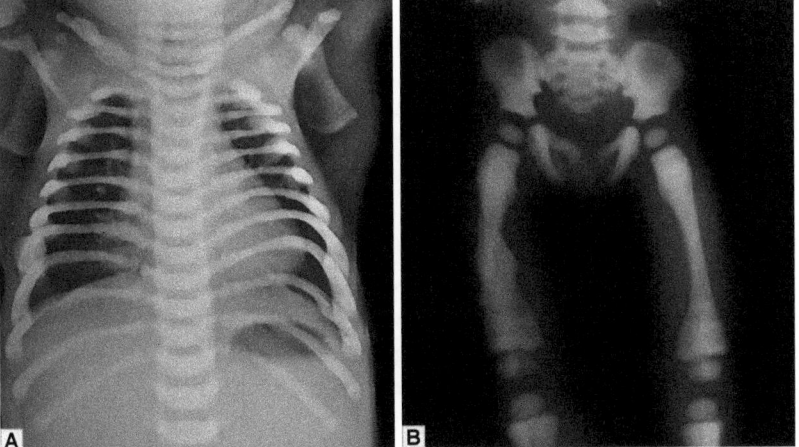

FIGS. 3A TO C: Achondrogenesis. Infantogram AP (B) and lateral (C), cropped thoracic region (C).
(A) Severe limb shortening of both upper and lower limbs;
(B) poor calvarial and vertebral ossification; and
(C) poor ossification of thoracic vertebral bodies (arrows), short thorax.

FIGS. 4A AND B: Osteopetrosis. Chest radiograph shows generalized increased bone density. (A) Sclerosis of ribs and vertebrae and (B) obliteration of marrow cavity, old fracture, and callus formation.

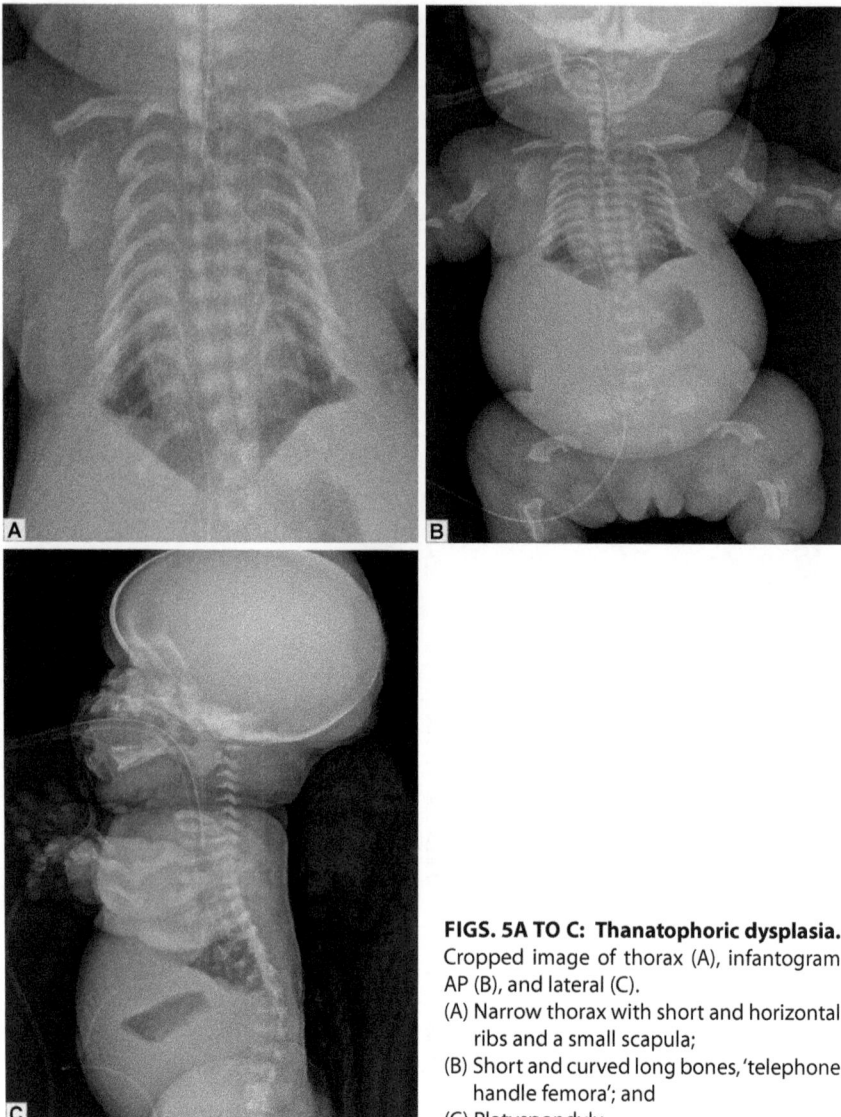

FIGS. 5A TO C: Thanatophoric dysplasia. Cropped image of thorax (A), infantogram AP (B), and lateral (C).
(A) Narrow thorax with short and horizontal ribs and a small scapula;
(B) Short and curved long bones, 'telephone handle femora'; and
(C) Platyspondyly.

Infections

A multitude of organisms can involve the chest wall depending on the immune status of the child. This may be involved by contiguous involvement from adjacent structures such as lung or nodes, etc.; or the primary site of involvement is the chest wall due to hematogenous spread.

Bacterial Infections

- It is a rare condition that typically involves the ribs or sternum.
- Most typically due to *Staphylococcus aureus*.
- Clinical findings are of acute infection including cellulitis.
- Radiograph is abnormal only after 7–10 days, consists of rib destruction, periosteal reaction, and overlying soft-tissue swelling **(Figs. 6A to D)**.
- CT or MRI remains the preferred imaging modalities.

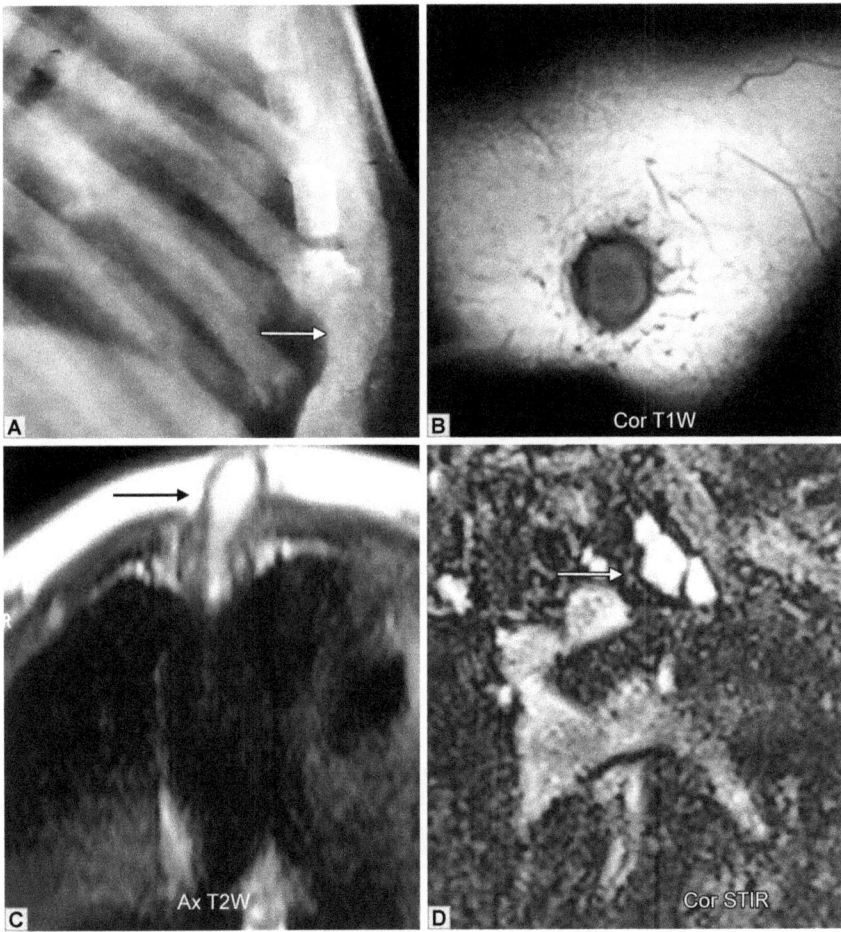

FIGS. 6A TO D: Sternal osteomyelitis. Chest X-ray (CXR) lateral (A) and MRI sequences (B to D). (A) Lytic destruction of the lower sternum (arrow); (B) hypointense marrow signal intensity in the sternum; (C) Axial T2W image shows sinus in the anterior chest wall with intrathoracic extension (arrow); and (D) short tau inversion recovery (STIR) coronal image shows mediastinal lymphadenopathy.

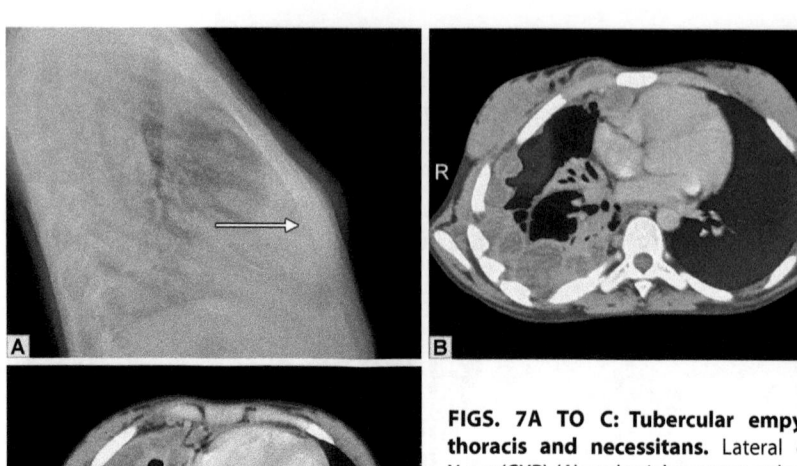

FIGS. 7A TO C: Tubercular empyema thoracis and necessitans. Lateral chest X-ray (CXR) (A) and axial contrast-enhanced computed tomography (CECT) chest (B and C) images—(A) opacity in the anterior chest wall and in the anterior lower mediastinum (arrow); (B) loculated fluid within the right pleural cavity with enhancement of pleural layers. Extension of the collection is seen into the right anterior chest wall involving the right costochondral junction.

Tuberculosis
- Constitutes <2% of all cases of tuberculosis
- Sternum, sternoclavicular joints, ribs, and spine
- Spine being the most frequent site with multilevel involvement; showing disk space loss, vertebral destruction, and paraspinal abscesses **(Figs. 7A to C)**. Also see Chapter 9.

Fungal Infections
- Seen in immunocompromised patient population.
- *Aspergillus* species account for up to 80–90%.
- *Mucor* species can also involve the chest wall by contiguous involvement from lungs; and may have an aggressive pattern of bone destruction **(Figs. 8A and B)**.
- Ribs involved by direct extension from an underlying pulmonary process.
- Imaging characteristics are nonspecific. Diagnosis is usually made in the appropriate clinical context and confirmed by either culture or histopathology.

Parasitic Infections
Unusual infections such as myocysticercosis can also involve the chest wall in children **(Figs. 9A and B)**.

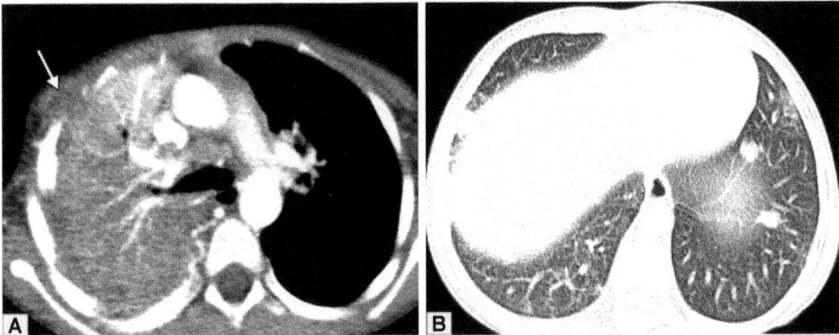

FIGS. 8A AND B: Invasive aspergillosis affecting the chest wall in a child with chronic granulomatous disease. Axial contrast-enhanced computed tomography (CECT) images. (A) Right upper lobe consolidation, with contiguous chest wall affection (arrow) and (B) well-defined nodules in left lower lobe.

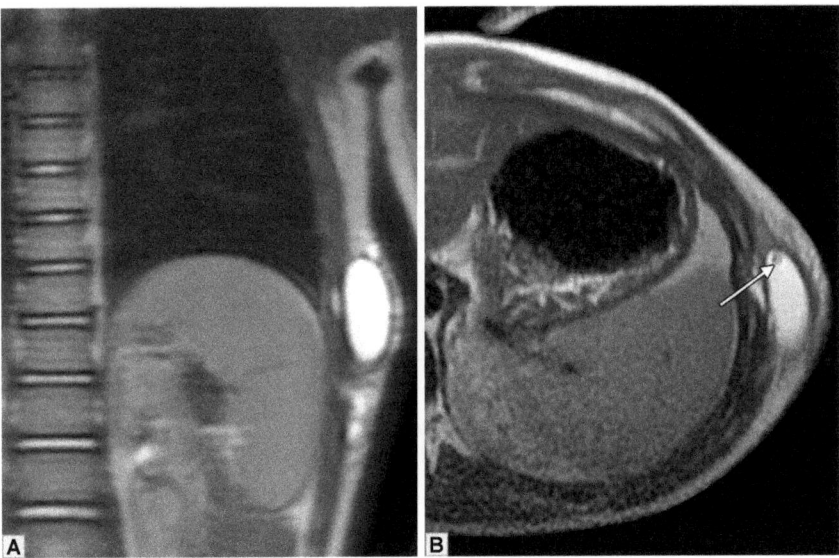

FIGS. 9A AND B: Chest wall cysticercosis. T2W coronal (A) and axial (B) images. (A) Well-defined hyperintense cystic lesion in subcutaneous plane of left lateral chest wall and (B) hypointense scolex within the cyst (arrow).

Trauma

Besides accidental trauma, chest is a common site of nonaccidental trauma due to child abuse.

Accidental Trauma
- Fracture of the ribs and sternum occurs less frequently due to elasticity of the pediatric chest wall.
- Metabolic bone diseases may predispose the patient to fracture, such as rickets or osteogenesis imperfecta.

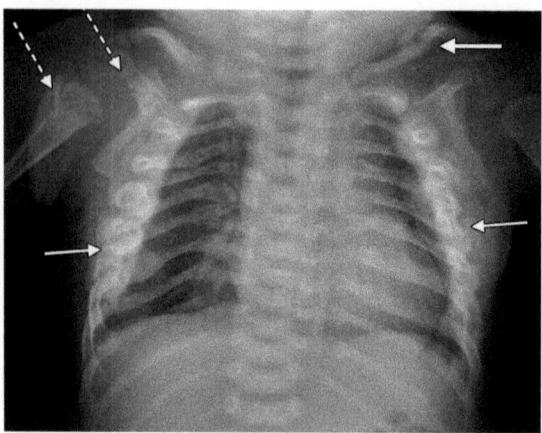

FIG. 10: Nonaccidental injury—multiple lateral rib fractures with callus formation (thin arrows); left-sided clavicle fracture (thick arrow); and right scapular and right humeral metaphyseal bucket handle fracture (dotted arrows).

Nonaccidental Trauma

- Combination of clinical history and imaging findings.
- Absence of major trauma, fractures of the ribs suggest nonaccidental trauma.
- Presence of multiple fractures at different temporal stages of healing (**Fig. 10**).

Metabolic Disorders

Chest wall manifestations of various metabolic disorders are described in **Table 3**.

TABLE 3: Thoracic wall manifestations of metabolic disorders.	
Disorder	**Manifestations**
Rickets	• Rachitic rosary • Expansion of the anterior rib ends at the costochondral junctions (**Fig. 11**) • Pectus carinatum • Harrison's sulcus—indrawing of the lower ribs
Scurvy	• Scorbutic rosary • Costochondral junction is more angular and has a sharper step-off • May relate to fracturing of the zone of provisional calcification during normal respiration
Osteomalacia	• Fuzzy trabeculae of bones • Pseudofractures • Vertebral endplate sclerosis
Hyperparathyroidism	• Resorption of lateral end of clavicles • Intracortical tunneling of the ribs • Brown tumors (expansile lytic lesions)

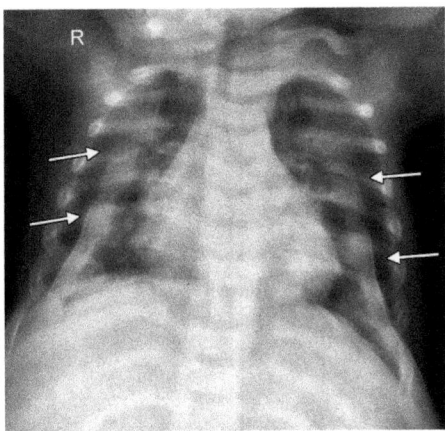

FIG. 11: Rickets—bulbous anterior ends of the ribs, giving rise to "rachitic rosary" (arrows).

Neoplasms

Osteochondroma

- Osteochondroma appears as an osseous protuberance in continuity with the surface of the originating bone.
- It may be sessile or pedunculated.
- CT is superior to radiography for showing the characteristic continuity of the cortex and medullary cavity with the osteochondroma.
- Cartilage cap (if calcified) can sometimes be seen on CT, but this structure is better visualized on MRI **(Figs. 12A to C)**.

Mesenchymal Hamartoma

- Lesion develops during fetal life, and is present at or shortly after birth.
- It consists of expansile intraosseous overgrowths of normal skeletal elements, including bone and hyaline cartilage.[2,3]
- Expansile chest mass that involves one or more ribs **(Figs. 13A to C)**.
- Speckled popcorn like calcifications.
- Secondary aneurysmal bone cyst formation showing fluid-fluid levels on imaging.
- Self-limited lesions that typically stop growing within the first year of life.
- Imaging features characteristic.
- Biopsy findings are variable, seldom diagnostic.
- Surgery indicated only in case of pressure symptoms.

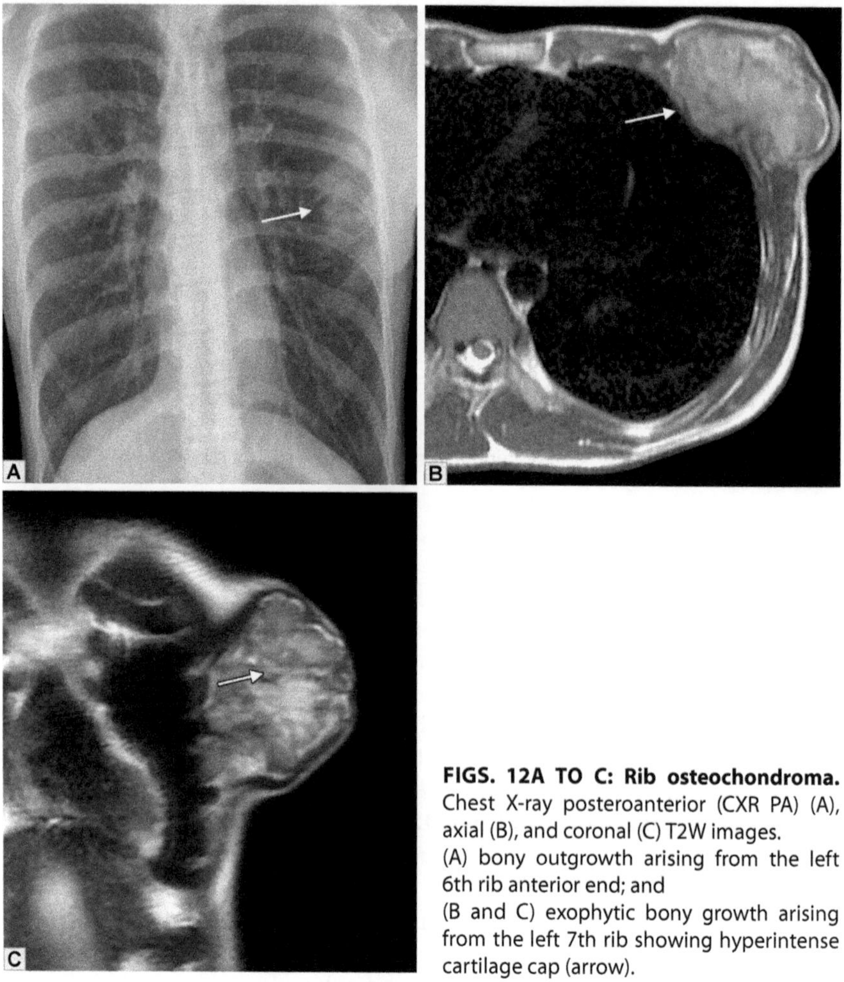

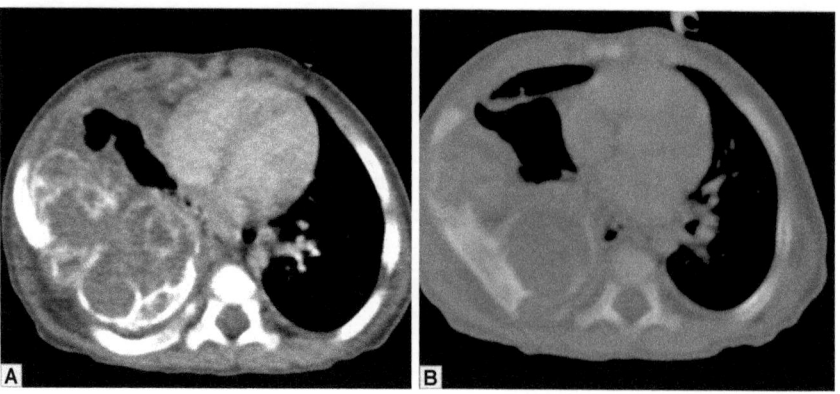

FIGS. 12A TO C: Rib osteochondroma. Chest X-ray posteroanterior (CXR PA) (A), axial (B), and coronal (C) T2W images.
(A) bony outgrowth arising from the left 6th rib anterior end; and
(B and C) exophytic bony growth arising from the left 7th rib showing hyperintense cartilage cap (arrow).

FIGS. 13A TO C: *Continued*

Continued

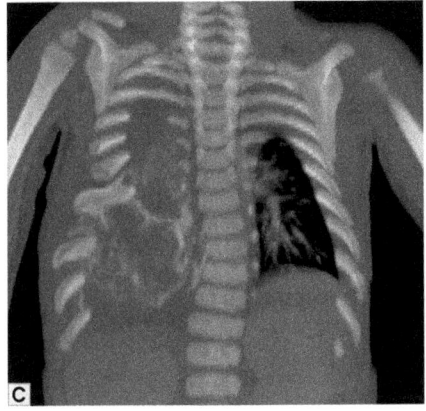

FIGS. 13A TO C: Mesenchymal hamartoma of chest wall. Axial contrast-enhanced computed tomography (CECT) (A and B) and coronal maximum intensity projection (MIP) image (C).
(A) enhancing soft tissue arising from right chest wall;
(B) bony expansion and expansile lesion arising out of right 7th rib;
(C) single rib involvement, well-defined bony lesion with narrow zone of transition.

Fibrous Dysplasia

- Typically, asymptomatic and found incidentally.
- Monostotic or polyostotic depending on the number of lesions.
- Expand and deform the bone, causing cosmetic deformity and mass effect on local structures **(Figs. 14A and B)**.
- Focal well-defined expansile intramedullary lesion with a ground-glass matrix.
- CT can detect amorphous calcifications within the lesion.
- On MRI, typically it is isointense to skeletal muscle on T1-weighted images and heterogeneously hyperintense on T2-weighted sequences and shows heterogeneous enhancement in active stage.

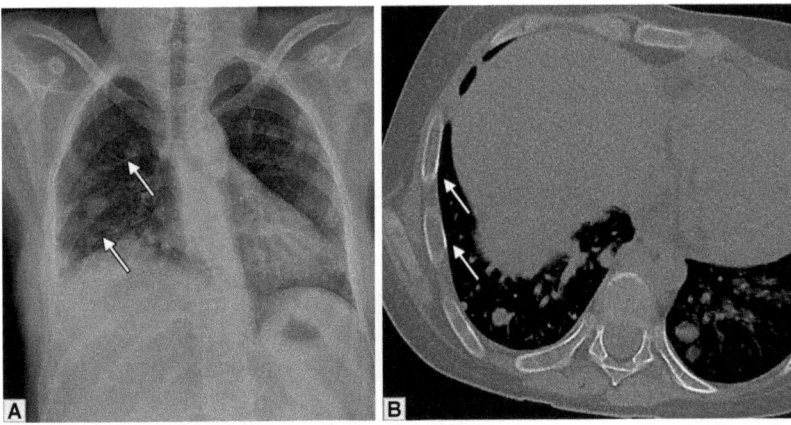

FIGS. 14A AND B: Polyostotic fibrous dysplasia in a patient with McCune–Albright syndrome. Chest X-ray posteroanterior (CXR PA) (A) and axial CT (B) image. (A) Expansion of multiple ribs on the right side with an internal ground glass matrix (arrows) and (B) medullary expansion of ribs on the right side with internal ground glass matrix.

Rhabdomyosarcoma
- High-grade mesenchymal tumors.
- Rapidly growing and painful.
- Bone involvement is less frequent and occurs later.
- Ultrasound shows a well-defined mass.
- CT can show the anatomic extent of the lesion as well as pulmonary metastases and bony metastases.

Ewing's Sarcoma Family of Tumors
- High-grade small round blue cell tumor
- It is the most common primary chest wall malignancy in this age group (and the third most common in older adults). This group is characterized by translocations between chromosomes 11 and 22 [t(11;22) (q24;q12)]. The group includes:
  - Ewing sarcoma of bone
  - Extraosseous Ewing sarcoma
  - Primitive neuroectodermal tumor (PNET) or Askin tumor
- Histologically, ESFT shows crowded sheets of round blue cells
- It has a slight male predominance, most are diagnosed within the second decade of life with rapidly growing chest wall masses, pain, neurologic symptoms, and fever.

Imaging:
- Ewing family tumors (EFTs) are large, heterogeneous masses with necrosis.
- There is usually no calcification.
- *Bone destruction*: The bone of origin (most frequently, rib) shows permeative bone destruction with or without sclerosis or periosteal reaction. CT also demonstrates the intrathoracic extension and invasion of adjoining structures **(Figs. 15A to F)**.
- On MRI, tumor usually shows contrast enhancement; necrosis and hemorrhage are better seen.
- The tumors are FDG avid.
- Treatment strategy for EFT is a combination of systemic chemotherapy and local therapy (surgery/RT) depending on the extent of resection that would be required.

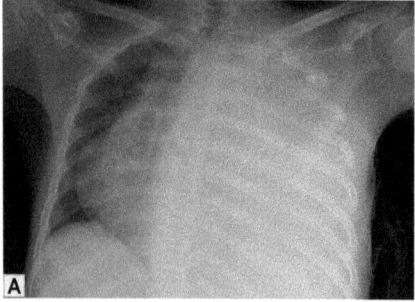 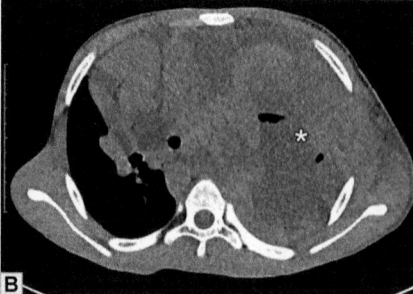

FIGS. 15A TO F: *Continued*

Continued

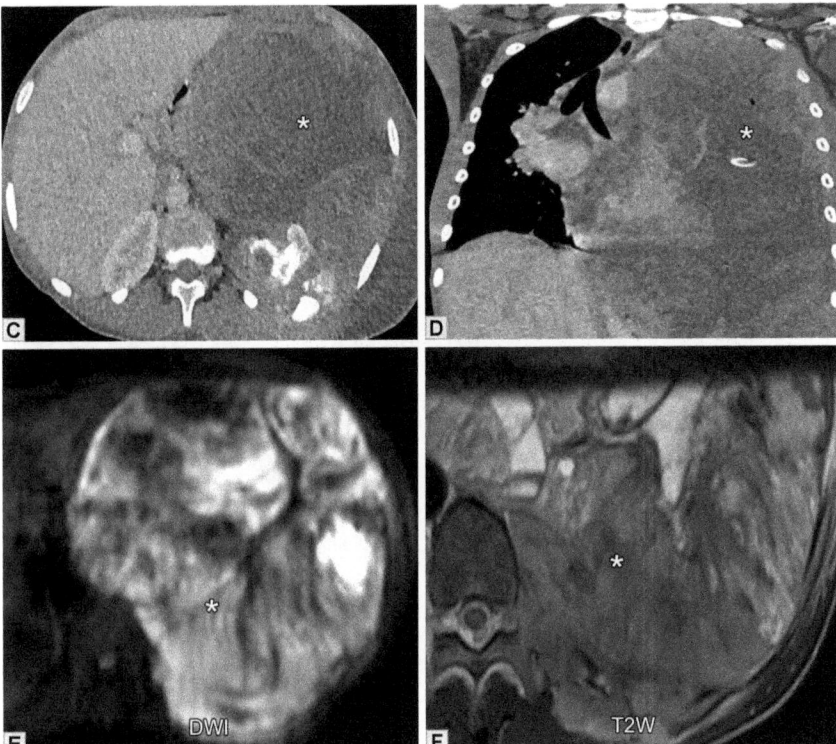

FIGS. 15A TO F: Ewing sarcoma of rib. Chest X-ray posteroanterior (CXR PA) (A), contrast-enhanced computed tomography (CECT) chest (B to D), Diffusion-weighted magnetic resonance (DWI) MR image (E), and T2W MR image (F). (A) Opaque left hemithorax with the contralateral tracheomediastinal shift. There is also a widening of ribs on the left side. (B to D) Large heterogeneously enhancing mass lesion in the left hemithorax (asterisk) causing a gross mediastinal shift towards the right side. The mass is showing central coarse calcification in continuity with rib. (E and F) The mass showed diffusion restriction (E), was heterogeneously hyperintense on T2W (F).

Extraskeletal Ewing Sarcoma

- This is rare as compared to Ewing tumor.
- Age of presentation varies between 20 months and 30 years.
- In contrast to bony ESFT, extraskeletal Ewing's tumor is seen equally in males and female, seen in older children and frequently affects the lower chest.
- Criteria for diagnosis of extraskeletal Ewing include:
  - No osseous involvement
  - No increased uptake in bone or periosteum

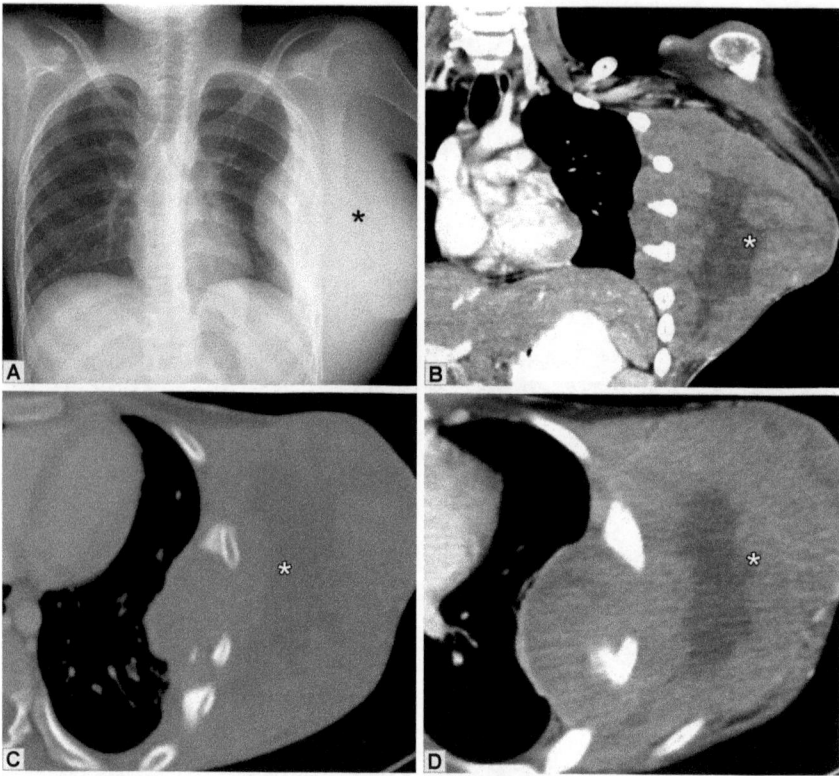

FIGS. 16A TO D: Extraskeletal Ewing tumor of the chest wall. Chest X-ray posteroanterior (CXR PA) (A), contrast-enhanced computed tomography (CECT) chest coronal (B), and axial (C and D) images. (A) Large soft tissue lesion (asterisk) along the left chest wall with intrathoracic extension. (B to D) Large soft tissue lesion (asterisk) involving left chest wall with intrathoracic extension and erosion of underlying ribs and thick periosteal reaction.

Imaging: Large soft tissue mass with underlying bone erosion, hyperostosis, cortical thickening, and osseous invasion can be seen **(Figs. 16A to D)**.

Metastatic Disease
- Most common malignant chest wall tumor
- Imaging appearance of metastatic disease involving the chest wall is often nonspecific **(Figs. 17A and B)**
- Typically presents as lytic lesions with overlying cortical disruption
- Neuroblastoma, rhabdomyosarcoma, lymphoma, or leukemia

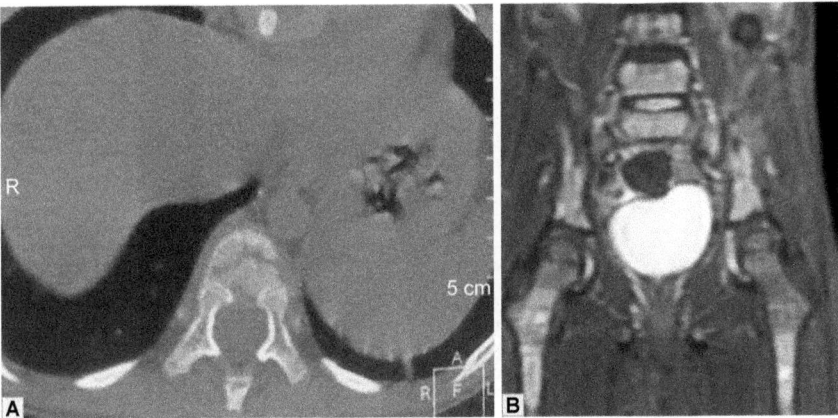

FIGS. 17A AND B: Neuroblastoma metastases. Axial computed tomography (CT) chest bone window (A) and magnetic resonance imaging (MRI) pelvis T2W fat suppressed image (B). (A) Lytic lesion involving thoracic vertebra with mild soft tissue and (B) hyperintense marrow lesions involving bilateral femora and pelvic bones.

Diffuse Periosteal Reaction of Thoracic Cage Bones in Children

Periosteal reaction/thickening involving the thoracic cage bones, especially the ribs can be seen in a host of physiological and pathological processes, and are listed in **Table 4**. Proper history taking and clinical evaluation often are contributory to the diagnosis.

TABLE 4: Causes of chest wall bony periosteal reaction.	
Condition	Clues to diagnosis
Physiological	Seen in infancy, self-limiting, and affected other long bones as well
Prostaglandin use	History of patent ductus arteriosus (PDA)
Caffey's disease/infantile cortical hyperostosis **(Fig. 18)**	Onset in early infancy presents with fever and irritability, usually self-limiting. Mandibular involvement and other flat bone involvement can be associated

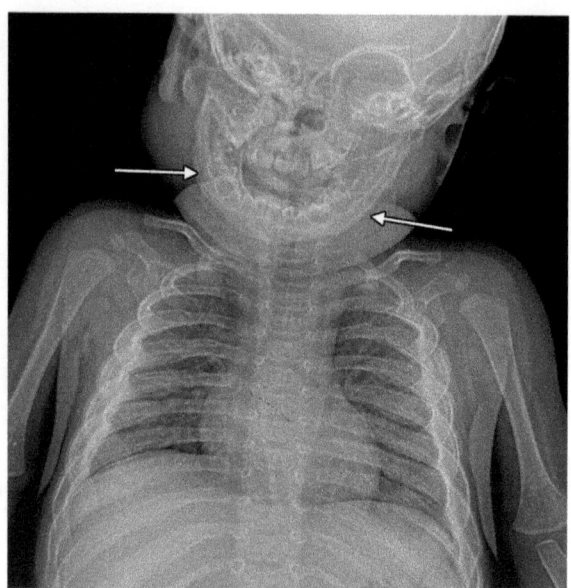

FIG. 18: Infantile cortical hyperostosis/Caffey's disease—diffuse periosteal reaction of bilateral lower ribs and hyperostosis of the mandible (arrows).

CONCLUSION

Chest wall lesions are common in the children; and can be either developmental, infectious, benign and malignant osseous, and soft tissue tumor. Imaging is extremely useful in the appropriate diagnosis as well as the extent of the lesion so that appropriate management can be done and unnecessary biopsies or surgeries can be avoided.

Other Related Chapter that can be Referred to:
- Chapter 24: Thoracic Tumors and Mimics: Part 2

REFERENCES

1. Baez JC, Lee EY, Restrepo R, Eisenberg RL. Chest wall lesions in children. Am J Roentgenol. 2013;200(5):W402-19.
2. Singh D. Imaging of chest wall and pleura. In Chawla A (Ed). Thoracic Imaging—Basic to Advanced. Singapore: Springer; 2019. pp. 325–60.
3. García-Peña P, Barber I. Pathology of the thoracic wall: congenital and acquired. Pediatr Radiol. 2010;40(6):859–68.

CHAPTER 26

Pleural Disorders: Imaging

Poonam Sherwani, Manisha Jana

- ❑ Imaging modalities
- ❑ Pleural pathologies
  - ➢ Pleural effusion
  - ➢ Pleural masses
  - ➢ Pleural thickening and nodular deposits
  - ➢ Pneumothorax
  - ➢ Hydropneumothorax
- ❑ Nonexpandable lung after drainage

INTRODUCTION

- Pleura is the serous membrane covering both hemithoraces and is composed of two layers—(1) visceral and (2) parietal layers, the former covering the lungs and fissural surfaces, the latter covering the thoracic cage and diaphragmatic surfaces.
- Vascular supply to the pleura is derived from intercostal and pulmonary vessels. The parietal pleura is innervated by intercostal nerves and hence is sensitive to a painful stimulus.
- Effusion is the most commonly encountered abnormality, others being pleural thickening and masses.

IMAGING MODALITIES

- Frontal chest radiograph [posteroanterior or anteroposterior (PA or AP)] depending on age of child is done initially.
- There is no role of lateral decubitus radiograph after the wide availability of ultrasound.
- Ultrasound has an important role in the evaluation of pleural abnormalities both for diagnosis, quantification, follow-up, staging, and guided interventions.
- Contrast-enhanced computed tomography (CECT) is required in selected situations based on underlying etiology.
- Magnetic resonance imaging (MRI) can be employed in the follow-up of infected pleural fluid collections (IPFC)/chronic empyema.

SECTION 9: Chest Wall and Pleural Disorders

■ PLEURAL PATHOLOGIES

The commonly encountered pleural pathologies are shown in **Flowchart 1**.

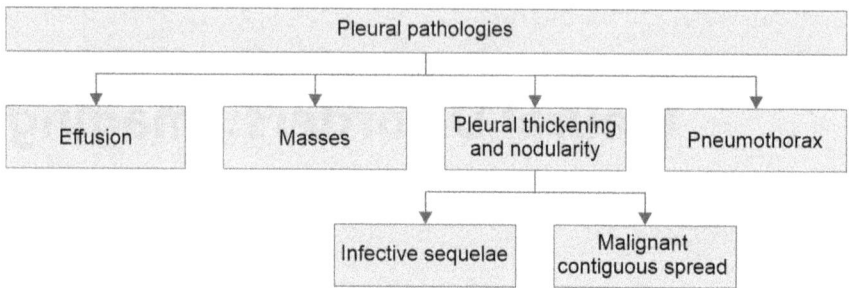

FLOWCHART 1: Broad classification of pleural pathologies.

Pleural Effusion

The terms transudate or exudate are used based on analysis of thoracentesis fluid and modified Light's criteria with common causes illustrated in **Flowchart 2**.

Radiograph

The radiographic features of free pleural effusion are listed in **Table 1**.

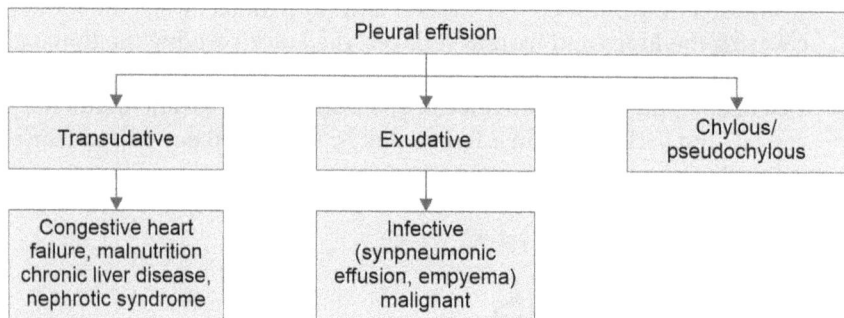

FLOWCHART 2: Common causes of pleural effusion.

TABLE 1: Signs of pleural effusion on radiograph (Figs. 1A and B).	
Signs on erect radiograph	**Signs on supine radiograph**
Increased density with concave upper margin (meniscus sign)	Increased opacity of hemithorax
Blunting of costophrenic angle	Superior mediastinal widening
Fluid within the fissures	Apical cap
	Fluid within the fissures

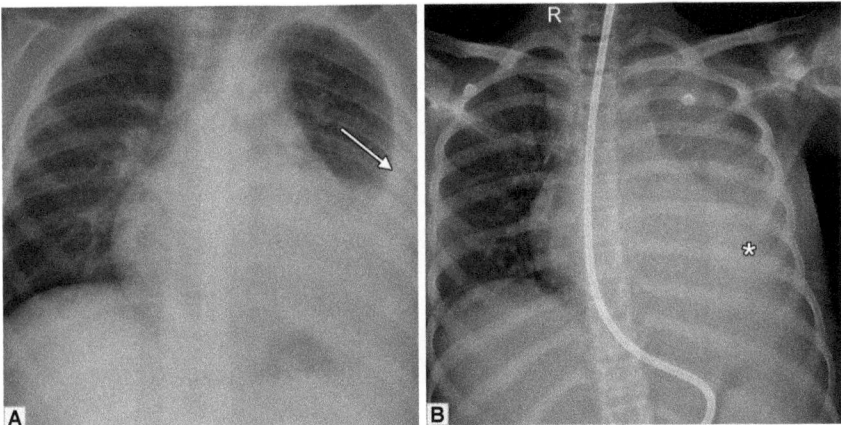

FIGS. 1A AND B: Free pleural effusion on erect (A) and supine (B) radiographs—Left costophrenic angle is blunted. Concave upper border which is medially slanting (meniscus sign, arrow in A). Homogeneous increased opacity in the left hemithorax (asterisk in B).

Ultrasound

Transudate/serous pleural effusion is seen as clear fluid, with no internal echoes on ultrasound or loculations. Some sonographic signs[1,2] are as follows:

- *Loss of mirror artifact:* There is artifactual mirroring of hepatic/splenic architecture above the hemidiaphragm as the lung descends in inspirations. With the presence of fluid, mirror artifact is lost.
- *Thoracic spine sign:* Due to free fluid, there is enhanced transmission through the pleura making the thoracic vertebral bodies visible. Normal, these are obscured by air-containing basal segments of the lungs.
- *Quad sign:* A quadrangular space formed by pleural free fluid where vertical boundaries are formed by two adjacent rib shadows and horizontal boundaries are formed by parietal and visceral pleura.
- *Sinusoid sign:* Respiratory variation in depth of effusion, as seen as a crest and trough of a wave in M-mode ultrasound **(Fig. 2)**.

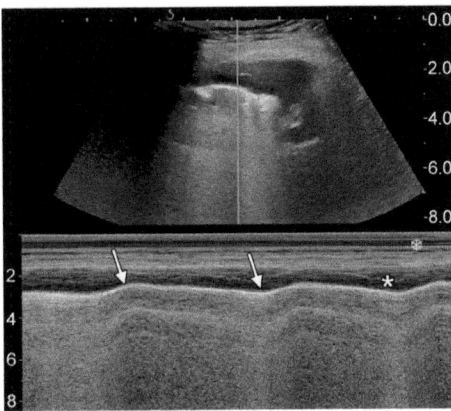

FIG. 2: Sinusoid sign—M-mode US showing to and fro movement of the lung toward the chest wall (arrows). The clear area (asterisk) denotes the pleural fluid.

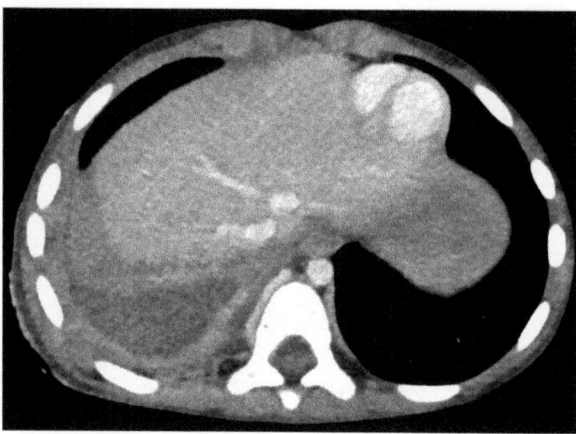

FIG. 3: Empyema right pleural cavity. CECT chest—enhancement of both parietal and visceral pleura, suggestive of split pleura sign.

Exudative pleural effusions are commonly infective (IPFC) or malignant. These show internal echoes on USG, loculations, and septations, underlying lung parenchymal abnormality (consolidation/collapse). The extent of these depends on the stage as discussed later in the chapter.

Contrast Enhanced Computed Tomography
- Transudative effusion is seen as clear crescent-shaped fluid with no pleural enhancement. Underlying lung is generally normal; passive atelectasis may be seen.
- Exudative effusion is associated with enhancement of visceral and parietal pleura on CECT **(Fig. 3)** and internal septations (better seen on ultrasound). "Split pleura sign" is seen on CECT when loculation develops. Infected pleural collections show pleural thickening and loculation. In cases of malignant effusion, the thickening is nodular.

Quantification of Pleural Effusion
Estimation of the amount of pleural fluid guides management decision. The various measurements used on different modalities are included.

Chest radiograph:
- *Blunting of costophrenic angle:* There is obliteration of costophrenic angle on frontal erect radiograph with >200 mL fluid within pleural cavity, while on lateral radiograph blunting is seen at ~50 mL of fluid.
- *Meniscus sign:* At >500 mL of free fluid within the pleura, effusion appears as a homogeneous opacity with a concave upper border which is lower medially than laterally, forming the pleural meniscus. No specific measurement parameters are available for children.
- Larger amount of pleural effusion can cause contralateral shift of the mediastinal structures.

Ultrasound and CT:
- Can detect pleural fluid as small as 5 mL.
- Methods for assessing the amount of fluid are listed in **Table 2**.

TABLE 2: Ultrasound methods of quantification of pleural effusion.[3-6]		
Method	Technique	Formula
Balik method	Supine position, with transducer perpendicular to chest posterolateral chest wall at end of expiration[4]	Pleural effusion in mL = maximum measured distance between parietal and visceral pleura (in mm) × 20
Eisenberg method	Supine position with transducer perpendicular to the chest wall at maximum inspiration[5]	Pleural effusion in mL = [maximum measured distance between lung and posterior chest wall (in mm) × 47.6] − 837
Goecke 2 method (Figs. 4A to D)	Sitting/erect position; USG image is obtained keeping probe longitudinally oriented along dorsolateral/posterolateral aspect of chest wall, and craniocaudal extent (X) and the lung base to mid-diaphragm distance/subpulmonary height (LDD) is measured. One can measure the volume of effusion using formula[3]	Estimated volume (EV) mL = (X + LDD) × 70
CT (Figs. 5A and B)	AP depth and AP quartile method on a supine axial CECT scan at maximum depth at midclavicular line[6]	• Depth < 3 cm or 0–25% of the hemithorax (first AP quartile): Mild • Depth 3–10 cm or 25–50% of the hemithorax (second quartile): Moderate • Depth > 10 cm or >50% (third and fourth quartile)

(AP: anteroposterior; CECT: contrast-enhanced computed tomography; LDD: lung to diaphragm distance)

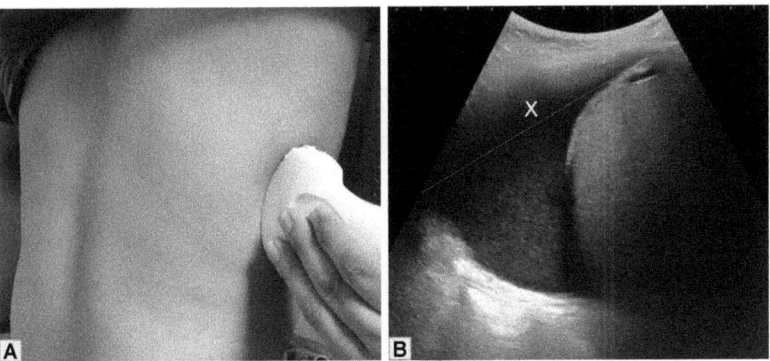

FIGS. 4A TO D: *Continued*

Continued

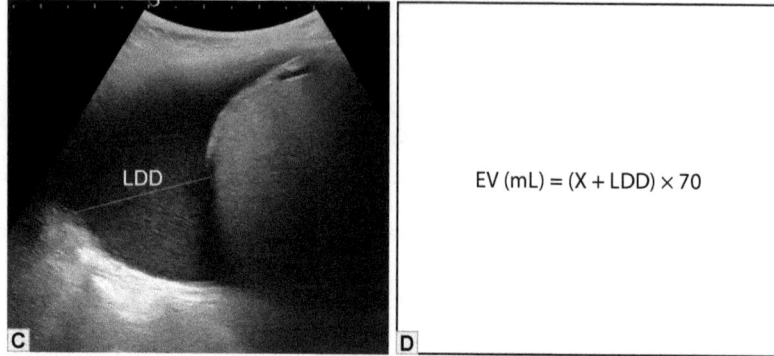

FIGS. 4A TO D: USG quantification technique—(A) probe position oriented longitudinally on dorsolateral aspect in erect/sitting position; (B) image showing measurement of X which is the craniocaudal extent in centimeter of the effusion measured in position A; (C) lung to diaphragm distance (LDD) which is the lung base to mid-diaphragm distance/subpulmonary height of the effusion (cm); and (D) formula used to calculate the volume, EV is the estimated effusion volume (mL) and 70 is the empirical factor/constant.

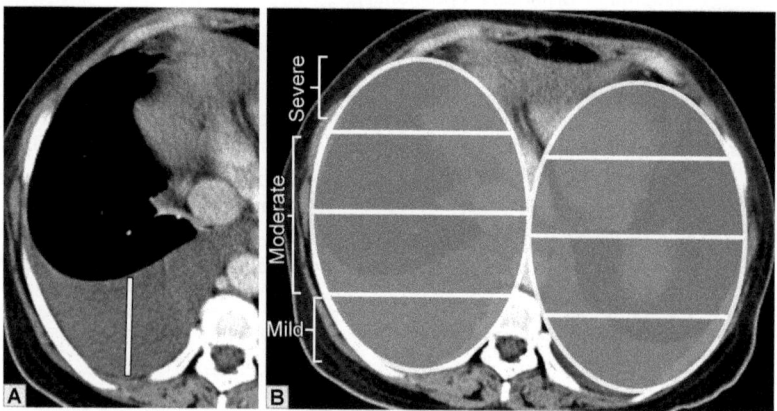

FIGS. 5A AND B: CT quantification of pleural effusion. (A) Measuring the anteroposterior (AP) depth of the pleural effusion at midclavicular line where the maximum fluid is seen. (B) Axial CT image with superimposed AP quartiles dividing the hemithorax to quantify the pleural effusion into mild, moderate, and severe categories. CT showing right moderate effusion since the fluid extends till the 25th–50th quartile of the hemithorax. Similarly on left side, there is mild pleural effusion since fluid extends till only 25th quartile of the hemithorax.

Special Situations

Loculated effusion:
- Loculations can occur due to adhesions, along the costal/mediastinal/diaphragmatic, or cervical pleura.
- Unlike free effusion, they have a sharply defined convex margin, and do not obey the gravitational rules.
- Loculation along fissures can give rise to "vanishing" or "phantom" tumor.

Subpulmonic effusion:
- Defined as free fluid in the infrapulmonary space, and is more common on right side.
- *Right:* Right hemidiaphragm is elevated with its peak shifted laterally.
- *Left:* Elevation of left hemidiaphragm with increased distance with the gastric air bubble **(Figs. 6A to C)**.
- The important differential is eventration of the diaphragm, however, in that case peak will be more medial than subpulmonic effusion.

Neonatal effusion:
- It can be seen in cases of transient tachypnea of newborn and neonatal group-B streptococcal pneumonia.
- Chylous effusion can occur either idiopathically or associated malformation.

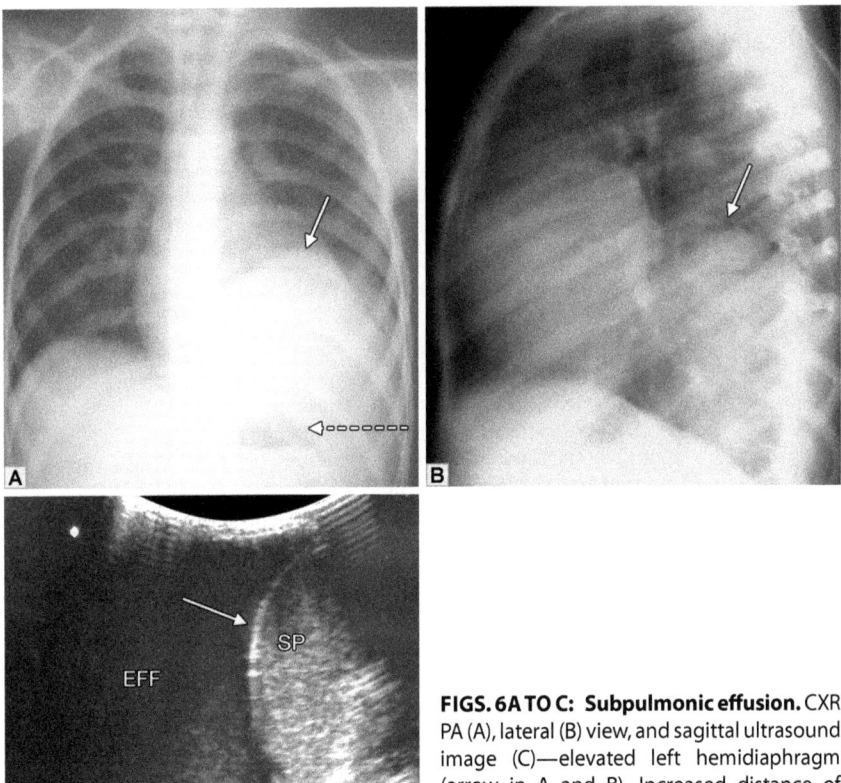

FIGS. 6A TO C: Subpulmonic effusion. CXR PA (A), lateral (B) view, and sagittal ultrasound image (C)—elevated left hemidiaphragm (arrow in A and B), Increased distance of diaphragm from the gastric bubble (dotted arrow), and Anechoic fluid collection (EFF) above diaphragm (arrow in C).

Infected Pleural Fluid Collection

Infected pleural fluid collections encompass both parapneumonic effusion and empyema. Parapneumonic effusion is defined as pleural fluid developing adjacent to pulmonary infection. Empyema is defined as the presence of pus within the pleural cavity. The stages of IPFC are listed in **Table 3**.

Management of IPFCs: The management of IPFC depends on quantity, patient's symptoms as well as stage. These stages have been described as exudative, fibrinopurulent, and organization; simple and complex (or complicated). IPFC is discussed subsequently.

- *Medical therapy*: Presence of IPFC in a pneumonia warrants admission and treatment with intravenous antibiotics. IPFCs can also be a reason for nonresponse of a child with pneumonia despite 48 hours of antibiotics.
- *Aspiration/drainage*:
    - Parapneumonic effusions are typically small volume, hence all procedures should be done under ultrasound guidance. Single-time aspiration is done for diagnostic purpose. However, large volume effusion causing respiratory compromise, persistent fever ± sepsis requires drainage. Repeated aspirations/thoracentesis should not be done for this purpose, instead a catheter/tube should be placed.

TABLE 3: Stages of infected pleural fluid collection.[7]		
Stage	Description	USG appearance (Figs. 7A to C)
Exudative	This is the early stage wherein the fluid has low WBC count	Anechoic clear fluid with few internal echoes. Floating thin septae may be present
Fibrinopurulent	In this stage, fibrin starts to get deposited on pleural surfaces leading to thickening and development of septae. These also result in loculation. The number of WBC cells also increases. When frank pus is present the term empyema is used, rest are termed as complex parapneumonic effusion as the number of WBCs within the fluid increases, it becomes thicker eventually forming pus	• Increase in internal echoes • Thick, fixed septae • Pleural thickening and loculations
Organizational/organizing stage	This stage is said to have been reached when a thick "fibrous peel" forms due to the fibroblasts. There is progressive volume loss and lung becomes nonexpandable "trapped". Several of these may result in chronic empyema	Thickened pleurae

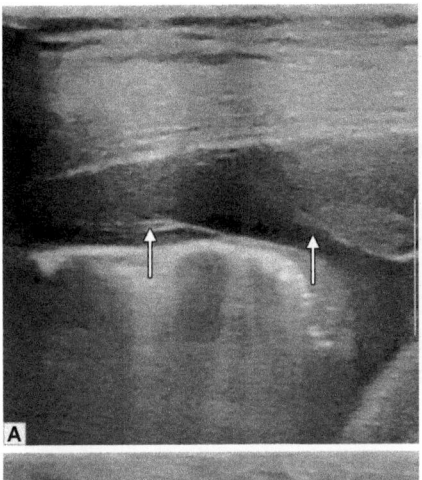
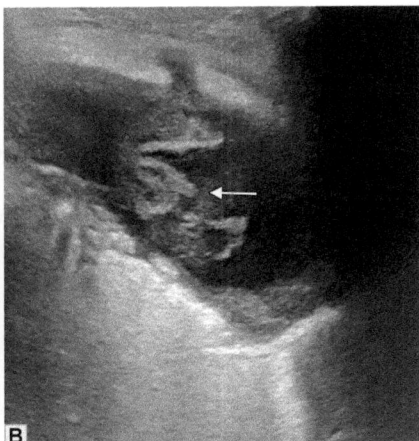
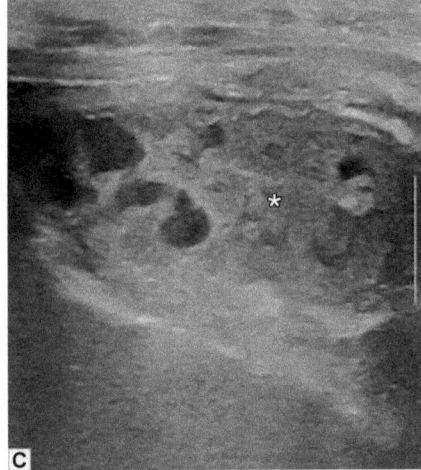

FIGS. 7A TO C: Stages of infected pleural fluid collection (IPFC) on ultrasonography (USG).
(A) *Exudative stage*: Anechoic fluid with a few thin mobile septae (arrows).
(B) *Fibrinopurulent stage*: Thick, fixed septations (arrow).
(C) *Organizing stage*: Thick, fibrinous content in the pleural cavity (asterisk).

- Assessing coagulation parameters and platelet count preprocedure is not advocated routinely, except in those with known risk factors. However, the choice depends on institutional protocols, and it may be prudent to do a basic international normalized ratio (INR) and platelet count.
- *Site of insertion*: In case of large bore chest tubes, the standard site of insertion is the mid axillary line (safe triangle). When placing smaller bore pigtail catheters, the site is chosen based on maximum collection. However, patient comfort should be borne in mind when choosing a site.
- *Technique*: Catheters need to be placed using Seldinger technique. Using a trocar-based system is strongly discouraged due to the risk of injury to the underlying lung when the sudden "give way" happens.

- **Tube care:**
  - Drainage catheter/tube should be immediately connected to a unidirectional flow system (underwater seal/Heimlich valve).
  - Underwater seal is to be kept lower than the level of patient's chest. Chest radiograph to be done postprocedure.
  - At one time up to 10 mL/kg of fluid can be removed, post which it should be clamped for 1 hour to prevent reperfusion edema.
  - Clamping of tube should not be done if bubbling is present. Further, if patient gets dyspneic it should be released, and radiograph repeated.
  - Monitor tube for blockage/kinking.
  - Flushing has to be done carefully as use of force can also lead to violation of inflamed pleura.
- *Intrapleural fibrinolytic therapy:*[7]
  - Intrapleural fibrinolytic therapy (IPFT) is used when despite adequate size, correctly placed tube, persistent collection present.
  - Aids in dissolving septae or loculations.
  - Streptokinase, urokinase, or tPA with DNAase has been used in adults.
  - In children, only urokinase has been studied adequately, and is hence recommended.
  - Dose of urokinase is as follows:
    - <10 kg body weight: 10,000 U in 10 mL saline
    - > 10 kg body weight: 40,000 U in 10 mL saline (0.9%). This dose is to be given BD (twice a day) × 3 days. In case of hemorrhagic return, the next dose can be withheld.
- *Surgery*: Surgery is indicated in case of inadequate response/persistent collection postdrainage. Chronic empyema is managed with decortication. Further, lung abscess should not be drained percutaneously. The child should be followed up till complete/near complete resolution of the IPFC.

Chylothorax

Chylothorax is discussed in the Chapter 20 on lymphatic disorders.

Pleural Masses

- Pleural masses encountered in children include pleuropulmonary blastoma, rarely neurogenic tumors (in neurofibromatosis setting), or solitary fibrous tumor.[1,2,6]
- For discussion on individual tumors, please see Chapters 23 and 24.

Pleural Thickening and Nodular Deposits

- Smooth thin pleural thickening can be seen after infection/empyema.
- Nodular pleural thickening is seen as soft tissue nodules or masses along the pleura, and suggest a malignant etiology **(Figs. 8A to C)**.[8] However, this distinction on imaging between benign and malignant causes is not absolute, and can show overlapping/atypical features.

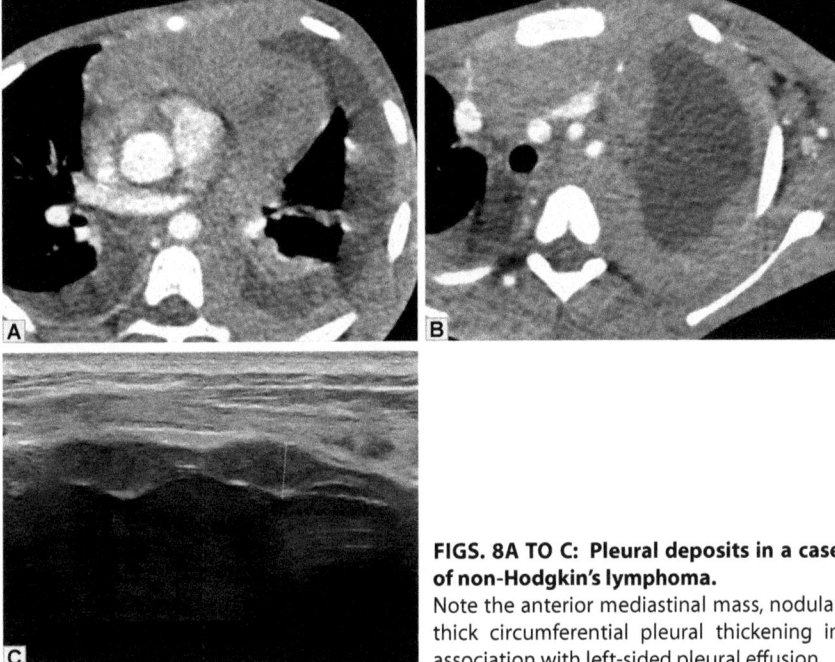

FIGS. 8A TO C: Pleural deposits in a case of non-Hodgkin's lymphoma.
Note the anterior mediastinal mass, nodular thick circumferential pleural thickening in association with left-sided pleural effusion.

- Further pleural thickening along the mediastinal surface or a thickness >1 cm suggests a malignant etiology.
- Pleural involvement in malignancies can either be contiguous or hematogenous.
- Contiguous extension in lymphoma **(Figs. 9A to C)** or mediastinal germ cell tumor are common causes in children.
- Hematogenous spread can be seen from a distant tumor.
- Usually associated with exudative pleural effusion.

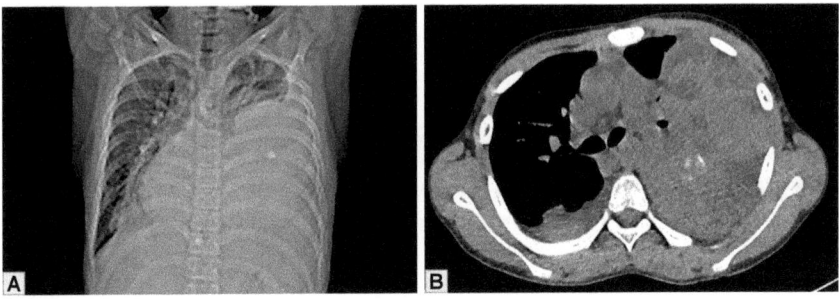

FIGS. 9A TO C: *Continued*

Continued

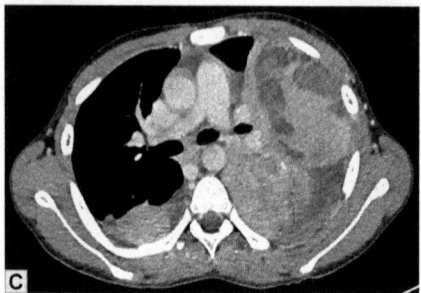

FIGS. 9A TO C: Contiguous pleural involvement in germ cell tumor. Computed tomography (CT) scout image (A), axial noncontrast CT (NCCT) (B), and contrast-enhanced CT (CECT) (C) images—opaque left hemithorax (A), pleural-based soft tissue attenuation nodules with foci of calcification (B), and heterogeneous enhancement (C).

Pneumothorax

Pneumothorax refers to a collection of air in the pleural cavity. Causes of pneumothorax are given in **Flowchart 3**.

Radiographs

The radiographic features are enlisted in **Table 4**. On radiographs, pneumothorax is seen as hyperlucent hemithorax with visible visceral pleural outline. There is lack of bronchovascular markings in peripheral fields.

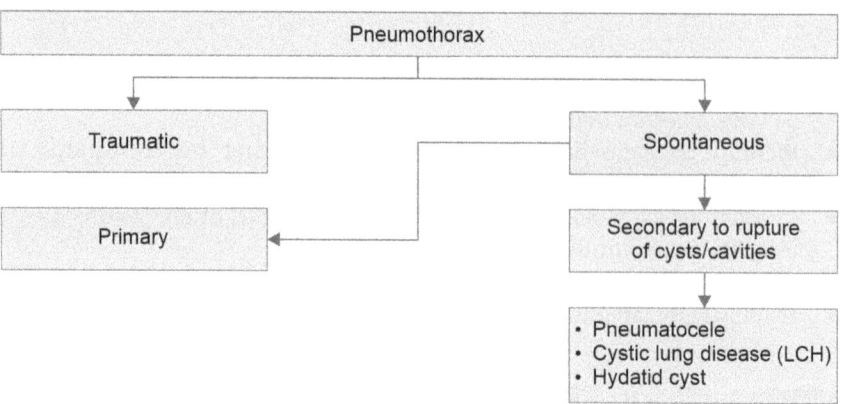

FLOWCHART 3: Causes of pneumothorax.

TABLE 4: Signs of pneumothorax on radiographs.	
Signs on erect radiograph (Fig. 10)	**Signs on supine radiograph (Figs. 11A to C)**
Lucency having a sharp margin with the underlying lung	Increased lucency of hemithorax
	Deep sulcus sign

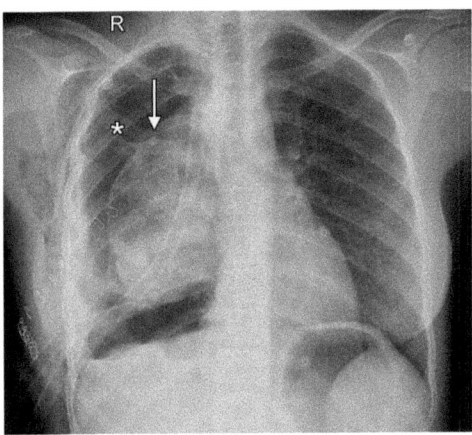

FIG. 10: Pneumothorax on erect chest X-ray (CXR)—pneumothorax (asterisk) with collapsed right lung (arrow).

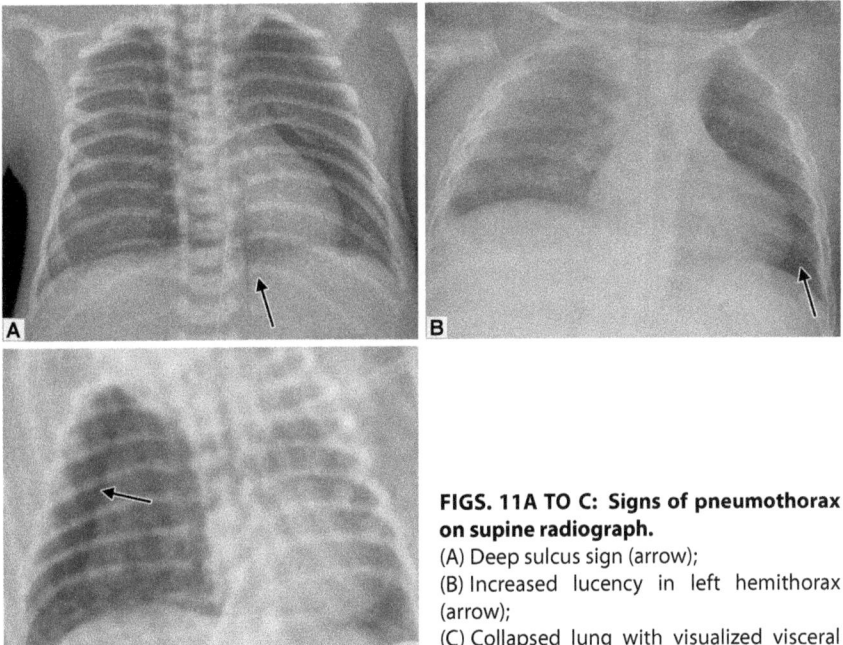

FIGS. 11A TO C: Signs of pneumothorax on supine radiograph.
(A) Deep sulcus sign (arrow);
(B) Increased lucency in left hemithorax (arrow);
(C) Collapsed lung with visualized visceral pleural margin (arrow).

Ultrasound

- On ultrasound, pneumothorax is seen as a loss of normal "lung sliding sign", in the presence of A lines.
- On M-mode ultrasound, it is seen as a "bar code" sign **(Fig. 12)**.
- "Lung point sign" is described as one specific ultrasound sign of pneumothorax, and is useful in quantification as well. It refers to the identification of a point where the pneumothorax ends and the lung sliding appears.

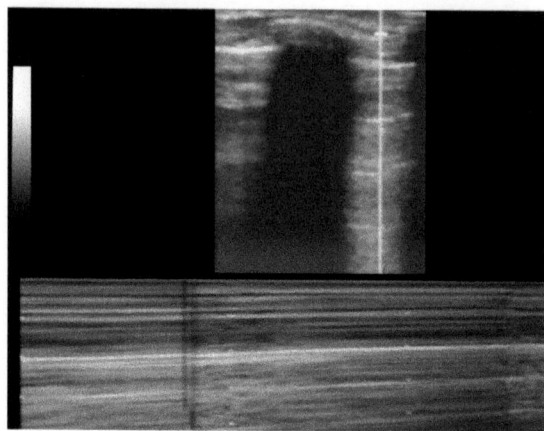

FIG. 12: Barcode sign on M-mode ultrasound.

Computed Tomography

- CT can detect even a small volume of pneumothorax. The added advantage is the ability to detect the underlying cause of pneumothorax **(Figs. 13A to C)**.
- CT is, however, seldom required for detection of pneumothorax, but for ascertaining the cause in spontaneous pneumothorax, NCCT suffices.
- CECT is required only for active infection.
- CT scan is more informative, if performed postdrainage so that the underlying lung is expanded and cysts/cavities can be detected.
- For the detection of small apical blebs, coronal reformat is necessary **(Figs. 14A to C)**.

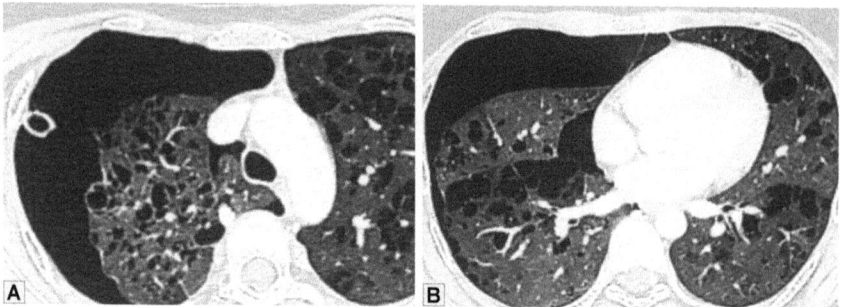

FIGS. 13A TO C: *Continued*

Continued

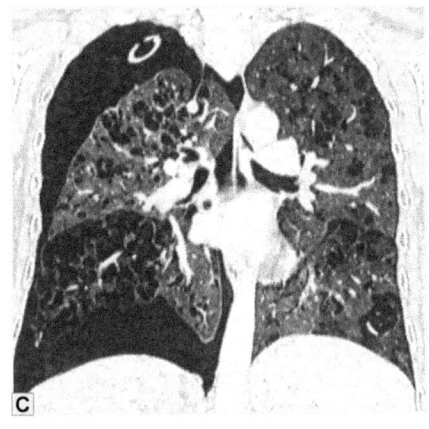

FIGS. 13A TO C: Pneumothorax in LCH.
Axial CT (A and B) and coronal MPR (C)—right-sided free pneumothorax and multiple variable sized cysts in both lungs.

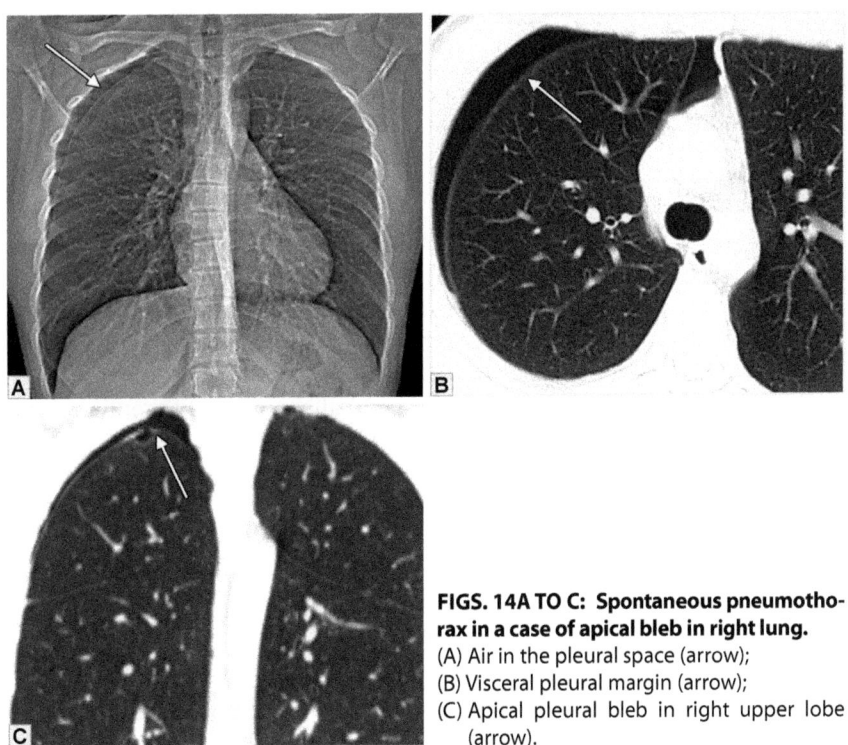

FIGS. 14A TO C: Spontaneous pneumothorax in a case of apical bleb in right lung.
(A) Air in the pleural space (arrow);
(B) Visceral pleural margin (arrow);
(C) Apical pleural bleb in right upper lobe (arrow).

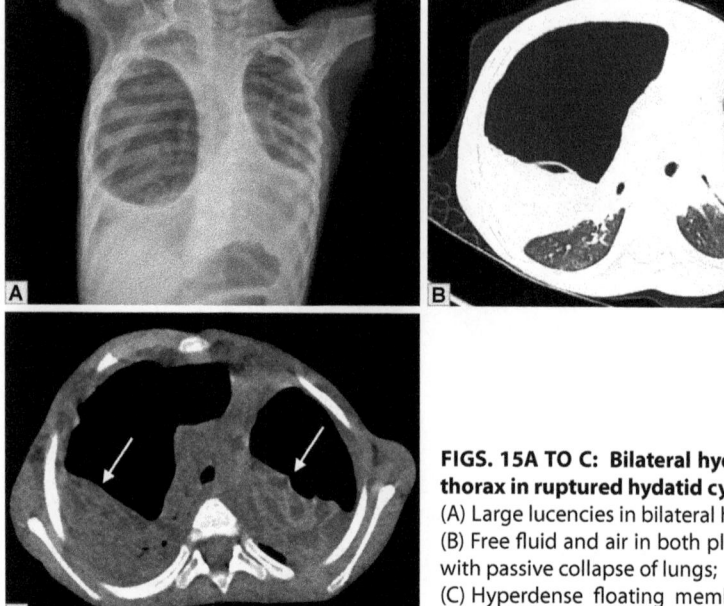

FIGS. 15A TO C: Bilateral hydropneumothorax in ruptured hydatid cysts.
(A) Large lucencies in bilateral hemithorax;
(B) Free fluid and air in both pleural cavities with passive collapse of lungs;
(C) Hyperdense floating membrane within the pleural fluid (arrows).

Hydropneumothorax

- Presence of both air and fluid in the pleural cavity can be iatrogenic (following, after or during surgery) or spontaneous **(Figs. 15A to C)**.
- Spontaneous hydropneumothorax results from rupture of underlying infected pneumatocele or abscess or even a bronchopleural fistula. When infected it is referred to as pyopneumothorax.
- Loculated hydropneumothorax can be challenging to differentiate from abscess/infected cavity:
  - Use of angle sign and epicenter of the lesion helps in differentiation.
  - Use of lateral radiograph and sagittal MPR on CT aids in differentiation **(Figs. 16A to C)**.
  - Pulmonary lesions tend to retain a round shape, while pleural collections extend anteroposteriorly.
- *Bronchopleural fistula (Figs. 17A to C)*:
  - This implies a communication of airway with pleural space. It can be secondary to either trauma/surgery or necrotizing infection (bacterial infection, tuberculosis, and septic emboli).
  - In postsurgical situation, it commonly develops 7–10 days after surgery. On radiographs, there is appearance of a large amount of air with contralateral mediastinal shift.
  - Postinfective bronchopleural fistula is associated with multiple air fluid levels and adhesions.

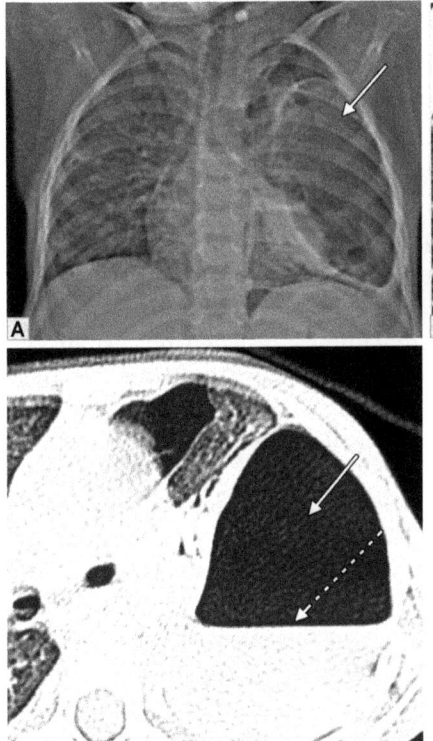
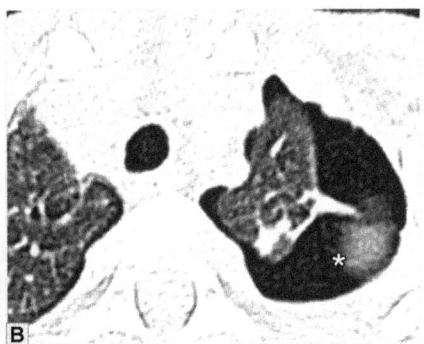
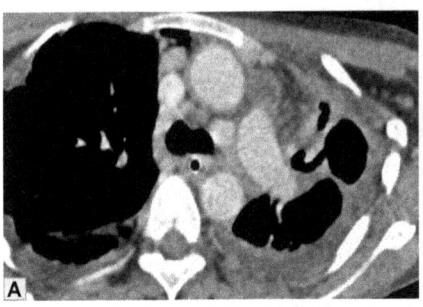

FIGS. 16A TO C: Loculated hydropneumothorax.
(A) Loculated pneumothorax (arrow);
(B) Free air in pleural cavity (asterisk);
(C) Loculated pneumothorax (arrow) with air fluid level (dotted arrow).

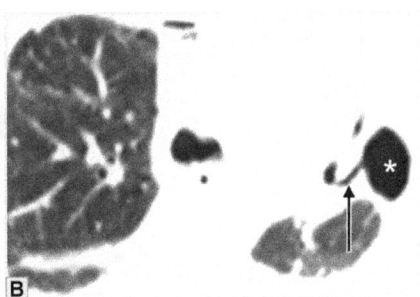
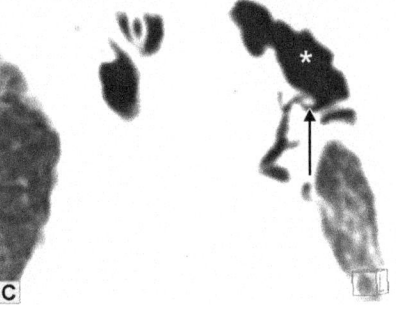

FIGS. 17A TO C: Infective bronchopleural fistula. Axial CECT (A and B), coronal MPR (C).
(A) Volume loss in left hemithorax with pleural thickening;
(B and C) Left apical cavity (asterisk) with bronchial communication (arrow).

NONEXPANDABLE LUNG AFTER DRAINAGE

This is a mechanical complication wherein the lung does not expand despite drainage with property placed adequately sized catheter.

The causes include:
- *Restriction by the visceral pleura*: Based on the duration, this can take two forms:
    1. *Lung entrapment*: When the lung is not expandable due to acute inflammation. the pleural fluid is exudative, and there is positive pleural pressure, causing contralateral mediastinal shift.
    2. *Trapped lung*: When there is pleural fibrosis, resisting lung expansion. The pleural fluid is transudative, but negative intrapleural pressure results in an ipsilateral mediastinal shift **(Figs. 18A and B)**.
- *Endobronchial obstruction*: This does not allow adequate air to enter lung for expansion.
- *End-stage lung fibrosis*: Herein the lung is incapable of full expansion.
- *Bronchopleural fistula (BPF)*: In BPF, due to continuous air leak, the pressure does not allow the underlying lung to expand.

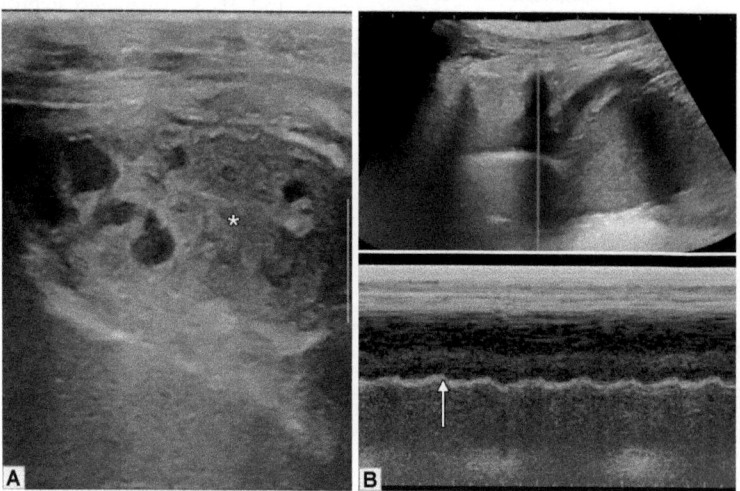

FIGS. 18A AND B: Trapped lung. B mode (A) and M-mode ultrasound (B)—thick fibrinous exudate in pleural cavity (asterisk) and reduced movement of the lung and visceral pleura (arrow).

CONCLUSION

Selection of ideal imaging modality is the key to evaluation of pleural pathologies. Ultrasound is a key imaging modality in pleural effusion, empyema, and thickening; whereas CT is invaluable in mapping the extent of disease in pleural thickening/empyema, pneumothorax, and pleural masses.

Other Related Chapters that can be Referred to:
- Chapter 1: Chest Radiograph: Basics and Role
- Chapter 24: Thoracic Tumors and Mimics: Part 2

REFERENCES

1. Maffey A, Colom A, Venialgo C, Acastello E, Garrido P, Cozzani H, et al. Clinical, functional, and radiological outcome in children with pleural empyema. Pediatr Pulmonol. 2019;54(5):525-30.
2. Efrati O, Barak A. Pleural effusions in the pediatric population. Pediatr Rev. 2002;23(12):417-26.
3. Ibitoye BO, Idowu BM, Ogunrombi AB, Afolabi BI. Ultrasonographic quantification of pleural effusion: comparison of four formulae. Ultrasonography. 2018;37(3):254-60.
4. Balik M, Plasil P, Waldauf P, Pazout J, Fric M, Otahal M, et al. Ultrasound estimation of volume of pleural fluid in mechanically ventilated patients. Intensive Care Med. 2006;32:318.
5. Eibenberger KL, Dock WI, Ammann ME, Dorffner R, Hormann MF, Grabenwoger F. Quantification of pleural effusions: Sonography versus radiography. Radiology. 1994;191:681-4.
6. Moy MP, Levsky JM, Berko NS, Godelman A, Jain VR, Haramati LB. A new, simple method for estimating pleural effusion size on CT scans. Chest. 2013;143(4):1054-9.
7. Bhalla AS, Jana M, Naranje P, Singh SK, Banday I. Challenges in image-guided drainage of infected pleural collections: A review. J Clin Interv Radiol ISVIR. 2022;6:131-40.
8. Jaworska J, Buda N, Ciuca IM, Dong Y, Fang C, Feldkamp A, et al. Ultrasound of the pleura in children, WFUMB review paper. Med Ultrason. 2021;23(3):339-47.

SECTION 10

Respiratory Emergencies

CHAPTER 27: Hemoptysis: Imaging and Interventions
CHAPTER 28: Thoracic Imaging in Intensive Care Unit

Respiratory Emergencies

CHAPTER 27

Hemoptysis: Imaging and Interventions

Priyanka Naranje, Ayush Jain, Ashu Seith Bhalla

- ❏ Etiology
- ❏ Imaging evaluation
  - ➢ Chest radiograph
  - ➢ Multidetector row computed tomography
  - ➢ Magnetic resonance imaging
  - ➢ Catheter angiography
- ❏ Specific etiologies
- ❏ Interventional radiology management of hemoptysis
  - ➢ Bronchial artery embolization
  - ➢ Pulmonary artery embolization

INTRODUCTION

- Hemoptysis in children is an infrequent symptom, and may vary from trivial to potentially life-threatening. It warrants careful assessment of the airways, parenchyma, and the pulmonary as well as systemic vasculature. Most cases are mild and are usually self-limiting. Massive hemoptysis is defined as a total volume of 8 mL/kg in 24 hours.[1] It can be life-threatening due to asphyxiation by flooding blood in the airways.
- In children, evaluation of hemoptysis is a diagnostic challenge due to lack of clear history and children often shallow their sputum.

ETIOLOGY

The spectrum of causes of hemoptysis in children is remarkably different from adults and imaging plays a pivotal role in evaluation of hemoptysis.
- In most cases, the source is from the systemic vasculature, and in about 5-10% of the cases from the pulmonary circulation.[2] Arterial source from systemic circulation is bronchial arteries (BAs) or nonbronchial systemic collaterals (NBSCs). These hypertrophy in presence of chronic inflammation or whenever there is narrowing/stenosis of pulmonary artery.

TABLE 1: Causes of hemoptysis in children.	
Broad categories	**Specific entities**
Active infection	Tuberculosis
	Necrotizing pneumonia
	Tracheobronchitis
	Infected bronchiectasis
Post-infective sequelae	Fibroparenchymal opacities
	Atelectasis
	Tractional bronchiectasis
	Postinfective cavities
Bronchiectasis	Cystic fibrosis
	Noncystic fibrosis
Congenital heart disease	
Foreign body	
Neoplasm	
Other causes	Interstitial lung diseases
	Vasculitis
	Diffuse alveolar hemorrhage
	Idiopathic

- The most common cause of hemoptysis in children is active infection (both tubercular and nontubercular), as opposed to adults, where postinfectious sequelae are most common **(Table 1)**.[3]
- Other important causes include bronchiectasis (including cystic fibrosis and noncystic fibrosis-related bronchiectasis), postinfectious sequelae, and congenital heart disease. Bronchiectasis related to cystic fibrosis is the most common cause in developed countries.[1]
- Rarely, interstitial lung disease, diffuse alveolar hemorrhage (DAH), and pulmonary vasculitis may result in hemoptysis. In few of the cases, even after extensive workup, no cause may be identified.

■ IMAGING EVALUATION

The various imaging modalities utilized are chest radiography, multidetector row computed tomography (MDCT), magnetic resonance imaging (MRI), and catheter angiography for therapeutic embolization of bleeding vessels.

Imaging in children with hemoptysis is performed to localize the site of bleeding, identify the source, and to ascertain the etiology.

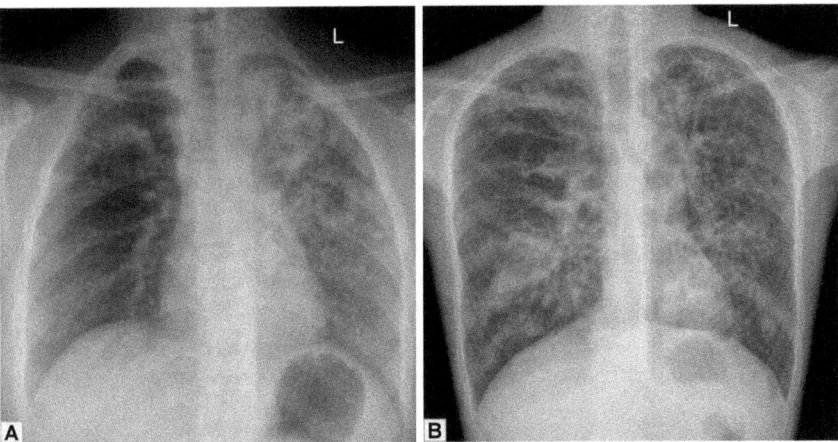

FIGS. 1A AND B: Chest radiographs—(A) Active tuberculosis involving the left upper mid zone with consolidation, nodules, and cavitations (B) case of cystic fibrosis with bronchiectasis both lungs.

Chest Radiograph

Chest radiograph is the initial radiological investigation, serving as a screening tool. It helps in lateralizing the site of bleeding and detecting parenchymal and pleural abnormalities. Parenchymal alveolar opacities with or without associated nodules and bronchial wall thickening may be seen in active infection, while fibroparenchymal opacities with bronchiectasis and cavities will be seen in old infective sequelae. Approximately, one-third of the children with hemoptysis may have a normal chest radiograph with eventual detection of a tracheobronchial cause in half of them, obviating the need for further imaging **(Figs. 1A and B)**.[4]

Multidetector Row Computed Tomography

Multidetector row computed tomography is the workhorse for imaging and planning management in children with hemoptysis. In addition to the information regarding the site and etiology, computed tomography angiography (CTA) is particularly helpful in identifying dilated pathological BAs, pseudo-aneurysms, and aberrant vessels.[5] CTA works as a roadmap for planning management in the form of bronchial or pulmonary artery embolization.

- CT technique involves acquisition of axial sections from the base of the neck to the level of the renal arteries, with injection of 2 mL/kg (300 mg/mL of iodine) of nonionic intravenous contrast media. In split bolus technique, adequate opacification of both the systemic and pulmonary vasculature achieved. *Split-bolus technique* involves administration of contrast using a pressure injector with an automated injection protocol where three-fourths of contrast administered at 3–5 mL/s, followed by one-fourth contrast at 1.5–3 mL/s followed by saline (volume equal to one-fourth of saline) at 1.5 mL/s.[3]

- Stepwise evaluation of MDCT images involves evaluation of the lung parenchyma, confirming the radiographic findings. In addition, fluid density material may be seen within the segmental bronchi with surrounding parenchymal consolidation, suggestive of hemorrhage. Tracheobronchial airway evaluation involves assessment for foreign bodies or endobronchial neoplasms that may be the cause of hemoptysis.
- The most common source of hemoptysis is from the BAs in 95% of the patients and hence, hypertrophied BAs (>2 mm in diameter) must be looked for. In 70% of the population, BAs arise from the descending thoracic aorta at the D5-D6 vertebral levels. Nonbronchial systemic arteries, including brachiocephalic, subclavian, axillary, internal mammary, and branches of inferior phrenic arteries may also result in hemoptysis **(Figs. 2A to F)**.
- Pulmonary artery abnormalities account for a minor proportion of all cases with hemoptysis, and the common abnormalities include pulmonary hypoplasia/aplasia, chronic thromboembolic disease, Rasmussen aneurysms, and pulmonary arterial hypertension secondary to congenital heart disease.[3]

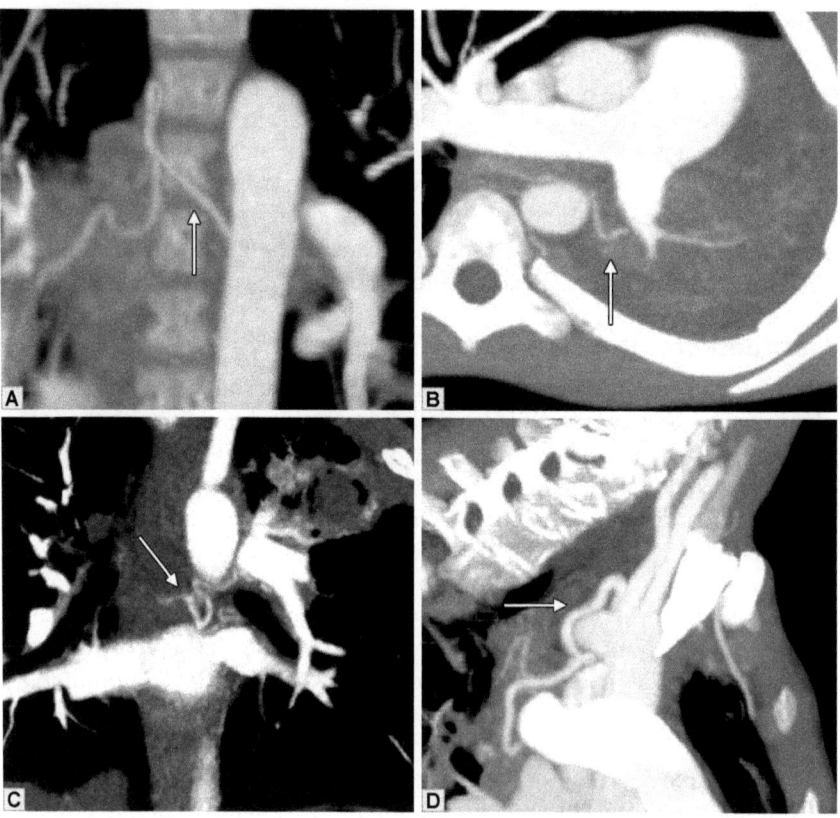

FIGS. 2A TO F: *Continued*

Continued

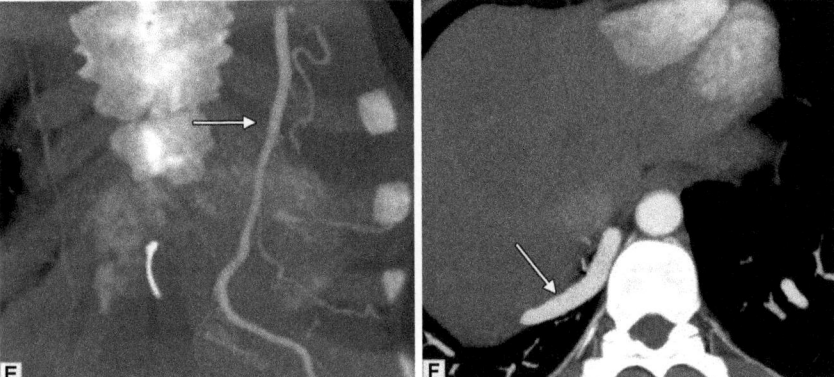

FIGS. 2A TO F: Bronchial arteries (BAs) and nonbronchial systemic collaterals (NBSCs)—(A) Orthotopic right intercostobronchial artery, (B) left bronchial artery, (C) common bronchial artery, (D) ectopic bronchial artery, (E) left internal mammary artery, and (F) right inferior phrenic artery.

Magnetic Resonance Imaging

Magnetic resonance imaging is not useful in acute hemoptysis, however, due to superior soft tissue contrast and radiation free, it can be used for evaluation of mediastinal, hilar pathologies, pulmonary arteriovenous malformation (PAVM), and congenital anomalies of pulmonary arteries.

Catheter Angiography

Invasive diagnostic catheter angiography is used when intervention is warranted for the purpose of embolization. It is not done for diagnostic purpose; but only when therapeutic intervention is planned. These are covered in this chapter later.

■ SPECIFIC ETIOLOGIES

The specific etiologies of hemoptysis are described here:
- *Acute lower respiratory tract infection*: Active infection in the form of tubercular, nontubercular necrotizing pneumonia, or tracheobronchitis leads to necrosis within the lung parenchyma and erosion of the blood vessels, leading to hemoptysis. Primary pulmonary tuberculosis is the most common type of tuberculosis infection in children. Necrotic lymph node causing erosion of vessel wall causing pseudoaneurysm can present with massive hemoptysis. Children with sequelae prior tubercular infection erosion of calcified nodes into vessels and trachea, bronchiectasis, or fungal infection in a cavity can result in hemoptysis. Chest radiograph will show pulmonary infiltrates, mediastinal lymphadenopathy, and pleural effusion as signs of active infection. CT findings include consolidation, ground glass opacity, cavity with shaggy walls, air fluid levels, pleural effusion, mediastinal lymphadenopathy, and complications such as empyema and bronchopleural fistula **(Figs. 3 and 4)**.

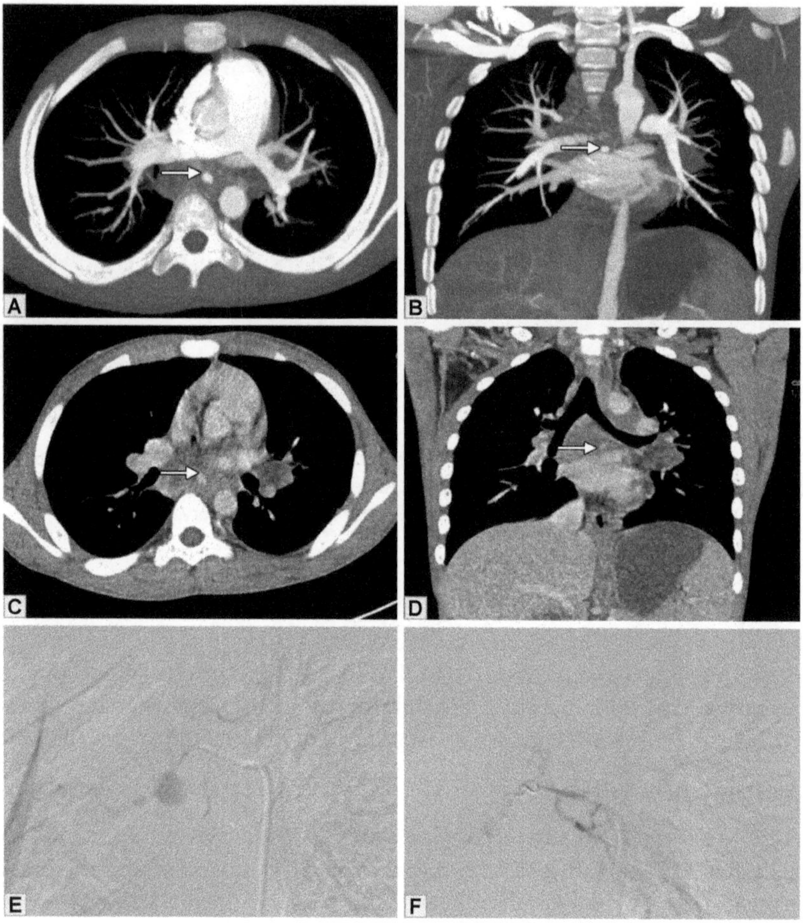

FIGS. 3A TO F: A 16-year-old boy with active mediastinal lymph nodal tuberculosis—(A and B) maximum-intensity projection (MIP) thick arterial phase image showing *pseudoaneurysm* (white arrow) from right bronchial artery, (C and D) multiple conglomerated necrotic mediastinal nodes in bilateral hilar and subcarinal location in venous phase, (E) digital subtraction angiography (DSA) image shows pseudoaneurysm from right bronchial artery, and (F) postcoil embolization of pseudoaneurysm.

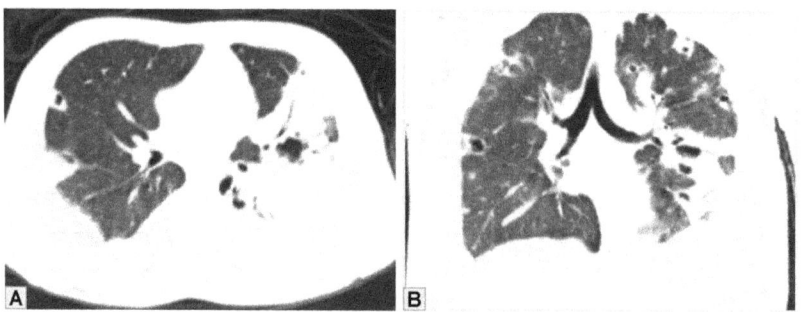

FIGS. 4A TO F: *Continued*

Continued

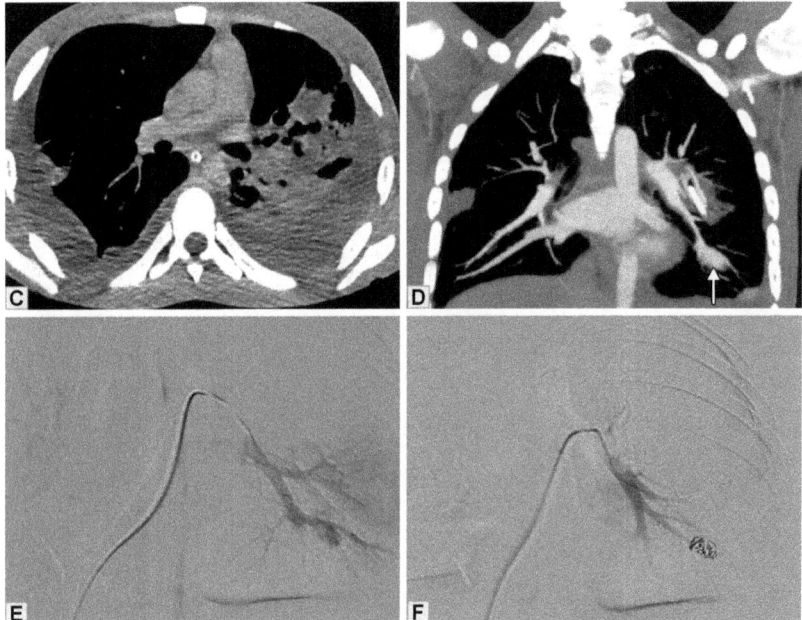

FIGS. 4A TO F: A 16-year-old boy with active staphylococcal necrotizing pneumonia— (A and B) lung window images showing multifocal consolidation with cavitations in both lobes and (C) soft tissue window shows bilateral pleural effusion, (D) subsequently the boy developed *pulmonary artery pseudoaneurysm* (white arrow) from lateral basal segmental branch of left descending pulmonary artery, and (E and F) digital subtraction angiography (DSA) images show pseudoaneurysm lateral basal segmental branch of left descending pulmonary artery from and postcoil embolization of pseudoaneurysm.

- *Bronchiectasis*: Bronchiectasis can occur secondary to infection, aspiration, cystic fibrosis, and ciliary dyskinesias. Chest radiograph will show tram track or parallel lines representing dilated bronchi. On CT imaging, bronchiectasis manifests with lack of normal bronchial tapering, bronchus is visible in the peripheral 1 cm of lung and >1 bronchoarterial ratio. Chronic inflammation and hypoxia promote proliferation of BA circulation leading to alteration in pulmonary hemodynamics. BA to pulmonary artery shunting results in increasing pressure in the pulmonary artery within bronchiectatic lung. Hypertrophied vascular channels weakened by the underlying chronic inflammatory process and mechanical stress erode and bleed into the airways **(Figs. 5A to D)**.
- *Post-infection sequelae*: Post-infection sequelae is one of the common cause of hemoptysis in children, and often requires radiological intervention. Tuberculosis is the commonest cause of chronic fibrotic and bronchiectatic changes **(Fig. 6)**.

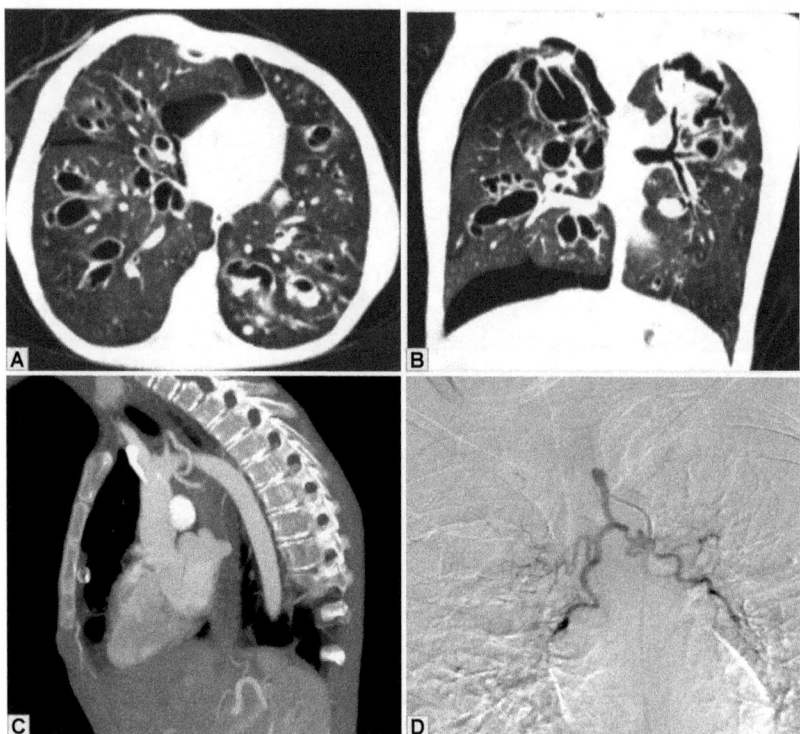

FIGS. 5A TO D: A 17-year-old patient with cystic fibrosis with massive hemoptysis—(A and B) lung window shows bilateral central cylindrical bronchiectasis, bronchial wall thickening, air-fluid level, and bilateral ground-glass opacity with right side pneumothorax, (C) sagittal maximum-intensity projection (MIP) thick image showing hypertrophied ectopic common bronchial artery origin from arch of aorta and dorsal vertebral kyphosis, and (D) digital subtraction angiography (DSA) image showing ectopic common bronchial artery showing parenchymal blush embolized with polyvinyl alcohol (PVA) particles.

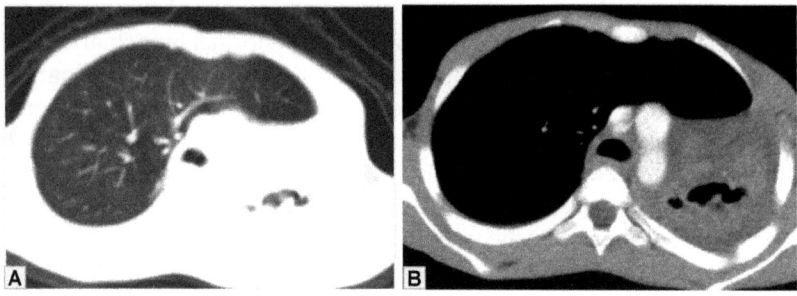

FIGS. 6A TO F: *Continued*

Continued

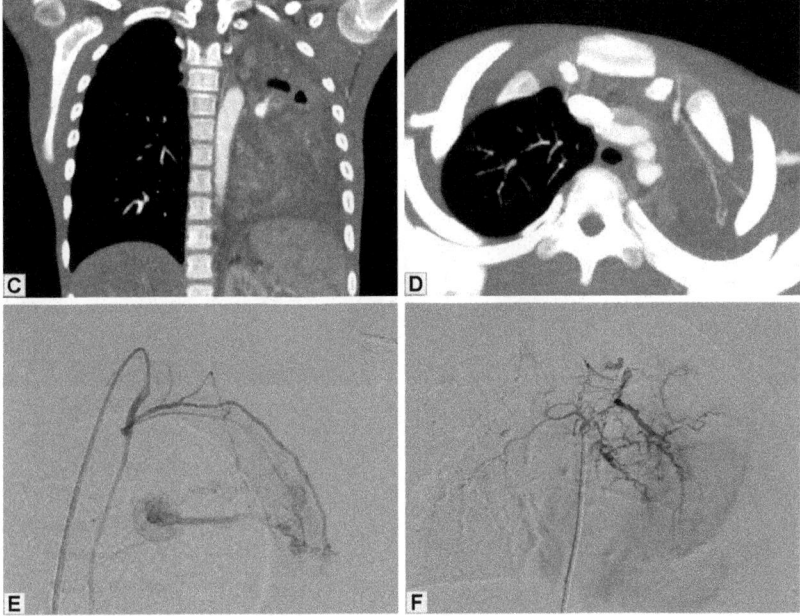

FIGS. 6A TO F: A 9-year-old boy with post-tubercular sequelae with hemoptysis—(A to C) fibrosis, collapse, and cavitation in left lung, (D) maximum-intensity projection (MIP) thick axial image showing hypertrophied branches from left internal mammary artery (IMA) supplying left lung fibroparenchymal thickening, (E) digital subtraction angiography (DSA) image hypertrophied branch of left IMA with pulmonary venous shunting, and (F) hypertrophied common bronchial artery embolized with polyvinyl alcohol (PVA) particles.

- *Congenital heart disease*: Hemoptysis in congenital heart disease are associated with pulmonary artery or venous stenosis/atresia. Hemorrhage results from hypertrophies and tortuous major aortopulmonary collateral arteries (MAPCAs). MAPCAs are nonregressed systemic to pulmonary embryologic connections from the aorta or its branches to the pulmonary arterial vasculature.
- *Proximal pulmonary artery interruption* is an uncommon developmental anomaly in children characterized by absence or termination of pulmonary artery within 1 cm of its origin. Interruption of right pulmonary artery is more common than left.[6] Lack of pulmonary arterial supply recruits systemic arteries from bronchial and NBSCs to perfuse the lung parenchyma. Hypertrophy and tortuosity of these arteries lead to vascular ectasia in the bronchial submucosa and rupture of ectatic vascular channels leads to hemoptysis. Diagnosis is made by absence/interruption of pulmonary artery and ipsilateral small volume lung, fine linear opacities and serrated thickening of pleura representing anastomosis of peripheral branches of the pulmonary artery with transpleural collateral vessels from enlarged intercostal and transpleural arteries

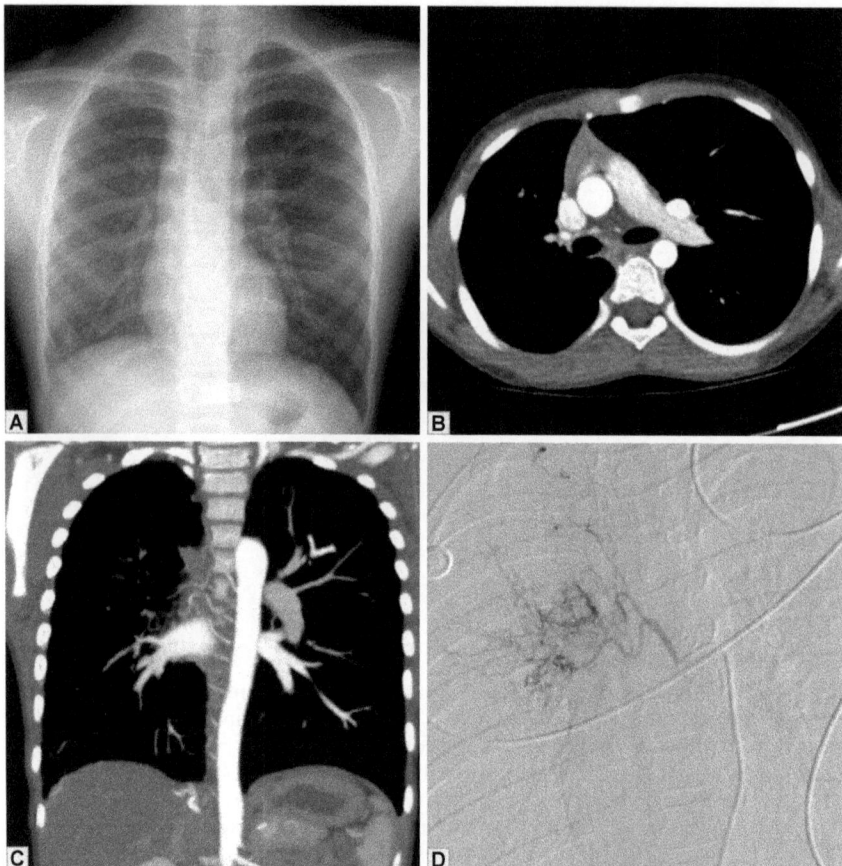

FIGS. 7A TO D: An 11-year-old girl with proximal pulmonary artery interruption presented with massive hemoptysis—(A) chest radiograph shows small volume right lung with reduced vascular marking on right side, (B and C) computed tomography (CT) images absent right pulmonary artery (B) and hypertrophied right intercostal bronchial trunk (RICBT) and posterior intercostal arteries on right side, and (C and D) digital subtraction angiography (DSA) imaging showing hypertrophied right intercostobronchial trunk (RICBT) during bronchial artery embolization (BAE).

and hypertrophied, tortuous bronchial and NBSCs from the branches of the intercostal, internal mammary, subclavian, and innominate arteries on CT scan. These patients may need pneumonectomy with ligation of collaterals for definitive management of hemoptysis **(Figs. 7A to D)**.
- *Pulmonary artery narrowing* from other causes may be congenital (pulmonary hypoplasia) or acquired (fibrosing mediastinitis and chronic pulmonary thromboembolism) will also result in hypertrophy of systemic collaterals resulting in hemoptysis.
- *Pulmonary arteriovenous malformations* are direct communication between the branches of pulmonary artery and veins without a capillary bed. PAVMs are commonly located in lower lobes and have very

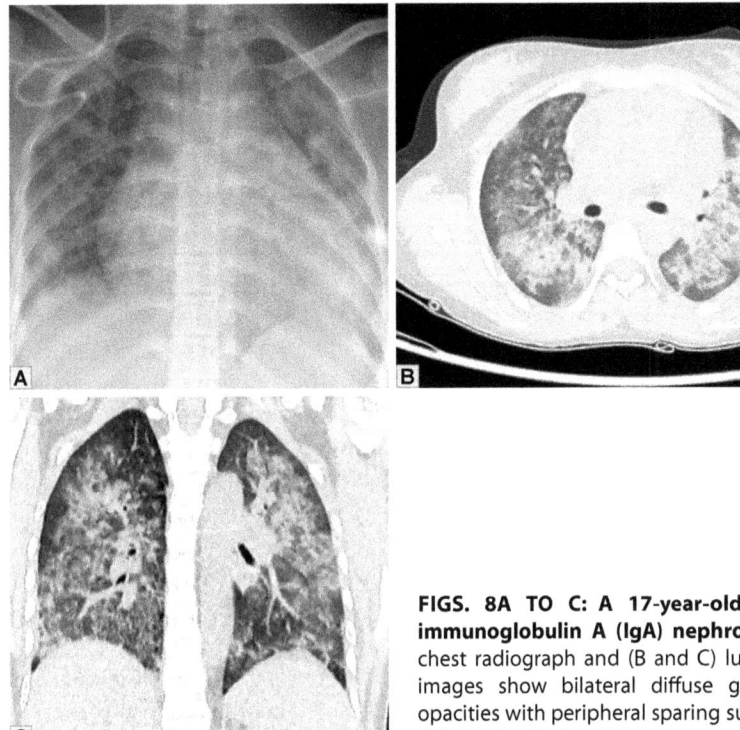

FIGS. 8A TO C: A 17-year-old girl with immunoglobulin A (IgA) nephropathy—(A) chest radiograph and (B and C) lung window images show bilateral diffuse ground-glass opacities with peripheral sparing suggestive of diffuse alveolar hemorrhage.

strong association with hereditary hemorrhagic telangiectasia.[7] Chest radiograph will show round or oval lobulated well-defined mass in lower lobe with radiating vessel to the hilum. MDCT can identify the connecting vascular feeder and drainage pathway more accurately.
- *Diffuse alveolar hemorrhage* is very uncommon in children. DAH results from bleeding from pulmonary vessels. DAH may present with hemoptysis, anemia, nonspecific respiratory symptoms, and hypoxemic respiratory failure. The causes of DAH include capillaritis, autoinflammatory diseases, cardiovascular diseases, coagulopathies, immunoallergic conditions, or by medical treatment/drug-induced lung injury.[8] In cases, where no underlying etiology of DAH found it is referred as idiopathic pulmonary hemosiderosis (IPH) **(Figs. 8A to C)**.
- *Idiopathic pulmonary hemosiderosis* is a rare cause of hemoptysis. IPH is characterized by triad of hemoptysis, anemia, and pulmonary hemosiderosis. Secondary hemosiderosis can be seen in systemic vasculitis and cardiac causes such mitral valve diseases. On imaging, diffuse or patchy ground-glass opacity seen in bilateral lower lobes sparing apices associated with interstitial thickening in some cases.
- *Foreign body*: In children <3 years of age, foreign body aspiration into the tracheobronchial tree can cause hemoptysis. Imaging helps in the localization of foreign body.

- *Neoplasms*: Bronchial neoplasm is a rare cause of hemoptysis in children. Bronchial carcinoids are the primary neoplasm in children. On imaging hilar or perihilar lobulated mass with obstructive changes in lung parenchyma such as atelectasis, consolidation, or hyperinflation.

INTERVENTIONAL RADIOLOGY MANAGEMENT OF HEMOPTYSIS

Life-threatening hemoptysis is defined as >8 mL/kg body weight in 24 hours. Initial management involves admission and immediate resuscitation. Evaluation for hemodynamic instability and airway compromise needs to be done, with assessment for coagulopathy and further correction. Drugs interfering with coagulation profile, including nonsteroidal anti-inflammatory drugs (NSAIDs) should be withheld. Bronchoscopic evaluation in selected children with suspected tracheobronchial source may be helpful in confirming the diagnosis, as well as local management by cautery/laser ablation of the bleeding vessel or by local injection of epinephrine. Balloon tamponade and unilateral bronchial intubation may also be performed.[9]

Bronchial Artery Embolization

- Being an invasive procedure with its own set of complications, bronchial artery embolization (BAE) is reserved for patients with severe life-threatening hemoptysis or when all other measures to control hemorrhage have been exhausted. It may also be performed for moderate chronic hemoptysis.
- The procedure is performed in general anesthesia for reduced motion and better image quality. Femoral route is preferred; however, radial approach may be used for difficult to cannulate BAs. In most patients, BAs originate between D5 and D6 vertebral levels, with a right-sided intercostobronchial trunk (ICBT) which supplies the right lung. On the left side, most commonly, two BAs are seen, arising directly from the descending aorta.[10]
- It is important to remember that the bronchial and spinal arteries have a common origin and hence, inadvertent embolization may result in paraplegia (as the vessels supply the anterior aspect of the cord). The largest of the anterior segmental medullary arteries is the artery of Adamkiewicz that has a characteristic hairpin configuration on angiogram.
- In patients with chronic lung disease, non-BAs are seen to supply the lungs and may be the source of hemoptysis. Hence, correlation with prior MDCT is helpful in identification and embolization of these nonbronchial systemic arteries **(Figs. 2 and 6)**.

- On bronchial angiograms, frank contrast extravasation is rarely seen. However, indirect signs of a vessel that are responsible for the hemorrhage include contrast blush in the surrounding parenchyma, along with an enlarged (>1.5 mm diameter) and tortuous BA.
- BAE is performed using polyvinyl alcohol (PVA) particles diameter of 350–500 μm.[10] Use of microcatheters for superselective catheterization is recommended to prevent nontarget embolization. BAE is effective in initial control of hemoptysis; however, recurrence is common. Hence, particles are preferred over coils, as coils once placed, prevent access to the vessel for repeat intervention.
- Neurological complication such as spinal cord ischemia occurs in <1% of BAE procedures. Postprocedure chest pain is the most common complication following BAE reported in half cases. Other minor complications include dysphagia and fever.[1,11]

Pulmonary Artery Embolization

Embolization of the pulmonary arterial branches is infrequently performed, and is indicated in patients with pseudoaneurysms as the cause of hemoptysis. Aneurysms of the pulmonary artery are more prone to rupture and hemorrhage, and hence glue embolization is the preferred **(Fig. 4)**.[12] Pulmonary artery AVMs (PAVMs) seldom become symptomatic in children; they usually present in young adults.

CONCLUSION

Hemoptysis in children is uncommon but can be life-threatening. Infection is the most common etiology of hemoptysis in children and MDCT is the imaging modality of choice for evaluation. Bronchial artery embolization is a life-saving process in the setting of hemoptysis.

Other Related Chapters that can be Referred to:
- Chapter 6: Congenital Lung Abnormalities
- Chapter 18: Pulmonary Artery Imaging

REFERENCES

1. Roebuck DJ, Barnacle AM. Haemoptysis and bronchial artery embolization in children. Paediatr Respir Rev. 2008;9(2):95-104.
2. Meena P, Bhalla AS, Goyal A, Sharma R, Kumar A, Srivastva DN, et al. Single-phase split-bolus dual energy computed tomography angiography for evaluation of hemoptysis: A novel application. J Thorac Imaging. 2018;33(6):366-76.
3. Shera TA, Bhalla AS, Naranje P, Meena P, Kabra SK, Gupta AK, et al. Role of computed tomography angiography in the evaluation of haemoptysis in children: Decoding the abnormal vessels. Indian J Med Res. 2022;155(3-4):356-63.

4. Stankiewicz JA, Puczynski M, Lynch JM. Embolization in the treatment of massive hemoptysis in patients with cystic fibrosis. Ear Nose Throat J. 1985;64(4):180-4.
5. Remy-Jardin M, Bouaziz N, Dumont P, Brillet PY, Bruzzi J, Remy J. Bronchial and nonbronchial systemic arteries at multi-detector row CT angiography: comparison with conventional angiography. Radiology. 2004;233(3):741-9.
6. Kieffer SA, Amplatz K, Anderson RC, Lillehei CW. Proximal interruption of a pulmonary artery. Am J Roentgenol Radium Ther Nucl Med. 1965;95(3):592-7.
7. Khurshid I, Downie GH. Pulmonary arteriovenous malformation. Postgrad Med J. 2002;78(918):191-7.
8. Susarla SC, Fan LL. Diffuse alveolar hemorrhage syndromes in children. Curr Opin Pediatr. 2007;19(3):314-20.
9. Yoon W. Embolic agents used for bronchial artery embolisation in massive haemoptysis. Expert Opin Pharmacother. 2004;5(2):361-7.
10. Walker CM, Rosado-de-Christenson ML, Martínez-Jiménez S, Kunin JR, Wible BC. Bronchial arteries: Anatomy, function, hypertrophy, and anomalies. Radiographics. 2015;35(1):32-49.
11. Yoon W, Kim JK, Kim YH, Chung TW, Kang HK. Bronchial and nonbronchial systemic artery embolization for life-threatening hemoptysis: A comprehensive review. Radiographics. 2002;22(6):1395-409.
12. Keeling AN, Costello R, Lee MJ. Rasmussen's aneurysm: A forgotten entity? Cardiovasc Intervent Radiol. 2008;31(1):196-200.

CHAPTER 28

Thoracic Imaging in Intensive Care Unit

Surabhi Vyas, Rakesh Lodha

- Imaging modalities
- Parenchymal abnormalities
  - Acute respiratory distress syndrome
  - Pulmonary edema
  - Infections
  - Diffuse alveolar hemorrhage
  - Acute interstitial pneumonia
- Pleural abnormalities
  - Pleural effusion
  - Pneumothorax
- Airway abnormalities
- Ventilator-associated air leak
- Lines and tubes

INTRODUCTION

Chest imaging forms the mainstay of diagnosis and follows-up of pediatric patients admitted in the intensive care unit (ICU). Critically ill patients undergo daily imaging for localization of various tubes and lines like endotracheal tube and also for assessment of volume status and chest pathologies. Imaging is primarily based on chest radiography (CXR) and ultrasonography (USG). In this chapter, an overview of common pediatric chest conditions associated with ICU stay will be elucidated.

IMAGING MODALITIES

- *Chest radiography*: CXR forms the mainstay of imaging in the ICU due to easy availability and portability. It is useful not only for pulmonary, pleural, and cardiac abnormalities, but also invaluable in assessment of position of various tubes and lines.
- *Ultrasonography*: Point-of-care USG has evolved over the last few decades to provide comprehensive assessment of pulmonary parenchymal abnormalities such as pulmonary edema and consolidation, but also for estimation and diagnosis of pleural effusion/empyema and pneumothorax. The role of USG aided by Doppler is essential in real-time guidance for various interventional procedures.

- *Computed tomography (CT)*: CT provides excellent cross-sectional assessment of the thorax with better visualization of mediastinal vascular structures with the use of intravenous contrast. In spite of the challenges of transportation of patients to the CT suite, CT is increasingly used for patients in ICU.
- *Magnetic resonance imaging (MRI)*: MRI has limited applications in chest evaluation of critical care patients.

PARENCHYMAL ABNORMALITIES

Acute Respiratory Distress Syndrome
- Diffuse alveolar damage (DAD) resulting from variety of insults, causing DAD, and requiring mechanical ventilation.
- Berlin definition—to standardize terminology used by intensivists and radiologists:
  - Acute onset of respiratory distress
  - Develops within one week of the clinical insult or new/worsening respiratory symptoms
  - Presence of bilateral pulmonary opacities on CXR
  - Respiratory failure not fully explained by cardiac failure or fluid overload

Categories of Severity (Based on PaO_2/FiO_2 Ratio at Positive End-expiratory Pressure or Continuous Positive Airway Pressure ≥5 cm H_2O)
- *Mild*: Arterial oxygen partial pressure/fractional inspired oxygen (PaO_2/FiO_2) ratio 200–300 mm Hg
- *Moderate*: PaO_2/FiO_2 ratio between 100 and < 200 mm Hg
- *Severe*: PaO_2/FiO_2 ratio < 100 mm Hg

Causes
- *Pulmonary/direct injury*: Pneumonia and aspiration
- *Extrapulmonary/indirect injury*: Sepsis, pancreatitis, major trauma, and multiple transfusions

Pathology
Diffuse alveolar damage, increased capillary and alveolar permeability, leads to edema (interstitial and alveolar), followed by a phase of fibrosis:

Three phases can overlap:
1. *Acute (exudative) phase*: Initial 7 days following insult; characterized by alveolar edema, interstitial inflammation, hemorrhage, and hyaline membrane formation.
2. *Subacute (proliferative) phase*: Proliferation of fibroblasts in the interstitium also in alveoli; proliferation of type II pneumocytes in alveoli. Conversion of alveolar exudates into cellular granulation tissue.
3. *Chronic (fibrotic) phase*: 2 weeks or more following injury. Diffuse parenchymal fibrosis with collagen deposition, bullae formation.

Chest Radiograph
- Chest radiograph can be normal in the first 24 hours—stage of early alveolar edema
- Over the next 2-3 days—extensive, bilateral air space opacification/consolidation ("White lung")[1]
- Homogeneous/patchy multifocal
- Picture similar regardless of the etiology
- *Radiographic criteria for diagnosis of acute respiratory distress syndrome (ARDS)*: Bilateral opacities (consistent with pulmonary edema), findings not explainable by pleural effusion, lung collapse, or nodules

High-resolution Computed Tomography
- CT is not an essential part of diagnostic criteria for ARDS, but when available implications of findings same as seen on CXR.
- *Acute phase*:
    - Normal initially, abnormalities appear after 12 hours
    - *Ground-glass opacities (GGOs)*: Dominant finding, diffuse, or patchy (geographic distribution)
    - *Consolidation*: Initially patchy, increase later in the exudative phase and become more homogeneous.
    - Apicobasal gradient may be seen, with more opacification seen in lung bases.
    - Areas of atelectasis may also be seen.
    - Lung morphology determines response to therapy.
- *Subacute phase* **(Figs. 1A to D)**:
    - Increasing consolidation in early phase, followed by appearance of interstitial fibrosis
    - Interlobular septal thickening superimposed on GGO—"crazy-paving pattern"
    - Bronchiectasis and bronchiolectasis
    - Severity of changes helps prognosticate.
    - Those with more severe changes likely to require more prolonged mechanical ventilation, with subsequent risk of its attendant complications.
- Chronic phase
- *Interstitial fibrosis increases*:
    - Coarse reticular fibrosis
    - Architectural distortion
    - Bronchiectasis, bronchiectasis with distortion of airways
    - Volume loss
    - Bullae
    - Severity of changes more in those with prolonged positive pressure ventilation
    - Morphological changes may persist in survivors even when imaging done months after the acute episode.

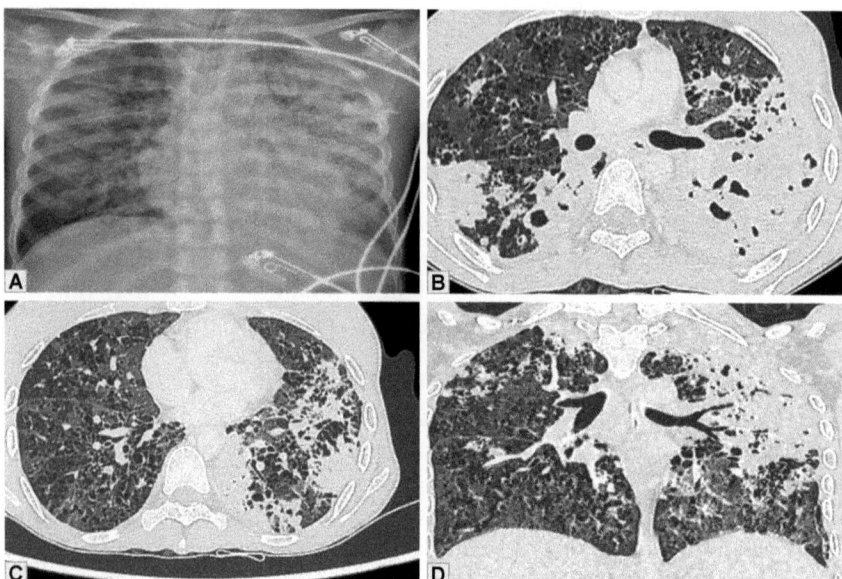

FIGS. 1A TO D: Pulmonary tuberculosis with acute respiratory distress syndrome (ARDS). Diffuse bilateral areas of consolidation and cystic change in a case of infection-induced ARDS.

Ultrasonography
- Aids in differentiation from hydrostatic pulmonary edema
- Heterogeneous distribution of abnormalities
- *B lines*: Well separated and discrete/coalescent
- *Areas of consolidation*: More in posterior regions, areas of sparing seen

Pulmonary Edema
- It may be cardiogenic or noncardiogenic.
- Pulmonary edema essentially refers to accumulation of fluid in the extravascular compartment of the lung.
- Common causes of cardiogenic pulmonary edema include ischemia, decompensation of heart failure, valvular dysfunction, or volume overload.
- Noncardiogenic pulmonary edema may be associated with pneumonia, sepsis, aspiration, or drowning.
- Up to 10% of patients with pulmonary edema may have multiple causes, e.g., ARDS with concomitant fluid overload or acute decompensated cardiac failure with associated lung injury.
- Paroxysmal nocturnal dyspnea or orthopnea suggests cardiogenic pulmonary edema. Signs and symptoms of infection, altered sensorium, witnessed aspiration, drowning, or multiple blood transfusions may indicate noncardiogenic cause.
- Engorged neck veins and peripheral edema may indicate fluid overload. S3 gallop is highly specific for left ventricular dysfunction. Other specific findings include murmurs of valvular stenosis or regurgitation.

Pathology
The mechanism includes hydrostatic edema (as in fluid overload/left ventricular failure); DAD and edema due to increased permeability but no DAD (e.g., high altitude pulmonary edema and transfusion-related acute lung injury). Two pathological phases are seen—(1) interstitial edema and (2) alveolar filling.

Laboratory Testing
- Electrocardiogram (ECG) findings, troponin levels, and serum brain natriuretic peptide (BNP) levels may be useful in differentiating cardiogenic pulmonary edema.
- Two-dimensional transthoracic echocardiogram is useful if history, physical examination, ECG, and chest X-ray do not establish the cause of pulmonary edema.
- Pulmonary artery catheterization, used to assess the pulmonary artery occlusion pressure, is considered the gold standard for determining the cause of acute pulmonary edema.

Imaging
Chest Radiograph
- Primary modality for diagnosis and follow-up
- *Early changes*: Enlargement of upper lobe pulmonary veins (due to diversion of blood flow)
- Airspace opacities with central/parahilar (bat wing distribution) **(Fig. 2A)**
- Kerley lines **(Fig. 3)**
- Pleural effusion

Computed Tomography
- High-resolution computed tomography (HRCT) not performed for diagnosis of hydrostatic pulmonary edema
- However, recognition of features necessary to allow differentiation from other causes
- *HRCT findings include*:
  - GGOs: Diffuse/patchy and parahilar. Gravitational predominance may be seen.
  - Differentiating feature from increased permeability edema, which has more subpleural and peripheral distribution.
  - In early cases, centrilobular ground-glass nodules may be seen, while areas of consolidation may be present in areas of more alveolar filling.
  - Smooth interlobular septal thickening, in conjunction with GGO, is characteristic of hydrostatic edema **(Fig. 2B)**. Focal nodularity, if seen, reflects dilated septal veins; often prominent in lung bases.
  - Peribronchovascular interstitial thickening appears as bronchial wall thickening or prominence of pulmonary vessels.
  - *Vascular prominence*: In cardiogenic pulmonary edema, pulmonary arteries and veins appear dilated. These include central vessels, intrapulmonary, centrilobular vessels as well as septal veins.

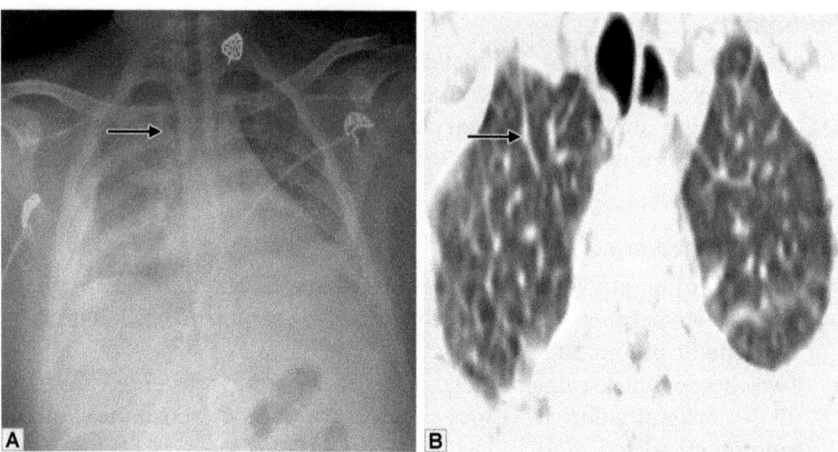

FIGS. 2A AND B: Pulmonary edema. Figure A shows enlarged cardiac silhouette with widened vascular pedicle (arrow) with prominent interstitial markings. Both costophrenic angles are blunted with rising meniscus due to pleural effusion. CT image shows the smooth interlobular septal thickening (arrow in B).

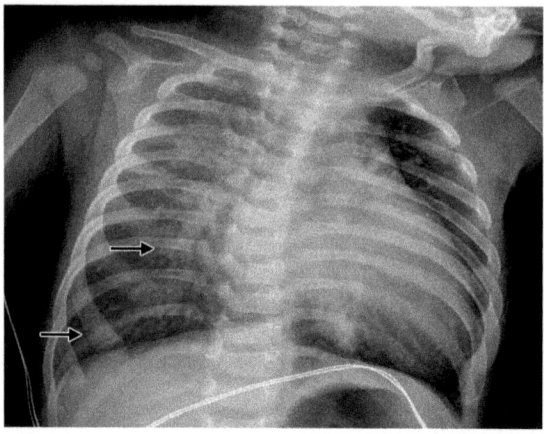

FIG. 3: Cardiogenic pulmonary edema. Perihilar and central air space opacities with Kerley A and B lines (arrows).

- *Pleural effusion*: Transudative pleural effusion, unilateral or bilateral with smooth fissural thickening.

Infections

- Infections such as pneumocystis, cytomegalovirus, influenza, atypical organisms (mycoplasma or chlamydia), or mycobacteria may have presentations similar to acute interstitial lung diseases (ILDs), or may cause acute exacerbations of preexisting ILDs.
- Ruling out infectious etiology, with use of bronchoalveolar lavage (BAL) should be a part of work-up of acute ILD.

The radiographic features of pneumonia include:[2,3]
- Patchy areas of consolidation and air space opacities, often with air bronchogram, without any volume loss, to differentiate these from atelectasis **(Figs. 4A and B)**.
- Pulmonary opacities in pneumonia are similar to those of pulmonary edema, however, the latter evolve within a matter of hours with therapy.
- In a patient with ARDS, a new or enlarging pulmonary opacity suggests pneumonia. However, radiography has poor diagnostic accuracy in identifying pneumonia in the setting of ARDS.
- Pneumonia can give rise to complications such as pulmonary abscess, empyema, and bronchopleural fistula **(Fig. 5)**.

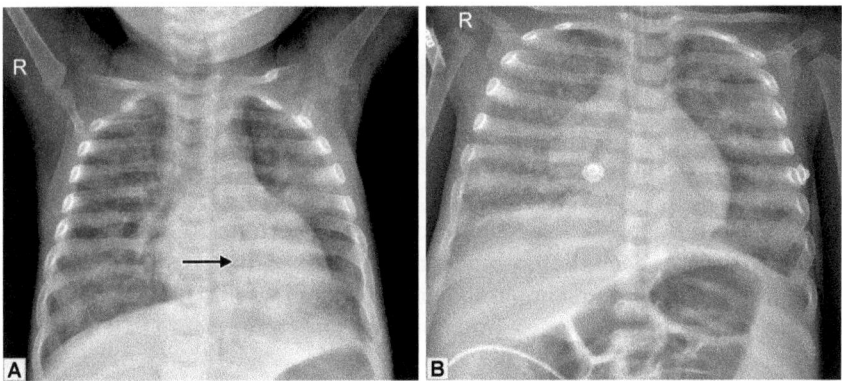

FIGS. 4A AND B: Pneumonia. Figure A shows left retrocardiac area of consolidation with air bronchogram (arrow in A). Follow-up radiograph (B) shows more diffuse involvement with diffuse areas of consolidation and air bronchogram in both lungs due to exacerbation.

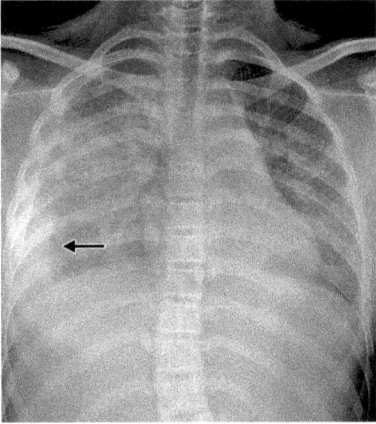

FIG. 5: Empyema with pneumonia. Right lung consolidation with right pleural collection due to empyema. Small patch of consolidation is also seen in the left paracardiac region.

Diffuse Alveolar Hemorrhage

- Diffuse alveolar hemorrhage (DAH) is a term used for diffuse bleeding from the pulmonary microcirculation (pulmonary arterioles, alveolar capillaries, and pulmonary venules) as a result of microvascular damage.
- Often a catastrophic clinical syndrome presenting with hemoptysis and dyspnea, which may progress to hypoxemic respiratory failure.
- Nonpulmonary signs and symptoms are those that accompany the underlying systemic disease.

Causes
Causes are broadly classified as immune and nonimmune causes:
- Nonimmune causes include endobronchial tumors, arteriovenous malformations or aneurysms, hemorrhagic pneumonia, infections, mitral valve disease, congestive cardiac failure, uremia, coagulopathies or thrombocytopenia, pulmonary veno-occlusive disease, or massive pulmonary embolism.
- Autoimmune DAH is due to capillaritis or endotheliitis; common etiologies being antineutrophil cytoplasmic antibodies (ANCA)-associated vasculitis, Goodpasture syndrome, systemic lupus erythematosus (SLE), or drugs (D-penicillamine and trimellitic anhydride).
- Other causes include immunocompromised status [postbone marrow transplant or acquired immunodeficiency syndrome (AIDS)] or idiopathic pulmonary hemosiderosis (unknown cause, sometimes associated with celiac disease).
- *Pathology*: Three different patterns have been described—associated with pulmonary capillaritis, bland alveolar hemorrhage with no vasculitis, and DAD related.

Diagnosis
- BAL fluid shows blood, with progressively more blood with serial aliquots. DAH should be considered if BAL cytology shows >20% hemosiderin-laden macrophages (on Prussian blue staining).
- Presumptive diagnosis of DAH can be made on the basis of clinicoradiologic, serologic, and BAL findings.
- BAL can also be utilized to rule out alternate infective etiology.
- Transbronchial lung biopsy may be used to diagnose pulmonary capillaritis, presence of granulomatous vasculitis, and immunofluorescent staining.
- Kidney biopsy can be done if required in patients with pulmonary renal syndromes.
- Thoracoscopic or surgical lung biopsy may be required to establish the cause if serologic testing or clinical history is unrevealing.
- Elevated serum creatinine or presence of active sediments in urine may point toward pulmonary-renal syndromes.

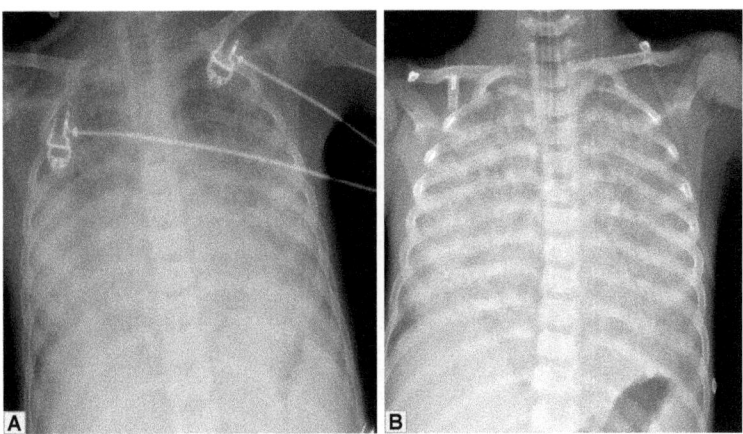

FIGS. 6A AND B: Diffuse alveolar hemorrhage. Bilateral lung consolidations which show worsening on follow-up radiograph (B) with diffuse involvement with confluent areas of consolidation in both lungs due to pulmonary hemorrhage.

- Markers of connective tissue disease such as antinuclear antibody (ANA), ANCA (either antiproteinase or antimyeloperoxidase), and antiglomerular basement membrane antibodies (anti-GBM antibodies) may point toward specific diagnosis. Investigations should include anti-tissue transglutaminase antibody (anti-tTG) IgA, and work-up for celiac disease.

Imaging
- *Radiography and HRCT*: Bilateral GGO/consolidation **(Figs. 6A and B)**; lobular appearance more in dependent areas
- In most cases, the pulmonary changes are reversible, except in those with DAD.

Acute Interstitial Pneumonia
- Synonym/earlier called Hamman–Rich syndrome
- *Pathology*:
  - Similar to ARDS, i.e., DAD
  - However, idiopathic—in patients who were otherwise healthy, with no known predisposing cause.
- *Clinical features:*
  - Dyspnea and rapidly progressing respiratory failure
  - Often preceded by a flu-like illness with symptoms such as fever and arthralgias
  - Poor prognosis

- *Imaging features:*
  - Similar to ARDS and vary according to the stage of the illness **(Fig. 7)**
  - Versus ARDS, acute interstitial pneumonia (AIP) more likely to have predominantly lower zones, symmetrical distribution of GGOs, and consolidation **(Table 1)**
  - With progression, the areas of involvement become more extensive.
  - Presence of bronchiectasis and bronchiectasis within the areas of increased attenuation are bad prognostic indicators, as these imply onset of fibrosis.
  - Residual abnormality in survivors—mild reticulation.

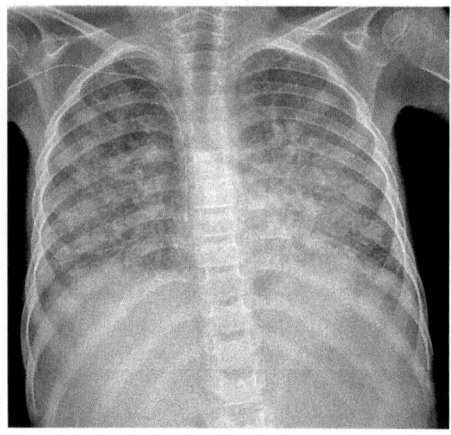

FIG. 7: Acute interstitial pneumonia. Extensive areas of ground-glass and reticular opacities in both lungs. Note is made of a peripherally inserted central catheter (PICC) line in situ.

TABLE 1: Differentiating features of ARDS, hydrostatic pulmonary edema, AIP, and DAH on imaging.

	ARDS	Hydrostatic pulmonary edema	AIP	DAH
Distribution of radiographic abnormality	Diffuse or patchy, geographical distribution	Central, perihilar, dependent areas, and "bat wing pattern"	Lower zone predominance, symmetrical	Central and dependent areas
Smooth interlobular septal thickening	Not common in acute phase	Commonly seen	Not common	Seen in intermediate phases
Pleural effusion	Not an essential finding	Commonly seen	Not common	Not common

(AIP: acute interstitial pneumonia; ARDS: acute respiratory distress syndrome; DAH: diffuse alveolar hemorrhage)

PLEURAL ABNORMALITIES

Pleural Effusion

Pleural effusion results from volume overload, synpneumonic with pneumonia or as a reactive process.

Radiographic findings reveal the following:
- While erect CXR easily reveals blunting of lateral CP angle due to pleural fluid, a supine radiograph reveals haze due to pleural fluid accumulating in the posterobasilar recess, which is the most dependent part **(Figs. 2 and 8)**. This is, however, a subtle finding, especially in thick set patients.
- The haze is seen without air bronchogram, thus differentiating it from basal consolidation.
- Obliteration of diaphragmatic contour is another finding.
- A loculated fluid along the fissure is usually seen as a wedge or biconvex homogeneous density.
- The amount of the pleural effusion also affects the radiographic appearance. An effusion of >500 mL usually creates a clearly visualized opacity. In patients with a history of trauma, or thoracic intervention, a sudden increase may point toward a hemothorax.[4]

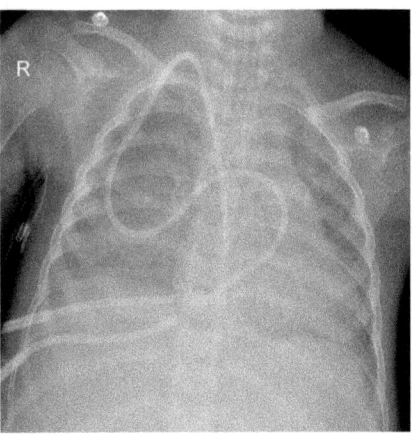

FIG. 8: Pleural effusion in supine radiograph. Diffuse haze in both lung fields with obscuration of diaphragmatic contour due to pleural effusion in a supine radiograph.

Pneumothorax

- Air in the pleural cavity can result from drainage procedures, catheter placements, or due to barotrauma in ventilated patients.
- As air rises to a nondependent area, the air lies along the anterior and medial aspects of the thorax in supine position.
- However, if there is associated subcutaneous emphysema, the identification of pneumothorax becomes difficult.
- The findings of pneumothorax on *supine* CXR include:
    - Hyperlucent anterior costophrenic sulcus **(Fig. 9)**
    - Hyperlucency over the upper abdomen
    - Sharp diaphragmatic contour **(Fig. 10)**

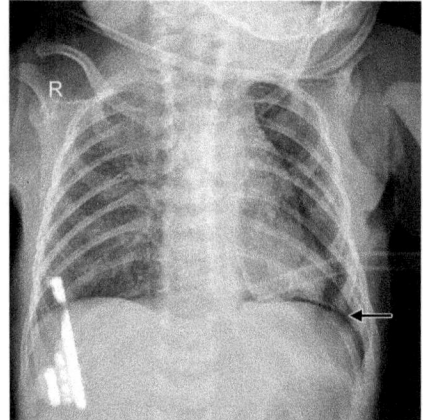

FIG. 9: Pneumothorax. Small left pneumothorax is seen as a hyperlucent area in the left costophrenic recess (arrow) with chest tube in situ.

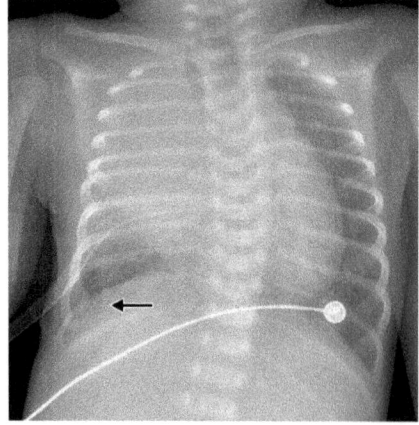

FIG. 10: Right pneumothorax with chest tube. Right CP angle pneumothorax (arrow) with sharp underlying diaphragmatic contour with chest tube in situ.

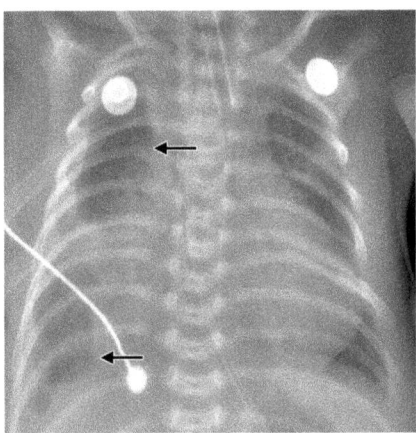

FIG. 11: Hydropneumothorax on supine radiograph. Image shows nondependent lucency (arrows) over right costophrenic sulcus and upper hemithorax with diffuse haze due to combination of fluid and air in the pleural cavity.

- Tension pneumothorax is indicated by flattened cardiac border, contralateral mediastinal shift, and widening of the depression of the lateral pleurodiaphragmatic sulcus, also known as "deep pleural sulcus sign".
- Combination of fluid and air both in the pleural space can complicate the imaging appearance. Hyperlucent nondependent area with diffuse-dependent haze is seen in a supine radiograph in such a case **(Fig. 11)**.
- Linear skin folds may be confused with pneumothorax, their continuation beyond the thoracic cage and unsharp appearance differentiates them from true pneumothorax.

AIRWAY ABNORMALITIES

- Various congenital and acquired conditions of the tracheobronchial tree can cause respiratory distress amongst pediatric population.
- Bronchiectasis, bronchiolitis, asthma, bronchial stenosis, and bronchial constriction being the common causes amongst this group.
- *Imaging features* vary from tram track such as branching lucencies, with surrounding consolidation, bronchial wall thickening, and air trapping **(Figs. 12 to 14)**.
- Secondary infection is also a common concern for these patients.

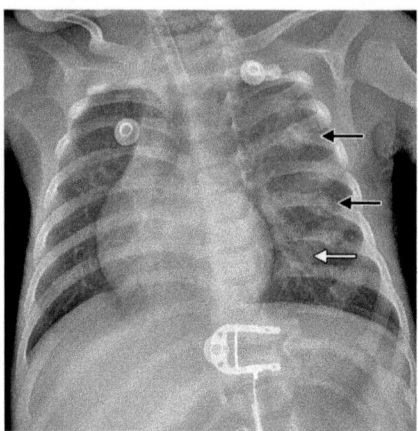

FIG. 12: Bronchiolitis. Perihilar opacities (white arrow) in a case of bronchiolitis with multiple old healed left-sided rib fractures (black arrows).

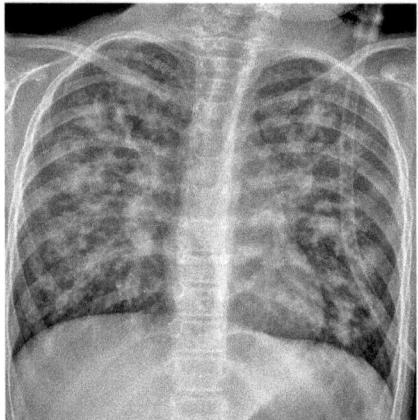

FIG. 13: Bronchopneumonia with bronchiectasis. Bronchiectasis with peribronchial areas of consolidation scattered in both lungs with relative peripheral lung sparing.

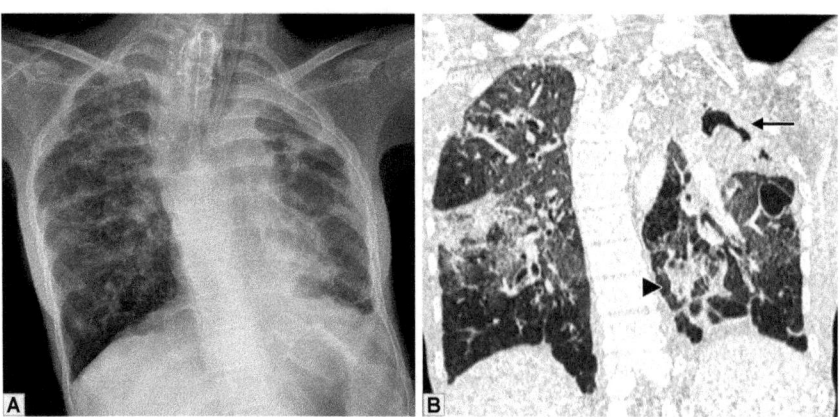

FIGS. 14A TO E: *Continued*

Continued

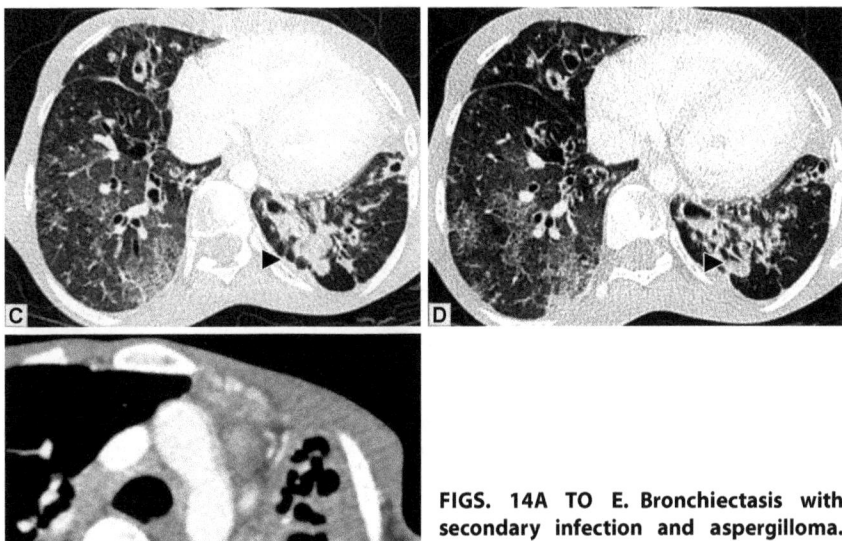

FIGS. 14A TO E. Bronchiectasis with secondary infection and aspergilloma. Postinfective fibroparenchymal changes in left lung with aspergilloma (black arrow) with bronchial wall thickening and intrabronchial contents (arrowhead in C). Patch of resolving pneumonia seen in the right lung. Tracheostomy tube in situ.

VENTILATOR-ASSOCIATED AIR LEAK

- Air leak is a hazard of invasive mechanical ventilation and is seen in 3-15% of patients.
- Patients with prolonged ventilation, higher peak inspiratory pressure (PIP) and those with a higher pediatric critical illness score (PCIS) are especially vulnerable.
- The air leak can occur into the pericardial, pleural, mediastinal, and subcutaneous spaces to cause pneumopericardium, pneumothorax, pneumomediastinum, and subcutaneous emphysema, respectively.
- Imaging features include presence of air in the above-mentioned spaces, which are well delineated on CXRs **(Figs. 15A and B)**. Small amount of air may be better visualized on CT.

LINES AND TUBES

Various lines and tubes used in the pediatric ICU are enumerated in the **Table 2** with pertinent radiological aspects.

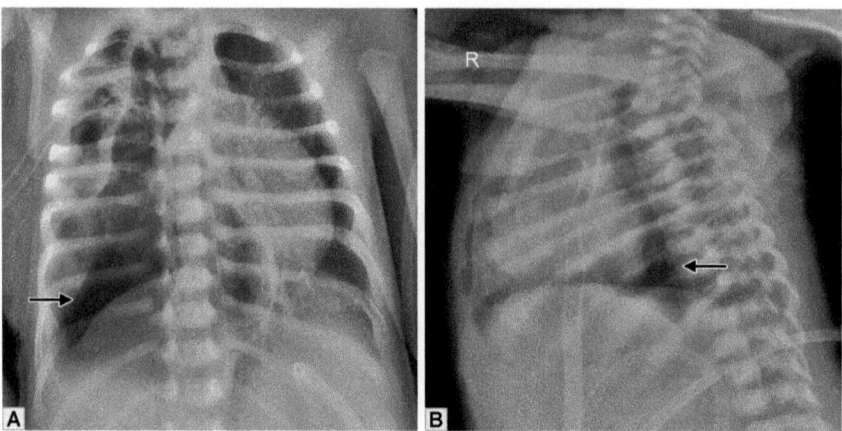

FIGS. 15A AND B: Pneumothorax and pneumomediastinum. Air outlining the right pleural cavity and the vertebral column (arrows) suggesting right pneumothorax and pneumomediastinum.

TABLE 2: Lines and tubes used in the intensive care unit with their key features.		
Lines and tubes	Optimum position	Key radiological pointers
Endotracheal tube	C7-T2, above the carina	Selective intubation of one bronchus can lead to contralateral lung collapse and ipsilateral hyperinflation **(Figs. 16A and B)**
Tracheostomy tube	Inflatable cuff position should be below the lower edge of cricoids cartilage	• Subcutaneous emphysema, pneumomediastinum, etc., may be seen due to air leak • Hyperinflation of the cuff can lead to tracheal injury and resultant stenosis **(Fig. 17)**
Intercostal drainage tube	In case of pleural effusion/empyema ideal position is 4/5 ICS. In case of pneumothorax drainage, second ICS in midclavicular line is optimum	Parenchymal or transdiaphragmatic positioning can occur which can lead to solid visceral injury **(Fig. 18)**
Nasogastric tube	Distal tip should be well in the proximal part of the stomach with anterior and left ward curve	Airway intubation may occur **(Fig. 19)**
Nasojejunal tube	Tip should lie in the midline or left paramidline in the mid jejuna loops	
Central venous catheter	PICC or central line provides venous access. The catheter tip should be at the cavoatrial junction at the trachea-bronchial angle/T6 vertebral level in chest radiograph	Atrial migration of the tip results in cardiac arrhythmias, thrombosis, and rarely perforation **(Figs. 20A to C)**

Continued

Continued

Lines and tubes	Optimum position	Key radiological pointers
ECMO	• VV ECMO—drainage cannula is seen in the common femoral vein, reinfusion cannula in the right IJV • VA ECMO—drainage cannula in the right atrium through right IJV, femoral vein or directly into the atrium, returning cannula to the thoracic aorta through the right carotid/femoral artery or aorta	Hemorrhage and hematoma formation may occur as local complication

(ECMO: extracorporeal membrane oxygenation; ICS: intercostal space; IJV: internal jugular vein; VA ECMO: venoarterial ECMO; VV ECMO: venovenous ECMO)

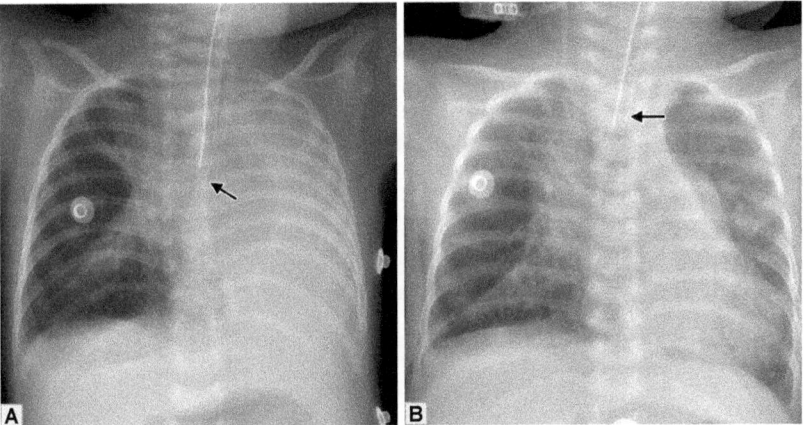

FIGS. 16A AND B: Malpositioned endotracheal tube. Endotracheal tube in right main bronchus (arrow in A) with left lung collapse. Follow-up radiograph (B) shows left lung expansion after repositioning of the tube in the trachea.

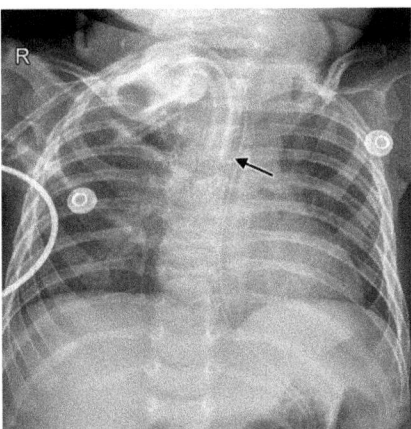

FIG. 17: Tracheostomy tube. A tracheostomy tube with tip positioned just proximal to the carina (arrow). Note is made of right paracardiac consolidation and multiple vertebral segmentation anomalies.

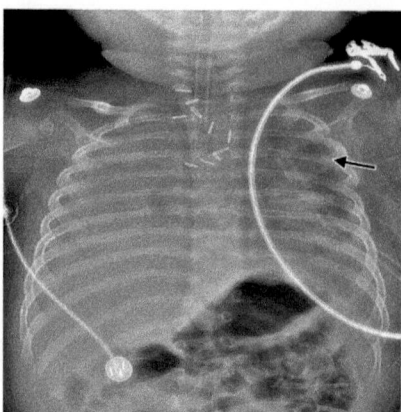

FIG. 18: Chest tube. Left-sided chest tube with pneumothorax (arrow) in a postoperative case of tracheopexy with white-out right hemithorax due to right lung hypoplasia. There is ipsilateral tracheomediastinal shift. Endotracheal tube is noted in situ with tip at D3 level.

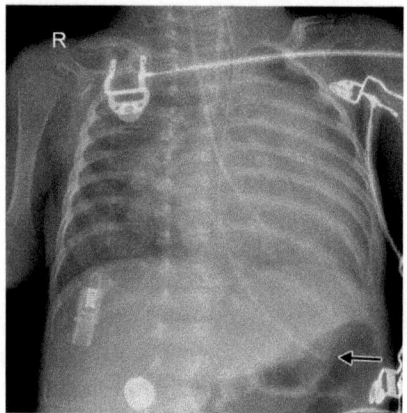

FIG. 19: Nasogastric tube. Nasogastric tube seen in situ with tip following the leftward curve in proximal stomach (arrow).

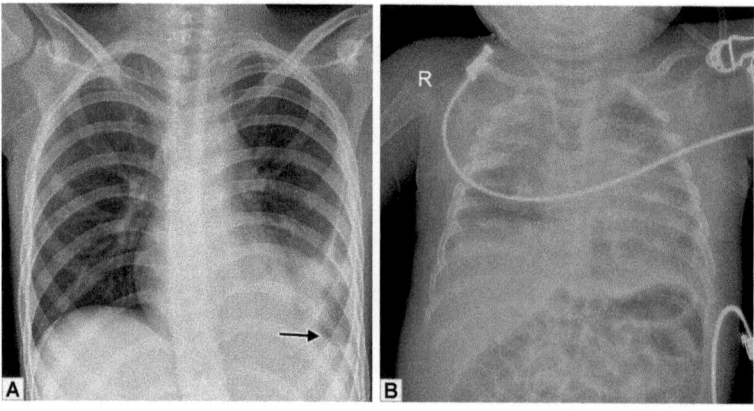

FIGS. 20A TO C: *Continued*

Continued

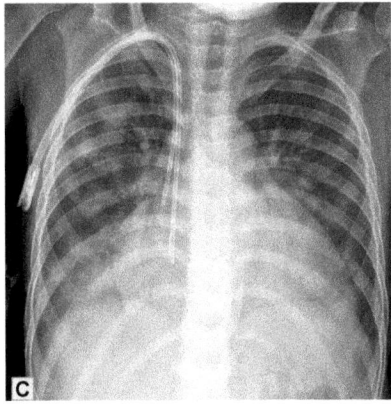

FIGS. 20A TO C: Central venous catheters.
PICC line (A) and central line (B) and double lumen venous catheter (C) noted in situ. Note made of loculated left hydropneumothorax and underlying lung collapse consolidation in (arrow in A).

■ CONCLUSION

Imaging of the thorax in the pediatric ICU is fraught with challenges. A clear clinical history with in-depth knowledge of various conditions, complication, and hardware is pertinent to achieve a comprehensive evaluation.

Other Related Chapters that can be Referred to:
- ❑ Chapter 7: Bacterial and Viral Chest Infections
- ❑ Chapter 26: Pleural Disorders: Imaging

■ REFERENCES

1. Gupta R, Nallasamy K, Williams V, Saxena AK, Jayashree M. Prescription practice and clinical utility of chest radiographs in a pediatric intensive care unit: A prospective observational study. BMC Med Imaging. 2021;21:44.
2. Foust AM, Phillips GS, Chu WC, Daltro P, Das KM, Garcia-Peña P, et al. International Expert Consensus Statement on Chest Imaging in Pediatric COVID-19 Patient Management: Imaging Findings, Imaging Study Reporting, and Imaging Study Recommendations. Radiol Cardiothorac Imaging. 2020;2(2):e200214.
3. Quasney MW, Goodman DM, Billow M, Chiu H, Easterling L, Frankel L, et al. Routine chest radiographs in pediatric intensive care units. Pediatrics. 2001;107(02):241-8.
4. Bird R, Braunold D, Matava CT. Chest trauma in children-what an anesthesiologist should know. Paediatr Anaesth. 2021;32(2):340-5.

SECTION 11

Reporting Formats Illustrative Cases and Self-assessment

CHAPTER 29: Reporting Formats and Illustrative Cases
CHAPTER 30: Self-assessment Module

CHAPTER 29

Reporting Formats and Illustrative Cases

Anuradha Singh

CASE 1

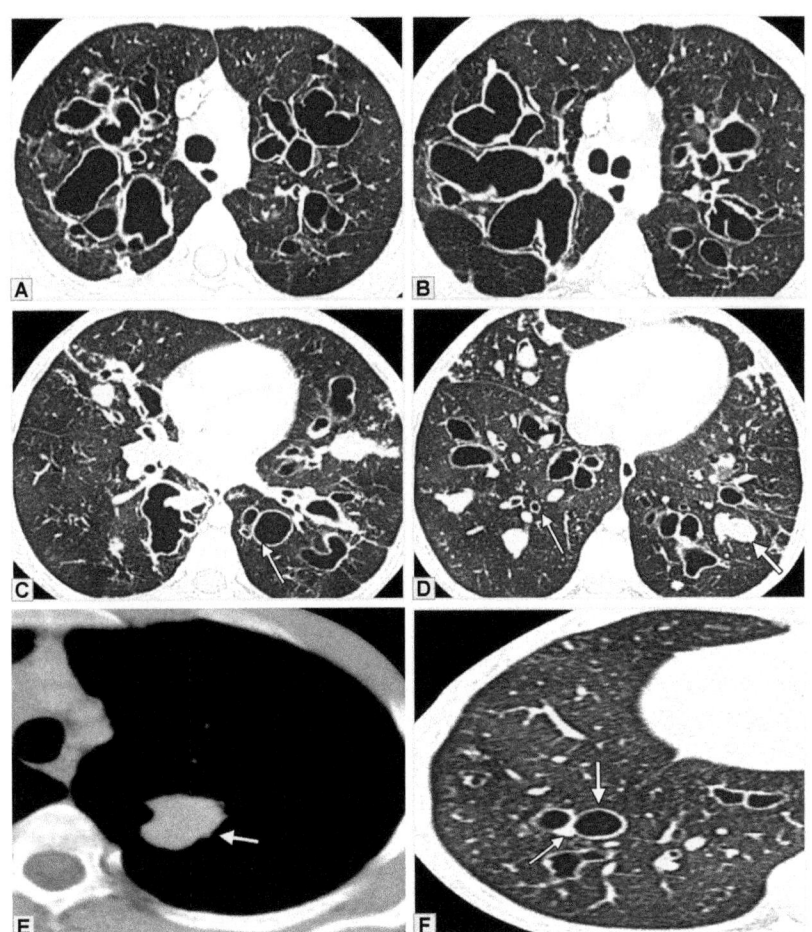

(A) Predominant finding: Bronchiectasis; **distribution**: Bilateral symmetrical (B and C) **morphology**: Varicoid, cystic (arrow); (D) mucus plugging (thick arrow), peribronchial thickening; (E) hyperdense mucus (density more than the adjacent paraspinal muscle); and (F) bronchoarterial ratio >1.5 (artery-thin arrow, bronchus-thick arrow).

SECTION 11: Reporting Formats Illustrative Cases and Self-assessment

Reporting Format for Bronchiectasis

Findings	Observations
• *Distribution:* * ○ Focal ○ Bilateral (symmetrical/asymmetrical) • *Distribution gradient (for diffuse involvement):* ○ Apical/basal ○ Central/peripheral • *Morphology*** (cylindrical/varicoid/cystic) • *Bronchoarterial ratio (BAR)***	Bilateral, symmetrical Apical > basal Central > peripheral Cystic >1.5
• Bronchial wall thickening (P/A)	P
• Air-fluid level (P/A)	A
• Retained mucus (P/A)	P (hyperdense)
• Tree in bud opacities (P/A)	A
• Fungal ball/Monod sign (P/A)	A
• Surrounding consolidation (P/A)	A
• *Central airways*: ○ Intraluminal lesion (P/A) ○ Stricture (P/A) ○ Bronchomalacia (P/A)	 A A A
• Lymph nodes (>1 cm in SAD, non-calcified): ○ Hilar ○ Mediastinal	 A A
MPA diameter (N/Abn)	N
Pleural effusion	A
Pleural thickening	A
Other findings	None
Summary	• Bilateral bronchiectasis • Upper lobe and central predominance • Hyperdense mucus
Conclusion (most probable etiology): • Infective (active disease/sequelae/acute on chronic disease) • Other etiologies (ABPA and CF)	ABPA
*Enlist lobes (RUL: right upper lobe; RML: right middle lobe; RLL: right lower lobe; LUL: left upper lobe, lingual; LLL: left lower lobe) **Most severe (cystic > varicoid > cylindrical, in decreasing order of severity) (A: absent; Abn: Abnormal; ABPA: allergic bronchopulmonary aspergillosis; CF: cystic fibrosis; N: normal; P: present) *Teaching point(s):* • *Distribution paramount importance*: Focal usually due to local causes and surgical candidates (if symptomatic). Bilateral usually due to systemic causes. • *Secondary changes of peribronchial thickening, air-fluid level, and aspergilloma*: May be responsible for exacerbation due to secondary infection or hemoptysis.	

CASE 2

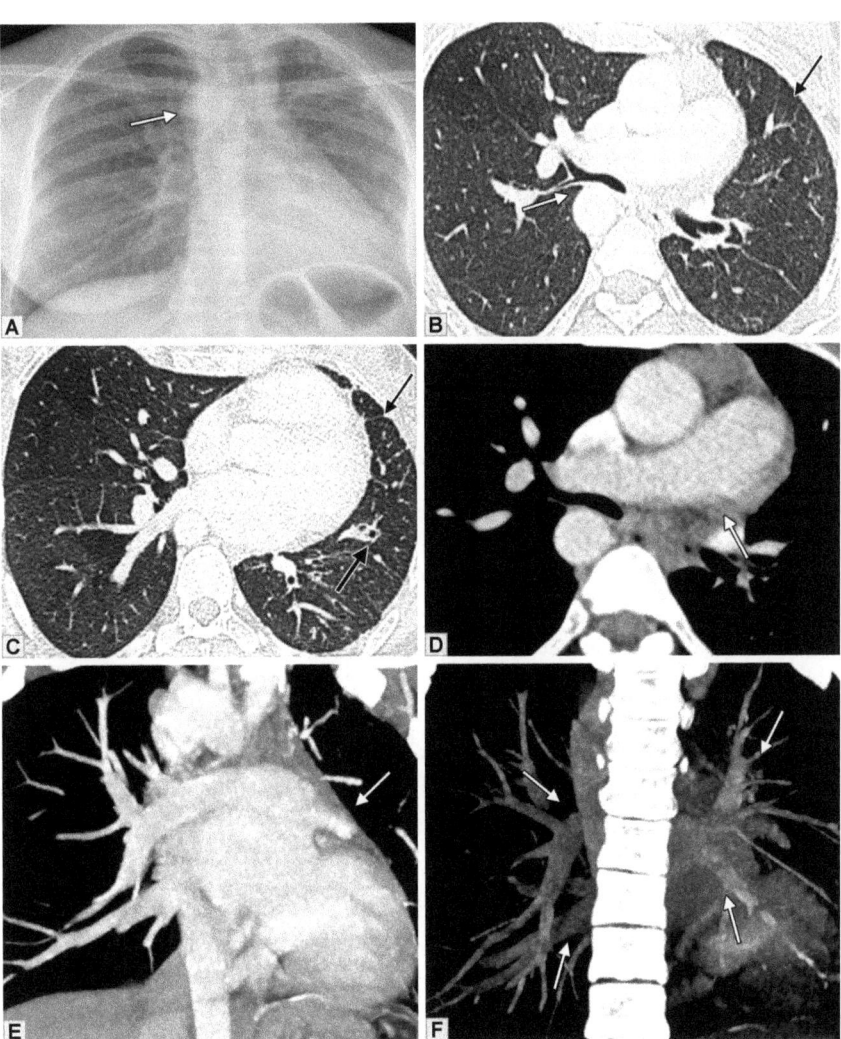

(A) Chest radiograph showing small left hemithorax with reticulonodular opacities and ipsilateral cardiomediastinal shift. Leftward displacement of trachea (arrow) due to right-sided aortic arch. (B and C) Lung window demonstrating increased peripheral coarse interlobular septal thickening (thin arrow) and mild bronchiectasis (thick arrow). (D and E) Mediastinal window and maximal intensity projection (MIP) showing absent left pulmonary artery. Note compression of right mainstem bronchus between right-sided descending thoracic aorta and right pulmonary artery. (F) All four pulmonary veins normal.

Reporting Format for Congenital Lung Abnormalities: Vascular Anomalies

Findings	Observations
• Hemithoracic volume (equal/small/expansion) • Density (equal/increased/decreased) • Mediastinal shift (no/ipsilateral/contralateral mediastinal)	• Left small • Slightly increased • Left

• *Vascular findings*:
  ○ Pulmonary artery (normal/hypoplasia/aplasia)
  ○ Pulmonary veins (normal/hypoplasia/atresia)
  ○ Any other aberrant vessel/vascular anomaly
	• Left pulmonary artery aplasia
	• Normal
	• Right-sided aortic arch (RAA)

• *Parenchymal findings*:
  ○ Hypoplasia/atelectasis/consolidation/hyperinflation
  ○ Other parenchymal changes
	• Left lung hypoplasia
	• Patchy coarse interlobular septal thickening, mild traction bronchiectasis

• *Airways*: ○ Patency (normal/atresia/compressed/tracheobronchomalacia)	Compression and malacia of the distal trachea and right main stem bronchus by RAA
Mediastinum	None
Extrathoracic findings	None
Skeletal	None
Any other	None
Summary	• Aplastic left pulmonary artery • Hypoplastic left lung • RAA leading to tracheobronchomalacia
Diagnosis (most probable)	Unilateral pulmonary artery atresia or proximal interruption of the pulmonary artery (PIPA)

Teaching point:
- Congenital lung anomalies are one of the conditions presenting with discrepant lung volumes or density (either global or focal) in childhood.
- A meticulous search for other congenital lung anomalies is warranted as they are frequently associated.

CASE 3

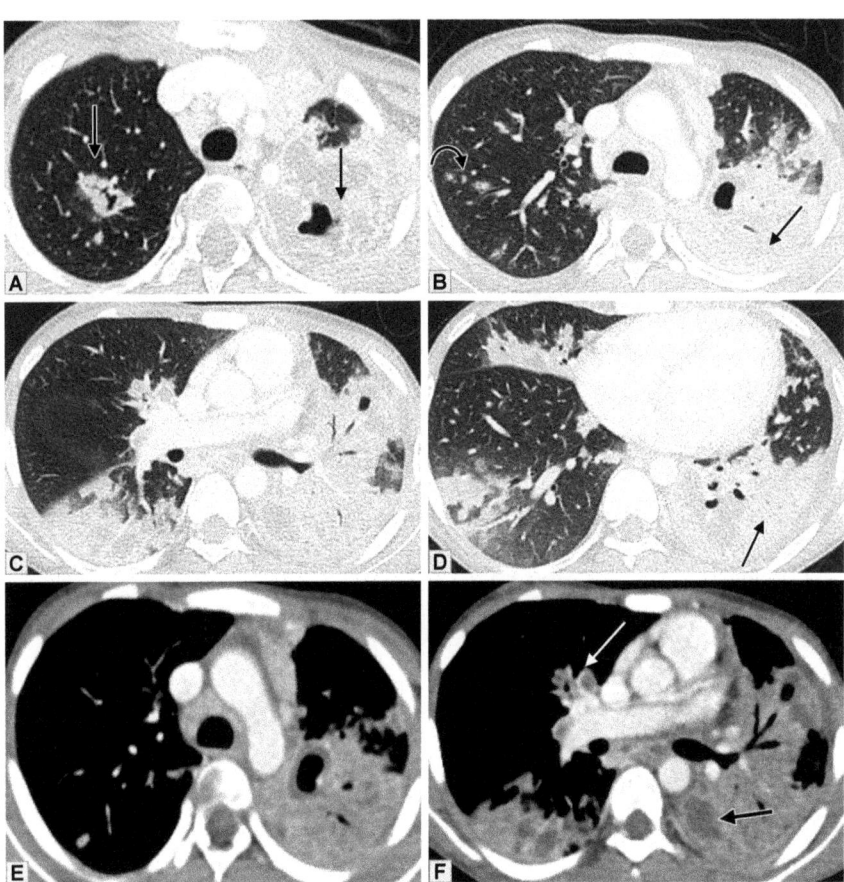

(A to D) Multifocal consolidation in bilateral lungs with air-bronchogram (thin arrow), thick-walled cavity in right upper lobe (thick arrow), centrilobular nodules (curved arrow in B). (E and F) Enlarged mediastinal and right hilar nodes, few showing necrosis (thin arrow). Note the consolidation shows areas of nonenhancement suggestive of necrosis with impending cavitation (thick arrow).

Reporting Format for Tuberculosis (TB)

Findings	Observations

Parenchymal findings:
• Consolidation
• Nodules**
• Ground-glass attenuation
• Cavity (thick-walled, active)
• *Fibroparenchymal opacities:*
  ○ Fibrocavitary changes
  ○ Fibrobronchiectatic changes
  ○ Aspergilloma formation*
• Bronchial wall thickening
• Atelectasis
• Ancillary findings
	P (multifocal, predominantly bilateral lower lobes)
	P (noncalcified in RUL, RML, and bilateral lower lobes)
	P (RLL)
	P (RUL, LUL, and LLL)
	A
	
	A
	A
	A
	A

Lymph nodes (size of the largest, non-calcified node, SAD): • Hilar • Mediastinal • Calcification • Necrosis • Perinodal fat stranding	 P (0.7 cm, right hilar) P (multicompartmental, largest 1.2 cm, 3A) None P (right hilar, subcarinal) P
Pulmonary artery (N/Abn) (MPA diameter)	N (21mm)
Pulmonary veins (N/Abn)	N
Pleural effusion (free/loculated)	A
Pleural thickening	A
Other findings	None
Summary	• Multifocal consolidation in bilateral lungs • Thick-walled cavities (bilateral upper and LLL) • Centrilobular nodules (RUL, RML, and bilateral lower lobes) • Necrotic mediastinal and hilar nodes
Conclusion: • Most probable etiology • Infective (active disease/sequelae/acute on chronic disease)	Infective (tuberculosis) Active

*Site
** Calcified/non-calcified
(A: absent; Abn: abnormal; N: normal; P: present; SAD: short-axis diameter)
Teaching point—identification of active infection (consolidation, nodules): Thick-walled cavity, consolidation, centrilobular nodules, and pleural effusion/empyema favor a diagnosis of active tuberculosis.

CASE 4

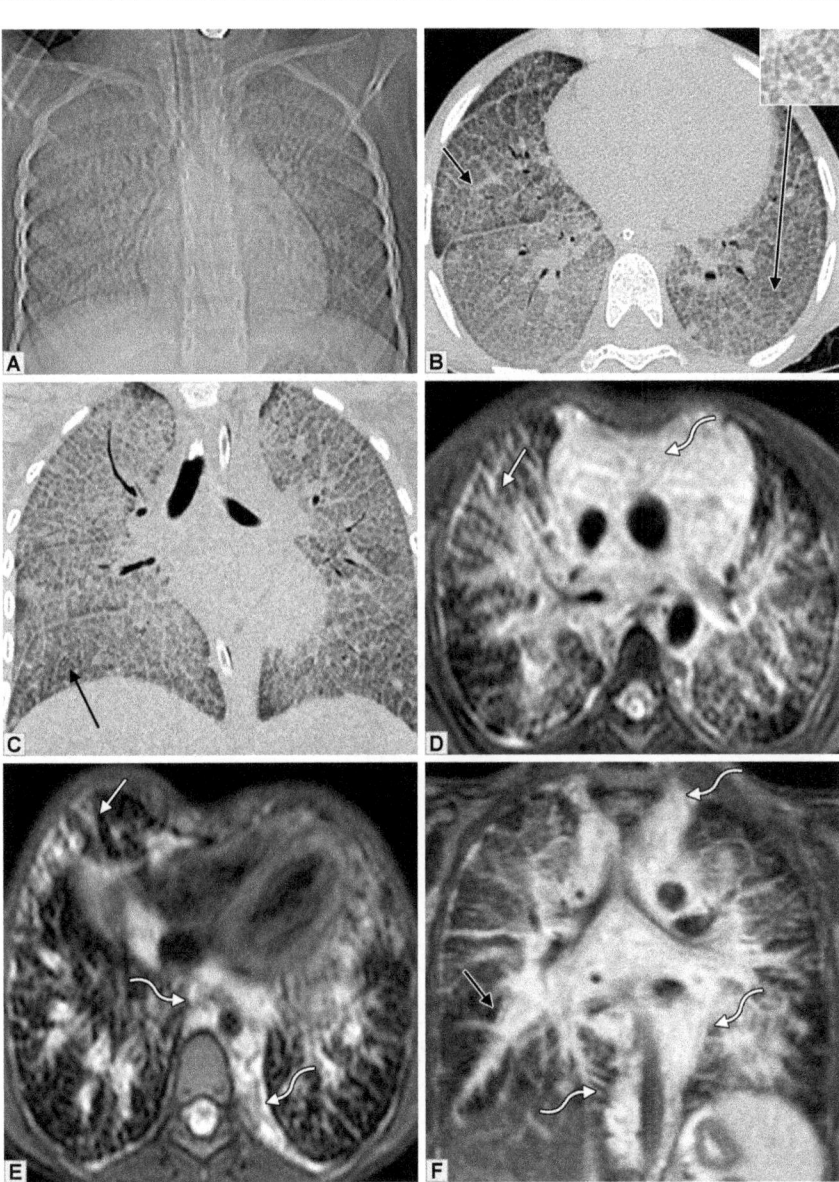

(A) Scout view of the chest CT shows reticulonodular opacities in bilateral lungs. (B and C) Lung window shows diffuse smooth interlobular (small arrow) and intralobular septal thickening (magnified in inset in B) involving entire lung with no gradient. Note smooth fissural thickening as well. (D to F) Half-Fourier acquisition single-shot turbo spin-echo (HASTE) images of the magnetic resonance imaging (MRI) shows T2 hyperintense septal thickening (arrows), bilateral minimal pleural effusion. Note the exuberantly prominent lymphatics in the mediastinum, visualized abdomen, and neck. This lymphangiectasia can be seen reflecting along the peribronchovascular interstitium (straight arrow in F).

Reporting Format for Pediatric Diffuse Lung Diseases (DLD)

Findings	Observations

• *Distribution:*
  ○ Bilateral (symmetrical/asymmetrical)
• *Distribution gradient (for diffuse involvement):*
  ○ Apical/basal
  ○ Central/peripheral
  ○ Anterior/posterior
  ○ Subpleural sparing
	Bilateral, symmetrical
	
	None
	None
	None
	None

Parenchymal /Interstitial abnormality:
• Ground-glass attenuation
• Consolidation
• Reticular opacities
• *Septal thickening:*
  ○ Interlobular
  ○ Intralobular
• Nodules (perilymphatic, centrilobular, random)
• Microcysts
• Macrocystic honeycombing
• Architectural distortion
• Traction bronchiectasis
• Bronchiolectasis
• Bronchial wall thickening
• Air-trapping/mosaic attenuation
	P (Diffuse)
	A
	P (Smooth)
	P (Smooth)
	P (Smooth)
	P (Smooth)
	A
	
	A
	A
	A
	A
	A
	P (Diffuse)
	A

Lymph nodes (size of the largest, noncalcified node, and SAD): • Size • Calcification/necrosis	None
MPA diameter (normal/abnormal)	Normal (22 mm)
Any obvious cardiac abnormality on CT/Echo	None
Pleural effusion	P (Minimal, bilateral)
Pleural thickening	None
Other findings	Diffuse peribronchial thickening, prominent lymphatics in the mediastinum, visualized abdomen, and chest

Continued

Continued

Findings	Observations
Summary: • *Predominant DLD pattern* (Fibrosing/nonfibrosing) • *Predominant pattern* (GGO/consolidation/septal thickening/mosaic-attenuation/cysts) • *Gradient*	Nonfibrosing Smooth inter and interlobular septal thickening Diffuse, no obvious gradient
Conclusion: • Most probable etiology • Pulmonary lymphatic disorders • Kaposiform lymphangiomatosis	Lymphatic disorders

*Disorders more prevalent in infancy (<2 years).
(A: absent; HSP: hypersensitivity pneumonitis; NEHI: neuroendocrine hyperplasia of infancy; NSIP: nonspecific interstitial pneumonia; P: present; PIG: pulmonary interstitial glycogenosis; OP: organizing pneumonia)

CASE 5

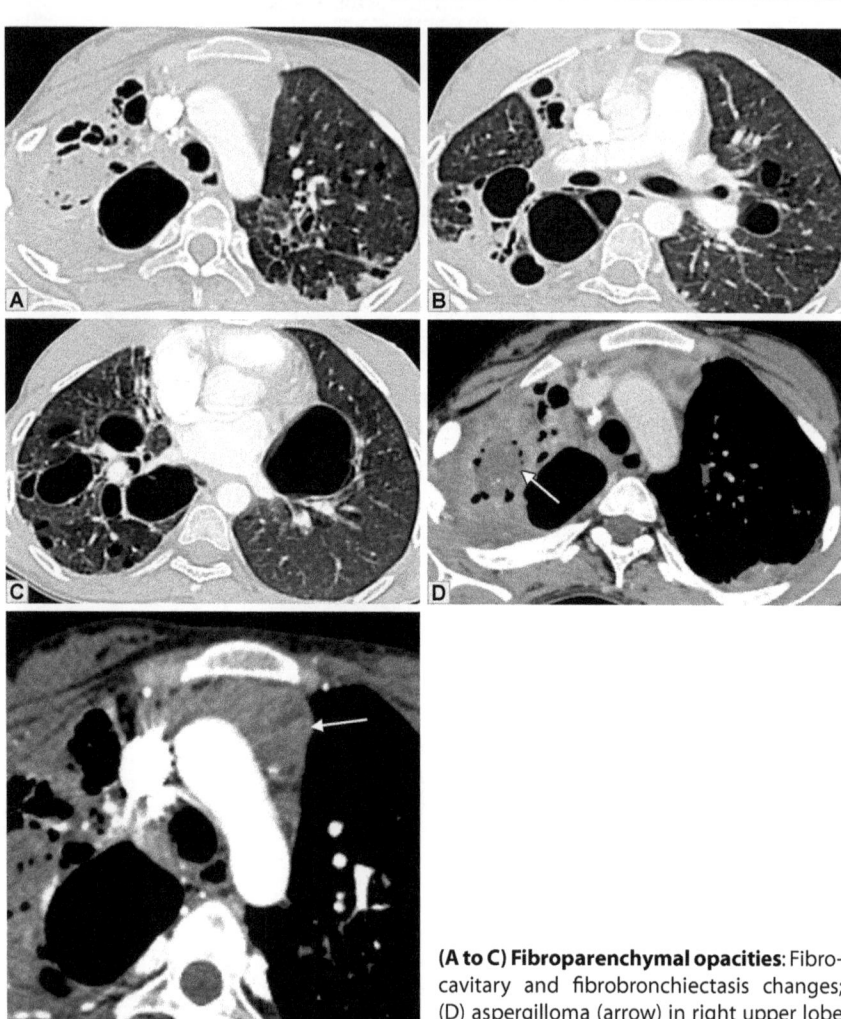

(A to C) Fibroparenchymal opacities: Fibrocavitary and fibrobronchiectasis changes; (D) aspergilloma (arrow) in right upper lobe (RUL); and (E) necrotic mediastinal lymph nodes (arrow).

Reporting Format for Hemoptysis

Findings	Observations
Parenchymal findings:	
• Consolidation	A
• Nodules	A
• Ground-glass attenuation	A
• *Fibroparenchymal opacities:*	
◦ Fibrocavitary changes	P
◦ Fibrobronchiectatic changes	P
◦ Aspergilloma formation*	P [right upper lobe (RUL), posterior segment]
• Bronchial wall thickening	A
• Atelectasis	P (RUL, RML)
• Ancillary findings	-
Lymph nodes (size of the largest, non-calcified node, SAD):	
• Hilar	P (1.2 cm, right hilar)
• Mediastinal	P (1.7 cm, 3A)
• Calcification	Few partially calcified
• Necrosis	P
• Perinodal fat stranding	P
Pulmonary artery (N/Abn):	N (22 mm)
• MPA diameter	
Pulmonary veins (N/Abn)	N
Pleural effusion	A
Pleural thickening	P, multifocal (bilateral upper hemithoraces, and right lower, maximum thickness ~4 mm)
Other findings	
*Thoracic angiographic findings:***	
• *Bronchial arteries*: Number (right, left, and common)	2 (right intercostobronchial trunk-1, left bronchial artery-1)
For each hypertrophied bronchial artery:	
◦ Right intercostobronchial trunk:	
– Origin (vertebral level, clock position)	Descending thoracic aorta, D5 vertebral level, 9 o'clock position
– Diameter at ostium	2.3 mm
– Course	Dilated and tortuous, traceable up to the right hilum and up to the wall of aspergilloma
• *Other hypertrophied systemic arteries:***	
◦ Collaterals from right supreme intercostal artery:	
– Origin	
– Diameter	Costocervical trunk
– Course	2.1 mm

Continued

Continued

Findings	Observations
○ Collaterals from internal mammary artery: 　– Origin 　– Laterality (R/L) 　– Diameter 　– Course	Tortuous course in the right apical region, traversing the right upper lobe fibrocavitary and fibrobronchiectatic lesions None significant
○ Collaterals from lateral thoracic artery: 　– Origin 　– Laterality (R/L) 　– Diameter 　– Course	 None significant
• Any other aberrant vessel	None
Summary	• Consolidation in RUL • Necrotic mediastinal and hilar nodes • Fibrocavitary and fibrobronchiectasis bilateral lungs (predominantly RUL, RLL, and LUL) • Aspergilloma (RUL) • Hypertrophied right intercostobronchial trunk and right supreme intercostal arteries
Conclusion (most probable etiology): • Infective (active disease/sequelae/acute on chronic disease) • Other etiology (ABPA, CF, CLA, etc.)	Infective Active on chronic disease

*Site (A: absent; Abn: abnormal; N: normal; P: present; SAD: short-axis diameter)

**May vary as per the site of the lesion/most involved segment in bilateral diseases. For example, IMA in upper lobe lesions, inferior phrenic artery in lower lobe lesions, lateral thoracic artery in lateral chest wall lesions.

(ABPA: allergic bronchopulmonary aspergillosis; BAE: bronchial artery embolization; CF: cystic fibrosis; CLA: congenital lung abnormalities)

Teaching points:

- *Identification of active infection (consolidation, nodules)*: Paramount importance as in case of hemoptysis, appropriate medical treatment should be initiated to control the underlying infection. BAE is only reserved in acute conditions if there is massive/life-threatening hemoptysis.
- *Identification of site of hemoptysis in diffuse conditions*: Presence of ground-glass density or aspergilloma may indicate the culprit site of bleeding.

CHAPTER 30

Self-assessment Module

Anuradha Singh

- Imaging modalities
- Congenital anomalies
- Neonatal respiratory distress
- Infections
- Airways
- Interstitial lung diseases
- Tumors including chest wall and pleura
- Interventions

■ IMAGING MODALITIES

Q.1. A toddler presented with fever and productive cough. The chest radiograph was unremarkable for any lung parenchymal findings but there was a concern for the widening of the superior mediastinum. A concern for physiological enlargement of thymus versus a mediastinal mass was raised. What should be the next best modality to proceed further?
a. Ultrasound
b. MRI
c. CT
d. ^{18}F-FDG-PET

Ans. a
Ultrasound is an easily available and radiation-free modality which serves as first-line screening tool for a suspected physiological large normal thymus in children versus an anterior mediastinal mass. The normal thymus on ultrasound is homogeneously hypoechoic with multiple internal echogenic foci and strands, classically referred as *"starry-sky appearance"*. The normal thymus lacks *any significant mass effect* on the surrounding structures and may *change its shape* on real-time ultrasonography (USG) with cardiac pulsations and respiration owing to its pliable nature. Furthermore, many a times on ultrasound of the neck or a computed tomography (CT) scan, a cervical extension of the thymus may mimic a mass. USG in such cases is very helpful by showing the continuity and echogenicity similar to the orthotopic thymus.

Q.2. A 6-year-old boy was on chemotherapy for non-Hodgkin's lymphoma (NHL). The child was responding well to the therapy; however, during one of the serial radiographs, there was evident widening of the anterior mediastinum. A concern for rebound thymic hyperplasia versus mediastinal recurrence was raised. Which of the following would be the best step for differentiating these two entities?
a. CT scan
b. MRI
c. ^{18}F-FDG-PET
d. Biopsy

Ans. b
Thymic hyperplasia is the enlargement of the thymic tissue following a period of stress or some preexisting conditions (sarcoidosis and hyperthyroidism). Morphologically, there is diffuse symmetric enlargement of the thymic tissue with a convex, nonlobulated margins. Moreover, it is homogeneous and lacks any necrosis or calcification. It conforms to the preexisting vascular structures without any significant mass effect. On the contrary, the malignancy is usually focal, asymmetric and may have necrosis or calcification. These morphological features, are however, not always reliable and can be appreciated on any cross-sectional modality. One peculiar feature of the true thymic hyperplasia is the retention of the native histological architecture with presence of *microscopic fat*. This *intravoxel fat* can be demonstrated on chemical shift imaging by showing signal drop on the opposed phase of the *chemical shift imaging on magnetic resonance imaging (MRI)*. Both the thymic hyperplasia and masses show uptake on fluorodeoxyglucose-positron emission tomography (FDG-PET). Although a cut-off of standardized uptake value of <3.4 is proposed for thymic hyperplasia, but it may not be always helpful. Biopsy is reserved as a problem-solving tool.

Q.3. Routine evaluation with MRI is indicated in mediastinal masses, *except*:
a. Tissue characterization
b. Posterior mediastinal masses
c. Anterior mediastinal masses
d. Suspected mediastinal invasion

Ans. c
Owing to its superior contrast resolution, MRI helps in better tissue characterization of microscopic fat, fluid, soft tissue, and hemorrhage within the lesions. Moreover, it better differentiates a cystic from a solid lesion on CT. MRI is better than the CT in assessment of spinal canal involvement in posterior mediastinal masses. Mediastinal invasion, especially cardiac involvement is better assessed on cine MRI. Although anterior mediastinal masses can also be better evaluated with MRI; however, they can be evaluated on CT too, if prolonged anesthesia or cost is constraints for MRI.

Q.4. In thymic lesions, all are the indications of MRI, *except*:
a. Indeterminate solid versus cystic masses on CT
b. Complex thymic cysts
c. Differentiating benign from invasive thymoma
d. Differentiating thymic hyperplasia from thymic neoplasm

Ans. c

At times, a cystic lesion may have pseudo-solid appearance due to hemorrhage or infection within. They may be of high attenuation (HU) on CT even on plain scan, thereby rendering the subtle enhancement difficult to appreciate. Similar to the evaluation of the complex renal cysts, wall and septal enhancement in the thymic cysts can be better appreciated on MRI. Invasive thymoma can be definitively diagnosed on histopathology by demonstrating capsular invasion. MRI is not much superior to the CT for demonstrating subtle mediastinal invasion; hence, not a routine indication to differentiate these entities. Based on the demonstration of microscopic fat in thymic hyperplasia, chemical shift imaging in MRI is a definite indication for this entity.

Q.5. Regarding chest ultrasound findings in neonates, which of the following statements is a *mismatch*?
a. Respiratory distress syndrome: Retrodiaphragmatic hyperechogenicity
b. Pneumothorax: Quad sign
c. Transient tachypnea of newborn (TTN): Double-lung point
d. Meconium aspiration syndrome (MAS): Consolidation with air-bronchogram

Ans. b

"Quad sign" is seen in pleural effusion in the longitudinal plane. It is constituted by two ribs, parietal and visceral pleura which are separated by the pleural fluid. On the M mode, corroboratory "sinusoid sign" is evident which refers to the undulating appearance of the pleural line reflecting the respiratory variation in the interpleural space between the parietal and visceral pleura.

"Retrodiaphragmatic hyperechogenicity" refers to the increased "B lines" behind the normal hyperechoic line of the diaphragm as seen on a *transhepatic or transplenic scan*. It is more pronounced at the lung bases. This sign has prognostic implications too, as its persistence beyond the day 9 of life is the earliest predictor for the subsequent development of bronchopulmonary dysplasia (BPD).

"Double lung point" is demonstrated in longitudinal plane and refers to the meeting point of the normal and abnormal point in TTN. Herein, the superior normally aerated lungs show expected findings of predominant "A lines" with widely spaces "B lines". On the other hand, the inferior fluid-filled lungs show abundant "B lines" with paucity of A lines.

CONGENITAL ANOMALIES

Q.6. A term neonate was found to have a hypoechoic lesion in the left suprarenal region on one of the antenatal ultrasonograms. There was no calcification within. All of the following remain differentials, *except*:
a. Neuroblastoma
b. Adrenal hematoma
c. Bronchopulmonary sequestration
d. Abscess

Ans. d

All except the option "d" are the differentials for an antenatally detected suprarenal lesion. Neuroblastoma and adrenal hematoma are usually diagnosed on a third trimester scan, whereas a bronchopulmonary sequestration (BPS) is usually diagnosed on a second-trimester scan.

Q.7. All of the following would be helpful in differentiating a BPS from neuroblastoma in a neonate, *except*:
a. Presence of a systemic feeding artery
b. Absence of calcification
c. Antenatal dating
d. Laterality of the lesion

Ans. d

Direct feeding artery from the descending thoracic aorta defines a sequestration. On the other hand, calcification, if present, favors a neuroblastoma. However, the most reliable clue on ultrasound remains the timing of the first detection of the lesion. Initial detection on a second trimester scan favors a sequestration, whereas fetal neuroblastoma is typically detected in the third trimester. Laterality of the lesion is not helpful, because, although left suprarenal region is a favored location for the sequestration, but not exclusive to this entity.

Q.8. Which of the following statements is *false* regarding a BPS?
a. Trivial risk of malignancy
b. Separate pleural investment in an extralobar sequestration
c. Arterial feeder from the lower lobe pulmonary artery in an intralobar sequestration
d. Systemic venous drainage in extralobar pulmonary sequestration

Ans. c

Bronchopulmonary sequestration refers to those congenital lung malformations (CLM) where there is a failure of tracheobronchial tree to establish a communication with the developing alveoli, latter nonetheless, remains dysplastic. They are the second most common CLM after congenital pulmonary airway malformation (CPAM). Presence of a separate pleural covering typifies this malformation into intra and extralobar types with the intralobar sequestration sharing the pleural covering of the native lung. Both these types derive direct systemic feeder from the aorta. Other differentiating features between these two types are enumerated in **Table 1**.

TABLE 1: Types and features of bronchopulmonary sequestration.		
Feature	Intralobar sequestration	Extralobar sequestration
Pleura	Shares with the native lung	Separate
Arterial supply	Systemic artery (aorta)	Systemic artery (aorta)
Venous drainage	Pulmonary veins (more likely)	Systemic veins
Recurrent infection	More	–
Most common radiographic finding	More likely to develop cystic changes	Focal opacity
Associated congenital malformations	–	More

Sharing of the pleura makes intralobar sequestration more precarious for recurrent lower respiratory infections. Consequently, it is more likely to develop cystic changes, consolidation, or there may be presence of air-fluid level. On the other hand, extralobar sequestration remains a focal opacity. Interestingly, it is not the respiratory symptoms, but the associated congenital anomalies which make their detection earlier than an intralobar sequestration. BPS may be associated with a type 2 CPAMs and these are referred as "hybrid lesions". Due to the associated dysplastic alveoli, there is a possible trivial risk of malignancy in these malformations.

Q.9. Regarding CLMs, which of the following statements is true?
a. Bronchial atresia is the most common
b. Type 1 CPAM have an increased risk for malignancy
c. Tubular opacity may be seen in congenital lung overinflation (CLO)
d. Bronchial atresia presents usually during infancy

Ans. d
Bronchopulmonary sequestration, CPAM, CLO, and bronchogenic cysts are the most common CLMs. Type 1 CPAM has increased risk of bronchioalveolar carcinoma. Tubular opacity radiating from the pulmonary hilum is seen in bronchial atresia. These tubular opacities suggest mucus impaction (mucocele) distal to the atretic bronchial segment. Compared to other CLMs, bronchial atresia may remain asymptomatic in most of the cases. The usual presentation in symptomatic cases is with recurrent infections or compressive effects.

Q.10. Regarding CPAMs, which of the following statements is *false*?
a. Type 1 CPAM is the most common
b. Type 4 CPAM may be associated with cancer predisposing genetic syndromes
c. Type 0 CPAM is incompatible with life
d. Type 2 can involve the entire lung

Ans. d
As per the Stocker classification, CPAMs are divided into five types (type 0 to 4). Certain peculiarities of these subtypes are enumerated in **Table 2**.

TABLE 2: Feature and types of congenital pulmonary airway malformations (CPAM).

Feature	Type of CPAM
Incompatible with life	Type 0
May involve entire lung	Type 0 and type 3
Associated with other congenital anomalies	Type 2 (renal anomalies, structural cardiac defects, sequestration) and type 3
Increased risk of malignancy	Type 1: Bronchoalveolar carcinoma
	Type 4: Pleuropulmonary blastoma
Risk of pneumothorax	Type 4

Type 4 CPAM may be associated with *DICER 1* mutation, a cancer predisposing syndrome which increases the risk of pleuropulmonary blastoma amongst other malignancies.

Q.11. Which of the following statements is *true* regarding CLMs?
a. A blind-ending bronchus on bronchoscopy is diagnostic of congenital bronchial atresia (CBA)
b. Congenital lobar overinflation (CLO) may remain asymptomatic till adulthood
c. Congenital diaphragmatic hernia (CDH) is the most common intrathoracic cause of secondary pulmonary hypoplasia
d. Symmetrically enlarged bilateral lungs with fluid-filled tracheobronchial tree and inverted bilateral hemidiaphragms on antenatal ultrasound can be seen in Turner's syndrome

Ans. c
On bronchoscopy, a blind-ending bronchus may be a normal variant and do not always suggest bronchial atresia. Hence, contrary to the other bronchial lesions, bronchoscopy is not diagnostic in establishing a diagnosis of *bronchial atresia*. Rather, its diagnosis needs to be substantiated by secondary lung parenchymal changes (hyperinflation) on a CT scan. *CLO* and *CBA* may have an imaging overlap of lung parenchymal hyperinflation. However, the bronchial obstruction in CBA is complete, whereas it is partial in CLO. The latter consequently causes more air-trapping due to ball-valve effect, hence, more compressive symptoms. This explains earlier presentation of CLO in the neonatal period with respiratory distress as compared to minimal symptoms in CBA. Moreover, dilated and atretic bronchus is seen in CBA and not CLO. CDH is the most common intrathoracic cause for secondary pulmonary hypoplasia whereas oligohydramnios is the most common extrathoracic cause. Symmetrical enlarged bilateral lungs, fluid-filled tracheobronchial tree, and inverted hemidiaphragms bilaterally are suggestive of pulmonary hyperplasia which occurs due to the obstruction to the outflow of the

fetal lung fluid. These findings are characteristic of congenital high airway obstruction syndrome (CHAOS) which may be due to laryngeal atresia, severe obstruction of trachea (atresia, stenosis, or web), or rarely due to vascular compression (double-aortic arch).

Q.12. Regarding "tracheoesophageal fistula" (TEF), which of the following statements is false?
a. "H-type" fistula may have communication between the larynx and esophagus in severe cases
b. "Pull back catheter esophagogram" is indicated for diagnosis in patients who are intubated
c. "Completely gasless abdomen" suggests type A or type B TEF
d. Successful passage of an enteric tube in the esophagus can be done in some of the subtypes of TEF

Ans. a
Communication between the larynx and esophagus is suggestive of laryngeal cleft with an altogether different management than TEF. Successful passage of enteric tube through the esophagus may be done in an " H-type " fistula which can happen as the fistula is small in size. Suspected cases of TEF are evaluated with a contrast swallow. However, *pulled back esophagogram* is indicated in those who are intubated or at risk of aspiration. There is better and more controlled distension of the esophageal lumen with the latter technique. "Completely gasless" abdomen is seen in the first two types of the TEF (types A and B), whereas the latter three subtypes (types C, D and E) have gas in the abdomen due to the communication of the distal esophagus with the trachea.

Q.13. Regarding foregut duplication cysts (FDCs), which of the following statements is false?
a. Bronchogenic cysts are the most common FDCs
b. Uncomplicated pulmonary bronchogenic cyst may have air
c. Wall thickening and air within the FDCs is suggestive of secondary infection
d. Incidentally detected asymptomatic FDCs need to be observed

Ans. d
Foregut duplication cysts included bronchogenic, esophageal, and neurenteric cysts. Of these, bronchogenic cysts are the most common which can occur in the mediastinum or lungs. Contrary to the bronchogenic cysts in the mediastinum, even *uncomplicated bronchogenic cysts in the lungs may have air*. FDCs have a smooth thin outer wall and internal fluid-contents. *Thick enhancing wall and air within the lesion* may suggest superimposed infection. All FDCs regardless of their symptoms are surgically resected to avert potential complications of infection, hemorrhage, mass effect, and rare risk of malignant transformation.

NEONATAL RESPIRATORY DISTRESS

Q.14. A neonate born at 37 weeks via cesarean section (performed due to maternal indications) had some respiratory difficulty soon after birth in the form of tachypnea and cyanosis. Chest radiograph showed streaky perihilar opacities which cleared spontaneously on day 3 of life. Which of the following statements is false regarding this condition?
a. Radiographic findings may be worse than the clinical status
b. Resolution of the radiographic findings within the next 48 hours
c. Cardiomegaly is a constant feature
d. Usually, a self-limiting condition

Ans. c

Respiratory distress in a term or near-term neonate is most likely due to the *TTN*. This entity is more commonly seen in the neonates born via cesarean section or difficult labor as there is delayed clearance of the fetal fluid from the lungs. The symptoms develop soon after birth and there is spontaneous clearance of the radiographic opacities in the next 48-72 hours. Quite characteristic of this entity is *clinicoradiological discrepancy*. Despite of a severe radiographic portrayal the neonate is "near-comfortable" clinically. Consequently, even with significant radiographic findings the child does not require any endotracheal intubation or ventilation. The radiographic findings at times may resemble pulmonary edema from the structural cardiac defects. However, usually a normal cardiac size and a rapid spontaneous recovery distinguish TTN from most of the congenital heart diseases.

Q.15. Regarding chest radiographic findings in TTN, which of the following statements is false?
a. Lung volumes are normal to increased
b. Distribution of radiographic findings may be asymmetric
c. Pleural effusion may be seen
d. Air-leak syndromes [pulmonary interstitial emphysema (PIE) and pneumothorax] may be seen

Ans. d

Streaky perihilar opacities and mild pleural effusion which may track into the fissure are the classically described radiographic findings in TTN. There may be lung hyperexpansion, thereby rendering the lung volumes normal to increased [c.f reduced lung volumes in respiratory distress syndrome (RDS)] leading to the flattening of the diaphragm. Significant progression may lead to the formation of alveolar opacities. However, despite of these exuberant radiographic findings, there would not be any endotracheal tube in the trachea which means the baby is doing fine clinically. This clinicoradiological discrepancy is the hallmark of this entity. Air-leak syndromes in a newborn may be seen in those who are on ventilation. It may also be seen if there is increased respiratory effort in a noncompliant lung with background fibrosis. In the context of the respiratory distress in a newborn, it may be seen in RDS or MAS.

Q.16. A 39-week-old neonate who was born via cesarean section presented with severe respiratory distress soon after the birth, eventually requiring ventilatory support. Which of the following would be the *most significant* aspect in further management?
a. History of antenatal glucocorticoids administration for fetal lung maturation
b. History of meconium-stained liquor
c. Immunization history
d. History of antenatal infection

Ans. b
Term neonates bon via cesarean are also prone to TTN. However, in contrast to the MAS, respiratory distress in the TTN is mild and the findings are self-limiting over the next 48–72 hours. Severe respiratory distress in near-term/term/post-term neonates is more suggestive of MAS. There would be history of meconium staining of the liquor which may be antenatal or intrapartum. In fact, prolonged contact with the meconium may cause staining of the fetal skin too. Interestingly, meconium staining of the liquor is seen in approximately 10–15% of the live births. However, only about 1–5% of these may develop MAS.

Q.17. Which of the following radiographic findings, if present, best differentiates TTN from MAS?
a. Asymmetrical lung opacities
b. Pleural effusion
c. Hyperinflated lungs
d. Pneumothorax

Ans. d
Except for the hyaline membrane disease (HMD) wherein the symmetrical distribution of the opacities is fairly characteristic of this entity. Rest all the other medical causes of respiratory distress (MAS, TTN, and neonatal pneumonia) in a newborn have asymmetric distribution. Pleural effusion and lung hyperinflation can be seen in both MAS and TTN. However, air-leak syndromes can complicate about 10% of MAS, whereas it is not seen in TTN. It may be due to either of the two reasons—complication of positive pressure ventilation or the mechanical occlusion of the peripheral small airways with the meconium plugs with distal alveolar rupture. Moreover, the rapid spontaneous recovery is the *most distinguishing* feature of TTN.

Q.18. A term-neonate presented with severe respiratory distress at birth. Chest radiograph showed opaque left hemithorax with rightward cardiomediastinal shift. A repeat radiograph after 12 hours showed multiple cystic lucencies in the left hemithorax with persistent compressive effects. Which of the following would be the most useful immediate step in further diagnosis?
a. Look for the paucity of the bowel gases in an abdominal radiograph
b. Left lateral decubitus radiograph

c. Cross-table lateral shoot through view
d. Further repeat frontal chest radiograph after 12 hours

Ans. a

Respiratory distress in a newborn with compressive symptoms is suggestive of a surgical cause. The major differentials for cystic bubbly lucencies in this context include CPAM and CDH. CDH can be ascertained by noting the paucity of bowel gases in the abdomen and looking for the diaphragmatic continuity. Fluid-filled bowel loops may appear opaque. Other methods to ascertain the diagnosis of CDH at the bedside include checking the position of the nasogastric tube or an ultrasound.

Q.19. A neonate born at 26 weeks of gestations developed nasal flaring, cyanosis, and tachypnea soon after birth with oxygen requirement. Which of the following statements is *incorrect* regarding the possible diagnosis?
a. Typical radiographic findings may lag the clinical features
b. Symmetrical distribution of the opacities on a chest radiograph is classical for this condition
c. PIE may develop during the hospital course
d. Pleural effusion may be present at initial presentation

Ans. d

A respiratory distress in a preterm neonate is suggestive of RDS which is a clinical diagnosis. Despite being symptomatic immediately after birth, maximum radiographic findings may take 12-24 hours to establish after the clearance of the fetal fluid from the lungs. *Even/symmetrical distribution* of the fine granular opacities is fairly typical of this condition. In fact, *uneven/asymmetrical distribution* of the findings may suggest alternative etiology. Air-leak syndromes (PIE, pneumothorax, etc.) is a known complication in these rigid and noncompliant lungs on a ventilatory support. Pleural effusion is not a feature of this entity, unless pulmonary edema develops due to relentless pulmonary hypertension. Apart from the clinical manifestation, the pulmonary edema would be manifested by sudden enlargement of the cardiac silhouette on a chest radiograph.

Q.20. The above neonate was managed on a positive pressure ventilation. However, he suddenly developed sudden diffuse opacification of bilateral lungs. All of these can be the cause, *except*:
a. Pulmonary edema
b. Pulmonary hemorrhage
c. Diffuse atelectasis
d. Pneumonia

Ans. d

Pulmonary edema can develop in the premature neonate due to fluid overload, patent ductus arteriosus, or decompensated pulmonary hypertension. Pulmonary hemorrhage may be suggested by the bleeding in the endotracheal tube. Diffuse atelectasis may be due to the decreasing ventilatory support, as these children are often on ventilator. Pneumonia is usually preceded by systemic symptoms and deranged laboratory parameters. Moreover, its onset is not sudden and the distribution of opacities is asymmetrical.

Q.21. A 28-weeker (ex-preterm) neonate presented with respiratory distress at birth. Chest radiograph later that day showed fine granular opacities classical for HMD. He was administered surfactant through the endotracheal tube and was put on ventilator. The child was doing fine clinically; however, a follow-up radiograph after two fays performed to check the placement of the central line showed asymmetrical patchy hyperlucency in bilateral lungs. A concern of usual evolution of the radiographic findings versus PIE was raised. Which of the following would be the *most* distinguishing feature to differentiate these two entities?
a. Clinical correlation
b. Checking the positive end-expiratory pressure (PEEP) of the ventilator settings
c. Follow-up evaluation with serial radiographs
d. Pneumothorax, if present, may support the diagnosis of PIE

Ans. a
Contrary to the fairly symmetrical even distribution of the granular opacities which are so characteristic of HMD, the resolving phase of this entity may not be homogeneous as always. The findings become uneven after surfactant administration as the alveoli may respond variably. Consequently, there would be patches of hyperexpansion mingling with patchy atelectasis. The radiographic findings may remain indistinguishable from PIE, especially in a child who is on ventilator. The best way to resolve this issue is a clinical correlation. In case of inhomogeneous opacities postsurfactant administration in an otherwise uncomplicated case, the child would be improving clinically. On the contrary, the babies with PIE will deteriorate clinically.

Q.22. An ex-preterm who had respiratory distress at birth and required ventilator support was discharged home. He required 6 L/min of oxygen supplementation at 2 months of postnatal life. All of the following are an expected finding on imaging at this stage, *except*:
a. Mosaic lung attenuation with areas of hyperexpansion intervened with segmental atelectasis
b. Subpleural triangular or linear opacities
c. Peribronchial thickening
d. Bronchiectasis is a constant finding

Ans. d
Persistent oxygen requirement even after 2 months of ex utero life in a preterm is suggestive of BPD, also known as chronic lung disease of prematurity. It is characterized radiographically by the heterogeneous lung opacities with areas of hyperexpansion and atelectasis. On CT, peribronchial thickening

and small subpleural triangular or linear opacities may be seen. These subpleural opacities are due to segmental/subsegmental opacities. The lung volumes are typically low in keeping with ensuing fibrosis. Despite of fibrosis, bronchiectasis is not a feature.

▰ INFECTIONS

Q.23. A 5-year-old boy presented with history of recurrent lower respiratory tract infections. His past history also included delayed passage of meconium at birth and recurrent abdominal pain. Which of the following is the *most* appropriate diagnosis?
a. Cystic fibrosis (CF)
b. Primary ciliary dyskinesia (PCD)
c. Kartagener's syndrome
d. Primary immunodeficiency syndrome (PID)

Ans. a
All the enlisted conditions can present with recurrent lower respiratory tract infections. However, the presence of abdominal symptoms is a pointer toward CF. It may present with meconium ileus at birth and later on pancreatitis can be a cause of abdominal pain. PCD (subtype Kartagener's syndrome) may have other symptoms including recurrent sinusitis, aural and nasal discharge, and infertility. Primary immunodeficiency may present with infection which is recurrent/prolonged/multiple or unusual sites. Such children may have poor gain weight or there may be failure to thrive.

Q.24. An 8-year-old boy presented with recurrent lower respiratory tract infection. Chest radiograph showed an opacity in the retrocardiac region with multiple cystic lucencies. Which of the following statements is *true*?
a. CT scan coverage to include the origin of celiac trunk
b. Immunodeficiency syndromes to be ruled out
c. Hydatid serology
d. Aspiration syndromes to be ruled out

Ans. a
In a child presenting with recurrent infection and an opacity in the left lower zone (LLZ)/retrocardiac region in a child presenting with recurrent pneumonia, sequestration remains the major concern. Due to the repeated infections or associated CPAM component (hybrid lesion), there may be cystic lucencies within. Diagnosis of sequestration rests on the demonstration of direct feeding artery from the aorta. This aberrant supply usually originates from the descending thoracic aorta, but at times the origin can be low from the abdominal aorta. Hence, in a case of suspected sequestration further work-up should be with a CT scan or MRI and care should be taken to include the coverage till the origin of celiac axis. Immunodeficiency and aspiration syndromes are also the causes for recurrent infection. However, they usually involve lower lobes bilaterally and with recurrent infection, bronchiectasis is a more common presentation.

Q.25. A 3-year-old presented with 3 days history of fever and productive cough. Chest radiograph showed a round mass in the right lower zone. All of the following are appropriate in further management, *except*:
a. Lateral chest radiograph
b. Interval chest radiograph
c. Sputum microscopy
d. CT scan

Ans. d
The age-group and the chest radiographic findings are quite suggestive of *round pneumonia*. This morphology is typically seen in children < 8 years of age because of the poorly developed pathways of collateral alveolar ventilation (pores of Kohn and channels of Lambert) resulting in the centrifugal spread of the inflammation. Most common etiology is *Streptococcus pneumoniae*. These usually measure > 3 cm in size. Its most important differential remains a neoplasm (primary or metastasis). Being a consolidation, the margins of the round pneumonia are irregular rather than being a perfectly round-shaped. Furthermore, it may not be perfectly round in some other radiographic projection (lateral view). As the malignancy remains the main concern, *the lesion should be followed with an interval chest radiograph performed after 4–6 weeks*. In a typical case (<8 years of age with febrile presentation), upfront CT is not required and hence, a lateral view along with an interval follow-up with the radiograph would solve the purpose.

Q.26. Which of the following statements is *true* about the round pneumonia?
a. Upper lobe predilection
b. Air-bronchogram frequently seen
c. Mass effect absent
d. Bone erosions may be seen

Ans. c
Round pneumonia is most commonly seen in the perihilar region or the posterior segments of the lower lobes owing to gravity-dependent preferential flow of the inhaled microorganisms. It is seen in <1% cases of pneumonia. Presence of air bronchogram (if present), absence of mass effect on adjacent vessels and bronchi and bone erosions differentiate this entity from an intrapulmonary mass lesion. For the obvious concerns of a mass lesion, these opacities are followed after a course of antibiotics with a chest radiograph at 4–6 weeks.

Q.27. A 17-year-old adolescent boy presented with low-grade fever and decreased appetite of 1 month of duration. He had notable headache and pharyngitis. No other systemic complaints. His blood work revealed mild leukocytosis (12,000). Chest radiograph revealed multifocal airspace opacities. Despite a 7-day course of intravenous antibiotics, there was no remarkable improvement. All of the following are the differential considerations, *except*:
a. Atypical pneumonia
b. Vasculitis

c. Malignancy
d. Acute eosinophilic pneumonia (AEP)

Ans. d

Prominent findings on the chest radiograph with lack of proportional pulmonary symptoms is indicating an atypical involvement. Subacute onset of symptoms, prominent extrapulmonary symptoms, and mild leukocytosis with lack of response toward the common antibiotics are subtle indicators toward an atypical infection. Their deviation from the usual clinical picture and radiographic findings makes them "atypical". Usually, implicated organisms in atypical infections include viral and bacterial (*Chlamydia, Mycoplasma, Bordetella* species, etc.). At the same time, with this symptomatology and a subacute onset, the patient needs to be worked up for other uncommon conditions with atypical presentation include connective tissue diseases (CTD), vasculitis, malignancy (low-grade or hematological malignancy), eosinophilic lung disease, and sarcoidosis. Even mycobacterium infection can have such atypical presentation in children. However, unlike the rest of the spectrum of the eosinophilic lung diseases with an insidious onset, *AEP has an acute onset* and remains indistinguishable from other causes of acute respiratory syndrome or severe community acquire pneumonia. Cigarette smoking is a proposed inciting event. AEP lacks peripheral eosinophilia is lacking and the diagnosis is established on demonstration of elevated eosinophil counts in bronchoalveolar lavage fluid or lung biopsy specimen.

Q.28. A 10-year-old HIV positive girl presented with high-grade fever, mild dyspnea, and anorexia of 5 days of duration. There were no other systemic complaints. Chest radiograph was unremarkable. Which of the following statements is *false* in further management?
a. CD4 count
b. History of antiretroviral and other prophylaxis therapy
c. Blood culture
d. No need of CT chest in view of unimpressive chest radiograph and radiation concerns

Ans. d

Pulmonary infections are a major cause of morbidity and mortality in an immunosuppressed/immunocompromised individual. Owing to its higher sensitivity, the threshold for performing a CT scan should be low. CD4 count and history of ongoing prophylaxis are also an important consideration as they help in narrowing the differential diagnosis amongst an exhaustive list of opportunistic pathogens.

Q.29. Regarding invasive fungal infection, which of the following statements is *false*?
a. Halo sign—early infection
b. Hypodense sign—intermediate stage
c. Air-crescent sign—worsening fungal infection
d. Bird nest's sign—more common in mucormycosis

TABLE 3: Radiological sign, findings, and prognostic significance of invasive fungal disease.

Radiological sign	Findings	Prognostic significance
Halo sign	*Center:* Consolidation *Periphery:* Ground-glass attenuation	Confers a better prognosis (possibly due to early diagnosis)
Hypodense sign	*Center:* Hypodense (nonenhancing) *Periphery:* Consolidation	• Seen a week prior to the air-crescent sign • Represents an intermediate stage
Air-crescent sign	*Center:* Crescent of air with a nodule in a cavity *Periphery:* Consolidation	• Represents healing • Seen in the recovery phase when neutrophil counts improve
Bird nest's sign	*Center:* Ground-glass attenuation with intersecting linear strands *Peripheral:* Consolidation	More suggestive of PM than IPA

(IPA: invasive pulmonary aspergillosis; PM: pulmonary mucormycosis)

Ans. c

Invasive pulmonary aspergillosis (IPA) and pulmonary mucormycosis (PM) are the two most dreadful pathogens in the spectrum of invasive fungal disease (IFD). Both these infections are seen in the context of immunocompromised/immunosuppression and portend a poor prognosis if not recognized early. Due to long waiting time in the culture reports and with nonspecific symptoms, the onus lies on to the radiologist to raise the red flag. Couple of radiological signs have been described in the IFD which along with their prognostic significance have been enlisted in **Table 3**.

All these signs are described on the *lung window* of a chest CT except the "hypodense sign". The hypodense sign is described on the *mediastinal window* of a contrast-enhanced CT scan.

Q.30. An 8-year-old girl presented with acute-onset high-grade fever with productive cough. CT chest showed consolidation with an evolving abscess in the right lower lobe. She also had history of recurrent upper respiratory tract infection, which grew *Aspergillus* species twice. At the age of 4 years, she had developed multiple small abscesses in the liver and spleen, the culture of which yielded *Staphylococcus aureus*. At the age of 6 years, she had history of discharging sinus in the right cervical region consequential to the suppurative lymphadenitis which yielded *Bordetella* species. The child should be investigated for which of the following conditions?
a. PIDs
b. HIV
c. Tuberculosis
d. Genetic syndrome

Ans. a

In the whole clinical context, the child is developing recurrent infection and those affecting multiple sites. It is highly suspicious for an underlying immunodeficiency state. Of note in this case is the recurrent infections with bacterial and fungal pathogens, which is quite suggestive of chronic granulomatous disease (CGD) which is characterized by the impaired phagocytic response of the neutrophils. This impaired function makes them susceptible to the infection with suppurative organisms and fungus. Infections in CGD may be recurrent, prolonged, multiple, or involve unusual sites. Usually, recurrent pulmonary infections and suppurative lymphadenitis predominates. Osteomyelitis and other deep-seated soft tissue infections may also be seen.

AIRWAYS

Q.31. Regarding bronchiectasis in children, which of the following statements are *false*?
a. Upper lobe predominant bronchiectasis in PCD
b. Most common cause is aspirated foreign body (FB)
c. Allergic bronchopulmonary aspergillosis (ABPA) is most commonly seen in the clinical backdrop of CF as compared to asthma in adults
d. Systemic etiology should be worked up if it is bilateral and fairly symmetrical

Ans. a

Upper lobe bronchiectasis—ABPA, CF, postcicatricial (TB, sarcoidosis, and postradiotherapy). Lower lobe bronchiectasis—aspiration, immunodeficiency syndromes. Bronchiectasis in PCD (subtype Kartagener's syndrome) predominates in bilateral lower lobes, right middle lobe, and lingula. FB is the most common cause of bronchiectasis in children, where it leads to focal bronchiectasis. Due to a structural intraluminal cause, bronchoscopy is the mainstay which serves the dual purpose of diagnostic as well as therapeutic investigation. ABPA is usually seen in the context of asthma in adults whereas in children, it is seen in the context of CF. Although, very difficult to identify as the CF itself causes bronchiectasis, superimposed ABPA should be suspected when the primary disease is not being controlled despite the best therapeutic measures. Imaging clues which may be helpful include transient pulmonary opacities (fleeting pulmonary opacities) in initial stages and the presence of inspissated high-attenuation mucus (HAM) (70–100 HU). This may be further be supported by serology tests (IgE levels, *Aspergillus* antigen detection). Systemic causes (infection, inflammatory, and immunodeficiency) usually lead to diffuse and bilateral bronchiectasis. It is important to identify this subset as the primary treatment in such cases is directed toward diagnosis and control of the primary pathology rather than aiming to treat bronchiectasis per se.

Q.32. A 1.5-year-old child, who was playing unsupervised, suddenly started choking. It settled after a while but there was a persistent wheezing. He was rushed to an emergency, where the chest radiograph showed doubtful hyperlucency of the left hemithorax. As the child was crying, an expiratory view could not be performed. What would be the *next* best alternative view?
a. Lordotic view
b. Paired decubitus view
c. Right lateral view
d. Left lateral view

Ans. b
There is a concern of FB aspiration in this child, which although remains undocumented as the child was playing unsupervised. However, the sudden development of the respiratory symptoms with asymmetrical hyperlucency heightens the suspicion. Radiopaque FB can easily be documented. However, the problem lies with a radiolucent FB which can be suggested and localized indirectly on a radiograph. A *completely obstructing* intraluminal FB would cause postobstructive atelectasis or consolidation. On the other hand, a *partially obstructing* FB causes air-trapping by limiting the airflow unidirectional (ball-valve mechanism). Chest radiograph performed in a crying child is inevitably an inspiratory acquisition. For confirmation of a FB, an expiratory view is needed, which at times is not possible in children. The alternative to an expiratory radiograph is a paired decubitus view. In the decubitus view, there is a partial collapse of the dependent lung which serves as a surrogate to expiration. Maintained transradiancy (lucency) in the dependent lung is suggestive of air-trapping, thereby, confirming the presence of FB. CT is incrementally being used in a suspected FB. Bronchoscopy remains the gold standard in diagnosis and serves therapeutic too.

Q.33. A 4-month-old infant girl presented with recurrent episodes of acute stridor which used to exacerbate on crying. The child was noticed to have multiple small reddish to bluish skin lesions distributed all throughout the body including the face. First noted at the age of 1.5 months, these lesions showed progressive increase in size. CT neck showed a polypoidal enhancing lesion in the subglottic airway. Which of the following is the most likely diagnosis?
a. Langerhans cell histiocytosis (LCH)
b. Hemangioma
c. Venous malformation
d. Papilloma

Ans. b
The history and clinical findings are consistent with infantile hemangioma. These are a true vascular neoplasm which are *not present at birth*, develop soon after and undergo a *proliferative phase* in the first year followed by *spontaneous regression* by the age of 5-6 years. In the airways, they are typically located in the subglottic airway, approximately 1-1.5 cm below the

true vocal cords. Subglottic hemangioma is usually associated with cutaneous hemangioma, especially those in the head and neck region.

Papilloma, on the other hand, is usually seen after the age of 5 years. LCH more commonly involves the lung interstitium over airways. Venous and lymphatic malformations are extremely rare tumors of the airways.

Q.34. A 3-year-old child was incidentally detected to have loss of the expected "shoulder configuration" of the subglottic airways which had a pointed configuration. Which of the following options would be the *next* step in further management?
a. Checking if epiglottis is thickened or not, on a lateral view
b. Clinically assess the child for any respiratory difficulty or cough
c. Checking the position of the vocal cords
d. Both b and c

Ans. d
Normal configuration of the subglottic airways:
- *Adult:* Shouldered margins
- *Children:* Much less angular configuration making shouldered margins less conspicuous

Subglottic airways can have a pointed configuration in croup where it has been described variously as *"steeple" or "pencil-point" sign*. However, even in normal children, the configuration of the subglottic airways can become pointed when the radiograph has been acquired with abducted vocal cords. Important clues to deem it a pathology versus normal would be suggested by checking the position of vocal cords on the AP radiograph. So, if the child is *symptomatic* and the vocal cords are in apposition (adducted), then it favors an abnormality.

INTERSTITIAL LUNG DISEASES

Q.35. A 11-year-old boy presented with low-grade fever, anorexia, and weight loss of 6 months of duration. Chest radiograph revealed lower lobe predominant reticulonodular opacities. CT chest additionally showed peribronchovascular thickening and few scattered thin-walled cysts and patchy multifocal ground-glass opacities (GGOs). What would be the *next* most significant step in further management?
a. HIV work-up
b. CTD profile
c. Sarcoidosis work-up
d. LCH evaluation

Ans. a
The imaging findings in this child are hinting toward a cystic lung disease in a background of prominent reticulonodular opacities. All these are suggestive of lymphoid interstitial pneumonia (LIP). It is usually secondary to some other conditions. In a child, it is more commonly seen in the context of HIV, whereas the adults should be worked-up for Sjogren's syndrome.

Q.36. A 16-years old HIV positive patient presented with subacute-onset breathlessness. No history of fever. His CD4 count was 150/cc. The patient was on prophylactic aerosolized medications (trimethoprim-sulfamethoxazole). Chest CT showed diffuse ground-glass attenuation in mid-lower lung predominance with relative subpleural sparing. Mild interlobular septal thickening was also present. No pleural effusion. His blood work revealed a hemoglobin of 12 mg/dL and a TLC of 11,000/cc. What is the most probable diagnosis?
a. Pulmonary edema
b. CMV pneumonia
c. Pneumocystis pneumonia
d. Diffuse alveolar hemorrhage

Ans. c
Pneumocystis pneumonia (PCP/PJP) is one of the life-threatening and AIDS-defining lesions in HIV positive individuals. In these individuals, it is usually seen with a CD4 count of <200/cc. Onset may be insidious with subacute-onset dyspnea and/or nonproductive cough. A high index for infection should be kept in these individuals and due to the overlapping imaging findings, the suspected microbial agent is best interpreted in the context pf CD4 counts. Although the aerosolized prophylaxis confers protection against contracting PCP but this is not absolute. Moreover, those who are on prophylaxis may tend to have some atypical features like an upper lobe predominance (owing to the poor ventilation of the upper lobes), nodules, consolidation, pleural effusion, or pneumatocele. In this context, for the ground-glass attenuation rest other options were also a differential consideration. Absence of pleural effusion makes pulmonary edema, a less likely possibility. CMV pneumonia is difficult to differentiate from PCP. It is seen with severe immunosuppression (CD4 count < 100 cc). CMV pneumonia has an inhomogeneous distribution of GGO, micronodules may be present and they lack of pneumatocele. Absence of any hemoptysis with relatively normal hemoglobin levels are against pulmonary hemorrhage.

Q.37. A term neonate presented with severe respiratory distress soon after birth. Chest radiograph showed diffuse haziness in bilateral lungs. The clinicoradiological picture closely mimicked surfactant deficiency disorders (SDD) as seen in a preterm baby and hence, exogenous surfactant was administered. Despite these measures, the symptoms did not improve. CT showed diffuse ground glass attenuation in bilateral lungs with interlobular septal thickening (crazy-paving pattern). Which of the following would be the next *best* step in further management?
a. Echocardiography
b. Biopsy and genetic testing for surfactant gene mutation
c. Chromosomal analysis to rule out Turner's syndrome
d. Bronchoalveolar lavage

Ans. b

Clinicoradiological features suggestive of *RDS* in a child otherwise a *term baby* should raise the suspicion of *genetic mutation in surfactant genes*. Moreover, the symptoms fail to improve even after surfactant administration and no other cause is found despite extensive work-up. The spectrum of surfactant gene mutations is characterized by impaired ability of pulmonary macrophages to clear the surfactant leading to a *pulmonary alveolar proteinosis (PAP)* kind of appearance on histopathology and CT scan. Commonly include surfactant genetic mutations include *SFTPB, SFTPC,* and *ABCA3* mutations.

Q.38. A 15-month-old boy presented with respiratory distress and a persistent tachypnea of 7 months of duration. No history of fever or any intercurrent infection. On examination, chest retractions were present, SpO_2 88% (on room air). No wheezing. CT showed patchy areas of GGOs interspersed with areas of mosaic attenuation. These GGOs were more pronounced in the right middle lobe and lingula. No bronchiectasis, consolidation, nodules, or cysts. Which of the following is the *most* probable diagnosis?
a. Neuroendocrine cell hyperplasia of infancy (NEHI)
b. Surfactant deficiency
c. Asthma
d. Bronchiolitis obliterans

Ans. a

All of these conditions can have the findings of GGO + air-trapping on CT. However, certain notable features of all these conditions are mentioned below:
- *NEHI*: GGO is primarily central with prominent involvement of the right middle lobe and lingula.
- *Surfactant deficiency*: Diffuse GGO (instead of patchy), septal thickening ± cysts.
- *Asthma*: GGO is not a prominent feature.
- *Bronchiolitis obliterans*: Bronchiectasis (especially central bronchiectasis with peribronchial thickening) is a primary feature.

Q.39. All of the following statements regarding NEHI is true, *except*:
a. Ground-glass densities in central lung characteristic feature
b. Septal thickening not a feature
c. Biopsy not needed in all cases
d. Steroid responsive

Ans. d

NEHI can be diagnosed on the basis of its characteristic clinical and radiological findings. It usually presents *after the age of 3 months with persistent tachypnea*, respiratory distress, crackles on auscultation, and hypoxemia. Clinically, it may mimic asthma; however, auscultatory findings negate a prominent airway disease. CT characteristically shows GGOs involving the *central lobes*. Usually, there is involvement of four or more lobes, *involvement of the right middle lobe and lingula are quite characteristic.* Mosaic attenuation (air-trapping) in a patchy or diffuse distribution is the next most common feature. Diffuse GGOs with septal thickening is a feature of SDDs amongst childhood ILDs. As per the American Thoracic Society guidelines (2015), biopsy can be obviated in a NEHI, if the clinicoradiological findings are fairly typical. However, if performed, it demonstrates only mild histological abnormalities. Immunohistochemistry shows abundance of *bombesin-positive neuroendocrine cells.* Unlike uncomplicated asthma, there is usually no response to steroids. Treatment is usually supportive with oxygen supplementation. Despite a long course, prognosis is usually good with spontaneous improvement as the child grows, usually by the age of 5 years.

Q.40. Regarding the key features in childhood ILD, which of the following statements is a *mismatch*?
a. Diffuse developmental disorders: Low-volume lungs with diffuse haziness
b. Pulmonary interstitial glycogenosis (PIG): Mosaic attenuation (air-trapping) with reticulations
c. Subpleural cysts: Trisomy 21
d. Surfactant deficiency disorders: Mosaic attenuation, septal thickening, and cysts

Ans. d
All these conditions (except incidentally detected isolated subpleural cysts in trisomy 21) can cause severe respiratory distress in a term or preterm neonate.

Diffuse developmental abnormalities usually present at or soon after birth. This includes acinar dysplasia, congenital alveolar dysplasia (CAD), and alveolar capillary dysplasia with malalignment of pulmonary veins. They cause low volume diffusely opaque lungs. Pulmonary artery hypertension is an accompaniment.

Pulmonary interstitial glycogenosis can be seen as an isolated abnormality or more commonly associated with other alveolar growth abnormalities. On CT, there is bilateral diffuse GGO or consolidation with interlobular septal thickening and presence of cysts.

Q.41. A 15-year-old boy presented with insidious onset fever, weight loss and breathlessness. He had prior history of pain in bilateral proximal upper and lower limbs for over 4 years. Chest CT showed multifocal consolidation in bilateral lungs predominantly involving the lower lobes in a peribronchovascular and subpleural distribution. Air bronchogram was present within these opacities with mild bronchial dilatation. What would be the *most likely* diagnosis?
a. Sarcoidosis
b. Eosinophilic pneumonia
c. Lymphoma
d. CTD

Ans. d

With a subacute-chronic onset, and the given imaging findings, the most likely diagnosis is organizing pneumonia. All these options can have these imaging findings. Most important distinguishing factor in this scenario is the presence of pain in bilateral proximal upper and lower limbs which is suggestive of an underlying connective tissue disorder, more specifically juvenile dermatomyositis.

Q.42. Which of the following is a *mismatch* pertaining to the *most commonly* seen ILD/pulmonary manifestation in a particular CTD in children?
a. Systemic sclerosis—NSIP
b. Dermatomyositis—organizing pneumonia
c. SLE—pleural effusion
d. Rheumatoid arthritis (RA)—UIP

Ans. d

Regarding the pulmonary manifestation/ILD of a CTD, all these options are a correct match for an adult. Despite UIP being most commonly seen in RA as compared to other ILDs, it is rarely seen in children, as this pattern takes time to establish. Hence, in children, RA most commonly has an LIP or bronchiolitis pattern.

Contrary to other CTDs, ILD is seen in <10% of the SLE patients. Its most common pulmonary manifestation including pleural effusion as a result of polyserositis.

■ TUMORS INCLUDING CHEST WALL AND PLEURA

Q.43. A 12-year-old girl presented with insidious-onset hoarseness, dysphonia, and mild dyspnea of 3 months of duration. No history of fever. Chest radiograph showed multiple nodules in bilateral lungs, few of which were showing cavitation. CT chest corroborated with the radiographic findings and showed these cavities to be thin walled. No significant mediastinal lymphadenopathy or pleural effusion. What would be the next step in further management?
a. Evaluation of larynx and tracheobronchial tree to rule our respiratory papillomatosis
b. Evaluation of paranasal sinuses, nasal septum, and renal function to rule out granulomatosis with polyangiitis (GPA)
c. Skeletal survey, ultrasound abdomen and skin examination to rule out LCH
d. Metastatic work-up

Ans. a

Insidious onset of symptoms with a prominent upper respiratory tract involvement is favoring juvenile respiratory papillomatosis (JRP) and GPA amongst the options provided. However, GPA is less commonly seen in this age group. Moreover, despite the upper respiratory tract involvement, symptoms (hoarseness, dysphonia, etc.) are not that pronounced. GPA usually leads to subglottic stenosis.

Respiratory papillomatosis, on the other hand, has a bimodal distribution—juvenile and adult forms. Juvenile form presents in <20 years age group and has a more aggressive/recurrent clinical course. Adults form presents in >20 years of age group and usually has a solitary lesion. The papillomas usually involve the larynx with the lesions confined to the glottis, subglottis, and the undersurface of the epiglottis. Tracheobronchial involvement (1–5%) and lung parenchymal involvement (about 1%) are even rarer. On CT, the papillomas appear as solitary or multiple lesions in the upper respiratory tract. Lung parenchymal involvement is in the form of multiple small nodules (2–3 mm in size) which may frequently cavitate into thin-walled cysts/cavities. Those papillomas obstructing the bronchi may cause distal atelectasis, consolidation, or bronchiectasis. Despite being a benign lesion, these lesions are notorious for their high recurrence rate (~90%) and a potential risk of malignant degeneration to a squamous cell carcinoma (1% in children). Hence, it is of utmost importance to evaluate the *central airways* in a young child with cavities, cysts, and nodules on CT so as to avoid mislabeling them as a "cystic lung disease" or vasculitis.

Q.44. A 10 years old boy was found to have a large mass in the mediastinum which was discovered incidentally during the chest radiograph performed for fitness test for a national level swimming championship. On CT, the mass was quite large and centered in the anterior mediastinum and extending anterior to the heart. It was insinuating between the mediastinum vascular structures without any significant mass effect. It was well marginated and had a large amount of macroscopic fat. There was some mildly enhancing soft tissue content within the mass in a whorled manner. No calcification or necrosis within it. No significant lymphadenopathy. What is the most probable diagnosis?
a. Thymolipoma
b. Teratoma
c. Lipoblastoma
d. Mediastinal lipoblastomas

Ans. a
Thymolipomas are rare, slow-growing, and encapsulated neoplasms of thymic origin. These are very pliable tumors which drape and insinuate in between the adjacent mediastinal structures, lung, and diaphragm. However, as they are encapsulated, fat planes with the adjacent structure are maintained. Moreover, as they enlarge, they *sag inferiorly in the anterior mediastinum*. As they usually *lack significant mass effect*, they are usually *detected incidentally* and reach a considerable size by the time they are diagnosed. Histologically, they are composed of mature adipose tissue and fibrous septa intermixed with thymic tissue. Imaging appearance is quite characteristics for the *"whorled appearance" of the thymic tissue with*

large amount of macroscopic fat. Rest all other options are the differential considerations for fat-containing mediastinal tumors too. Teratoma and lipoblastoma usually have mass effect. Moreover, about 25% of mediastinal teratoma can have calcification. Mediastinal lipomatosis is the benign proliferation of mediastinal fat which lacks any soft tissue component or calcification within.

Q.45. Which of the following statements is *true* regarding mediastinal germ cell tumor (GCT) in children?
a. Most common site in the body
b. Screening for Down's syndrome in non-seminomatous GCT
c. May present paraneoplastic syndrome
d. More likely to be symptomatic in infants and young children

Ans. d
Mediastinum is the third most common site for GCT in children after sacrococcygeal region and central nervous due to the persistence of the fetal germ cell precursors there. Non-seminomatous GCT are more likely to be associated with Klinefelter syndrome with a magnificent increase of 19 times than the general population. GCT usually lacks paraneoplastic syndrome as their cell of origin is germ cells. Owing to the relatively small thoracic size in young children, these tumors are more likely to be symptomatic and presenting with respiratory distress.

Q.46. Regarding mediastinal GCT, which of the following statements is a *mismatch*?
a. Fat-fluid level or teeth in the lesion: Mature teratoma
b. Metastatic at presentation: Non-seminomatous GCT
c. Solid enhancing component in a teratomas: Immature teratoma
d. Well-encapsulated tumor: Seminoma

Ans. d
Presence of macroscopic fat, cystic components, and calcification are characteristic of mediastinal teratoma. Fat-fluid level or a tooth suggest a mature teratoma. On the other hand, presence of enhancing solid component and invasive features favor immature teratoma. All the mediastinal GCTs *except teratoma* lack a capsule and show invasive features with the adjacent structures. Moreover, non-seminomatous GCTs are more likely to be metastatic at presentation.

Q.47. Regarding anterior mediastinal lymphoma in children, which of the following statements is *true*?
a. Mostly NHL
b. Associated pleural effusion is more common in Hodgkin's disease (HD) than NHL
c. The primary mass can be necrotic even without treatment
d. Compressive effect on the trachea is not a contraindication for anesthetic purposes as the masses are soft

Ans. c
In children, NHL are more common (60%) than HD. However, contrarily, mediastinal involvement is more common in HD (60–70%) than NHL (50%), thereby making the HD most common anterior mediastinal mass in children. Pulmonary involvement and pleural effusion are more common in NHL (50–75%) than HD (5%). Large lesions and aggressive NHL can be necrotic even without treatment. Compression of the trachea to >50% has the potential risk of airway obstruction during sedation or anesthesia.

Q.48. As compared to the mature teratoma, immature teratoma is more likely to have these features, *except*:
a. Increased soft tissue content
b. Increased calcification
c. Less cystic content
d. Presence of metastasis

Ans. b
Immature teratoma is more likely to have increased soft tissue component with less calcification and cystic contents as compared to the mature teratoma. Moreover, immature teratoma may show invasive features and metastasis.

Q.49. Which of the following statements regarding ganglion tumors versus nerve sheath tumors in the mediastinum are *false*?
a. More vertically oriented: Ganglion tumors
b. More likely to have calcification: Nerve sheath tumor
c. More likely to be capsulated: Nerve sheath tumor
d. Remodeling of the posterior chest wall including ribs: Nerve sheath tumor

Ans. b
Ganglion tumors (neuroblastoma, ganglioneuroblastoma, and ganglioneuroma) are more likely to be vertically oriented than the nerve sheath tumors (schwannoma and neurofibroma). Ganglion tumors usually span *three to five vertebral bodies* and their plane of growth is parallel to the vertebral column in keeping with the course of the autonomic nervous system chain. On the other hand, nerve sheath tumors usually span *one-two vertebral bodies* and then their plane of maximum growth is perpendicular to the vertebral column. Nerve sheath tumors are more likely to be encapsulated (unless malignant). Benign nerve sheath tumors cause bony remodeling of the adjacent bones including ribs splaying and widening of the neural foramina. On the contrary, due to their aggressive nature, ganglion tumors (especially neuroblastoma) are more likely to cause bone destruction. Calcification is more likely to be present in the ganglionic tumor (neuroblastoma 30–50%, ganglioneuroma 20%) than the nerve sheath tumors (schwannoma 10%).

Q.50. Regarding pulmonary neoplasms, which of the following statements is *false*?
a. Metastasis is the more common than the primary malignancy

b. Pulmonary metastasis is more common in neuroblastoma than Wilms's tumor
c. For evaluation of pulmonary metastases, no need for contrast administration on CT
d. In testicular GCT, pulmonary metastasis is more common if there is retroperitoneal involvement than in its absence

Ans. b

Pulmonary metastasis constitutes 80% of all lung tumors and 95% of the lung malignancies in children. Secondaries from the Wilm's tumor and osteosarcoma are the most common cause of pulmonary metastasis. For detection of thoracic metastasis, contrast is indicated if the extrapulmonary involvement is suspected. Otherwise, for the evaluation of pulmonary metastasis no contrast is needed. In Wilm's tumor, pulmonary metastasis is present in 12–15% of cases at the time of diagnosis. On the contrary, it is seen in <5% of neuroblastoma and that too, in advanced disease with widespread dissemination. In testicular GCT, pulmonary metastasis is seen in 50% of cases with retroperitoneal involvement and 10% of cases without any retroperitoneal involvement.

Q.51. Regarding bronchial carcinoids, which of the following statements is *false*?
a. Peripheral carcinoids are more common than the central ones
b. Metastasis is more common with atypical carcinoids
c. Carcinoid syndrome is more common with liver metastasis
d. Nearly one-third of the carcinoids shows calcification

Ans. a

Central carcinoids because of the location becomes symptomatic early and presents with cough, wheeze, hemoptysis, or recurrent pneumonia. They may be inferred indirectly on a radiograph with distal atelectasis or consolidation. Peripheral carcinoids comprise nearly 25% of all carcinoids and are usually an incidental detection on the radiographs. Histologically, carcinoids are classified into typical and atypical carcinoids. Typical carcinoids are less aggressive, slow growing, and low-grade malignancy with little tendency for invasion. On the other hand, atypical carcinoids more commonly lead to hilar or mediastinal lymphadenopathy (30–70%) as compared to the typical carcinoids (5–20%). Unlike their name, carcinoid syndrome is rarely seen with the localized disease and more commonly seen, if they are >5 cm in size. Carcinoid syndrome is seen in nearly 80% of cases with liver involvement.

Q.52. A 12-year-old boy presented with sudden enlarging lesion in the right upper back over a duration of 2 months. CT chest showed a large heterogeneously enhancing soft tissue mass in relation to the right scapula and posterior ribs. No calcification. Which of the following would be the *most* useful step toward further diagnosis?
a. Evaluating the osseous structures for any involvement
b. Evaluating lymphadenopathy or pulmonary metastasis

c. Examining for any cutaneous stigmata of neurofibromatosis
d. Hematological work-up for lymphoma

Ans. a
Ewing' sarcoma (EWS) or peripheral primitive neuroectodermal family of tumors (PNETs) are the most common chest wall neoplasms in children. These may masquerade an infective lesion in their presentation and even on blood investigations. On imaging, they are solid noncalcified masses with a large soft tissue component. Key to their diagnosis is to meticulously identify the osseous involvement which is usually disproportionate or subtle compared to the large soft tissue component. Assessing lymphadenopathy and pulmonary metastasis would be helpful in staging but can be seen with any malignant tumors such as osteosarcoma. Malignant presentation of a peripheral nerve sheath tumor is usually seen in a preexisting lesion and is suspected with rapid painful enlargement. Lack of any calcification with the lesion usually goes against osteosarcoma. Rhabdomyosarcoma can have similar presentation but osseous involvement is usually a late feature. Moreover, it is a primarily soft tissue tumor with secondary bone involvement as opposed to the EWS, where the tumor is primarily of osseous origin.

Q.53. Which of the following statements is *false* about inflammatory myofibroblastic tumor (IMT)?
a. Most common primary lung tumor in children
b. Predilection for the lower lobes
c. Pleural effusion is a feature
d. Lymph nodal metastasis common

Ans. d
IMTs are the most common primary lung tumors in children. They are usually slow growing neoplasms which have nonspecific constitutional features. They are usually large, lobulated masses with a predilection for lower lobes. Necrosis may be seen and up to 25% of cases may have coarse calcification. These tumors are more prone for local recurrence (~14% recurrence rate) than metastasis. Lymphadenopathy is usually not seen.

Q.54. Regarding pleuropulmonary blastomas (PPB), which of the following statements is *false*?
a. CPAM a risk factor
b. Usually lack calcification
c. Screening for *DICER1* gene mutation
d. Metastasis an early feature

Ans. d
Pleuropulmonary blastomas are rare intrathoracic tumor in children which can have a pleural or pulmonary origin, usually seen in children < 6 years of age. These are categorized into three types which represent a continuum in their progression:
1. *Type 1*: Exclusively cystic (uni or multilocular cyst)
2. *Type 2*: Mixed solid-cystic

3. *Type 3*: Solid
Up to two-thirds of the cases may have mutation in the *DICER1* gene which is a tumor suppressor gene, thereby, making these individuals prone to *DICER1* syndrome.

They are more common on the right side with a medial location. They usually lack calcification and intraspinal extension.

They usually present with a large mass when they are diagnosed owing to the nonspecific clinical presentation. Chest wall invasion is uncommon. They may metastasize to the lungs or brain.

■ INTERVENTIONS

Q.55. Regarding endovascular management of vascular malformations, which of the following statements is *false*?
a. Communication with the deep venous system is a contraindication for sclerosant injection in a venous malformation
b. Caution advised in the sclerotherapy for the malformations of head and neck
c. Microcystic lymphatic malformations are not amenable for sclerotherapy
d. Arteriovenous fistula (AVF) is more receptive to embolotherapy than arteriovenous malformation

Ans. a
An initial phlebogram is performed prior to the sclerosant injection in a venous malformation to look for the drainage into the deep venous system. If a deep draining vein is present, then a tourniquet should be tied distal to the intended site of puncture, in order to avoid sclerosant reaching there. *Sclerosant should be injected with caution at anatomically difficult sites or closed spaces.* This is because the postprocedural edema may exert compressive symptoms and may lead to compartment syndrome (as in palmar surface of hands) or airway compromise in the neck vascular malformations. As suggested by their name, microcystic malformations have a pseudosolid appearance on USG and MRI and do not have any sizeable potential spaces to inject the sclerosant.

Arteriovenous malformations are notorious for recurrence if treated only by embolization and their definitive treatment is resection. However, if large, or if involving surgically difficult site, then preoperative embolization is done to reduce their size and the subsequent hemorrhage. However, the intent in such cases is to embolize as close to the nidus as possible because proximal embolization would aggravate it by collaterals recruitment. On the other hand, embolization can cure an AVF. While angioembolization of AVF, target is to embolize the fistulous communication and the draining vein through transarterial or transvenous route.

Index

Page numbers followed by *b* refer to box, *f* refer to figure, *fc* refer to flowchart, and *t* refer to table.

A

Abdominal situs inversus 223*f*, 288*f*
Aberrant right subclavian artery 275*f*
Abnormal bronchial branching pattern 221
Abnormal mucociliary clearance, causes of 287*t*
Abscess 249, 289
　deep organ 176*f*
　formation 254
　hepatic 169*f*
　peritonsillar 246
　prevertebral 254*f*
　pulmonary 485
　retropharyngeal 246, 247*f*, 248, 254*f*, 255*f*
　splenic 175
Accidental trauma 433
Achondrogenesis 429*f*
Acidosis, metabolic 67
Acinar dysgenesis, bilateral 64
Acinetobacter 170
Acquired immunodeficiency syndrome 48, 130, 153, 156, 159*f*, 173
Acute inflammatory response, causes of 302
Acute pulmonary arterial thrombus 321*f*
Acute respiratory distress syndrome 106, 228, 184, 480, 482*f*, 488
　diagnosis of 481
Adaptive immunity, disorders of 158, 158*t*
Adenocarcinoma 413
　fetal 413
Adenoid
　hypertrophy 251, 252*f*
　nasopharynx ratio 251
Adenoiditis 248*f*
Adenoma 273
Adenopathy, abdominal 175
Adenosine deaminase 161, 175
　deficiency 167

Adenovirus 102
　pertussis tuberculosis 301
Adipocytes, immature 419
Agenesis 259
　pulmonary 78, 78*t*, 260*f*, 261, 261*f*, 266*f*
Air
　bronchogram 12*f*, 27*f*, 36, 505
　　lack of 110*f*
　crescent sign 117, 118, 122
　extrapleural extension of 10*f*
　leak 192
　　ventilator-associated 493
　space opacities 105
　trapping 289, 291, 298, 301
Airway 70, 386, 528
　abnormality 47, 54, 71, 491
　anomalies 70, 77
　branching anomalies of 218, 259
　centric fibrosis 189
　complications 218, 218*t*
　compression 218
　　extrinsic 274
　development anomalies of 259
　disease 44
　　small 296, 297*f*, 299, 303, 304*f*
　infections, healing of 293
　inflammation 291
　invasive aspergillosis 120, 121*f*, 225
　large 152, 259
　lesion 417
　　inflammatory 270
　malacia 269
　obliteration of 248*f*
　obstruction syndrome, congenital high 77
　pathologies 50
　splints, external 269
　subglottic 414*f*
　symptoms 254
　tumors 413
Alara, principles of 92

Allergic bronchopulmonary aspergillosis 48, 116, 123, 284, 286, 294, 512
   staging of 126
Alleviate right ventricular pressure 313
Alpha-fetoprotein 396
Alveolar damage, diffuse 480
Alveolar epithelial cells 102
Alveolar hemorrhage 184, 209f
   diffuse 175, 185, 466, 475, 475f, 486, 487f, 488
Alveolar microlithiasis, pulmonary 215
Alveolar proteinosis, pulmonary 181, 184, 185, 195, 206
Anechoic fluid 451
Aneurysmal bone cyst formation, secondary 418
Aneurysms 486
Angioinvasive aspergillosis 117
Angiosarcoma 370
Anomalous pulmonary venous drainage 81
Anomalous single pulmonary artery 333
Anterior mediastinal
   cystic mature teratoma 390f
   mass 7, 360, 360f, 362, 363
   mature teratoma 389f
Anterior mediastinum 387, 391f, 393
   pathologies of 363t
Antibody deficiency 157
Antineutrophil cytoplasmic antibodies 208
Aorta 31, 314f, 381
   abdominal 90
   arch of 274
   ascending 223f
   reversal of 231f
Aortic arch 7, 79f, 166, 288f
   anomalies 175
Aortopulmonary collateral arteries 231
Aplasia 78, 78t, 166, 167f, 261, 468
   pulmonary 78
Arterial diameter, reduced 313
Arterial vasodilation, pulmonary 313
Arteriovenous malformation 33, 84, 91, 230, 417, 486
   pulmonary 83, 231, 232f, 313, 318, 334, 469, 474
Arteritis 319, 213
Artery
   innominate 275f
   pulmonary 19f, 71, 78, 84f, 88, 207, 207f, 221, 224f, 231f, 266, 274, 307, 308, 311-313, 314f, 315f, 316, 317, 331, 381, 474f, 506, 511

Arthritis, juvenile idiopathic 209
Arytenoid cartilage 240f
Ascaris lumbricoides 113
Ascites 344f
Askin tumor 438
Aspergilloma 122, 493f, 502, 510, 512
   simple 122
   wall of 511
Aspergillosis 116, 121, 129t, 321f
   chronic pulmonary 116, 121
   invasive 123, 129, 433f
Aspergillus 117, 127, 145, 169, 377
   fumigatus 123, 124
   nodule 123
Aspiration 303, 480
   syndrome 112
Asthma 303, 304f
   overlaps, severe 303
Ataxia 168
   telangiectasia 168, 168f
Atelectasis 225, 234
Atresia
   pulmonary 308, 309
   tracheal 77, 259
Atrial septal defect 231f, 326
Autoimmune disorders 165, 297, 298
Autosomal recessive disorder 215
Azoospermia
   causes of 288
   triad of 288

B

Bacteremia 106
Bacteria 292, 377
   encapsulated 163
Barcode sign 34, 455, 456f
Barky cough 269
Barry-Perkins-Young syndrome 288
B-cell lymphoma, large 402f
Bechet's disease 313, 319, 320f
Beta-human chorionic gonadotropin 395
Bhalla scoring system 291
Bilateral lower lobe
   aspiration pneumonitis 221f
   bronchiectasis 171f
Bilateral upper lobar fibrosis 142f
Biopsy 375
Bird's nest sign 127, 128f, 129
Black pleura sign 215
Blastoma, pleuropulmonary 385, 387, 408, 409f, 410f
Blastomyces dermatitidis 126, 133

Bleomycin 352
  sclerotherapy 353*f*
Blood
  flow, pulmonary 230
  toxicity 354
Bone
  Ewing sarcoma of 438
  marrow 354
  morphogenetic protein receptor 315
Bourneville disease 387
Bowel diseases, inflammatory 300
Brachiocephalic vein 31
Brain natriuretic peptide, serum 483
Breast 168
Breath 123
Bridging bronchus 80, 267*f*
Bronchi 18
  bilateral hyparterial 224*f*
  central 413
  lack of distal tapering of 281
  major 152, 381
Bronchial angiograms 477
Bronchial artery 465, 469*f*, 470*f*, 511
  embolization 476, 512
  enlargement 285
  hypertrophy of 285, 302*f*, 511
Bronchial atresia 49, 73, 74*f*, 87*f*, 91, 263*f*
  congenital 73
Bronchial branching
  anomalies of 265*f*
  disorders of 264
Bronchial bud development, disorders of 261
Bronchial fibrosis 271
Bronchial neoplasm 476
Bronchial varix 333
Bronchial wall thickening 291, 298
Bronchiectasis 14*f*, 48, 125, 152, 163, 170*f*, 175, 279, 281*f*, 284*f*c, 285*f*, 286*t*, 288, 288*f*, 289, 298, 301, 466, 471, 492*f*, 493*f*, 501, 502
  bilateral central 112*f*
  central 291*f*
  chest radiographic signs of 280*b*
  diffuse 283
  distribution of 283, 284*t*
  etiologies of 283
  extensive 283
  mild 302*f*
  morphology of 125
  pathogenesis of 289*f*c
  post-foreign body 293, 294*f*

postinfective 292, 293*f*
post-tubercular 152*f*
severe forms of 279
severity of 281, 291
signs of 280, 280*f*
types of 282, 283*f*
Bronchiolectasis 297, 297*f*, 298
Bronchioles 296
Bronchiolitis 296, 303, 492*f*
  acute 298
  viral 273*f*
  bronchiectasis-associated 298
  chronic infectious 299
  constrictive 298, 300
  fibrotic 300
  infectious 299*f*, 301
  inflammatory 297, 298
  obliterans 102, 198, 199*f*, 300
  types of 298*t*
  viral 12
Bronchoalveolar lavage 200
  use of 484
Bronchocele 112*f*, 280*f*
Bronchoesophageal fistula, congenital 262
Bronchomalacia 267
  vascular 269*f*
Bronchopleural fistula 108, 458, 460, 485
Bronchopneumonia 105, 140, 492*f*
Bronchopulmonary sequestration, types of 517*t*
Bronchus 78
  tracheal 77, 265, 266*f*
Bruton's agammaglobulinemia 164
Bulky disease 402
Bullae 481
Burkholderia 169
  cepacia 293, 377

C

Caffey's disease 442*f*
Calcium 405
Callus formation 434*f*
Cancer predisposition syndromes 386
Candida 116, 227
  albicans 126, 132
Cannula 39*t*
  sites of 39
Carbon monoxide 206
Carcinoid 273, 417
  tumor 274*f*

Carcinoma
  esophagus 17
  mucoepidermoid 386, 417
  nasopharyngeal 371*f*
Cardiac chamber 381
Cardiac defects 88, 175
Cardiac diseases, congenital 217
Cardiac failure 94
  congestive 234, 486
Cardiac systems 217
Carina
  level of 248
  low position of 266, 267*f*
Cartilage 405
Castleman's disease 369, 370
  multicentric 161, 162
Catheter angiography 469
Causative organism 158, 174
Cavitary lesions, bilateral 151*f*
Cavitation, parenchymal 139
Cavities, postinfectious 115
Cavopulmonary blood flow 233
Cells, inflammatory 298
Cellular bronchiolitis 298, 299, 299*f*, 300
  causes of 300
Cellular growth 353
Central airway 258
  abnormalities 48, 258
  anomalies, classification of 259*t*
  imaging 258
Central nervous system 133, 180
Central vascular anomalies 229
Central venous catheters 497*f*
Centrilobular nodules 101, 120, 188*f*, 200, 297, 298, 299*f*, 301
Cerebral abscess 83
Cervical
  lymph nodes 247*f*
  lymphadenitis 146
  lymphadenopathy 402
Cervicothoracic extension 375*f*, 399*f*
Chest
  infection 76*f*, 77*f*, 97, 99, 156, 164*f*
    bacterial 99
    recurrent 86*f*
    viral 99
  radiograph 3, 90, 101*f*, 102, 103, 117, 137, 140, 141, 145-147, 166, 173, 260, 261, 263, 266, 271, 273, 274, 277, 280, 296, 307, 308, 359, 466, 467, 467*f*, 479, 481, 483
    pediatric 5
    type of 4

retractions, presence of 59
tube 496*f*
tuberculosis 136
tumors
  pediatric 385
  spectrum of 385
  wall 23, 33, 136, 386, 388
    bony periosteal reaction, causes of 441*t*
    cysticercosis 433*f*
    deformity 419*f*
    extraskeletal Ewing tumor of 440*f*
    imaging 425
    involvement 151
    lesions, classification of 426*t*
    lipoblastoma of 420*f*
    manifestations 434
    mass 54, 417, 418
    mesenchymal hamartoma of 418, 419*f*, 437*f*
    muscles 25*f*
    pathologies 425
    plexiform neurofibroma of 418*f*
    tumors 417
    X-ray 62*f*, 63*f*, 66*f*, 67*f*, 75-77, 79, 84, 87, 91, 399, 400
Childhood diffuse lung disease, classification of 192*b*
Chlamydia 484
Cholangiopancreatography 340, 341
Chondroid pattern 419*f*
Chondroma 405
  pulmonary 406*f*
Chromosomal abnormalities 194
Chronic granulomatous disease 127, 153, 161, 169, 169*f*, 176*f*, 433*f*
Chronic obstructive pulmonary disease 206
Chylothorax 345, 452
  bilateral 346*f*
  idiopathic 346
  isolated neonatal 347
Chylous
  ascites 343*f*
  effusion 344*f*
Cidofovir 417
Ciliary dysfunction, primary 218
Ciliary dyskinesia, primary 286, 287*f*, 288
Cisterna chyli, anatomy of 339
Clavicle fracture 434*f*
Cleft
  lip 241
  palate 241

Index 545

Coccidioides immitis 126, 133
Coccidioidomycoses 172
Coil embolization 231
Collagen vascular disorder 208, 209
Collapse 30, 125
Common variable immunodeficiency 160, 161, 163-165, 175, 214, 284, 294, 299
Complement deficiency 158, 171
Complete pulmonary vein atresia 331*f*
Complete tracheal rings 218
Complex cardiac malformation 325
Complex cystic lesions, assessing solid component of 362
Complex lymphatic
 anomalies 353
 malformations 350
Complex pleural fluid 35*f*
Computed tomography 46, 75-77, 79, 84, 87, 92, 101, 138, 143, 166, 456, 480, 483
 angiography 44, 220, 308, 309, 323, 467
 contrast-enhanced 44, 145, 148, 173, 239, 243, 244, 247, 248, 250, 253, 254, 256, 260, 261, 263, 267-269, 271, 272, 274, 275-277, 443, 446, 447
 halo sign 118
 high-resolution 40, 41, 181, 182, 184, 186, 188-190, 196, 197, 210, 296, 481, 483
 multidetector 414, 466, 467
 noncontrast 274
 role of 92, 362
 scan 38
Congenital anomalies 69, 259, 309, 469, 516
Congenital lobar
 emphysema 70
 hyperinflation 70, 91
 overinflation 63, 63*f*, 64*f*
Congenital lung
 abnormalities 69, 198, 504, 512
 anomalies 69, 71*t*, 91, 94, 504
  categorization of 70
 lesions 28
Congenital peribronchial myofibroblastic tumor 386, 388, 413
Congenital pulmonary airway
 malformations 28, 49, 64, 65*f*, 74, 76, 87, 91, 108
 types of 518*t*
Conglomerate homogenous mass 365*f*
Connective tissue disorders 209*t*, 298, 300
Continuous diaphragm sign 10*f*

Continuous positive airway pressure 269, 480
Cor triatriatum 228, 325
Coronary sinus 325
Coronavirus disease 2019 102
Corrosive injury 256*f*
Corticosteroids 115
Corynebacterium 377
Costocervical trunk 511
Costophrenic angle, blunting of 446
Costophrenic sulcus 491*f*
Cough 245
 acute-onset 200*f*
 nonproductive 130
 recurrent 219*f*, 224*f*
Craniofacial syndromes 241
Crazy paving sign 104, 184
C-reactive protein 106
Crohn's disease 300
Cryptococcus 116, 172
 neoformans 126, 132
Cystic anterior mediastinal masses 363*fc*, 364*f*
Cystic bronchiectasis 12*f*, 112*f*, 125*f*
Cystic fibrosis 47, 112*f*, 115, 122, 171*f*, 288, 289*b*, 289*fc*, 290-292*f*, 467*f*, 472*f*, 512
Cystic lung disease 122, 186, 282
Cystic medial necrosis 317
Cystic middle mediastinal mass 371*f*
Cystic posterior mediastinal mass 373*f*
Cysts 376, 376*t*
 acquired 29
 bronchogenic 7, 49, 67*f*, 71, 89, 94*f*, 110, 369, 376
 congenital 29
  laryngeal 244*f*
  craniocaudal extent of 277*f*
 dominant diffuse lung disease 186
 duplication 277*f*, 369, 376
 mediastinal 89
 neurenteric 32, 89
 peribronchovascular 214
 rupture of 211
 ruptured dermoid 391*f*, 392*f*
 ruptured hydatid 458*f*
 subcarinal bronchogenic 89*f*
 thin-walled 108
 thymic 367, 375
 tiny subpleural 215
 vallecular 242
Cytomegalovirus 102, 158, 167, 484

D

Deep sulcus sign 455
Dengue virus 377
Dermatomyositis 208, 209
Dermoid cyst 364f, 375, 391f, 393f
Dextrocardia 288f
Diabetes mellitus 156
  uncontrolled 115
Diaphragm 16, 23, 33, 81
Diaphragmatic excursion 34f
Diffuse infiltrative lymphocytosis
  syndrome 161, 162
Diffusion-weighted imaging 50, 292, 362, 400
DiGeorge syndrome 7, 166
Digital subtraction angiography
  clips 345
  role of 94
Dilated pulmonary vessels 333
Dipeptidyl peptidase 294
Disseminated intravascular coagulation 106
Distal bronchiectasis 271f, 283
Distal lung collapse 274f, 276f
Distal trachea 219
Distal tracheostomy in situ 256f
Diverticulum, tracheal 266, 266f
Doughnut sign 361f
Down's syndrome 113f, 195f
Doxycycline 352
Dynamic air bronchogram 29, 30, 36
Dysplasia
  bronchopulmonary 193, 194f, 267, 269
  congenital lymphatic 347
  fibrous 437
  frontonasal 241
Dyspnea 130, 204f, 219f, 223f
  acute-onset 209f
  paroxysmal nocturnal 482

E

Eccentric thrombus 320f
Echocardiography 308, 314
Ectoderm 388
Ectopic bronchial artery 469f
Edema
  acute pulmonary 483
  cardiogenic pulmonary 484f
  interstitial 483
  noncardiogenic pulmonary 482
  pulmonary 12, 184, 225, 228, 234, 481, 482, 484f

Eisenmenger's syndrome 229, 230
Electrocardiogram 53
Embolism, pulmonary 43f
Embolization, technique of 351
Embryonic fat 419
Emphysema
  compensatory 11
  obstructive 10
Empyema 106, 485, 485f
  loculated 151f
  necessitans 33, 152f
  reliable sign of 107
Encephalocele 241
Endemic fungi 116
Endocrine neoplasia, multiple 387
Endoderm 388
Endothelial cells 102
  apoptosis of 315
Endotheliitis 486
Endotracheal tube 495f, 496f
  malpositioned 495f
Endovascular embolization 86, 418
Entomophthoromycosis 251
Eosinophilia 203t, 204f
  tropical pulmonary 203, 204f
Epiglottis 245
Epiglottitis 245, 246
Epstein-3Barr virus 158, 377
Erythema nodosum 213
Erythrocyte sedimentation rate 106
Esophageal atresia 66
Esophageal lung 263f
Esophagus 381
Ewing's sarcoma 253f, 420, 438
  extraosseous 438
  extraskeletal 439
Ewing's tumor 252
Expiratory rhonchi 269
Extracorporeal membrane oxygenation 331, 495
Extralobar sequestration 86, 517
Extraparenchymal lesion 21
Extrapleural lesions 20
Extrinsic compression 276

F

Fallot tetralogy 218, 226f, 230
False vocal cords, level of 240f
Fast spin echo 54, 341
Fat 405
  suppression 342
Febrile illness, acute 109
Feeding artery 232f

Felson's method 358*f*
Felson's system 358, 359*t*
Fever 130, 245
  high-grade 223*f*
Fibrinous pleural septations 107
Fibroblasts 413
Fibrobronchiectatic lesions 512
Fibrocavitary stage 122
Fibrocytes, interstitial 102
Fibroelastosis
  pleuroparenchymal 234
  pleuropulmonary 234
Fibroparenchymal opacities 467, 510
Fibrosarcoma
  congenital 420
  infantile 420
Fibrosing mediastinitis 369, 379, 381*f*
  secondary effects of 381*t*
Fibrosis 255, 256, 353
  interstitial 481
  peribronchial 154*f*
  peribronchovascular 201*f*
  pulmonary 215
Filamin A 180, 194
Fissure, minor 12*f*
Fistula 270
  formation 255, 255*f*
  infective bronchopleural 459*f*
  tracheoesophageal 66, 220
Flaccid trachea 268
Flip angle 341
Fluid 458
  bronchogram 30, 36
  fluid levels 418
Fluoroscopy 5
Follicular bronchiolitis 163, 188*f*, 214, 214*f*
Fontan circulation 233
Fontan procedure 229*f*
Fontan surgery 224
Foreign body inhalation 5*f*, 271
Frank contrast extravasation 477
Fungal
  disease, invasive 527*t*
  infection, pulmonary 116
Fungi 132, 133
  affecting respiratory tract 116
  classification of 116
Fusarium 116
  solani 126, 133
Fusobacterium 377

G

Galactomannan, serum 121
Ganglioneuroblastoma 372, 386
Ganglioneuroma 372, 373*f*
Gastroesophageal reflux 113*f*
  disease 112, 269
Gastrointestinal abnormalities, multiple 192
Gastrointestinal tract 85, 156, 158, 163
Gaucher's disease 207*f*
Generalized lymphatic
  abnormality 347
  anomaly 348*f*
Generalized lymphoproliferative disorders 163
Genitourinary abnormalities 192
Germ cell tumor 386, 388, 454*f*
  nonseminomatous 365*f*, 395, 396, 397*f*
Ghon's complex 149*f*
Ghon's focus 149*f*
Glossoptosis 241
Glottis 239*f*
Gloved finger opacities 124
Goiter
  congenital 252
  mediastinal extension of 375
Goodpasture syndrome 208, 486
Gorham–Stout disease 350
Granulocyte
  disorders of 169
  macrophage colony-stimulating factor 186, 196
Granulomatosis 210, 211*f*
  bronchocentric 303
Grave's disease 366
Great vessels 9
Ground-glass
  attenuation nodules 200*f*, 201*f*
  density 512
  halo 285*f*
  nodules 232*f*, 298
  nodules, multiple 316
  opacity 101, 128*f*, 162*f*, 180, 182*f*, 184-186, 187*f*, 196, 197, 202, 203, 205-210, 224, 230, 297, 330, 481
  diagnosis of 48
  diffuse 316
Growth abnormalities 192, 193
Gynecomastia 395

H

Haemophilus influenzae B 104
Half-Fourier single-shot turbo spin echo 341, 507
Halo sign, reversed 118, 128*f*, 129
Hamartoma 405
    congenital mesenchymal 388
    infantile cartilaginous 418
    mesenchymal 418, 419*f*, 435, 437*f*
    pulmonary 405, 406*f*
Hamartomatous lesion 64
Hantaviruses 377
Heart 9
    disease, congenital 67, 80, 82, 217, 230, 313, 466, 473
    hypoplasia 330
Hemangioma 33, 241, 388, 405, 413, 415*f*, 417
    infantile 252, 413
    multiple intrapulmonary 407*f*
    subglottic 242, 245*f*, 252, 273, 413, 414*f*
Hemangiomatosis, pulmonary capillary 315, 316, 316*f*
Hematopoietic stem cell transplantation 133, 185
Hemithorax 15*f*, 503
    bilateral 458
Hemoptysis 44, 79, 81*f*, 94, 117, 211*f*, 230, 231, 465
    causes of 466, 466*t*
    evaluation of 465
    interventional radiology management of 476
Hemoptysis, life-threatening 476
Hemorrhage 184, 205*f*, 249, 396
    acute alveolar 205*f*
    pulmonary 28, 208, 208*f*, 225, 229, 487*f*
    recurrent pulmonary 204, 205*f*
Hemosiderin-laden macrophages 204
Hemosiderosis 366
    Hemosiderosis, idiopathic pulmonary 204, 205*f*, 475
Hepatic abscesses, multiple 159*f*
Hepatic vein 87, 328
Hepatoblastoma 385
Hepatopulmonary syndrome 206, 318, 319*f*
Hernia, congenital diaphragmatic 16*f*, 66, 66*f*, 182*f*
Herpes simplex virus 158
Heterogeneous opacification 232*f*
Heterotaxy syndromes 221
Hilar angle sign 18
Hilar enlargement, causes of 18*t*
Hilar mass 17, 18, 18*f*, 19*fc*
    bilateral lobulated 320*f*
Hilum
    bronchi of 18
    convergence sign 18, 19*f*, 360
    overlay sign 360
Histopathology electron microscopy 286
Histoplasma capsulatum 126, 133, 172, 377
Histoplasmosis 377
Hodgkin's lymphoma 161, 400, 402
Homocystinuria 427
Homogenous soft tissue 380
H-type tracheoesophageal fistula 260, 261*f*
Human chorionic gonadotropin 396
Human herpes virus 161
Human immunodeficiency virus 48, 115, 133, 161, 173, 187, 188, 214
    infection 173
Human metapneumovirus 102
Human papillomavirus disease 415
Human parainfluenza virus 102
Hyaline membrane disease 59, 60*f*
Hybrid lesions 74, 87, 87*f*
Hydatid cyst, chronic cavities of 122
Hydropneumothorax 458, 491*f*
    bilateral 458*f*
    loculated 459*f*
    spontaneous 458
Hydrops 347
Hydrostatic pulmonary edema 488, 488*t*
Hyperdense floating membrane 458
Hypereosinophilic syndrome 203
Hyper-immunoglobulin syndrome 161, 166, 171
Hyperinflation, obstructive 112*f*
Hyperintense cartilage cap 436
Hyperostosis, infantile cortical 442*f*
Hyperparathyroidism 434
Hypersensitivity pneumonitis 200, 200*f*, 201*f*, 298, 303, 509
Hypertension
    chronic central venous 224
    persistent pulmonary 66
    pulmonary 79, 225
        arterial 199*f*, 205-207, 468
Hyperthermia 67
Hypodense sign 118
Hypoechoic solid mass 32*f*

Hypogenetic lung syndrome 87, 328
Hypointense mass 393
Hypopharynx 248, 256*f*
  level of 243*f*
Hypoplasia 78*t*, 88, 166, 259
  generalized 77
  pulmonary 11, 66, 78, 78*f*, 182*f*, 193, 193*f*, 198, 262, 262*f*, 308, 309, 331*f*, 468
Hypotonia, pharyngeal 241
Hypoxia 197

I

Iatrogenic strictures 241, 270
Immune
  deficiencies 297
  disorders 208
  dysregulatory diseases 157
  mediated diseases 366
  reconstitution inflammatory syndrome 153
Immunity, innate 158, 158*t*
Immunocompromised host 48, 156, 298
  disorders of 192, 214
Immunodeficiency 158, 176*f*, 283, 286
  disorder 158*t*
    primary 115, 153, 156, 157, 157*t*, 161*t*, 163, 166, 174, 299
    severe combined 157, 161, 167, 175, 299
Immunoglobulin 161
  nephropathy 475*f*
Infections 33, 44, 93, 158, 160, 225, 234, 249, 283, 300, 317, 334, 426, 430, 484, 524
  acute 50
  bacterial 225, 377, 431
  chronic 50
    pulmonary 48
  fungal 115, 126, 132, 132*f*, 432
  metastatic 106
  mycobacterial 174
  parasitic 432
  pulmonary 160*t*
  routes of 155
  secondary 491, 493*f*
  viral 292
Inferior vena cava 83, 232*f*, 233, 326, 328
  enlargement 314
Inflammation
  tracheal 269
  vicious cycle of 283

Influenza 484
  viruses 377
Inguinal nodes 345
Injury
  extrapulmonary 480
  indirect 480
  inhalational 300
  nonaccidental 434*f*
Innate immunity, disorders of 158, 158*t*
Innominate artery 275*f*
  compression syndrome 275*f*
Intensive care unit 22, 479
Intercostal space 495
Intercostobronchial trunk 476
Internal airway stents 269
Internal jugular vein 339, 495
International Thymic Malignancy Interest Group 358, 370
Interstitial disease, chronic 12
Interstitial hemosiderin deposition 204
Interstitial lung disease 44, 50, 54, 156, 161, 163, 190, 192, 195*t*, 209, 210, 530
  acute 484
  childhood 179, 191, 192
Intervening septae 419
Intestines 288
Intrabronchial rupture 392*f*
Intracardiac anomalies, excellent visualization of 309
Intralobar sequestration 84, 86, 86*f*, 517
Intraluminal airway obstruction 259, 271
Intranodal contrast injection, technique of 342
Intrapleural fibrinolytic therapy 452
Intrathoracic extension 419*f*
Intrinsic airway
  abnormalities 259, 270
  obstruction 273
Invasive pulmonary aspergillosis 116, 117, 527
Inverted mucus
  impaction signal 125, 291
  sign 48*f*
Ipsilateral pulmonary artery 78*f*

K

Kaposi's sarcoma 160, 161, 174
Kaposiform lymphangiomatosis 348, 349*f*
Kartagener's syndrome 286, 288*f*
Kawashima procedure 232*f*
Kerley lines 484*f*
Klebsiella 170
  pneumonia 104

L

Langerhans cell histiocytosis 14, 187*f*, 188, 211, 212*f*, 213, 213*f*
Large airway 152, 259
  dimension of 267
Laryngeal airway obstruction, causes of 242*t*
Laryngeal atresia 77
Laryngeal web 241, 242, 243*f*
Laryngitis 245
Laryngocele, external 244*f*
Laryngomalacia 241, 242
Laryngotracheobronchitis 245*f*, 246
Larynx 240*f*, 241, 245, 256*f*, 416
Left inferior pulmonary vein 327, 329
Left internal mammary artery 469*f*, 473*f*
Left lower lobe bronchus 272*f*
Left lower pulmonary vein 323
  atresia 332*f*
Left main bronchial
  compression 94*f*
  lumen 274*f*
Left main bronchus 89*f*, 145*f*, 266
Left parapharyngeal space neuroblastoma 253*f*
Left pulmonary artery 79*f*, 193*f*, 218, 269*f*, 274, 302*f*, 310, 320, 327
Left pulmonary vein 327
Left upper lobe agenesis 224*f*
Leishmania donovani 172
Lesions, congenital 67, 376
Leukemia 400
Leukocyte adhesion defect 170, 170*f*
Lichtheimia 126
Ligamentum arteriosum 219
Lip 174
Lipid-laden macrophages 201
Lipiodol 351
Lipoblastoma 388, 419, 420
Lipoblastomatosis 388, 419, 420
Lipoblasts 419
Lipoid pneumonia 113
  exogenous 201, 202*f*
Lipoma 388
Liver 175
Lobar bronchus, irregular 272*f*
Loeffler syndrome, parasitic 203
Low flow vascular malformation 250*f*
Lower lobe 188*f*
  bronchiectasis 156
  pulmonary vein 328*f*

Lower respiratory tract 111
  infection 156, 469
Ludwig's angina 246, 248*f*
Lung 10, 23, 26, 70, 352, 386
  abscess 106
  asymmetric hyperinflated 197*f*
  attenuation 227
  bilateral 505
  biopsy, role of 211
  changes 199*f*
  collapse 273*f*, 495*f*
  diffusing capacity of 206
  disease 59, 185*fc*, 187*fc*, 189
    chronic 89*f*, 193, 279, 476
    diffuse 179-184, 186, 188, 191, 508
  disorders 217
  entrapment 460
  fibrosis 201*f*
    end-stage 460
  fungal infections of 115
  hyperinflated 180, 180*fc*, 181*f*, 290*f*
  hypoplasia of 88, 496*f*
  involvement 207*f*
  masses 402
  morphology determines 481
  neoplasms 30
  nodules 54
    multiple 159*f*
  normal anatomy of 47*f*
  parenchyma 224, 410*f*
    abnormalities 71
    complications 108
    damage of 117
  perfusion 50
  point sign 455
  segment 63
    multiple 299
  sliding sign 455
  tissue 78, 78*f*
    absence of 78
  volume, normal 182, 183*fc*
Lymph nodal enlargement, lobulated 18*f*
Lymph node 7, 18, 31*f*, 136, 141, 147, 337, 342*f*, 364, 506, 508, 511
  central hypoechoic 276*f*
  multiple necrotic mediastinal 149*f*
  necrotic mediastinal 510
  tubercular 149
Lymphadenopathy 146, 147*b*, 148*f*, 169, 369
  intrathoracic 149*f*
  metastatic 371*f*

paratracheal 137*f*, 154*f*
tubercular 150*f*, 276*f*
    mediastinal 51*f*
    right hilar 139*f*
Lymphangiectasia 228
Lymphangiography 340
    conventional 228
    intranodal conventional 345
Lymphangioleiomyomatosis 387, 407, 408
Lymphangiomas, thin-walled 407
Lymphangiomatosis, diffuse pulmonary 405, 407
Lymphatic 381
    anomalies 337, 347
    channels 350*f*
    disorders 509
    disruption 354
    duct 338, 339*f*
        central hypoechoic 340
        embolization 350
    embolization procedures 345
    hyperperfusion syndrome 229*f*, 234
    malformation 345, 347, 350, 353*f*
    obstruction 190*f*
    perfusion, abnormal 346*f*
    prominent 508
    system 337
        normal anatomy of 338*f*
    vessel 338
        disorders 345
Lymphocytic infiltrative disorders 214
Lymphocytic interstitial
    pneumonia 160, 162, 209, 214
    pneumonitis 215*f*
Lymphoid
    enlargement 251
    hyperplasia 163, 366
    interstitial pneumonia 162*f*, 186, 187
    tissue, bronchus-associated 298
Lymphoidal enlargement 251
Lymphoma 334, 365*f*, 370, 379, 379*t*, 400, 402, 402*t*
    non-Hodgkin's lymphoma forms of 400
    primary effusion 161
Lymphoproliferative disorder, benign 298
Lysosomal storage disorders 206*fc*

M

Macrocyclic contrast agents 53
Macroglossia 241
Macrophages, disorders of 169

Magnetic resonance
    angiography 53, 54
    cholangiopancreatography 343, 344
    imaging 46, 47, 53, 54, 139, 145, 149, 279, 309, 399, 400, 443, 466, 469, 480
        dynamic contrast-enhanced 343, 344
    sequences 53
    lymphangiography 340
Major aortopulmonary collateral arteries 231
Malformations, congenital lymphatic 49, 51, 112
Malignancy
    development of 74
    risk of 74
Malignant 386, 417, 420
    airway tumors 417
    chest wall masses 420
    neoplasms 408
    peripheral nerve sheath tumor 386, 387, 399, 400*f*
Mandible, hyperostosis of 442*f*
Marfan disease 427
Masses 251, 273, 276, 284, 375
    cardiac 370
    characterization of 49
    extraparenchymal 19
    hyperechoic 414*f*
    intrabronchial 273
    lesion 30
    malignant 334
    mediastinal 7*f*, 19*f*, 32, 54, 360*t*, 359*b*, 362, 375, 403*f*, 405
    multi-compartmental 373, 374*f*, 374*t*, 375*f*, 401*f*
    pulmonary 21*t*
    vascular 375
Massive hemoptysis 465, 472*f*
Mature connective tissue 405
Mature teratoma 391*f*, 395*b*
    magnetic resonance imaging features of 392*b*
Maximum intensity projection 93, 232*f*, 263, 328, 329, 331, 334, 342, 437*f*
McCune–Albright syndrome 437*f*
Mechanical ventilation 268
Meconium aspiration syndrome 28, 61, 62, 62*f*
Mediastinal fibrosis 313, 321*f*, 334, 357, 369

Mediastinal lymph node 31
 disease 139
 enlarged 276
 tuberculosis 470f
Mediastinal lymphadenopathy 31f, 146, 234, 378t
 noninfectious causes of 377
Mediastinal lymphoma 32, 32f
Mediastinal mass 7f, 19f, 32, 54, 360t, 359b, 362, 375, 403f, 405
 detection 51
 lobulated 32f
 signs of 359
Mediastinal soft tissue, multi-compartmental 321
Mediastinum 6, 17, 23, 31, 357, 386, 504
 compartments of 357, 358t
 division of 358f
Meniscus sign 15f, 445f, 446
Mesenchymal cell proliferation 198
Mesenchymal tissues, primary 418
Mesoderm 388
Metabolic disorders 434
 thoracic wall manifestations of 434t
Metaphyseal dysplasia 175
Metastasis 50, 370
Metastatic disease 440
Microcatheters 351
Micrognathia 241
Microsporum 126
Microsurgical techniques 417
Middle mediastinal mass 7, 360, 361f, 369, 369b, 370t
Midface hypoplasia 241
Miliary nodules 144
Minimum intensity projection 77, 145, 263, 266, 267, 271, 273, 275-277, 328
Minor fissure, upward displacement of 12f
Mitogen-activated protein kinase pathway 354
Mitral regurgitation, congenital 219f
Mitral valve
 disease 486
 prolapse 427
Monocyte, disorders of 169
Monod sign 122
Moraxella catarrhalis 293
Morquio syndrome 427
Mosaic attenuation 281, 303
Mucociliary clearance
 apparatus 286
 defects 286
 disorders of 283

Mucoid impaction 281
Mucormycosis 126, 128, 129, 129t
 pulmonary 128, 128f, 527
Mucosa, inflammation of 100
Mucus
 abnormal 287
 impaction 290f
 plug 273, 286, 289, 501
 obstruction 13f, 273, 273f
Multilocular appearance 32
Multilocular thymic cysts 163
Multiorgan failure 106
Multiple vertebral segmentation anomalies 495f
Mural inflammation 334
Mycobacteria 484
 nontuberculous 292, 377
Mycobacterial diseases 172, 173
Mycobacterium
 avium intracellulare 299
 tuberculosis 299
Mycoplasma 225, 301, 484
 pneumonia 99
Myofibroblasts 413
Myxoid stroma 419

N

Naclerio's V sign 15f
Nasogastric tube 496f
Nasopharyngeal airway 252f
 obstruction, causes of 241
Nasopharynx 241, 248, 251
N-butyl-2-cyanoacrylate glue 351
Neck 156
 lateral radiograph of 239f, 248f
 veins, engorged 482
Necrosis 396
Neonatal lymphatic flow disorders 345, 347
Neoplasms 30, 33, 435, 466, 476
 benign 405
 hematolymphoid 401f
 high-grade 401f
 mesenchymal 50f
Nerve
 damage 353
 sheath tumors 399
Neuroblastoma 110, 372, 385, 397, 398f
 metastases 441f
Neuroendocrine cell hyperplasia 180, 181f, 197, 197f, 509
Neurofibroma 372, 418

Neurofibromatosis 387, 400, 418
    setting of 399
Neutropenia
    cyclical 170
    episodes of 171*f*
Nocardia 169
    infection 171
Nodal enlargement 376
Nodular lung disease 188*fc*
Nodules
    dominant diffuse lung disease 187
    larger 145
    multiple 118, 211*f*
        cavitating 13*f*
    pulmonary 13
Nonbronchial systemic collaterals 465
Noncavitary disease 140
Noncontrast computed tomography 40, 273, 364
    protocols 40
Nonhemorrhagic disease 208
Non-Hodgkin's lymphoma 161, 375*f*, 400, 402, 453*f*
Nonspecific interstitial
    pneumonia 185, 189, 509
    pneumonitis 195, 208, 209
Nonsteroidal anti-inflammatory drugs 476
Nontuberculous mycobacterial infection 122
Noonan syndrome 427
Normal pulmonary vein 335*f*
    anatomy 324*f*
Noxious fumes 302

O

Obstruction
    endobronchial 460
    endoluminal 274*f*
    extrinsic 320
Opacification, pulmonary 12
Opacities, pulmonary 485
Opportunist fungi 116
Organ transplants 156
Organic foreign body 271, 272*f*
Orogastric tube 67*f*
Oropharynx 241, 248
Osler-Weber-Rendu syndrome 83
Osteochondroma 435
    infantile 418
Osteogenesis imperfecta 427
Osteomalacia 434

Osteomyelitis 175
    multifocal tubercular 172
    sternal 431*f*
Osteopenia 175
Osteopetrosis 429*f*
Ostium secundum 231*f*
Ovarian cancers 168

P

Pancreas 288
    fatty replacement of 171*f*
Pancreatic fatty atrophy 176*f*
Pancreatitis 480
Pancreatoblastoma 385
Papilloma 273, 415
    malignant transformation of 416
Papillomatosis, recurrent respiratory 386, 415, 416*f*, 417*f*
Paracoccidioides brasiliensis 126
Paradoxical embolism 230
Paralysis, diaphragmatic 33
Paranasal sinuses 164*f*
Parapharyngeal spaces 249
Parapneumonic effusion 106, 450
Parenchyma 153
    pulmonary 261
Parenchymal abnormality 90, 480, 508
Partial anomalous pulmonary venous connection 82*f*, 324-327, 329
Patent ductus arteriosus 218, 269*f*
Pectus
    carinatum 233, 427, 428*f*
    excavatum 426, 427*f*
Pediatric central airway diseases 277
Pelvic bones 441*f*
Peribronchial thickening 289, 291, 292*f*, 501
Pericardial infiltration 401*f*
Pericardium 136
Perihilar opacities 492*f*
Perilymphatic nodules 144, 162*f*, 188*f*
Peripheral airways, visualization of 281
Peripheral fine lymphatic ducts 337
Peripheral pulmonary blood vessels 229
Pertussis 292
Phaeohyphomycosis 133
Phagocytic disorders 157, 158, 169, 170
Phantom tumor 20*f*
Pig bronchus 265
Plastic bronchitis 218, 224, 228, 345, 346
Platelets, defective 168
Platyspondyly 430

Pleura 23, 34, 136, 443
　serrated thickening of 309
Pleural cavity 458
Pleural complications 106, 233*t*
Pleural disorders 443
Pleural effusion 14, 139, 150, 159*f*, 233, 444, 448*f*, 484, 489, 502, 506, 508, 511
　causes of 444*fc*
　larger amount of 446
　quantification of 446, 447*t*
　signs of 14*t*, 444*t*
Pleural fluid 458
　collection 150, 175, 450
Pleural involvement 150
Pleural lesions 20
Pleural masses 21*t*, 452
Pleural pathologies 444
　classification of 444*fc*
Pleural space 14
Pleural thickening 452, 502, 506, 508, 511
Plexiform neurofibroma 399, 399*f*, 418*f*
Pneumatoceles 175
　large 172*f*
Pneumocystis 484
　jirovecii 126, 130, 167, 377
　　infections 166
　　　pneumonia 130, 130*b*, 131, 174
Pneumomediastinum 10, 10*f*, 192, 494*f*
Pneumonia 61, 109, 110*f*, 111, 480, 485, 485*f*, 509
　acute
　　eosinophilic 203
　　interstitial 102, 487, 488, 488*f*
　bacterial 104, 106
　chronic 111
　　eosinophilic 203
　community acquired 12*f*
　desquamative interstitial 184, 185, 195
　eosinophilic 203
　fulminant 110
　hemorrhagic 486
　infectious 125
　lobar 104
　multilobar 104
　necrotizing 106
　neonatal 61, 61*f*
　nonresolving 112*f*
　progressive 110
　recurrent 111, 113*f*, 174
　　pneumococcal 159*f*
　viral 100, 101*f*, 102, 106
Pneumonitis
　bleomycin-induced 353
　chronic 195

Pneumothorax 5*f*, 14, 35*f*, 61, 62, 93, 192, 454, 455*f*, 459, 472*f*, 490, 490*f*, 494*f*, 496*f*
　causes of 454*fc*
　signs of 15*f*, 15*t*, 454*t*, 455*f*
　spontaneous 457*f*
Poland syndrome 11, 11*f*
Polidocanol 352
Polyangiitis 210, 211*f*
Polymyositis 208, 209
Polyostotic fibrous dysplasia 437*f*
Polysplenia 232*f*
Polyvinyl alcohol 477
　particles 473*f*
Popcorn calcification 405
Portal vein 87
Positive end-expiratory pressure 480
Posterior mediastinal mass 7, 360, 372, 372*t*, 373*f*
　signs of 361*f*
Posterior mediastinum 388
　immature teratoma of 394*f*
Postinfectious bronchiolitis obliterans 199*f*, 301, 301*f*
Postintubation tracheal stricture 270*f*
Post-transplant lymphoproliferative disorder 234
Protein
　deficiency 195*t*
　synthesis 353
Proximal pulmonary artery interruption 473
Pseudoaneurysm 129*f*, 470*f*
Pseudocarina, formation of 80*f*
Pseudomass 20*f*
Pseudomonas 170, 298
　aeruginosa 293, 377
Pulmonary agenesis 78, 78*t*, 261, 261*f*, 266*f*
　aplasia-hypoplasia complex 78
Pulmonary artery 19*f*, 71, 78, 84*f*, 88, 207, 207*f*, 221, 224*f*, 231*f*, 266, 274, 307, 308, 311-313, 314*f*, 315*f*, 316, 317, 331, 381, 474*f*, 506, 511
　abnormalities 307, 468
　　classification of 308*t*
　aneurysms 317, 317*f*
　catheterization 483
　congenital anomalies of 469
　dilatation of 199*f*, 215*f*, 335*f*
　embolization 477
　hypertension 161, 230, 231*f*, 269*f*, 285, 308, 313, 314, 314*fc*, 315, 315*f*, 316, 326, 335
　imaging 307

measurement of 314*f*
narrowing 474
occlusion pressure 483
proximal interruption of 11*f*, 79, 308, 309, 310*f*, 504
pseudoaneurysm 471*f*
sling 80, 219, 267*f*, 310
stenosis of 465
Pulmonary consolidation 110
differentials of 30*t*
Pulmonary edema 12, 184, 225, 228, 234, 481, 482, 484*f*
causes of 483
Pulmonary function tests 206
Pulmonary interstitial
edema 60
glycogenolysis 184*f*, 198, 198*f*, 509
Pulmonary lymphatic 228
perfusion syndrome 225, 228, 345
Pulmonary lymphoid hyperplasia complex 174
Pulmonary mucormycosis 128, 128*f*, 527
complications of 129*f*
Pulmonary vein 71, 83, 233, 323, 325, 331, 332*f*, 333, 381, 506, 511
anomalies 81, 335
acquired 334
classification of 324*t*, 325*t*
congenital 325
atresia 325, 330
disorders of 324
imaging 323
misalignment of 192
obstructive syndrome 324, 334
stenosis 82, 325, 332
thrombosis 333
Pulmonary veno-occlusive disease 189, 315, 316, 335*f*
Pulmonary venous connection, type of 87

Q

Quad sign 445

R

Rachitic rosary 435*f*
Radiological sign 527
Rapamycin inhibitor, mechanistic target of 353
Rasmussen aneurysms 468
Regional right ventricular function 309

Renal infections 175
Respiratory distress
causes of 67
medical causes of 59
neonatal 59, 68, 260, 520
surgical causes of 62
syndrome 26, 26*f*, 28, 59, 69, 196*f*
Respiratory failure 192
Respiratory syncytial virus 100, 101, 158, 167, 225
Respiratory systems 217
Respiratory tract 210
infections, recurrent 220
lower 111
primordial 260
Reticular fibrosis 481
Reticular pattern 189
Reticulogranular opacities 60
Reticulonodular opacities 503, 507
diffuse 60*f*
Retrocardiac mass 361
Retrognathia 241
Retroperitoneal lymph nodes, enlarged 169*f*
Retroperitoneum 350*f*
Retropharyngeal lymphatic malformation 251*f*
Retropharyngeal space 248, 249
Retrosternal lucency, loss of 360
Rhabdomyoma 370, 388
Rhabdomyosarcoma 385, 420, 438
Rheumatoid arthritis 300
Rhinorrhea 245
Rhizopus 126
Ribs 25*f*
bulbous anterior ends of 435*f*
Ewing sarcoma of 439*f*
fracture 433, 492*f*
multiple lateral 434*f*
osteochondroma 436*f*
posterior 398*f*
sclerosis of 429*f*
Rickets 427, 434, 435*f*
Right inferior
phrenic artery 469*f*
pulmonary vein 327, 331
Right lower
lobe 65*f*
pulmonary veins 323
sternocostal joints 428*f*

Right lung 457*f*
 agenesis 78*f*
 hyperinflation 219
 hypoplasia 220
Right lymphatic duct 339
Right main bronchus 272*f*, 311, 328*f*, 495*f*
Right middle lobe 63, 311
 collapse 287*f*
Right pulmonary artery 193*f*, 262*f*, 274, 310*f*, 320, 320*f*, 327
Right upper lobe 77*f*, 125*f*, 311, 511
 fibrocavitary 512
Rokitansky protuberances 388
Rosai–Dorfman disease 369, 370

S

Salmonella typhi 172
Sarcoidosis 122, 188*f*, 213, 300, 369, 379, 379*t*
Scedosporiosis 116
Scedosporium 126
Schwannoma 372
Scimitar syndrome 87, 88*f*, 221, 328, 328*f*
Scimitar vein 328*f*
Sclerosis
 progressive systemic 208
 systemic 209, 210*f*
 tuberous 387, 408
Sclerotherapy 352, 353
 role of 352
Scoliosis 400*f*
Scurvy 434
Seashore sign 25*f*, 34
Segmental stenosis 77
Seldinger technique 451
Seminoma 395
 characteristic of 395
Sepsis 480
Septic emboli 13*f*, 227
Sequestration 49, 69
 pulmonary 28*f*, 73, 84, 87, 91
Severe acute respiratory syndrome coronavirus 2 102
Short-limb dwarfism 175
Short-tau inversion recovery 47, 54, 292, 341, 343, 344, 346
Shred sign 36
Shwachman–Diamond syndrome 171, 171*f*, 176*f*
Signet ring sign 281, 282*f*
 use of 281

Silhouette sign 7*f*, 16, 17*f*, 360
Simple lymphatic malformations 352
Sinonasal tract 245
Sinusitis 288
 concomitant 129
 recurrent 164*f*
Sinusoid sign 445, 445*f*
Sirolimus 353
Sjögren's syndrome 209, 214, 300
Skeletal abnormalities 67, 175
Skeletal dysplasia 428
 thoracic manifestations of 428*t*
Skin 156
 ulceration 353
Small airway disease 296, 297*f*, 299, 303, 304*f*
 signs of 297*t*
Small caliber pulmonary arteries 232*f*
Sodium tetradecyl 352
Soft tissue 420
 components 394
 lateral 249
 lesions, benign 417
 mass, large 248*f*
 neck 414
 opacity 252*f*
Solid anterior mediastinal masses 364*fc*, 365*f*
Solid middle mediastinal mass 371*f*
Solid nodules, multiple 416*f*
Solid organ transplantation 117, 133
Spectral attenuated inversion recovery 341
Spiglottis 239*f*
Spindle cells 413
Spine sign 360
Spleen 337
Splenectomy 159*f*
Splenic abscess 175
 multiple 169*f*
Splenic granuloma formation 169
Split pleura sign 107, 446*f*
Split-bolus technique 467
Squamous cell carcinoma 417
Staphylococcal necrotizing pneumonia 471*f*
Staphylococcal pneumonia, recurrent 172*f*
Staphylococcus 169
 aureus 105
Starry sky
 appearance 8
 pattern 367*f*

Steeple sign 245f
Stenosis 77, 256, 259, 465
  congenital subglottic 242, 243f
  postintubation subglottic 256f
  pulmonary 230, 308, 313
  subglottic 218, 221, 241, 255, 259
Sternal lytic lesion 149f
Steroid therapy 156
Stomach, proximal 496f
Stratosphere sign 35f
Streptococcus 377
  milleri 377
  pneumoniae 104
Streptokinase 452
Stridor 59
Stroke 83
Subclavian vein 339
Subpleural parenchymal
  bands 309
  focus 149f
Subpulmonic effusion 449, 449f
Superior mediastinal syndrome 401
Superior pulmonary vein 222f
Superior vena cava 87, 222f, 232f, 326, 327, 329, 360, 381
  syndrome 401
Supraglottitis 246
Surfactant dysfunction disorders 192, 194
Surfactant protein 181, 195
  deficiency disorder 196f
Surgery 354
  cardiac 234
Sweat
  chloride test 171f
  electrolyte measurement 288
Swelling 418
Swyer–James–Macleod syndrome 11, 102, 293f, 301, 302f
Systemic lupus erythematosus 185, 189, 208, 209f, 366, 486

T

Tachypnea 197
  transient 27, 27f, 28, 61
Takayasu's arteritis 313, 319, 320f
T-cell
  acute lymphoblastic leukemia 400, 402
  disorders 166
  functions 165
  leukemias 168

Telangiectasia
  conjunctival 168
  hereditary hemorrhagic 83
  microvascular 233
Tension pneumothorax 491
Teratomas 388
  benign mature 375
  immature 393, 394f, 395b
Thanatophoric dysplasia 430f
Thoracic
  aorta, descending 320f, 468, 511
  cage 233, 443
  disease 398
  duct 339
    drainage of 340
  mass lesion, localization of 16
  neuroblastoma, features of 397b
  situs inversus 288f
  spine sign 445
  tumors 385-387, 387t, 405
    pediatric diffuse 386t
  vertebral bodies, poor ossification of 429
Thorax, generalized increased
  translucency of 10
Thromboembolic disease, chronic 468
Thromboembolism, pulmonary 44, 230, 313, 320, 322
Thromboendarterectomy, pulmonary 54
Thymic
  aplasia 166, 167f
  evaluation 52f
  hyperplasia 362, 366, 367, 367f, 367t
  hypoplasia 167f, 176f
  mass 367
Thymolipoma 365f
Thymoma 362
Thymus 8
  abnormal 31
  aplasia of 166
  enlarged 275
  hyperdense 366, 366f
  normal 8f, 31, 365, 365t
  starry-sky appearance of 25f
Tissue, subcutaneous 25f
Tonsillitis, acute 246, 248f
Total anomalous pulmonary venous
  connection 81, 324, 325
    subtypes of 325t
  return 228

Toxic fume
  exposure 302
  inhalation of 298
Trachea 31, 152, 219f, 239f, 245, 254, 267, 381, 416
  anomalous division of 265
  anterior displacement of 277f
  lateral displacement of 277f
  lower 261f
Tracheal bud, development of 259
Tracheal lumen 267
Tracheal stenosis 80, 220, 255
  congenital 260f, 266
Tracheal web 259
Tracheitis 245, 246
Tracheobronchial tree 224f
Tracheobronchomalacia 218, 220, 267
  primary 268f
Tracheobronchoscopy 269
Tracheoesophageal fistula 66, 220
  repair of 294
Tracheoesophageal septum development, disorders of 260
Tracheomalacia 267
Tracheostomy tube 495f
  in situ 493f
Transcription-polymerase chain reaction 103
Trauma 317, 426, 433
  nonaccidental 434
Tree-in-bud
  appearance 214f
  nodules 286
  opacities 144
Tricuspid
  atresia 230
  regurgitation 314
Trisomy 194
Troponin levels 483
Tubercular empyema thoracis 432f
Tuberculosis 122, 136, 138, 144, 145, 152f, 153, 170f, 173f, 174, 270, 284, 292, 299, 321f, 376, 377, 379, 379t, 432, 506
  congenital 155
  drug-resistant 154, 154f
  extrapulmonary 146
  miliary 141f
  pediatric 3, 138b
  pleural 151f
  post-primary 142
  primary 142

  pulmonary 137f, 140, 482f
  thoracic 149f
Tumors 44, 252, 376, 387, 534
  cells 396
  congenital 385
  dysembryonic 385
  dysontogenetic 385
  embryonal 385
  endobronchial 486
  high-grade mesenchymal 438
  inflammatory myofibroblastic 386, 411, 412f
  mediastinal 388
  mesenchymal 276, 413
  neurogenic 7, 372
  pediatric 386
  primary pulmonary 405
  primitive
    neuroectodermal 438
    neuroendocrine 387
  pulmonary 405
  sites of 419
  slow-growing 395
  solitary fibrous 386
  thoracic 385-387, 387t, 405
Tympanic membrane perforation 202f
Tyrosine kinase inhibitors 354

U

Ulcerative colitis 300
Ultrashort echo time imaging 47, 53
Ultrasonography 22, 28, 75, 90-92, 138, 142, 146, 479, 482
  appearances, normal 24
  role of 362
Ultrasound 244, 445, 455
  chest 22
Unilateral pulmonary artery atresia 504
Univentricular heart physiology 231
Upper airway 239, 254, 257, 258
  abnormalities 241
  imaging 239
  infections 245, 246t
  obstruction 241
    causes of 241
Upper esophageal region 66
Upper pulmonary vein 323, 329
Upper respiratory tract 111
Upper thoracic esophagus 275f
Uremia 486
Urokinase 452

V

Varicella-zoster virus 377
Varicoid 501
Varicose 282
 bronchiectasis 291f, 293f
Varix, pulmonary 325, 332, 333
Vascular anomalies 71, 78, 84, 93, 504
Vascular complications 285
 pulmonary 230t
Vascular compression, sites of 219f
Vascular endothelial growth factor
 inhibitors 354
Vascular malformation 33, 249, 375
Vascular ring 10, 219
Vasculature, pulmonary 229, 231
Vasculitis 208f, 300, 366
 necrotizing 210
Vasodilation, pulmonary 319
Vein, pulmonary 71, 83, 233, 323, 325, 331, 332f, 333, 381, 506, 511
Vena cava
 inferior 83, 232f, 233, 326, 328
 superior 87, 222f, 232f, 326, 327, 329, 360, 381
Venoarterial extracorporeal membrane oxygenation 495
Venovenous collaterals 230, 233
Venovenous extracorporeal membrane oxygenation 495
Ventilation, chronic 269
Ventricular septal defect 218
Vertebrae, sclerosis of 429f
Vessels
 abnormal 330t
 pulmonary 18, 30
Video-assisted thoracic surgery 138
Visceral larva migrans 203
Visceral pleural margin 457
Vocal cord 242
 paralysis 241, 242
Volume rendering technique 232f, 425
von Recklinghausen disease 387
Voriconazole prophylaxis 129

W

Waldeyer's ring 251
Wegener's granulomatosis 208, 210
Wheeze 59, 123
 persistent 80f
White blood count 106, 354
Wilms tumor 385
Wiskott–Aldrich syndrome 168

X

X-linked agammaglobulinemia 164, 165, 284, 294

Y

Young's syndrome 288

Z

Zero echo-time 53

EU GSPR Authorised Reprsentative
Logos Europe, 9 rue Nicolas Poussin
1700, La Rochelle, France
Phone: +33 (0) 6 67 93 73 78
E-mail: contact@logoseurope.eu

www.ingramcontent.com/pod-product-compliance
Ingram Content Group UK Ltd.
Pitfield, Milton Keynes, MK11 3LW, UK
UKHW050427150426
5217IPUK00019B/1275